58

ADVANCED NURSING PRACTICE
An Integrative Approach

ADVANCED NURSING PRACTICE
An Integrative Approach

Ann B. Hamric, MS, RN
Doctoral Candidate, University of Maryland School of Nursing, and Assistant
Professor, Louisiana State University Medical Center School of Nursing, New
Orleans, Louisiana

Judith A. Spross, MS, RN, OCN, FAAN
Doctoral Candidate, Boston College School of Nursing, and Clinical Nurse
Specialist, Cancer Rehabilitation and Pain Management, Braintree Hospital
Rehabilitation Network, Braintree, Massachusetts

Charlene M. Hanson, EdD, RN, CS, FNP, FAAN
Professor and Project Director of the Family Nurse Practitioner Program,
Georgia Southern University, Statesboro, Georgia

W.B. SAUNDERS COMPANY
A Division of Harcourt Brace & Company
Philadelphia   London   Toronto   Montreal   Sydney   Tokyo

W.B. SAUNDERS COMPANY

A Division of Harcourt Brace & Company

The Curtis Center
Independence Square West
Philadelphia, Pennsylvania 19106

Library of Congress Cataloging-in-Publication Data

Advanced nursing practice: an integrative approach / [edited by] Ann B. Hamric,
Judith A. Spross, Charlene M. Hanson. — 1st ed.

　　p.　　cm.

ISBN 0–7216–5894–6

1. Nurse practitioners.　　2. Midwives.　　3. Nurse anesthetists.　　I. Hamric,
Ann B.　　II. Spross, Judith A.　　III. Hanson, Charlene M.　　[DNLM:
1. Specialties, Nursing—methods.　　2. Nurse Clinicians.　　3. Nurse
Practitioners.　　4. Nurse Midwives.　　5. Nurse Anesthetists.
WY 101 A244 1996]

RT82.8.A384 1996　　610.73—dc20

DNLM/DLC　　　　　　　　　　　　　　　　　　　　　　　95-6050

ADVANCED NURSING PRACTICE: AN INTEGRATIVE APPROACH　　　　　ISBN 0–7216–5894–6

Printed in the United States of America.

Last digit is the print number:　　9　　8　　7　　6　　5　　4　　3

CONTRIBUTORS

Anne-Marie Barron, MS, RN, CS
Senior Lecturer, Division of Nursing
    Studies, Curry College, Milton,
    Massachusetts

**Jeri L. Bigbee, PhD, RN, CS,
FNP, FAAN**
Associate Professor and Director,
    Family Nurse Practitioner Program,
    Samuel Merritt College, Oakland,
    California

**Deborah McCaffrey Boyle, MSN,
RN, OCN**
Oncology Clinical Nurse Specialist, The
    Cancer Center at Fairfax Hospital,
    Falls Church, Virginia

Sarah Jo Brown, PhD, RN
Nurse Educator, Thetford, Vermont

**Karen A. Brykczynski, DNSc,
RN, CS, FNP**
Associate Professor, University of Texas
    at Galveston School of Nursing,
    Galveston, Texas

Ellen B. Clarke, MSN, RN
Doctoral Student, Harvard University
    Graduate School of Education,
    Cambridge, Massachusetts

**Margaret W. Dorroh, MN, RN,
CNM, FNP-C**
Certified Nurse-Midwife, Family Nurse
    Practitioner, and Director, Family
    Health & Birth Center, Inc.,
    Savannah, Georgia

**Susan E. Davis Doughty, MSN,
RN, CS, NP**
Nurse Practitioner, Women to Women,
    Yarmouth, Maine

**Margaret Faut-Callahan, DNSc,
CRNA, FAAN**
Professor and Program Director, Nurse
    Anesthesia Program, Rush University
    College of Nursing, Chicago, Illinois

**Shirley A. Girouard, PhD, RN,
FAAN**
Director of Program Planning and
    Evaluation, National Association of
    Children's Hospitals and Related
    Institutions, Alexandria, Virginia

Elizabeth M. Grady, PhD, RN
Organizational Development
    Consultant, Belmont, Massachusetts

Diane L. Hanna, MS, RNC, FNP
Nurse Practitioner and Clinical
    Instructor, Medical College of
    Virginia/Virginia Commonwealth
    University, Richmond, Virginia

Doreen C. Harper, PhD, RN, CS, ANP, FAAN
Associate Professor and Director of
    Community Partnerships and Faculty
    Practice, George Mason University
    College of Nursing and Health
    Science, Fairfax, Virginia; and
    Adjunct Associate Professor and
    Director, Nurse Practitioner Program,
    The George Washington University
    School of Medicine and Health
    Sciences, Washington, DC

Kerry V. Harwood, MSN, RN
Oncology Clinical Nurse Specialist and
    Director, Cancer Patient Education
    Program, Duke University Medical
    Center, Durham, North Carolina

Carole A. Kenner, DNS, RNC
Professor and Chair, Parent-Child
    Nursing Department, College of
    Nursing and Health, University of
    Cincinnati, Cincinnati, Ohio

Terry Boyle Kenyon, MSN, RNC, NNP
Neonatal Nurse Practitioner, Sinai
    Hospital of Baltimore, Baltimore,
    Maryland

Michael Kremer, MSN, CRNA
Doctoral Candidate, Rush University
    College of Nursing, Chicago, Illinois

Sharon L. Krumm, PhD, RN
Director of Nursing, Johns Hopkins
    Oncology Center, Baltimore,
    Maryland

Judy Wright Lott, DSN, RNC, NNP
Neonatal Nurse Practitioner Director,
    Children's Hospital Medical Center,
    Cincinnati, Ohio

Vicky A. Mahn, MS, RN
System Associate for Quality and
    Clinical Case Management,
    Carondelet Health Care, Tucson,
    Arizona

Beverly L. Malone, PhD, RN, FAAN
Dean, School of Nursing, North
    Carolina Agricultural and Technical
    State University, Greensboro, North
    Carolina

Deborah B. McGuire, PhD, RN, FAAN
Edith Folsom Honeycutt Chair in
    Oncology Nursing and Associate
    Professor, Nell Hodgson Woodruff
    School of Nursing, Emory University,
    Atlanta, Georgia

Diane Kaschak Newman, MSN, RNC, CRNP, FAAN
President and Adult Nurse Practitioner,
    Access to Continence Care &
    Treatment, DKN & Associates, Inc.,
    Philadelphia, Pennsylvania

Sheila F. Norton, MSN, RN, CNM
Doctoral Student, Harvard University
    Graduate School of Education,
    Cambridge; and Certified Nurse-
    Midwife, Harvard Pilgrim Health
    Care, Medford, Massachusetts

Judith D. Polak, MSN, RNC, NNP
Neonatal Nurse Practitioner, University
    of West Virginia, Morgantown, West
    Virginia

Juanita Reigle, MSN, RN, CCRN
Practitioner/Teacher, University of
    Virginia Health Sciences Center and
    School of Nursing, Charlottesville,
    Virginia

Allison Weber Shuren, MSN, RN, CCRN, CPNP
Former Pediatric Nurse Practitioner/
Clinical Nurse Specialist, Division of
Pediatric Surgery, Children's Hospital
Medical Center, Cincinnati, Ohio;
Presently Juris Doctor Candidate,
University of Michigan Law School,
Ann Arbor, Michigan

Margretta Madden Styles, EdD, RN, FAAN
President, International Council of
Nurses, and President, American
Nurses Credentialing Center, Largo,
Florida

Diana L. Taylor, PhD, RN, FAAN
Associate Professor and Director,
Women's Primary Care Program,
University of California, San
Francisco School of Nursing, San
Francisco, California

Patricia White, MS, RN, CS
Assistant Professor, Graduate School
of Health Studies, Graduate
Nursing, Simmons College, Boston;
and Adult Nurse Practitioner,
Norwood Medical Associates,
Norwood, Massachusetts

PREFACE

These are times of uncertainty and rapid change in both the health-care system and the nursing profession. The health-care reform initiatives of the early 1990s mobilized the nursing profession to re-examine all advanced nursing practice roles. The nursing profession highlighted advanced practice nurses as key providers who could meet the needs of many Americans for primary health care and illness management (American Nurses Association, 1993). The American Nurses Association recognizes four advanced nursing practice roles: the clinical nurse specialist, the nurse practitioner, the nurse anesthetist, and the nurse-midwife. As the profession rallied around advanced nursing practice as a response to the need for reform, considerable discussion and debate arose around merging the clinical nurse specialist and nurse practitioner roles. Another recurrent theme has focused attention exclusively on the nurse practitioner role. We believe it is time for a thorough exploration of advanced nursing practice and its definition, competencies, and roles. To fully understand the meaning of advanced nursing practice and its potential contributions to shaping the future of health care, the contributions of all advanced nursing practice roles, whether established or evolving, must be considered. It is also essential to identify the opportunities for advanced practice that can be envisioned in a future health-care system where advanced practice nurses and all nurses participate more fully, visibly, and equitably with medical and other colleagues.

TERMINOLOGY

Consistent terminology has been used throughout the book in referring to advanced nursing practice (ANP), the advanced practice nurse (APN), and particular ANP roles (clinical nurse specialist [CNS], nurse practitioner [NP], certified nurse-midwife [CNM], and certified registered nurse anesthetist [CRNA]). In the literature generally and in clinical arenas, the terms "advanced nursing practice" and "advanced practice nursing" are used interchangeably. Other than in Chapter 2, no distinctions are intended between these terms. For the sake of clarity and consistency, we have chosen to use the former term. Thus the practice is designated ANP and the nurse is designated APN.

Additionally, throughout the book, persons with health-care needs will be variously referred to as individuals, patients, clients, or consumers. These terms should also be viewed as being interchangeable. The differences reflect the differing preferences of our authors as well as differing terminology in the literature.

PURPOSE

This is a new book for a new time. For readers familiar with Hamric and Spross's earlier work on the CNS, it is important to underscore that this book is a new text and not another edition of that earlier work. This book is considerably different in emphasis and scope, as it addresses *all* ANP roles and the broad issues important to advanced nursing practice. Even though some of the authors and chapter titles are the same, the contents of the chapters are quite different in this volume, as they have been reworked to enlarge their focus to include all APNs and to be consistent with the book's central concept of advanced nursing practice. The editors' experiences as APNs, educators, administrators, and leaders on the front lines shaping advanced nursing practice over the past 20 years have informed the ideas presented here.

Advanced Nursing Practice: An Integrative Approach represents a comprehensive, in-depth exploration of advanced nursing practice as well as the varied and evolving roles that APNs assume in the health-care system. Distinguishing features include the integration of literature from all of the ANP roles and a holistic, inclusive, and unified vision of advanced nursing practice consistently applied throughout the text.

This book is grounded in a conviction that advanced nursing practice must have a definable and describable core even as it must have differing roles to enact the varied practices that APNs undertake. **All of the advanced practice roles described in this book are beneficial to the health of patients.** These ANP roles are also crucial to the continuing evolution and strengthening of the nursing profession. Rather than debate whether the CNS and NP roles should separate or merge, the position here is that *both* separate *and* blended NP and CNS roles, in addition to other ANP roles, are valuable and needed in an increasingly complex health-care system. Rather than ignore CRNAs and CNMs in the description of advanced practice, this book explicitly includes these roles and their related literature in every chapter. Rather than promote only one role as "the" ANP role, as some nursing leaders are doing with the blended CNS/NP role or the NP role in its primary care and acute care forms, we support variety, diversity, and continued permutations of existing ANP roles so long as they remain within the umbrella concept of advanced nursing practice (described in Chapter 3), and titles are kept consistent. The reality is that no one nurse can master all the practice roles currently being enacted by APNs. There is danger in any one role claiming to be "all things to all people" and ignoring the contributions of other ANP roles to health care.

This vision of advanced nursing practice is consistent with the Report of the American Association of Colleges of Nursing Task Force on the Essentials of Master's Education for Advanced Practice Nursing (American Association of Colleges of Nursing, October, 1995). It described CNS, NP, CRNA, and CNM roles as having "equal relevance to advanced practice" (p. 3), even as the Association recognized that advanced practice roles continue to evolve.

ORGANIZATION

Advanced Nursing Practice: An Integrative Approach is organized into four major parts. In Part I, Historical and Developmental Aspects of Advanced Nursing Practice, the history of advanced nursing practice is traced. Conceptualizations of advanced nursing practice are described and analyzed, and a core definition of advanced nursing practice is developed. As noted, this definition is followed throughout the book, giving conceptual clarity and consistency to the discussions. Issues in ANP education are identified, and a curricular plan is proposed. Role development literature from all of the advanced practice roles is described, and key themes and issues are identified.

In Part II, Competencies of Advanced Nursing Practice, the eight core competencies that define advanced nursing practice are examined as they are enacted in practice. These competencies include expert clinical practice, expert coaching and guidance, consultation, research skills, clinical and professional leadership, collaboration, change agent skills, and ethical decision-making skills.

In Part III, Advanced Practice Roles: The Operational Definitions of Advanced Nursing Practice, the varied job roles assumed by APNs are described and differentiated from one another. These include the established ANP roles of CNS, primary care NP, CNM, and CRNA, as well as the evolving roles of ANP case manager, acute care NP (ACNP), and the blended CNS/NP.

The final section, Part IV, Issues in the Continuing Evolution of Advanced Nursing Practice, describes faculty practices, deals with health policy and legislative and regulatory issues, provides strategies for developing markets for advanced nursing practice, and describes the realities of program and practice management. The critical issue of administrative support and justification for advanced practice is also discussed. Data from ANP evaluation and research literature are summarized and commonalities identified in the chapter on evaluating the processes and impact of advanced nursing practice. Finally, we use the themes from the first chapter on the history of advanced nursing practice to reflect upon future challenges and opportunities for APNs.

AUDIENCE

This book is intended for practicing APNs in all roles, graduate students, educators, administrators, and leaders in the nursing profession. For practicing APNs, the book contains both theoretical and practical content to guide role implementation. Individuals interested in strengthening or changing their roles will find many strategies for accomplishing these changes. The book will be useful to graduate students studying for any advanced practice role throughout their program of study. Indeed, we believe the book will be most useful if students begin reading content in initial core courses and continue to use the book in later ANP and functional role courses. For educators, the book will serve as a comprehensive curricular resource in preparing APNs for practice. It also serves as a guide to standardize core education for advanced practice. Nursing administrators will appreciate the descriptions of various ANP roles and the strategies for justifying and supporting ANP positions. For nursing leaders, this book is a clarion call to come to common ground regarding our understandings of advanced nursing practice and the roles APNs assume, so that we speak with authority and consistency to policy makers, to other disciplines, and to one another.

APPROACH

We have sought to describe advanced nursing practice at its best, as it is being enacted by APNs throughout the country. Certainly we recognize that there is much work to be done: not all ANP students are educated to practice with the competencies described herein; too many nurses are in ANP roles without the necessary credentials or competencies, so that true advanced practice is not demonstrated; and there is too much "alphabet soup" in role titles (for example, the ACNP is variously called tertiary care NP, critical care NP, pediatric intensivist, and so on and so on).

Creating this book has been an immensely challenging undertaking. One of the early learnings was how disparate and separated different ANP groups are—integrating and incorporating the perspectives of all the ANP specialties was difficult. The literature from the various advanced practice specialty groups is also unfortunately separated, and clinicians and educators tend to read only their own group's literature. In addition, not all groups have addressed the core concept of advanced practice or the competencies of APNs in a complete or consistent manner. One of the major contributions of this book is the attempt at synthesis regarding advanced nursing practice. Adopting this integrative approach, as challenging as it has been, has immeasurably enriched this understanding of advanced nursing practice.

Our approach is unified around core criteria and competencies but flexible enough to accommodate emerging ANP roles. There is no doubt that roles will continue to evolve as nursing continues to mature in its understanding and enactment of advanced nursing practice. But advanced nursing practice must be distinct, recognizable, and describable if it is to continue to exist. As the AACN Task Force Report (1995) noted, "The greater concerns for consumer confidence, quality graduate education, and clear outcomes mandate that a more coherent and consistent set of curricular standards be articulated. Moreover, titling must be simplified and specifically relevant to the core clinical competencies that an advanced practice nurse brings to the health care delivery process" (pp. 2–3). It will be clear to the reader that the diverse roles described in Part III, while they share the core criteria and competencies of advanced nursing practice, are different and distinct from one another in their role enactment. This should be a cause for celebration, as nursing recognizes its strength and range in meeting client needs.

We are convinced that advanced nursing practice is absolutely essential to improving the health and well-being of the citizens of this nation! Advanced practice nurses can and must be active participants in solving some of the pressing problems in health-care delivery being experienced as we move into the 21st century.

Ann B. Hamric
Judith A. Spross
Charlene M. Hanson

REFERENCES

American Association of Colleges of Nursing. (1995, October). *The essentials of master's education for advanced practice nursing.* Report from the Task Force on the Essentials of Master's Education for Advanced Practice Nursing. Washington, DC: Author.

American Nurses Association. (1993). Primary health care: The nurse solution. *Nursing Facts.* Washington, DC: Author.

ACKNOWLEDGMENTS

We could not have undertaken such an ambitious work without the efforts and experience of our contributors. In making a commitment to the vision of advanced nursing practice we sought to portray, the contributors became involved with us in a creative enterprise. We are most grateful to these colleagues for their insights into the components of advanced nursing practice and the issues shaping its evolution. Each chapter reflects many interactions between contributors and editors and between contributors and their colleagues. Contributors often consulted with each other to ensure that their work reflected the breadth of advanced nursing practice.

We also thank the colleagues with whom we have consulted, debated, and otherwise shared the intense work of developing these chapters. We are grateful to the many graduate students and APNs with whom we have had contact over our careers. Whether participating in a class or a continuing education offering, or being precepted in the clinical area, these individuals challenged our thinking and sustained and enlarged our vision of advanced nursing practice.

Finally, we are grateful for the support of Thomas Eoyang, Vice President and Editor-in-Chief of Nursing Books at the W.B. Saunders Company. Thomas's patience, persistence, and unfailing confidence in our ability to complete this book are some of the main reasons it moved from idea to completion. The production staff at the W.B. Saunders Company, in particular Tina Rebane and Denise LeMelledo, also earn kudos for grace under fire in producing the book in record time.

CONTENTS

PART I
HISTORICAL AND DEVELOPMENTAL ASPECTS OF ADVANCED NURSING PRACTICE

PART II
COMPETENCIES OF ADVANCED NURSING PRACTICE

PART III
ADVANCED PRACTICE ROLES: THE OPERATIONAL DEFINITIONS OF ADVANCED NURSING PRACTICE

HISTORICAL AND DEVELOPMENTAL ASPECTS OF ADVANCED NURSING PRACTICE

CHAPTER 1

History and Evolution of Advanced Nursing Practice

Jeri L. Bigbee

INTRODUCTION

This chapter focuses on the historical development of four established advanced practice roles, specifically nurse anesthetists (CRNAs), nurse-midwives (CNMs), clinical nurse specialists (CNSs), and nurse practitioners (NPs). It is acknowledged that other advanced nursing roles, such as case managers, exist and are evolving. However, these four major roles were selected for review because of the depth of the historical information available. The history of each of the four advanced nursing practice (ANP) roles will be examined, including significant professional and educational developments, inter- and intra-professional struggles, and legal and legislative advances. In addition, the broader historical context that has shaped the nursing profession, including gender, health manpower, and other sociopolitical issues will be discussed.

The evolution of the term "advanced" in relation to nursing practice is unclear. The use of the related term "specialist" in nursing can be traced back to the turn of the century, when postgraduate courses were offered by hospitals. Using an apprenticeship model, these courses were offered in a variety of specialty areas, including anesthesia, tuberculosis, operating room, laboratory, and dietetics. Some of these areas of specialization, such as dietetics, actually broke off to form new professions (Bullough, 1992). In the first issue of the *American Journal of Nursing*, an article by Dewitt (1900) entitled "Specialties in Nursing" addressed the development of specialized clinical practice within the profession. At that time the term was used to designate a nurse who had completed a postgraduate course in a clinical specialty area or who had extensive experience and expertise in a particular clinical area. With the increasing complexity of health-care knowledge and technology and enhanced professional sophistication, specialization became a force in the twentieth century. By 1980 the American Nurses Association (ANA) declared, "Specialization in nursing is now clearly established" and contended that "Specialization is a mark of the advancement of the nursing profession" (American Nurses Association, 1980, p. 22). Early in the evolution of the NP role during the 1960s and 1970s, the term "expanded" or "extended" role was used throughout the literature, implying a horizontal movement to encompass expertise from medicine and other disciplines. The more contemporary term, "advanced," suggests a more hierarchical movement encompassing increasing expertise within nursing rather than expansion into other disciplines. Several progressive state nursing practice acts, such as the one in Washington, included the term "advanced practice nurse" (APN) in the 1970s and 1980s to delineate CRNAs, CNMs, CNSs, and NPs. This regulatory influence promoted the contemporary use of the term "advanced" and served to demonstrate the commonalties of the various advanced practice specialties.

NURSE ANESTHETISTS

HISTORICAL REVIEW

Nurse anesthesia is the oldest advanced nursing specialty. Since the mid-1800s, with the advent and development of anesthesia agents and care, nurses have been involved in administering anesthesia. Major advances in anesthesia science paved the way for the development of the CRNA role. Nitrous oxide was the first anesthesia agent identified in the mid-1800s. This anesthetic agent was adopted initially by

American dentists. About the same time ether and chloroform were widely used as anesthesia agents for surgical procedures. The concurrent advancement in antiseptic surgery and anesthesia promoted the growth of hospitals, because surgeries were becoming too complex to be conducted in the home.

Diers (1991) noted that "anesthesizers" were originally often unpaid or minimally paid surgeons in training who were logically most interested in the surgical procedure and not the anesthesia care. Under this system there was no incentive for physicians to become full-time anesthetists. So, in order to provide surgeons with the anesthesia care needed, nurses were recruited and trained. These early nurse anesthetists were readily accepted, because the nurse offered more stability over time and would solely concentrate on the anesthesia process versus the medical intern, who would tend to focus more on the surgical procedure. These first nurse anesthetists were religious sisters who did not expect any remuneration, which also contributed to their early acceptance. Gender was also an issue that promoted early female nurse anesthetists, whose practice was justified because of their "gentle touch" (Olsen, 1940).

The first nurse anesthetist was Sister Mary Bernard at St. Vincent's Hospital in Erie, Pennsylvania, in 1877 (Bankert, 1989). In the late 1800s the Sisters of the Third Order of St. Francis established a network of hospitals throughout the Midwest through contracts with the Missouri Pacific Railroad. One of these hospitals was the Mayo Clinic, where all anesthesia was administered by nurses. The "mother of anesthesia," Alice Magaw, was an early nurse anesthetist at Mayo who reported and published an accounting of her work. By 1906, she had participated in over 14,000 surgical cases without one anesthesia-attributable death (Thatcher, 1953). Her visionary evaluative research is paralleled by the early work of nurse-midwife Mary Breckinridge and speaks to the importance of evaluative research in the early development of the advanced specialties. Magaw contended that hospital-based anesthesia services, which at the time included only nurse anesthetists, should remain separate from nursing service administrative structures, because it was a specialized field requiring education and recognition not possible under a nursing department (Thatcher, 1953). This early move away from nursing service reflected the alienation of nurse anesthesia from mainstream nursing still seen today.

Historically, because of the trauma-related nature of anesthesia practice, nurse anesthesia has been greatly influenced by and involved with the American military and major wars. During World War I, hospital-sponsored medical units provided anesthesia care on the battlefield, resulting in reduced mortality. World War I served to greatly enhance the visibility and public enthusiasm for nurse anesthetists. However, this growing acceptance of nurse anesthetists became an increasing concern for physician anesthetists.

Physicians began specializing in anesthesia practice around the turn of the century. Interestingly, female physicians were the initiators, because the low pay and status of anesthesia practice made it unattractive to male physicians. These women were active in the establishment of the Association of Anesthetists of the United States and Canada in the early 1920s (Bankert, 1989). Although they shared a great deal with nurse anesthetists in terms of gender discrimination and stereotyping, the early women physician anesthetists unfortunately were actively opposed to nurse anesthetists. The medical journal *Anesthesiology* was established in 1940, further strengthening medicine's claim to anesthesia practice. By the 1950s increasing numbers of male physicians specialized in anesthesiology, and women's leadership in the field declined.

World War II served to institutionalize the nurse anesthetist role even further with the military clarifying the position and elevating the status of the nurse anesthetist. Nurse anesthesia was declared a clinical nursing specialty within the military nursing structure with unique pay and assignments (Bankert, 1989). Immediately after the end of the war in 1945, the American Association of Nurse Anesthetists (AANA) initiated their certification program. This formal credentialing of CRNAs was far ahead of the other nursing specialties, and was a significant benchmark in the history of advanced practice.

In the post-war period, the close association of nurse anesthesia with the military continued. The Army established nurse anesthesia educational programs, including one at Walter Reed General Hospital, which graduated its first class in 1961, consisting of all men. Soon after, the Letterman General Hospital School of Anesthesia in San Francisco also graduated an all-male class. This significant movement of males into nurse anesthesia is unparalleled in any of the other advanced nursing specialties. Not surprisingly, nurse anesthetists played an active role in the Vietnam War, providing vital services in the prompt surgical treatment of the wounded. Of the ten nurses killed in Vietnam, two were male nurse anesthetists (Bankert, 1989). Currently, CRNAs in the United States administer 65% of the anesthesia nationally (American Association of Nurse Anesthetists, 1989) and at least 70% in rural areas (Bankert, 1989).

ORGANIZATIONAL DEVELOPMENT

The nurse anesthesia specialty was highly successful in building a strong national presence early in its history. The AANA was established in 1931 by Agatha Hodgins, who served as the organization's first president. At the first meeting of the association, the group voted to affiliate with the ANA, but were rebuffed by the ANA. Thatcher (1953) contended that the ANA's refusal was based on their fear of assuming legal responsibility for a group that could be charged with practicing medicine. Men were first admitted to the AANA in 1947, reflecting the growing role and acceptance of men in the specialty. This opening of the professional organization to men was followed by special efforts of the American military to increase the number of male nurse anesthetists. As indicated in Table 1–1, as of 1994, there were 26,530 CRNAs, 97% of whom were members of the AANA (American Associa-

TABLE 1–1. NUMBER OF ADVANCED PRACTICE NURSES IN THE UNITED STATES

Title	Total Number	% Currently in Nursing	% Nationally Certified
CRNAs	25,238*	86.3	100
CNMs	7,405†	85.9	66.0
CNSs	58,185	86.5	13.5
NPs	48,237	88.4	58.0

*As of 1994, the American Association of Nurse Anesthetists estimates that there are 26,530 CRNAs (American Association of Nurse Anesthetists, 1995).
†As of 1995, the American College of Nurse-Midwifery estimates that of the 5,200 CNMs nationally, approximately 4,000 (77%) are practicing as CNMs (American College of Nurse-Midwives, 1995).
(From U.S. Department of Health and Human Services, Division of Nursing. (1992). National Sample Survey of RNs, 1992; American Nurses Association. (1993). *Advanced practice nursing: A new age in health care, nursing facts.* Washington, D.C.: American Nurses Publishing.)

tion of Nurse Anesthetists, 1995). Nurse anesthesia remains unique among the advanced nursing specialties in its success in attracting a significant percentage of males (approximately 40% of practicing CRNAs are male). This success has been influenced by historical efforts to recruit males, the close relationship with the American military, and the relatively high salaries available to nurse anesthetists.

EDUCATIONAL DEVELOPMENT

Educationally, nurse anesthesia training initially involved informal apprenticeship programs operated within hospitals. The first official postgraduate course was offered at St. Vincent's Hospital in Portland, Oregon, in 1909, consisting of 6 months of instruction under the direction of Agnes McGee (Thatcher, 1953). Subsequently, a postgraduate course in anesthesia for Sisters only was established at one of the Sisters' hospitals, St. John's Hospital in Springfield, Illinois, in 1912, admitting the first secular nurse in 1924. This early connection between nurse anesthesia and women's religious communities certainly affected future gender issues within the specialty, particularly slowing the acceptance of increasing numbers of male nurse anesthetists. By the onset of World War I, there were five postgraduate schools of nurse anesthesia in the United States. At the well-established Lakeside Hospital program in Cleveland, critical experimentation with combined nitrous oxide/oxygen administration, as well as the first use of morphine and scopolamines as adjuncts to anesthesia, was conducted with the participation of nurse anesthetist Agatha Hodgins. In 1952 an accreditation program to monitor the quality of anesthesia programs was established under the AANA. By 1972 there were 208 schools of anesthesia, most of which were small, graduating approximately 800 nurse anesthetists each year (Bullough, 1992).

Despite early advances in credentialing, nurse anesthesia education has only recently joined mainstream graduate nursing education. Because of their historical "step-child" relationship with nursing, nurse anesthesia programs, if they were associated with educational institutions, were often housed in schools of medicine or allied health, similar to some early NP programs. The first master's degree nurse anesthesia program was established at the University of Hawaii in 1973. By 1980 there were four master's programs in nurse anesthesia, growing to 17 in 1990 and 85 in 1995 (American Association of Nurse Anesthetists, personal communication, 1995). The AANA mandated a baccalaureate degree for certification in 1987, and a master's degree will be required in 1998.

INTER- AND INTRA-PROFESSIONAL DYNAMICS

Inter-professional conflict has been an ever-present dynamic for CRNAs, intensifying as medical anesthesiologists increased their control over anesthesia practice. These struggles were often played out in the courts and state legislatures in the early 1900s and ultimately served to establish the legal basis of the practice of nurse anesthesia. In 1911 the New York State Medical Society unsuccessfully declared that the administration of an anesthetic by a nurse violated state law (Thatcher, 1953). In response, the Ohio State Medical Board passed a resolution in 1912 specifying that only physicians could administer anesthesia, which culminated in action taken against the Lakeside Hospital program as the "chief source of the nurse-anesthetist abuse." This action was also unsuccessful but resulted in nurse anesthetists amending the Ohio Medical Practice Act, protecting the practice of nurse anesthesia.

Shortly after, the Kentucky attorney general ruled that the administration of anesthesia fell within the practice of medicine, resulting in the first landmark court case. A suit was filed against the State Board of Health by a Louisville surgeon and nurse anesthetist team, Louis Frank and Margaret Hayfield. Initially the court ruled in favor of the State Board; however, on appeal the decision was reversed, and the appeals court ruled in 1917 that nurse anesthesia was not the practice of medicine. Legal challenge then moved to California, where nurse anesthetist Dagmar Nelson was sued by the Anesthesia Section of the Los Angeles County Medical Association for practicing medicine without a license. Nelson argued successfully that the Medical Association had no standing to sue. In response, a physician, William Chalmers-Frances, filed a similar suit against Nelson in 1936, which again resulted in a judgment for Nelson. The ruling was appealed, and in 1938 the California Supreme Court supported the decision, stating that Nelson was not practicing medicine because she was supervised by the operating surgeon (Thatcher, 1953). Thus the Frank et al. v. South et al. (1917) and Chalmers-Frances v. Nelson (1936) cases provide the critical legal basis of nurse anesthesia practice.

The relationship between organized nurse anesthesia and anesthesiology has reflected these historical inter-professional struggles. Between 1947 and 1963 there was no official communication between the AANA and the American Society of Anesthesiologists (ASA), because of the ASA's stand that only physicians could be involved in anesthesia education (Bankert, 1989). In 1972, after years of negotiation, the AANA and the ASA issued the Joint Statement on Anesthesia Practice, which promoted the concept of the anesthesia team. However, in 1976 the ASA Board of Directors voted to withdraw support from the 1972 statement, preferring one that explicitly maintained physician control and leadership.

Over the years challenges from physician anesthesia groups have continued, particularly in relation to malpractice policies and most recently in relation to antitrust and restraint of trade issues, similar to those experienced by CNMs. Oltz v. St. Peter's Hospital (1986) established the standing of CRNAs to sue for anticompetitive damages when anesthesiologists conspire to restrict practice privileges. A second case (Bhan v. NME Hospitals, Inc., et al., 1985) established the right of CRNAs to be awarded damages as a result of exclusive contracts.

Legislatively, the AANA led a long and complex effort to secure third-party reimbursement under Medicare beginning in 1977. They were finally successful in 1989. In relation to modification of state nursing practice acts to reflect nurse anesthesia practice, historical activity has been limited. This may be explained by the legal view of nurse anesthesia as performing a dependent function under physicians in the administration of anesthesia. In 1972, over a century after the inception of nurse anesthetists, only four state practice acts specifically mentioned them.

NURSE-MIDWIVES

HISTORICAL REVIEW

Nurse-midwifery was the second major advanced nursing specialty to develop historically, but its history is commingled with the ancient practice of midwifery. In the United States, as in most other parts of the world, deliveries were assisted by traditional (lay) midwives until the turn of the century. Midwives were imported to the United States with the slave trade in 1619 (Robinson, 1984) and later with waves of European immigration. Midwives were respected and rewarded community members in early Native American, colonial, and pioneer communities. However, by the early 1900s, midwives in America were discredited because of religious attitudes, economic demands, replacement by physicians, inadequate education, lack of organization, influx of immigrants, and the low status of women (Varney, 1987). Most early midwives were educated in England, where midwifery was controlled by the Church of England, which placed moralistic and church doctrine restrictions on practice. In early Puritan communities, midwives were suspected of witchcraft, especially if birth defects occurred.

During the 1700s and 1800s, major advancement in nursing and medical science greatly enhanced the scholarly basis of obstetrical practice. Improved technology produced improved outcomes related to cesarean sections, obstetric anesthesia, and puerperal fever. These scientific advancements excluded the midwife because of her limited education and lack of professional organization. Immigration patterns, which peaked in the late 1800s, produced culturally isolated ethnic communities in urban areas that used "old country midwives" who were untrained, similar to "granny midwives" in the South whose practice was passed on through generations of women within families. Their practice focused on home remedies, prayer, and patience (Varney, 1987). By the late 1800s European obstetrical trends had changed, making it fashionable to use male midwives (physicians), and soon this trend was reflected in the United States. At that time physicians made a concerted effort to gain control over birthing as a means of recruiting patients and increasing income (Fox, 1969). Concurrently, the status of women was an increasingly volatile issue in turn-of-the-century America. Swenson (1968) contended that the status of women was at a "low ebb" with women seen as economically exploitable but socially and politically incompetent. These negative views particularly undermined the status of American midwives, as well as the profession of nursing.

Between 1900 and 1920 the health status of the American population, particularly with regard to perinatal health indicators, was poor. Midwives were falsely blamed for the poor maternal-child health outcomes of the period. Maternal and infant mortality rates were high because of inadequate hospital resources for the treatment of complicated deliveries, the inadequate preparation of physicians related to obstetrics, the lack of attention to prenatal care, and the inadequate education, regulation, and supervision of midwives. A 1906 study conducted by the New York City Health Department indicated that 40% of the births in the city were attended by 3,000 untrained midwives (Varney, 1987). In response, the Children's Bureau and the Maternity Center Association were established to promote improved maternal and child health and welfare. The Children's Bureau, established in 1912 and spearheaded by nursing leader Lillian Wald, conducted studies of infant and maternal mortality, conclusive of the importance of early and continuous prenatal care. In 1921 the Sheppard-Towner Act was passed, allocating federal funds to be administered by the Children's Bureau to provide improved maternal-child care. The impetus behind the increasing attention on public health and the passage of the Sheppard-Towner Act of 1921 was based on national security concerns. In the post–World War I sociopolitical climate, supporting the health of women and children was viewed as essential to maintain national security, particularly in ensuring an adequate supply of healthy soldiers (Tom, 1982). Interestingly, over time organized medicine withdrew its support of this legislation because programs were not under physician control, and the legislation lapsed (Diers, 1991).

Negative attitudes related to traditional midwives peaked around 1912, with heated debates surrounding issues of midwife licensing and control. Concurrently, medicine was assuming ever-increasing control of obstetrical care with a mass movement away from home births. Several states passed laws granting legal recognition of midwives with regulatory controls, resulting in the establishment of midwifery schools. Public health nurses were involved as instructors in these midwifery schools.

A landmark in nurse-midwifery history was the establishment of the Maternity Center Association (MCA) in 1918 in response to a study conducted by the New York City health commissioner, which also indicated the need for comprehensive prenatal care. The MCA served as the central organization for a network of community-based maternity centers throughout the city, providing education and administrative support to the centers. In 1921 their efforts narrowed, demonstrating the provision of comprehensive maternity care in just one district. The MCA also collaborated with the Henry Street Visiting Nurse Association, identifying the need to prepare nurses to provide maternity services. These groups proposed the establishment of a school of nurse-midwifery, which was tabled because of strong opposition from medicine, nursing, and city officials. This opposition was related to professional turf issues as well as the increasingly discredited public view of traditional midwifery.

Meanwhile, in England, traditional midwives were being replaced by nurse-midwives with the emergence of nursing education. In 1925 Mary Breckinridge, a registered nurse and British-trained nurse-midwife, established the Frontier Nursing Service (FNS), which would serve as a futuristic model of advanced nursing practice in nurse-midwifery as well as later for NPs. In an economically depressed rural mountain area of Kentucky, Breckinridge established a network of clinics to serve the Appalachian women and children, using imported British midwives traveling on horseback (Breckenridge, 1952). Outstanding evaluation data were maintained from the outset, and when analyzed by the Metropolitan Life Insurance Company in 1951, they indicated that 8,596 births were attended, 6,533 in the home, since 1925 (Varney, 1987). The FNS maternal mortality rate of 1.2 per 1,000 was significantly lower than the national average of 3.4 per 1,000 over the same period. General primary health care and dental services were also provided to the population.

Early nurse-midwifery graduates either practiced with the MCA or the FNS or became involved in public health programs, which often included teaching and supervising indigenous midwives in rural areas. Many early graduates were not able to practice clinical nurse-midwifery because of limited opportunities, so they assumed roles in nursing education and administration. In the late 1950s and 1960s nurse-midwives made efforts to practice in hospitals, where 70% of births took place, bringing with them models of family-centered maternity care that would revolutionize maternity care. However, barriers to practice were formidable. In 1963, only 11% of CNMs who responded to a national survey were practicing midwifery. This proportion increased to 23% by 1967; however, about one in four of these CNMs were practicing abroad through church and international health organizations. Within the United States, the proportion of CNMs actually practicing midwifery was highest in areas with strong educational programs, specifically New Mexico, Kentucky, and New York City (American College of Nurse-Midwives, 1968).

In the late 1960s and early 1970s nurse-midwifery finally turned the corner, experiencing rapidly increasing demand. This dramatic change was due in part to the increased visibility and involvement of the women's movement in birthing issues, which resulted in increased consumer recognition and demand for nurse-midwifery services. In addition, sociopolitical developments, including the increased utilization of CNMs in federally funded health projects, the official recognition of CNMs by the American College of Obstetricians and Gynecologists in 1971, and the increased birth rate due to baby boomers reaching adulthood coupled with inadequate supplies of obstetricians, served to foster the rapid blossoming of CNM practice. Although in 1971 only 36.9% of CNMs who responded to an American College of Nurse-Midwives (ACNM) survey were in clinical midwifery practice, by 1977 this percentage had increased to 50.7%, with the majority practicing in the Southwest, Southeast, and Southern Appalachia, often in rural areas. Also in the early 1970s the first nurse-midwifery private practice was instituted, leading to the rapid "discovery" of midwifery services by middle- and upper-income families. By 1977 approximately 26% of all practicing CNMs were engaged in private practices.

The more recent expansion of nurse-midwifery practice and education has been influenced by factors similar to those affecting the other advanced specialties, including the shortage of physicians, the availability of federal funding, and changes in nurse practice acts. In addition, the women's movement, including the demands for sensitive and caring approaches to women's health care, has fueled the success of nurse-midwifery in the United States. By mid-1982 there were almost 2,600 CNMs, with the majority located in the East Coast. The percentage of nurse-midwives in midwifery practice increased to 67% in 1982. As shown in Table 1–1, as of 1995, of the current 5,200 CNMs nationally, approximately 4,000 (77%) are practicing as CNMs (American College of Nurse-Midwives, 1995). The 1992 National Sample Survey of RNs also indicated that only 66% of CNMs are nationally certified (American Nurses Association, 1993). This surprisingly low figure may reflect CNMs engaged in non-midwifery roles as well as non-mandatory certification requirements. As Varney (1987) stated, "Nurse-midwifery had become not only acceptable but also desirable and demanded. Now the problem was that, after years during which nurse-midwives struggled for existence there was nowhere near the supply to meet the demand" (p. 31). This pattern is also seen within the evolution of other advanced practice nursing specialties.

ORGANIZATIONAL DEVELOPMENT

Historically, nurse-midwives have been highly active and well organized since the 1920s. The American Association of Nurse-Midwives (AANM) was founded in 1928, originally as the Kentucky State Association of Midwives, an outgrowth of the FNS. Nationally, nurse-midwives first organized as a section within the National Organization of Public Health Nurses in the mid-1940s. When that organization was subsumed within the ANA and the National League for Nursing, the maintenance of a distinct section to address the needs of nurse-midwives was not possible. As a result, the American College of Nurse Midwifery was incorporated in 1955 as an independent specialty nursing organization. In 1956, the AANM merged with the College, forming the American College of Nurse-Midwives (ACNM). Beginning with a charter membership of 124, the College grew to 860 members in 1975, 2,434 in 1984, and 5,200 in 1995 (American College of Nurse-Midwives, personal communication, 1995). This relatively young organization made major progress in a relatively short time, including the establishment of an accreditation process in 1962, implementation of a certification examination and process in 1971, and the publication of a professional journal (*Journal of Nurse-Midwifery,* formerly the *Bulletin of the*

American College of Nurse Midwifery, begun in 1955). In recent decades some have argued that nurse-midwifery has moved away from nursing and attempted to establish itself as a separate profession (Diers, 1991). Although RN licensure is required for initial certification under the ACNM, continued licensure is not required (except by state regulation). Since certification was begun in 1971, approximately 4,000 nurse-midwives have been certified by the ACNM.

In 1962 the ACNM established the definitions of the nurse-midwife and nurse-midwifery. These definitions clearly emphasized that the role was an "extension" of nursing practice (American College of Nurse-Midwives, 1962). These definitions of practice and philosophy were revised in 1978, reflecting more of an emphasis on the distinct midwifery and nursing origins of the role (American College of Nurse-Midwives, 1978a, 1978b). Thus, CNMs are unique from other APNs in that they conceptualize their role as the combination of two disciplines, nursing and midwifery.

The ACNM has been active historically in policy formation related to some controversial areas. In 1971 the College approved a statement prohibiting CNMs from performing abortions. The College also issued a statement in 1980 allowing CNMs to practice in a variety of settings, including hospitals, homes, and birthing centers.

EDUCATIONAL DEVELOPMENT

Educationally, the first nurse-midwifery training program was established in 1932 in connection with the Maternity Center of New York City. Named the School of the Association for the Promotion and Standardization of Midwifery, this program was also known as the Lobenstine Midwifery School. The impetus for creating this program was to prepare public health nurses to work as instructors and supervisors of traditional midwives as well as nurses with limited obstetrical training. The school was operated in connection with the Lobenstine Midwifery Clinic and attended 7,099 deliveries between 1932 and 1958, producing a maternal mortality rate of 0.9 per 1,000 births as compared with a rate of 10.4 per 1,000 for the same geographic area (Varney, 1987). Between 1933 and 1959 the Maternity Center Association School of Nurse-Midwifery graduated 320 students.

The second formal nurse-midwifery training program was established by the FNS in 1939. With the advent of World War II, the FNS faced a crisis when many of the British nurse-midwives returned to their homeland. As a result, the Frontier Graduate School of Midwifery was established in 1939. This historic school had graduated 460 nurse-midwives by 1976 and continues today as the Frontier School of Midwifery and Family Nursing. In the 1930s through 1960s several nurse-midwifery educational programs were established throughout the country, including Tuskeegee, Philadelphia, and New Mexico, although some operated only briefly. In 1955 there were three certificate and two master's degree programs; by mid-1982 there were 11 certificate and 14 master's degree programs, consistent with the trend toward master's preparation reflected in the other advanced practice specialties (Adams, 1983). As of 1995 there were 44 CNM educational programs, including 31 master's programs, 10 certificate programs, and 3 pre-certification programs (American College of Nurse-Midwives, personal communication, 1995). The pre-certification programs provide nurses practicing as traditional midwives with portions of a nurse-midwifery curriculum, making them eligible to sit for national certification.

INTER- AND INTRA-PROFESSIONAL DYNAMICS

Like nurse anesthesia, nurse-midwifery has been highly active in the legal and legislative arenas, often related to inter-professional struggles. As nurse-midwives reached increasing levels of acceptance and demand, inter-professional conflicts increased, with medicine perceiving CNMs as a competitive threat. This conflict was manifested by state legislative battles over statutory recognition of CNMs, denial of hospital privileges, attempts to deny third-party reimbursement, and malpractice insurance struggles. As a result, in 1980 an investigative congressional hearing was conducted regarding the problems of CNMs, specifically restraint-of-trade issues, involving the Federal Trade Commission. In two cases, one in Tennessee and one in Georgia, the Federal Trade Commission obtained consent orders against hospitals and insurance companies that attempted to limit the practice of CNMs (Diers, 1991). Third-party reimbursement was first approved in 1980 for CNMs in the Civilian Health and Medical Program of the Uniformed Services (CHAMPUS) for military dependents and Medicaid. From a state regulatory perspective, as late as 1963 only three states and New York City legally authorized CNM practice. By 1984 all states had recognized nurse-midwifery within state laws or regulations (Varney, 1987).

One unique legal issue relates to the contention of CNMs that they represent the combination of two disciplines, nursing and midwifery. Legally, this has resulted in several interesting cases involving nurses practicing midwifery who were not educated as nurse-midwives (Leggett v. Tennessee Board of Nursing, 1980; Leigh v. Board of Registration in Nursing, 1984; Smith v. State of Indiana ex rel. Medical Licensing Board of Indiana, 1984). In all cases midwifery and nursing were found to be separate disciplines. However, there has never been a case of a CNM being sued for practicing medicine without a license, a legal challenge that both CRNAs and NPs have been forced to confront (Diers, 1991).

The history of nurse-midwifery in America certainly reflects significant inter-professional struggle and some intra-professional tension as evidenced by early organizational efforts. CNMs, however, have consistently promoted an interdisciplinary perspective as reflected in the 1971 joint statement of the ACNM, the American College of Obstetricians and Gynecologists, and the Nurses' Association of the American College of Obstetricians and Gynecologists. In this statement, the three groups supported the development and utilization of CNMs in obstetrical teams "directed by a physician." This dated concept of physician-directed teams will certainly be challenged as CNMs develop increasingly independent practice models.

CLINICAL NURSE SPECIALISTS

HISTORICAL REVIEW

The historical development of CNSs has followed quite a different pattern from other advanced nursing specialties. According to Hamric (1989) the role of the CNS "originated for the purpose of improving the quality of nursing care provided to patients" (p. 3). Historically there is disagreement as to the origin of the CNS concept. According to Peplau (1965) the title originated in 1938. In 1943, Reiter (1966) first coined the term "nurse clinician" to designate a nurse with advanced clinical competence and recommended the preparation of such clinicians in graduate educational programs. Norris (1977) contended that the CNS concept was first introduced in 1944 in connection with the Committee to Study Postgraduate Clinical Nursing Courses of the National League for Nursing Education. Smoyak (1976) traced the origin of the concept to a national conference of directors of graduate programs that was held in 1949 at the University of Minnesota. During this period, the dominant view of nursing education was that the diploma was the preferred basic preparation for professional nursing, a stance that greatly limited the growth of graduate programs. Thus, until the second half of the twentieth century, graduate nursing education focused primarily on functional rather than clinical specialization, with students concentrating on administration, education, or supervision. According to Sills (1983) this trend was influenced by the following: the orientation of nursing's early leaders in graduate nursing education at Teachers College, Columbia University; the increased emphasis on in-patient hospital care in the post–World War II era; and the resultant shift in the delivery of nursing care from a private duty to a supervisory model within the hospital administrative structure. The conservative gender attitudes related to the roles of women that predominated during the mid-century period also served to inhibit the emergence of innovative and autonomous leadership roles in clinical nursing.

The evolution of the CNS role is expansive because of the multiple specialties represented. The historical development of psychiatric CNSs is thus presented as an example, because theirs is the oldest and one of the most highly developed CNS specialties. Peplau (1965) contended that the development of areas of specialization is preceded by three social forces: (1) an increase in specialty-related information, (2) new technological advances, and (3) response to public need and interests. All of these forces clearly helped shape the development of the psychiatric CNS role. The first American training program for psychiatric nurses was opened in 1880 at McLean Hospital in Massachusetts (Critchley, 1985). Nursing's role in mental health care at the time was basically providing custodial care and supervision of ancillary physical care providers under the direction of physicians (Goodnow, 1938). In the early 1900s the specialty area of psychiatric nursing emerged, largely because of the leadership of Linda Richards. Between 1900 and 1930, psychiatry changed dramatically as a result of increasing scholarship, including the influence of Freud and Sullivan. It was in this period that the first psychiatric text, *Nursing Mental and Nervous Diseases,* was published in 1920 by Harriet Bailey and served as the primary resource in the field for over 30 years. Sullivan's classic writings in psychiatry beginning in the 1930s had a dramatic effect on psychiatric nursing. The emphasis on interpersonal interaction with patients and milieu treatment supported the movement of nurses into a more direct role in the psychiatric care of hospitalized patients. Technological advances during this period, including insulin, chemotherapy, and electroshock therapies, supported the growing emphasis on interpersonal therapy, with nurses serving a direct, active role in treatment. Sociopolitically, World Wars I and II produced increased public recognition of mental health concerns because of war-related psychiatric problems in returning soldiers (Critchley, 1985). Thus, the stage was set in the late 1930s and 1940s for psychiatric nursing to make major strides in developing a specialized direct-care role. By 1943 three postgraduate programs in psychiatric nursing were established, but more developed soon, including the first master's program at Rutgers in 1954. The National Mental Health Act in 1946 designated psychiatric nursing as a core discipline; as a result, funding for graduate and undergraduate educational programs and research became available. During the late 1940s and 1950s the scholarship in psychiatric nursing blossomed, including the classic writings of Peplau, who proposed the first conceptual framework for psychiatric nursing. This growth in the psychiatric nursing body of knowledge provided the support for psychiatric nurses to begin exploring new leadership roles in the care of mental health clients in both in-patient and out-patient settings. The expansion of the psychiatric CNS role in outpatient mental health was greatly enhanced by the Community Mental Health Centers Act of 1963 as well as the growing interest in child and adolescent mental health care during the 1960s. By 1970 a cadre of graduate-prepared psychiatric CNSs assumed roles as individual, group, family, and milieu therapists and obtained direct third-party reimbursement for their services. Soon after, psychiatric nurses led the way in identifying minimal educational and clinical criteria for CNSs and the establishment of national specialty certification through the ANA (Critchley, 1985).

The impressive development of the psychiatric CNS role helped initiate the growth of other CNS specialty areas. Following the enactment of the Nurse Training Act (NTA) (Title VIII of the Public Health Service Act) in 1965, attention to clinical specialization in graduate education increased, in contrast with the prior emphasis on education and administration. The NTA was instrumental in the development of master's programs emphasizing clinical specialization in schools of nursing. In the development of these new clinically focused graduate programs, nursing faculty members were instrumental in further developing and defining the role of the CNS. This specialist would provide a high level of specialized nursing care as well as serve as change agent in hospital settings through role modeling and consultation with other providers (Christman, 1991).

As with the other advanced nursing specialties, the development of the CNS role included early evaluation research that served to validate and promote the innovation. Landmark studies by Georgopoulos and his colleagues (Georgopoulos & Christman, 1970; Georgopoulos & Jackson, 1970; Georgopoulos & Sana, 1971) evaluated the effect of CNS practice on nursing process and outcomes in in-patient adult health-care settings. These and other evaluative studies (Ayers, 1971; Girouard, 1978; Little & Carnevali, 1967) demonstrated the positive effect of the introduction of the CNS in relation to nursing care improvements and functioning. More recently, McBride (1987) and her associates similarly demonstrated that nursing practice, particularly in relation to documentation, improved as a result of the introduction of a CNS in an in-patient psychiatric setting. Increasingly, evaluation of the CNS role has also focused on client outcomes (e.g., Brooten et al., 1986; Linde & Janz, 1979; Pozen et al., 1977), which provide even stronger data supporting the contribution of the CNS role.

Employment opportunities for CNSs, particularly in non-psychiatric specialties, were initially limited, so like CNMs, many early CNS graduates assumed roles in administration or education. Over time, the role became more institutionalized, especially in large health-care institutions and in the professional and educational communities. As a result, the CNS role became accepted by and included in the practice arena relatively rapidly and without significant controversy, as noted by the National Commission on Nursing (1983) and the Task Force on Nursing Practice in Hospitals (McClure, 1983). However, by the mid-1980s, some concerns related to the future of the CNS role were surfacing in light of the increasing concern with health-care cost containment (Hamric, 1989). Currently, CNSs make up the largest ANP group, totaling 58,185 in 1992 (American Nurses Association, 1993) (see Table 1–1).

ORGANIZATIONAL DEVELOPMENT

Organizationally, CNSs have actively participated in independent specialty nursing organizations as well as councils within the ANA that reflect their particular clinical area of interest. Certification of CNSs began in the mid-1970s under the ANA and has increased in specialty organizations over time. This process has been somewhat slow because of the multiple specialties of CNSs. Complicating the situation is the fact that certification has been available primarily at the basic specialty level, rather than the advanced level. For example, in oncology, basic certification has been available for several years through the Oncology Nursing Society (ONS). In 1995 the first certification examination for advanced practice in oncology nursing was administered by the ONS. For some specialties no certification at either the basic or the advanced level is available. This may explain why only a small percentage of CNSs are nationally certified (13.5%), according to the National Sample Survey of RNs conducted in 1992 (American Nurses Association, 1993) (see Table 1–1).

Historically, legislative or regulatory turmoil relative to the CNS has been limited, although psychiatric CNSs were early leaders in seeking third-party reimbursement and changes in state nursing practice acts to recognize APNs. Currently, not all state nursing practice acts specifically recognize the CNS role.

EDUCATIONAL DEVELOPMENT

As previously discussed, psychiatric nursing was the first nursing specialty to initiate clinical preparation at the master's level. According to Critchley (1985), this emergence was directly influenced by the effect of nurses returning from World War II, who were eligible to pursue advanced education under the G.I. Bill. Early educational programs were developed in psychiatric nursing and other specialties, often in connection with universities, although graduate degrees were not conferred. As noted earlier, Peplau established the first master's program in psychiatric nursing at Rutgers University in 1954. This is considered the first CNS educational program. The expansion of the Professional Nurse Traineeship Program to include CNS students in 1963 served as a major impetus for the development and expansion of graduate programs preparing CNSs. By 1984 the National League for Nursing (NLN) accredited 129 programs for preparing CNSs (National League for Nursing, 1984). NLN (1994) data indicate that CNS programs are the most numerous of all the master's nursing programs nationally, serving over 11,000 students. The largest area of specialization is adult health/medical surgical. Recent data indicate declines in the demand for CNS graduate programs with the rapid growth of NP educational programs (National League for Nursing, 1994).

INTER- AND INTRA-PROFESSIONAL DYNAMICS

The relative ease with which the CNS was incorporated into the health care system contrasts with the experience of the other advanced nursing specialties. This could be due to the fact that the CNS role did not represent a radical change in the organization or power dynamics of health care delivery patterns but was incorporated within existing nursing organizational structures. The CNS role was an innovation born out of mainstream nursing and enjoyed the strong support of nursing leaders. Territoriality struggles related to perceived turf encroachment with other disciplines, particularly medicine, were less public, occurring more quietly within institutions. The initial establishment of CNS preparation at the graduate level was also probably a positive factor in reducing controversy.

From an intra-professional perspective, however, the CNS role produced some highly controversial dynamics. The introduction of a CNS may be interpreted by staff as a criticism of staff performance, resulting in suspicion and hostility toward the CNS. Woodrow and Bell's (1971) experience confirmed the isolation and rejection encountered by many CNSs, especially initially. Christman (1991) wrote as follows:

> For many years nurses received their advanced preparation under such rubrics as education, management, or supervision. This advanced preparation usually was devoid of clinical content . . . . This may be one of the reasons that nurse specialists threaten nurse managers, who do not have extensive clinical training, and why they are down played or underemployed by these administrators . . . . In breaking new ground at the graduate level, the nurse specialist was perceived as a threat to the status quo because she took as her model the full professional role in its broadest sense. (pp. 111–112)

These intra-professional struggles were faced first by psychiatric CNSs historically, who were successful in delineating the differences between generalist and advanced practice within psychiatric nursing, thereby promoting collaborative intra-professional practice.

NURSE PRACTITIONERS

HISTORICAL REVIEW

NPs developed somewhat later than CNSs, again with very different dynamics. In the late 1950s and early 1960s discussion about the expansion of nursing functions increased, especially as related to domains of practice traditionally seen as "medical" (McGivern, 1986). Growing out of the role of the public health nurse as the closest example of a broad scope of practice with a relatively high degree of autonomy, examples of innovative practice emerged in settings such as rural nursing, occupational settings, and venereal disease clinics (Kalisch & Kalisch, 1986). Early experiments with role expansion in the United States and Canada also focused on chronic illness management, reflecting a physician extender perspective (Lewis and Resnick, 1967). A major impetus for NP development was the shortage of primary care physicians, which was acute in the 1960s and 1970s. The trend toward medical specialization drew increasing numbers of physicians away from primary care, leaving many areas underserved. Socially and politically the United States was engaged in a period of rapid change related to the Vietnam War, domestic unrest, and movements promoting racial and gender equity. The consumer movement was at its height, demanding accessible, affordable, and sensitive health care. The women's movement also increased the awareness of nurses and of society that nurses were undervalued and underutilized. In health-care delivery, costs were increasing at an annual rate of 10% to 14% (Jonas, 1981). One innovation growing out of the shortage of physicians and the Vietnam War was the introduction of the physician assistant role in the 1960s. Nursing leaders were not generally supportive of this new role, contending that nurses were more logical health professionals to assume a more direct role in primary health care. Thus, the NP role emerged in a unique context in response to needs within the population, the nursing profession, and the health-care delivery system. The development of the NP role was fueled by an increasing emphasis on primary health care in the 1970s and 1980s (McGivern, 1986). The focus was on ambulatory, interdisciplinary, and family-centered care as exemplified by demonstration projects such as the Yale Family Care Project and the Martin Luther King Health Care Center in New York.

Growing out of this period of social change, the NP role rapidly made a major impact on nursing and health-care delivery. Loretta Ford (1991), one of the originators of the NP concept, wrote in retrospect, "The nurse practitioner movement is one of the finest demonstrations of how nurses exploited trends in the larger health care system to advance their own professional agenda and to realize their great potential to serve society" (p. 287). Ford contended that the NP concept initially took hold because of the political perception of the NP as a physician substitute in a climate of physician shortage. However, "the movement thrived because the foundation of the nurse practitioner was deeply rooted in the enduring values and goals of professional nursing" (Ford, 1991, p. 287).

The landmark event marking the birth of the NP role was the establishment of the first pediatric NP program by Loretta Ford and Henry Silver at the University of Colorado in 1965. This demonstration project, funded by the Commonwealth Foundation, was designed to prepare professional nurses to provide comprehensive well-child care as well as to manage common childhood health problems. Family dynamics and community cultural values were strongly emphasized. A study evaluating the project indicated that pediatric NPs were highly competent in assessing and managing 75% of well and ill children in community health stations. In addition, pediatric NPs increased the number of clients served in private pediatric practice by 33% (Ford & Silver, 1967). This strong evaluation data, similar to that collected by innovators in the other advanced practice specialties, demonstrates the importance of concurrent research activities with the development of new ANP roles. This first pediatric NP program shifted the focus of NP practice from the care of medical illness to the strong family-oriented health promotive approach. It was a post-baccalaureate certificate program including a 4-month intensive educational and practical training period, followed by a 20-month period of concentrated training and practice in community-based health stations, often in rural areas. Interestingly Ford (1991) saw the development of the pediatric NP as a reclaiming of the nurse's role in well-child care, which was lost in the 1930s when the American Academy of Pediatrics claimed that well-child care was the domain of pediatricians rather than public health nurses.

The emergence of the NP role attracted considerable attention from professional groups and policy makers. Health policy groups, such as the National Advisory Commission on Health Manpower, issued statements in support of the NP concept (Moxley, 1968). In the early 1970s, Health Education and Welfare Secretary Elliott Richardson established the Committee to Study Extended Roles for Nurses. This group of health-care leaders was charged with evaluating the feasibility of expanding nursing practice (Kalisch & Kalisch, 1986). They concluded that extending the scope of the nurse's role was essential to providing equal access to health care for all consumers. The committee urged establishment of innovative curricular designs in health science centers with increased financial support for nursing education. They also advocated commonality of nursing licensure and certification, including a model nursing practice law suitable for national application. In addition, the report called for further research related to cost-benefit analyses and attitudinal surveys to assess the impact of the new role. The report resulted in increased federal support through the Maternal and Child Health Service, Regional Medical Programs, and the Division of Nursing of the U.S. Public Health Service. This federal support, as well as support through private funding agencies, stimulated the rapid development of educational programs for family NPs, adult NPs, pediatric NPs, rural NPs, emergency NPs, and OB/GYN NPs. Numerous research studies that evaluated the role of the NP were conducted, both within nursing and outside the profession. These studies consistently demonstrated the efficacy and effectiveness of NPs in collaborative practice with physicians.

By 1984 approximately 20,000 graduates of NP programs were employed, for the most part in settings "that the founders envisioned" (Kalisch & Kalisch, 1986, p. 715): outpatient clinics, health maintenance organizations (HMOs), health departments, community health centers, rural clinics, schools, occupational health clinics, and private offices. However, only 12% of all NPs were employed in remote or satellite clinics, often because of problems securing physician collaboration. As of 1992, there were 48,237 NPs nationally, 88.4% currently practicing in nursing, which is the highest of all the ANP specialties (American Nurses Association, 1993).

ORGANIZATIONAL DEVELOPMENT

Organizationally the ANA Commission on Nursing Education functionally described the NP role in 1972. The NLN's Council of Baccalaureate and Higher Degree Programs immediately endorsed the NP role description. Nevertheless, considerable controversy regarding the educational preparation of NPs and their role within nursing versus medicine continued within the profession. The Primary Health Care Nurse Practitioner Council was established within the ANA. Several independent NP organizations also developed in the 1970s and 1980s, including the National Association of Pediatric Nurse Associates and Practitioners and the American Academy of Nurse Practitioners. Organizationally, however, NPs remained rather fragmented at a national level until concerted efforts at combining forces began in the 1990s. Since the 1970s, credentialing of nurse practitioners has also been somewhat disorganized, with certification offered through multiple specialty organizations with varying requirements. As of 1992, 58% of NPs were nationally certified (American Nurses Association, 1993).

EDUCATIONAL DEVELOPMENT

The development of NP education was controversial. Like nurse anesthesia and nurse-midwifery, early NP education did not develop for the most part within the mainstream of nursing education. Based on the Colorado project, new programs rapidly developed, including some "mutations" as called by Ford (1991), that shifted from a nursing to a medical model with little consistency in academic standards. Over time, however, NP programs were increasingly institutionalized within major schools of nursing at the graduate level. By 1990 there were 135 master's degree and 40 certificate NP programs (Bullough, 1992). The majority of the certificate programs focused on women's health care. Most NP leaders support the master's degree as the educational requirement for NP practice. However, a vocal contingent remains within the NP community that advocates for continued certificate programs as a more effective means to prepare NPs to meet the needs of underserved populations. This view is similarly voiced within the CNM community (Rooks, Carr, & Sandvold, 1991). Currently, NP educational programs are proliferating rapidly in response to increasing demand. Between 1992 and 1994 the number of institutions offering NP programs increased from 78 to 158, resulting in a total of 384 NP programs (National Organization of Nurse Practitioner Faculties, 1995).

INTER- AND INTRA-PROFESSIONAL DYNAMICS

The legal and legislative history of NPs has been stormy. In 1971, Idaho became the first state to officially authorize an expanded role for nurses with a focus on NPs. The control and regulation of NP practice was often shared between state boards of nursing and medicine initially, moving to mainly nursing boards in the 1980s and 1990s. Prescriptive authority was and is a particularly volatile legislative issue. Most states that allow prescriptive authority specify it as a delegable function under the physician. A few states, including Oregon and Washington, have passed independent prescriptive authority.

Inter- and intra-professional relationships surrounding the NP role have also been controversial. Initially, there was considerable intra-professional resistance from the nursing community, which viewed NPs as not practicing nursing (Ford, 1982). Martha Rogers (1972), one of the most outspoken opponents of the NP concept, argued that the development of the NP role was a ploy to lure nurses away from nursing to medicine and thereby undermine nursing's unique role in health care. This view divided nurse leaders and educators, resulting in barriers to the establishment of NP educational programs within mainstream nursing education. NPs were increasingly accepted by nursing over time as they proved to provide a high quality of care using a nursing approach. The increasing move toward NP educational standardization at the master's level has also served to reduce intra-professional tension.

Inter-professional conflicts with organized medicine and to a lesser extent with pharmacy have centered on control issues and the degree of independence the NP is allowed. These conflicts have intensified as NPs have moved beyond the "physician extender" model to a more autonomous one. In 1980 a landmark case, Sermchief v. Gonzales (1983), was brought against two women's health-care NPs charged with practicing medicine without a license by the Missouri medical board (Doyle & Meurer, 1983). The initial ruling was against the NPs, but on appeal the Missouri Supreme Court overturned the decision, concluding that advanced nursing functions may evolve without statutory constraints (Wolff, 1984). This case supported the development of liberalized state nursing practice acts that addressed advanced practice in generalized wording. Such practice acts are important in affording future development of advanced nursing practice roles and functions.

In 1986 NPs faced a new challenge in the form of a liability insurance crisis. Major malpractice insurance carriers threatened to drop coverage for NPs or to dramatically increase rates (Pearson, 1987). This crisis was actually preceded by a similar crisis for CNMs in 1985. The national NP organizations were successful in quickly meeting the challenge, negotiating reasonable coverage for NPs in various types of practice settings. An outgrowth of this crisis was increased sophistication within the NP community regarding the importance of maintaining accurate claims data related to NP practice. These data have proved highly effective in demonstrating the low risk of NPs for malpractice actions.

Over time the territorial and legal struggles faced by NPs have changed, similar to the experience of other advanced practice specialties. Most recently legislative efforts to secure third-party reimbursement and maintain nursing's control over NP practice have been active areas. In addition, restraint-of-trade issues are being addressed as NPs are increasingly viewed as a competitive threat by other providers, particularly physicians.

SUMMARY AND CONCLUSIONS

The preceding historical review of the development and evolution of advanced nursing practice makes it clear that the various specialties have areas of commonality. Recurrent themes and dynamics are apparent, including the impact of societal forces, dynamic inter- and intra-professional struggles, and the importance of organizational, educational, and research development.

Societal forces have clearly influenced the development of advanced nursing practice. Gender issues have affected all the specialties to some degree because of the unique position of nursing as a female-dominated profession. In nurse anesthesia, the increasing acceptance of males in the specialty has been a challenge. Within nurse-midwifery, the status of women and their health was a powerful force in the establishment and development of the specialty. Among CNSs and NPs, gender biases have impeded attempts to assume an autonomous role in the male-dominated health-care system. Changing societal attitudes toward women have promoted advanced nursing practice; however, gender-related conflicts have also contributed to intra- and inter-professional tensions. A second powerful societal influence is the impact of wars and the relationship between advanced nursing practice and the American military. Each of the four nursing specialties reviewed were influenced in some significant way by the major wars of the twentieth century. Historians have noted that major social changes often follow periods of war, and this phenomenon is certainly demonstrated in the history of advanced nursing practice. In general, wars have served as catalysts to promote the development of advanced nursing practice, education, and professional organization.

The powerful influence of inter-professional struggles is also apparent in all the advanced specialties, with the possible exception of CNSs. The historical struggles between nursing and medicine are long standing, particularly in relation to nurse anesthesia and nurse-midwifery. Most of these tensions revolve around issues of control, autonomy, and economic competition. The resulting legal and legislative battles for the most part have proved positive for nursing and have helped to institutionalize the APN roles.

Similarly, struggles within the nursing community have been characteristic of the evolution of all the advanced practice specialties. CRNAs, CNMs, and to some extent NPs have developed parallel to mainstream nursing, with CNSs developing more within the mainstream. These intra-professional struggles are understandable in relation to the fact that each of the advanced nursing specialties represented innovations that shook the status quo of the nursing establishment as well as the health-care system. CRNAs, CNMs, and NPs perhaps presented the most unsettling innovations for some because they challenged the boundaries between nursing and medical practice. But each specialty has struggled for acceptance and recognition with nursing colleagues at individual practice, institutional, and larger professional levels. These territorial struggles will continue, particularly as the health-care delivery system changes. History teaches us that these issues must be assertively confronted through strong and proactive organizational efforts. Organizational unity and consensus among all the advanced nursing specialties should be a goal to enhance political and legislative effectiveness. Fortunately, over time, the intra-professional tensions seem to be lessening for all the advanced practice specialties, perhaps as the inter-professional struggles intensify.

Within the development of each of the advanced nursing specialties, several common themes emerge. The critical importance of strong national organizational leadership has been clearly demonstrated to enhance the growth and protection of the specialty. Based on the experience of the two oldest specialties, nurse anesthesia and nurse-midwifery, the process of establishing an effective national organization has taken a minimum of three decades. The newest advanced practice specialties, NPs and CNSs, are still struggling with their organizational development. The specialty organizations have also historically played a critical role in the creden-tialing process for individuals within the specialty, with nurse anesthesia and nurse-midwifery being most developed. The strength, unity, and depth of the organiza-tional development of the two oldest advanced nursing specialties should serve as a model for the younger developing specialties.

Along with organizational development, the establishment of credible and stable educational programs is a crucial step in the evolution of advanced nursing specialties. Historically, advanced practice training programs have moved from informal, institutionally based models with a strong apprenticeship approach to more formalized graduate education models housed in nursing units within institu-tions of higher education. Clearly, the national commitment among most nursing leaders and educators is that preparation for advanced nursing practice should be at the master's level. If current trends continue, this commitment will be realized by the turn of the century. Ensuring consistency and quality across programs, a process that is complemented by strong specialty organizations, is a related vital issue for all the advanced practice specialties.

The history and evolution of advanced nursing practice has also demonstrated the importance of evaluative research to document the contribution of the specialty to health care and client well-being. The early APNs were particularly visionary in their inclusion of evaluative studies within their development processes. This re-search clearly served to promote the growth and acceptance of the specialties using facts and measurable outcomes.

With the rapid changes in nursing and health care it is clear that the ANP specialties will continue to evolve and diversify. Current examples of these newly evolving roles include the case manager and the acute care nurse practitioner. The beauty of the concept of advanced nursing practice is the inherent flexibility and creativity to quickly adapt to changing health-care needs. As new advanced practice roles emerge, the historical trends and struggles of the "older siblings" can certainly provide guidance and support in terms of current and future strategies. Close collaboration and support among all the advanced practice specialties are neces-sary to promote the dynamic evolution of all the roles.

In summary, the history and evolution of advanced nursing practice indicate that these nursing leaders were clearly the vanguard of the development of modern nursing. Their position as trail blazers was neither safe nor comfortable in terms of attacks from within and beyond. As a result of their concerted and dedicated "pushing of the limits" through strong collective action, the profession of nursing and health care as a whole has benefited immeasurably.

ACKNOWLEDGMENT
The author thanks Rhonda Ramirez, RN, for her assistance in the preparation of this chapter.

REFERENCES

Adams, C. J. (1983). *Nurse-midwifery: Health care for women and newborns.* New York: Grune & Stratton.

American Association of Nurse Anesthetists. (1989). *Guidelines for nurse anesthesia practice.* Park Ridge, IL: American Association of Nurse Anesthetists.

American Association of Nurse Anesthetists. (1995). Personal communication.

American College of Nurse-Midwives. (1962). Definition of a Certified Nurse-Midwife. Washington, D. C.: ACNM.

American College of Nurse-Midwives. (1968). Descriptive data, Nurse-Midwives–U.S.A. Washington, D. C.: ACNM.

American College of Nurse-Midwives. (1978a). Definition of a Certified Nurse-Midwife. Washington, D. C.: ACNM.

American College of Nurse-Midwives. (1978b). Philosophy. Washington, D. C.: ACNM.

American Nurses Association. (1980). *Nursing: A social policy statement.* Kansas City, MO: ANA.

American Nurses Association. (1993). *Advanced practice nursing: A new age in health care, nursing facts.* Washington, DC: American Nurses Publishing.

Ayers, R. (1971). Effects and development of the role of the clinical nurse specialist. In R. Ayers (Ed.), *The clinical nurse specialist: An experiment in role effectiveness and role development.* Duarte, CA: City of Hope National Medical Center.

Bankert, M. (1989). *Watchful care: A history of America's nurse anesthetists.* New York: Continuum.

Bhan v. NME Hospitals, Inc. et al. (1985). 772 F. 2nd 1467 (9th Cir.).

Breckenridge, M. (1952). *Wide Neighborhoods: A Study of the Frontier Nursing Service.* New York: Harper.

Brooten, D., Kuman, S., Brown, L. P., et al. (1986). A randomized clinical trail of early hospital discharge and home follow-up of very-low-birth-weight infants. *New England Journal of Medicine, 315,* 934-939.

Bullough, B. (1992). Alternative models for specialty nursing practice. *Nursing and Health Care, 13*(5), 254-259.

Chalmers-Frances v. Nelson. (1936). 6 Ca. 2nd 402.

Christman, L. (1991). Advanced nursing practice: Future of clinical nurse specialists. In L. H. Aiken & C. M. Fagin (Eds.), *Charting nursing's future: Agenda for the 1990s* (pp. 108-120). New York: J. B. Lippincott.

Critchley, D. L. (1985). Evolution of the role. In D. L. Critchley & J. T. Maurin (Eds.), *The clinical specialist in psychiatric mental health nursing* (pp. 5-22). New York: John Wiley & Sons.

Dewitt, K. (1900). Specialties in nursing. *American Journal of Nursing, 1,* 14-17.

Diers, D. (1991). Nurse-midwives and nurse anesthetists: The cutting edge in specialist practice. In L. H. Aiken & C. M. Fagin (Eds.), *Charting nursing's future: Agenda for the 1990s* (pp. 159-180). New York: J. B. Lippincott.

Doyle, E., & Meurer, J. (1983). Missouri legislation and litigation: Practicing medicine without a license. *Nurse Practitioner, 8,* 41-44.

Ford, L. C. (1982). Nurse practitioners: History of a new idea and predictions for the future. In L. H. Aiken (Ed.), *Nursing in the 80s* (pp. 231-248). Philadelphia: J. B. Lippincott.

Ford, L. C. (1991). Advanced nursing practice: Future of the nurse practitioner. In L. H. Aiken & C. M. Fagin (Eds.), *Charting nursing's future: Agenda for the 1990s* (pp. 287-299). New York: J. B. Lippincott.

Ford, L. C., & Silver, H. K. (1967). The expanded role of the nurse in child care. *Nursing Outlook, 15*(8), 43-45.

Fox, C. G. (1969). Toward a sound historical basis for nurse-midwifery. *Bulletin of the American College of Nurse-Midwives, 14,* 76.

Frank et al. v. South et al. (1917). *Kentucky Reporter 175,* 416-428.

Georgopoulos, B. S., & Christman, L. (1970). The clinical nurse specialist: A role model. *American Journal of Nursing, 70,* 1030-1039.

Georgopoulos, B. S., & Jackson, M. M. (1970). Nursing Kardex behavior in an experimental study of patient units with and without clinical specialists. *Nursing Research, 19,* 196-218.

Georgopoulos, B. S., & Sana, M. (1971). Clinical nursing specialization and intershift report behavior. *American Journal of Nursing, 71,* 538-545.

Girouard, S. (1978). The role of the clinical nurse specialist as change agent: An experiment in preoperative teaching. *International Journal of Nursing Studies, 15,* 57-65.

Goodnow, M. (1938). *Outline of nursing history* (6th ed.). Philadelphia: W. B. Saunders.

Hamric, A. B. (1989). History and overview of the CNS role. In A. B. Hamric & J. Spross (Eds.), *The clinical nurse specialist in theory and practice* (2nd ed., pp. 3–18). Philadelphia: W. B. Saunders.

Jonas, S. (1981). *Health care delivery in the United States.* New York: Springer.

Kalisch, P. A., & Kalisch, B. J. (1986). *The advance of American nursing* (2nd ed.). Boston: Little, Brown and Company.

Leggett v. Tennessee Board of Nursing (1980). 612 *South Western Reporter,* 2nd, 476.

Leigh v. Board of Registration in Nursing (1984). 481 N.E. 2nd 401 (Ind. App.).

Lewis, C. E., & Resnick, B. A. (1967). Nurse clinics and progressive ambulatory patient care. *New England Journal of Medicine, 277*(3), 1236-1241.

Linde, B. J., & Janz, N. M. (1979). Effect of a teaching program on knowledge and compliance of cardiac patients. *Nursing Research, 28,* 282-286.

Little, D. E., & Carnevali, D. (1967). Nurse specialist effect on tuberculosis. *Nursing Research, 16,* 321-326.

McBride, A. B., Austin, J. K., Chesnut, E. E., et al. (1987). Evaluation of the impact of the clinical nurse specialist in a state psychiatric hospital. *Archives of Psychiatric Nursing, 1,* 55-61.

McClure, M. L., Poulin, M. A., Sovie, M. D., & Wandelt, M. A. (1983). *Magnet hospitals.* Kansas City, MO: ANA.

McGivern, D. (1986). The evolution of primary care nursing. In M. Mezey & D. McGivern (Eds.), *Nurses, nurse practitioners: The evolution of primary care.* Boston: Little, Brown and Company.

Moxley, J. (1968). The predicament in health manpower. *American Journal of Nursing, 68,* 1490.

National Commission on Nursing (1983). *Summary Report and Recommendations.* Chicago: The Hospital Research and Educational Trust.

National League for Nursing (1984). *Master's education in nursing: Route to opportunities in contemporary nursing, 1984–1985.* New York: National League for Nursing.

National League for Nursing (1994). *Nursing Datasource 1994: Volume KK graduate education in nursing advanced practice nursing.* New York: National League for Nursing.

National Organization of Nurse Practitioner Faculties (1995). Nurse Practitioner Program Number of Institutions Specialty Tracks by State. New York. Washington, D. C.: NONPF.

Norris, D. M. (1977). One perspective on the nurse practitioner movement. In A. Jacox & C. Norris (Eds.), *Organizing for independent nursing practice* (pp. 21-33). New York: Appleton-Century-Crofts.

Olsen, G. W. (1940). The nurse anesthetists: Past, present and future. *Bulletin of the American Assoication of Nurse Anesthetists, 8*(4), 298.

Oltz v. St. Peter's Community Hospital (1986). CV 81-271-H-Res, Montana District Court.

Pearson, L. J. (1987). The liability insurance crisis: Address it now or pay later. *Nurse Practitioner, 12*(6), 6-15.

Peplau, H. E. (1965). Specialization in professional nursing. *Nursing Science, 3,* 268-287.

Pozen, M. W., Stechmiller, J. A., Harris, W., et al. (1977). A nurse rehabilitator's impact on patients with myocardial infarction. *Medical Care, 15,* 830-837.

Reiter, F. (1966). The nurse-clinician. *American Journal of Nursing, 66,* 274-280.

Robinson, S. (1984). A historical development of midwifery in the black community: 1600–1940. *Journal of Nurse-Midwifery, 29*(4), 247-250.

Rogers, M. E. (1972). Nursing: To be or not to be. *Nursing Outlook, 20,* 42-46.

Rooks, J. P., Carr, K. C., Sandvold, I. (1991). The importance of non-master's degree options in nurse-midwifery education. *Journal of Nurse-Midwifery, 36,* 124-130.

Sermchief v. Gonzales (1983). 660 S.W. 2nd 683.

Sills, G. M. (1983). The role and function of the clinical nurse specialist. In N. L. Chaska (Ed.), *The nursing profession: A time to speak* (pp. 563-579). New York: McGraw-Hill.

Smith v. State of Indiana ex rel. Medical Licensing Board of Indiana (1984). 459 NE. 2nd 401 (In. App. 2 Dist).

Smoyak, S. A. (1976). Specialization in nursing: From then to now. *Nursing Outlook, 24,* 676-681.

Swenson, N. (1968). The role of the nurse-midwife on the health team as viewed by the family. *Bulletin of the American College of Nurse-Midwives, 13,* 125.

Thatcher, V. S. (1953). *A history of anesthesia: With emphasis on the nurse specialist.* Philadelphia: J. B. Lippincott.

Tom, S. A. (1982). Nurse-midwifery: A developing profession. *Law, Medicine and Health Care, 10,* 262-266.

Varney, H. (1987). *Nurse-midwifery* (2nd ed.). Boston: Blackwell Scientific Publishing.

Wolff, M. A. (1984). Court upholds expanded practice roles for nurses. *Law, Medicine and Health Care, 12,* 26-29.

Woodrow, M., & Bell, J. (1971). Clinical specialization: Conflict between reality and theory. *Journal of Nursing Administration, 1,* 23-27.

CHAPTER 2

Conceptualizations of Advanced Nursing Practice

Margretta Madden Styles

INTRODUCTION

Fundamental to the sound progress of any practice field is the development of a common language and conceptual framework for communication and for guiding and evaluating practice, policy, theory, research, and teaching. Such a foundation is particularly crucial at this stage in the development of advanced practice nursing. In this chapter, some of the conceptual impediments to developing a shared understanding of advanced practice nursing are identified, working definitions are proposed, and conceptual models to serve the above purposes are explored.

CONCEPTUAL CONUNDRUMS IN ADVANCED PRACTICE NURSING

Currently, there appear to be two general areas of conceptual confusion or uncertainty in the evolution of advanced practice nursing. The first is the shunned, but essential, distinction between *advanced practice nursing* and *advanced nursing practice.* The second conceptual hazard is a quagmire filled with slippery (i.e., inconsistently used and defined) terms of reference. A core, stable vocabulary, a *lingua franca,* is needed for definition and model building. These two conceptual problems are briefly described below.

ADVANCED PRACTICE NURSING AND ADVANCED NURSING PRACTICE

It is the view of this author that advanced practice nursing includes, but is not synonymous with or limited to, advanced nursing practice. The distinction between these terms is perhaps best grasped through an analogy: advanced practice nursing is to advanced nursing practice as nursing (or the nursing profession) is to nursing practice. *Nursing* and *advanced practice nursing* are the broader terms, describing the fields of occupation. At the core of the field is the practice (the work of the field), but also included in the field are the supportive and derivative factors associated with practice and practitioners.

There is confusion when these terms are used interchangeably, as becomes apparent when one examines a range of conceptual frameworks, some dealing with the field, some dealing with the practice, and some focusing on selected aspects of both. Most of the frameworks deal with advanced nursing practice (ANP), which is the focus of the remainder of the chapter.

A CORE VOCABULARY FOR CONCEPTUAL FRAMEWORKS

The basic elements or building blocks of conceptual models in the advanced practice nursing literature are variously domains, theories, roles, subroles, competencies, functions, activities, skills, abilities, and others. The problem in comparing, refining, or developing models is that these terms are used with no universal meaning or frame of reference; occasionally, no definition at all is offered, or the meaning seems uncertain or inconstant. In laying the foundation for their nurse practitioner (NP) model, Shuler and Davis (1993) stated that "one of the greatest barriers to using nursing models in practice relates to vocabulary and communication within the models" (p. 11). This instability and inconsistency in terminology are pointed out as various models are introduced in this chapter. It is rightly anticipated that conceptual models of the field and its practice change over time. However, it would assist such evolution and its comprehension if scholars and practitioners in the field could agree on the use and definition of fundamental terms of reference.

THE NATURE, PURPOSES, AND COMPONENTS OF CONCEPTUAL MODELS

What is a conceptual model? What purposes does it serve? What are its components? There are a number of answers to these questions in the nursing literature. In describing nurse-midwifery, Carveth (1987) drew heavily from various expert sources to arrive at the clear, comprehensive explanation of a conceptual model paraphrased as follows:

A conceptual model is that which orders, clarifies, and systematizes selected components of the phenomenon (i.e., advanced nursing practice) it serves to depict. The model then becomes a tool for interrelating concepts in a way in which the concepts can be better understood and explained. The term *conceptual framework* is often used synonymously with *conceptual model*, as is the case in this chapter. Conceptual models are abstract and untestable, unlike theories, which are less abstract and are able to be tested.

Conceptual frameworks serve many purposes. In professional role identity and function, conceptual models help practitioners organize their beliefs and knowledge about their professional roles and practice and provide a sound base for further development of knowledge. In research, the conceptual model provides structure to the development of theory in relation to the concepts being studied. In education, conceptual models assist curriculum planning in the identification of important concepts and the relationships among them and in the selection of experiences to enhance student learning and their application of these relationships. In clinical practice, conceptual models allow practitioners to see the bigger picture so that holistic and comprehensive care is provided.

The components of conceptual frameworks are concepts and relationships (i.e., concepts in meaningful configuration) that reflect assumptions about the philosophy, values, and practices of a profession. Carveth (1987) identified three schools of conceptual models in nursing, which she classified according to their foci and their derivation from other disciplines. *Interactionist* models are derived from social psychology and focus on the gestalt of the individual. *Developmental* models are derived from developmental psychology and focus on concepts of change and growth and levels of development. *Systems models* are derived from physics and sociology and focus on the integrity of the system through structure and organization. The conceptual frameworks reviewed in this chapter are variously derived from these three schools.

Holt (1984) defined a conceptual framework as "a network or an interrelationship of concepts that provides a rationale for action" (p. 446). She posited that conceptual frameworks need several types of concepts:

- Concepts that explain the nature of the unit (be it a cell, a person, a community, or a world);

- Concepts that identify the goal of the unit;
- Concepts that describe the "normal" sequential growth and development of the unit;
- Concepts that explore the deviation from the expected developmental pattern;
- Concepts that describe other units in the universe and the environment in which the units exist; and
- Concepts that address relationships—internal and external.

It has been said that conceptual models reflect assumptions about the philosophy, values, and practices of the profession. Two key assumptions guide the present discussion of conceptualizations of advanced nursing practice. The first is that advanced nursing practice will reach its full potential to the extent that identified conceptual components are appropriately addressed. The second assumption is that the development and strengthening of advanced nursing practice will lead to two *goals:*

1. A maximum social contribution of the advanced practice nurse (APN) to the health-care needs of society and
2. The actualization of practitioners of advanced practice nursing.

FOUNDATIONAL FACTORS THAT SUPPORT ADVANCED NURSING PRACTICE

The term *factor* does not customarily appear in any formal sense as a concept or building block in conceptual models. *Factor* is a nonesoteric term that appears widely throughout public discourse; it is not the proprietary claim of a particular discipline. The dictionary defines factors as conditions that bring about a result; in mathematics, factors are quantities that form a product when they are multiplied together. As the term is used herein, *factors are conditions that in combination lead to a result.* The result is the fullest development of advanced nursing practice, as put forth in the aforementioned assumptions and goals. The term *factor* is generous, permitting conditions or qualities of a different nature to be clustered.

There are several types of conditions that form the essential platform that supports a profession or occupational field. Thirteen of these foundational factors can be identified as supports for advanced nursing practice. These foundational factors are both internal and external to the field, as recognized by Roy and Martinez (1983) in their systems framework for clinical nurse specialist (CNS) practice.

Within the external environment, these conditions create opportunities for the field, for example,

1. The health needs of the people,
2. The openness to innovation and new administrative structures of the health delivery system,
3. The health policy of the government, and
4. The status of and fluidity within the health workforce situation.

The history of the field of advanced practice nursing discloses many of these "opportunity factors." Ford (1982; cited in Mezey & McGivern, 1993) noted that society's needs and nursing's potential led to the development of the first NP program in 1965. The shortage of primary care physicians, described in some areas as a contributing factor, was seen by Ford as the opportunity, and not the reason, for the new role.

Within the environment of the greater nursing profession, some significant conditions that have contributed to the development of advanced practice nursing are

5. The strength of the profession to advocate and advance a new area of practice;
6. Necessary manifestations of the profession's sanction and support for the development of advanced specialties, such as lobbying for favorable governmental laws and policies; and
7. Nursing's willingness to grant a special status and privilege to a segment of its members and to delegate certain powers of self-determination to the group, as reflected, for example, in credentialing policies.

Within the environment of advanced practice nursing are various conditions that have, in particular, contributed to the quality of advanced nursing practice and enabled its growth. Principal among them are conditions relating to the characteristics of the practitioners themselves. Within this category are such factors as the practitioners'

8. Proper role identity and understanding of the field,
9. Positive values and attitudes,
10. Advanced education, and
11. Substantial experience.

A very useful framework for analyzing the role and attitude transformation that occurs as a practice field develops has been provided by Thibodeau and Hawkins (1994). They administered two instruments to NPs to determine correlations among (1) role attitudes and values, (2) confidence about practice knowledge and skills, and (3) orientation to a medical or nursing model to guide practice. A direct positive correlation was found between level of confidence and degree of nursing orientation.

Role theory provided the framework for articulating the research questions and analyzing the results of the Thibodeau and Hawkins (1994) study. Specifically, Oda (1977) identified three phases for specialized nursing role development: role identification, role transition, and role confirmation (also see Chapter 5 for discussion of role development models). The practitioners studied appeared to have reached the stage of role confirmation. Role development frameworks should be extremely useful in efforts to trace over time the role identity of nurses in advanced practice, a critical enabling factor in the continuing evolution of advanced nursing practice.

Two final conditions critical to the continued growth of advanced nursing practice are

12. The development and dissemination of a significant research base for the practice and
13. The existence of an organization to mobilize the practitioners and enable them to exert control over the standards and influence of the field, pro-

mote the development of a literature and sound educational programs, and represent the field within the external environment.

These thirteen foundational factors are essential conditions if the overall field of advanced nursing practice is to develop and credible practice is to take root and flourish.

CONCEPTUALIZATIONS OF ADVANCED NURSING PRACTICE

As explained above, practice conditions are supported by environmental opportunities and internal and external professional advocacy. They are further derived from the expertise (attitudes, education, knowledge, and experience) of practitioners and from research in the field. *Practice is the central, the clinical, work of the field.* Practice is the reason for which the field was created. Maximizing that work in terms of its development and impact is the reason why the conditions discussed above are so important.

What are the characteristics of advanced nursing practice? How does it differ from other nursing practice? What is its scope and purpose? What knowledge and skills are required? Within what roles does this practice occur?

Scores of writers have written on this subject from a variety of different angles. As mentioned earlier, comparisons are difficult, because terms of reference and their meanings vary according to the type of framework used and the level of analysis performed. In broad and mixed terms, advanced nursing practice, as compared with basic level nursing, is most commonly characterized as

- specialized, in terms of focus and population served;
- expanded, in terms of knowledge and skills;
- complex, in terms of clinical challenges and clinical judgment; and
- independent, in terms of decision making.

Practitioners must be highly educated and experienced to practice within a field so characterized. Though they may practice in a variety of roles—CNS, NP, certified nurse-midwife (CNM), certified registered nurse anesthetist (CRNA), case manager, and others—what characterizes the practice is knowledge and expertise, clinical judgment, skilled and self-initiated care, and scholarly inquiry, not job description, title, or setting (Diers, 1985; see also Chapter 6).

In the conceptual frameworks reviewed in this section, the term *role* is used loosely and variably, sometimes seemingly describing functions, such as management or teaching or research, and sometimes taking a psychological or sociological perspective on developing social roles or selves in relation to environment. Dictionaries, adding to the confusion, use the terms *role, function, occupation,* and *duties* to define one another. In this discussion, *role* is used only in a concrete sense, to refer to titles appearing in legal documents, certification programs, or job descriptions. For example, from this perspective the CNS, NP, CNM, CRNA, and case manager are advanced practice roles.

Turning now from consideration of who engages in advanced nursing practice and in what capacity to consideration of models depicting the practice itself, one sees that such practice models could serve a variety of purposes. They could serve as a template against which (1) levels of practice can be distinguished; (2)

educational programs can be developed and evaluated; (3) knowledge and behaviors can be measured for certification purposes; (4) practitioners can understand, examine, and improve their own practice; (5) job descriptions can be developed; and (6) progress in a field can be traced for historical purposes. Models can also be used in the identification of and as a context for researchable questions and for theory development.

The ultimate usefulness of particular practice models will be assessed according to the extent they serve one or more of these purposes and to the degree to which they provide some clarity about and direction to the field. And the purposes served will be determined by the concepts explicated within the framework. For example, frameworks that depict configurations of knowledge are applicable to test construction and curriculum content. Frameworks that depict configurations of competencies are useful in examining behavior and in role development.

From the present review of a number of frameworks it can be seen that *competency* may be the most commonly used concept in explaining nursing practice and advanced nursing practice. Again, meanings are not consistent.

BENNER'S MODEL OF EXPERT PRACTICE

Many of the models use, adapt, and refine Benner's (1984) seminal work, *From Novice to Expert*. In using an interpretive approach to identifying and describing clinical knowledge in interviews with expert clinicians, Benner defined two key terms (pp. 292–293):

Competency: An interpretively defined area of skilled performance identified and described by its intent, function, and meanings.

Domain: A cluster of competencies that have similar intents, functions, and meanings.

Through the analysis of clinical exemplars discussed in the interviews, Benner derived a group of competencies. Clustering the competencies resulted in further identification of seven domains of expert nursing practice. Within her lexicon, these domains are a combination of roles, functions, and competencies, although the three have not been precisely differentiated. The seven domains and competencies associated with each domain are listed in Table 2–1.

In a later work, Benner (1985) more directly described ANP expertise in discussing the CNS. She saw CNS expertise as a hybrid of practical knowledge gained from frontline clinical practice and sophisticated skills of knowledge utilization. The CNS has in-depth knowledge of a particular clinical population and grasps in theory and practice the illness and disease trajectory of that patient population.

FENTON'S AND BRYKCZYNSKI'S EXPERT PRACTICE DOMAINS OF THE CLINICAL NURSE SPECIALIST AND NURSE PRACTITIONER

Fenton (1985) and Brykczynski (1989) each independently applied Benner's model of expertise at the ANP level in examining the practice of CNSs and NPs, respectively. In a later publication, Fenton and Brykczynski (1993) compared their earlier research findings to identify similarities and differences between CNSs and NPs. They used Benner's understanding of the concepts of domains, competencies, roles, and functions. Fenton and Brykczynski verified that nurses in advanced

TABLE 2–1. BENNER'S DOMAINS OF NURSING PRACTICE

Domain: The Helping Role

The healing relationship: Creating a climate for and establishing a commitment to healing

Providing comfort measures and preserving personhood in the face of pain and extreme breakdown

Presencing: being with a patient

Maximizing the patient's participation and control in his or her own recovery

Interpreting kinds of pain and selecting appropriate strategies for pain management and control

Providing comfort and communication through touch

Providing emotional and informational support to patients' families

Guiding a patient through emotional and developmental change; providing new options, closing off old ones

Channeling, teaching, mediating:

    Acting as a psychological and cultural mediator

    Using goals therapeutically

    Working to build and maintain a therapeutic community

Domain: Administering and Monitoring Therapeutic Interventions and Regimens

Starting and maintaining intravenous therapy with minimal risks and complications

Administering medications accurately and safely: monitoring untoward effects, reactions, therapeutic responses, toxicity, and incompatibilities

Combating the hazards of immobility; preventing and intervening with skin breakdown, ambulating and exercising patients to maximize mobility and rehabilitation, preventing respiratory complications

Creating a wound management strategy that fosters healing, comfort, and appropriate drainage

Domain: Effective Management of Rapidly Changing Situations

Skilled performance in extreme life-theatening emergencies: rapid grasp of a problem

Contingency management: rapid matching of demands and resources in emergency situations

Identifying and managing a patient crisis until physician assistance is available

Domain: The Diagnostic and Monitoring Function

Detection and documentation of significant changes in a patient's condition

Providing an early warning signal: anticipating breakdown and deterioration prior to explicit confirming diagnostic signs

Anticipating problems: future thinking

Understanding the particular demands and experiences of an illness: anticipating patient care needs

Assessing the patient's potential for wellness and for responding to various treatment strategies

Domain: The Teaching-Coaching Function

Timing: capturing a patient's readiness to learn

Assisting patients to integrate the implications of illness and recovery into their lifestyles

Eliciting and understanding the patient's interpretation of his or her illness

Providing an interpretation of the patient's condition and giving a rationale for procedures

The coaching function: making culturally avoided aspects of an illness approachable and understandable

Domain: Monitoring and Ensuring the Quality of Health Care Practices

Providing a backup system to ensure safe medical and nursing care

Assessing what can be safely omitted from or added to medical orders

Getting appropriate and timely responses from physicians

Domain: Organizational and Work-Role Competencies

Coordinating, ordering, and meeting multiple patient needs and requests; setting priorities

Building and maintaining a therapeutic team to provide optimum therapy

Coping with staff shortages and high turnover:

    Contingency planning

    Anticipating and preventing periods of extreme work overload within a shift

    Using and maintaining team spirit; gaining social support from other nurses

    Maintaining a caring attitude toward patients even in absence of close and frequent contact

    Maintaining a flexible stance toward patients, technology, and bureaucracy

(Excerpted from *From novice to expert* by Patricia Benner. Copyright © 1984 by Addison-Wesley Publishing Company. Reprinted by permission; as it appeared in Fenton, M. V. (1985). Identifying competencies of clinical nurse specialists. *Journal of Nursing Administration, 15*(12), 31–37.)

practice were indeed experts and identified some additional domains and competencies, as outlined in Figure 2–1.

    In considering the applications of Benner's model and the Fenton refinements to CNS practice, Spross and Baggerly (1989) made recommendations for further development. With some modification, these apply to advanced nursing practice

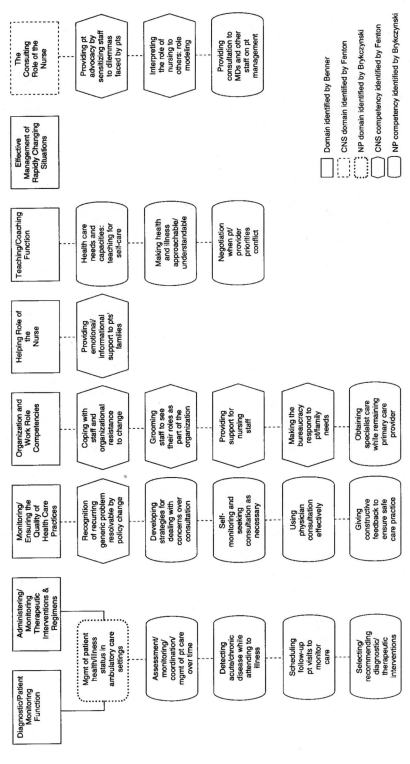

FIGURE 2-1. Expert practice domains of the clinical nurse specialist (CNS) and nurse practitioner (NP). (From Fenton, M. V., & Brykczynski, K. A. (1993). Qualitative distinctions and similarities in the practice of clinical nurse specialists and nurse practitioners. *Journal of Professional Nursing, 9,* 313–326. Used with permission.)

in general. Needed are (1) further application of the model to advanced nursing practice; (2) extension of the teaching/coaching domain to teaching nurses; (3) comparison of the non-master's-prepared clinician's competencies and the advanced practice nurse's (APN's) competencies to further elucidate components of expert versus advanced practice; and (4) student experience with ethnographic methods to enable graduates to address Benner's challenge to uncover the knowledge embedded in practice (Spross & Baggerly, 1989).

In an examination of NP conceptualizations conducted for the National Organization of Nurse Practitioner Faculties (Zimmer et al., 1990), a further reworking occurred to facilitate use of the domains as a framework for primary care NP curricula. The original six domains were collapsed to five:

1. Management of client health/illness status in ambulatory care settings,
2. Monitoring and ensuring of the quality of health care practices,
3. Organizational and work role competencies,
4. Helping role, and
5. Teaching-coaching function.

These domains were seen as a beneficial organizing framework for NP curricula development because they described the lived experience of NP practice, offered a way to organize a large amount of content while retaining a primary health-care focus, and allowed for individual NP faculties to overlay other nursing frameworks as desired (Price et al., 1992).

CALKIN'S MODEL OF ADVANCED NURSING PRACTICE

Benner and her colleagues derived their framework from the data upward. They began by collecting samples of nursing practice, to which they applied their interpretive expertise. Others have taken a more deductive approach, first developing a theoretical rationale to explain particular phenomena. In this manner, Calkin (1984) developed a model for nurse administrators to use in determining how to distinguish advanced nursing practice in personnel policies. She proposed that this be accomplished by matching (1) patient responses to health problems (as nursing is defined in the American Nurses' Association 1980 Social Policy Statement) to (2) the skill level and (3) knowledge level of nursing personnel. Three curves were overlaid on a normal distribution chart. Calkin depicted the skills and knowledge of novices, experts-by-experience, and APNs in relation to knowledge required in caring for a range of patients (Figure 2–2).

Calkin (1984) illustrated the application of this framework in explaining how APNs perform under three different sets of circumstances: when there is a high degree of unpredictability; when there are new conditions or a new patient population or new sets of problems; and when there are a wide variety of health problems, requiring the services of "specialist generalists," as she called them. She defined what APNs do in terms of functions. For example, when patients' health problems

---

FIGURE 2–2. Patient responses correlated with the knowledge and skill of beginning practitioners, experienced nurses, and advanced practice nurses. (From Calkin, J. D. (1984). A model for advanced nursing practice. *Journal of Nursing Administration, 14*(1), 25–27. Used with permission.)

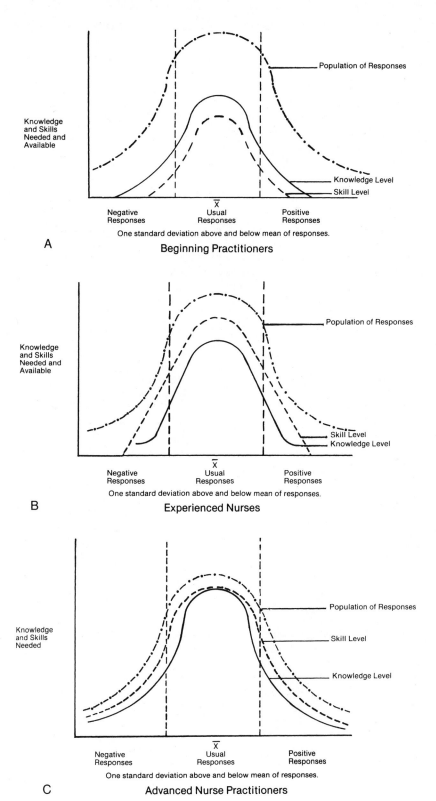

Knowledge and Skills Needed and Available

Population of Responses

Knowledge Level

Skill Level

Negative Responses

$\overline{X}$
Usual Responses

Positive Responses

One standard deviation above and below mean of responses.

A

Beginning Practitioners

Knowledge and Skills Needed and Available

Population of Responses

Skill Level

Knowledge Level

Negative Responses

$\overline{X}$
Usual Responses

Positive Responses

One standard deviation above and below mean of responses.

B

Experienced Nurses

Knowledge and Skills Needed

Population of Responses

Skill Level

Knowledge Level

Negative Responses

$\overline{X}$
Usual Responses

Positive Responses

One standard deviation above and below mean of responses.

C

Advanced Nurse Practitioners

FIGURE 2–2 *See legend on opposite page*

may elicit a wide range of human responses with continuing and substantially unpredictable elements, the ANP functions are to

- Identify and develop interventions for the unusual by providing direct care;
- Transmit this knowledge to nurses and, in some settings, to students;
- Identify and communicate needs for, or carry out research related to, human responses to these health problems;
- Anticipate factors that may lead to the presence of unfamiliar responses; and
- Provide anticipatory guidance to nurse administrators when the changes in the diagnosis and treatment of these responses may require altered levels or types of resources (Calkin, p. 28).

A principal advantage of Calkin's model is that the skills and knowledge of the practitioner are placed in the direct context of patient needs. The model, however, has been left for others to test. It does provide a framework for scholars to use in studying the function of APNs in a variety of work situations. It should also be a useful conceptualization for administrators who must maximize a multi-level nursing workforce and thus need to rationalize the use of APNs.

SHULER'S MODEL OF NP PRACTICE

Shuler's NP practice model is a systems model that is wellness oriented and definitive in terms of how NP-patient interaction, patient assessment, intervention, and evaluation should occur (Shuler & Davis, 1993). It was derived from a number of disciplines and is most ambitious in embracing myriad theoretical constructs within an internal-external-input-throughput-output systems framework. The elements include (1) the four concepts of nursing's metaparadigm (person, health, nursing, and environment), (2) nursing process, (3) a table of humanistically based assumptions about patients and students, and (4) a table of theory concepts underlying practice model constructs. The model appears to be, in fact, a network or system of frameworks.

Shuler's model is intended "to impact the NP domain at four levels: theoretical, clinical, educational, and research" (Shuler & Davis, 1993, p. 17). Its scope and intent are enormous; the model is perhaps best utilized when single constructs are isolated and addressed, though visualized within the larger whole. The most helpful subframework for clinicians, teachers, theoreticians, and researchers to use in identifying elements of practice may be the model constructs and underlying theory concepts presented in Table 2–2.

MODELS FOR NURSE-MIDWIFERY AND NURSE ANESTHESIA PRACTICE

Models of CNM and CRNA practice are available to amplify and clarify the picture of advanced nursing practice, although their scopes are delimited and specific to these two advanced roles. Official statements of CNM and CRNA organizations describe these practices.

The model of the American College of Nurse-Midwives (ACNM, 1992) includes core competencies, defined as the fundamental knowledge, skills, and behaviors expected of a new graduate. These competencies are categorized within the following management and care framework:

TABLE 2–2. MODEL CONSTRUCTS AND UNDERLYING THEORY CONCEPTS INCLUDED
IN SHULER'S MODEL OF NURSE PRACTITIONER (NP) PRACTICE

Theoretical Practice Model Constructs	Wholistic Patient Needs	NP/Patient Interaction	Self-Care	Health Prevention	Health Promotion	Wellness
Underlying Theory Concepts	Basic needs Wellness activities Health/Illness Psychological health Family Culture Social support Environmental health Spirituality	Contracting Role-Modeling Self-Care activities Teaching/ Learning Communication Problem-Solving Decision-Making	Wellness activities Preventive health activities Health promotion activities Compliance Problem-Solving Teaching/ Learning Contracting Culture Family Social support Environmental health	Primary prevention Secondary prevention Tertiary prevention Preventive health behavior Family Culture Environmental health	Health promotion behavior Wellness Family Culture Environmental health Social support	Self-Care activities Wellness activities Disease prevention activities Health promotion activities Family Culture Social support Environmental health Spirituality Contracting Teaching/Learning

(From Shuler, P. A., & Davis, J. E. (1993). The Shuler nurse practitioner practice model: A theoretical framework for nurse practitioner clinicians, educators, and researchers, part I. *Journal of the American Academy of Nurse Practitioners,* 5(1), 11–18. Used with permission.)

> Nurse-Midwifery Management
>> Primary management
>> Collaboration (co-management)
>> Referral
> Components of Nurse-Midwifery Care
>> Preconception care
>> Antepartum care
>> Interpartum care
>> Postpartum care
>> Neonatal care
>> Family planning/gynecological care
>> Professional aspects (ACNM, 1992)

The specific competencies under each heading are stated in terms of behaviors of the CNM in performing the functions outlined. Associated areas of knowledge are listed for many of the competencies. These competencies have been developed principally as guidelines for educational programs in the field. They should prove useful also to clinicians in developing and evaluating their practice and as a broad template for their certification program.

The American Association of Nurse Anesthetists (1992) listed 11 functions as summarizing the scope of CRNA practice in *Guidelines and Standards for Nurse Anesthesia Practice.* These 11 functions fall within the general areas of (1) preanesthetic preparation and evaluation; (2) anesthesia induction, maintenance, and emergence; (3) postanesthesia care; and (4) perianesthetic and clinical support functions. An example function from the category preanesthetic preparation and evaluation states that CRNA scope of practice includes "performing and documenting a preanesthetic assessment and evaluation of the patient, including requesting consultations and diagnostic studies; selecting, obtaining, ordering, or administering preanesthetic medications and fluids; and obtaining informed consent for anesthesia" (AANA, 1992, p. 2). Twelve standards for practice are largely descriptive of structure and process, within the Donabedian (1966) model of patient care evaluation (i.e., structure, process, and outcome criteria). The standards are for practitioners and peers to use in evaluating examples of specific practice.

FUTURE DEVELOPMENT

Further work is needed to clarify and harmonize the conceptual basis of advanced nursing practice. This review of various ANP models points out at least four striking areas for future development in model building and testing.

First, for some time cross-matching of frameworks has been going on to contrast, compare, and combine the role of CNS and NP. Now is the time for the focus to shift toward bringing the practice of all APNs, including CNMs and CRNAs, into conceptual unity. This is not to suggest that the practice is identical for all, but that the common elements should be identified and differences noted (see Chapter 3 for further discussion of this important recommendation). The mélange of terms, constructs, concepts, and levels of abstraction, as mentioned before, makes this an imposing challenge.

Second, attention should be directed to the "scope" dimension of advanced nursing practice. Among its other features, advanced nursing practice is specialized. Most of nursing's specialties have statements of scope, often with associated competencies or functions. At this stage in the evolution of advanced nursing, it would be helpful to devise, test, and use a conceptual framework for comparing and contrasting respective scopes of practice for advanced practice specialties. This is being done at the higher level of analysis, that of the NP and CNS (Fenton & Brykczynski, 1993; Williams & Valdivieso, 1994). Sometime soon, the respective scopes of practice in the various specialties within advanced practice roles must be addressed and a rationale articulated for further development and refinement. The American Nurses' Association's work in developing uniform formats and scopes and standards in cooperation with various specialty organizations should serve as a good platform for launching the project.

Third, the relationship of advanced nursing practice to medical practice is either a theme or an undercurrent throughout most models (e.g., Thibodeau and Hawkins' [1994] role identification; Ford's [1982] explanation of the origins of the NP role; and multidisciplinary partnerships and joint practice models [Brown, 1983]). Furthermore, it is an important issue in the contemporary debates about authority for practice, direct reimbursement, and "junior doctors." The relationship of advanced nursing practice to medical practice must be identified as a significant issue that requires ongoing attention.

The related issue of authority for practice deserves mention. Many in nursing would prefer the word *autonomy* instead of *authority*. The author, however, prefers authority as the broader and more descriptive term. *Authority is the right to act, to take action, to make decisions, even to command.* The higher authority of nurses in advanced practice derives from the recognition of their expertise by the public, regulatory bodies, the health policy arena, the health care system, and the greater profession. Authority is not just received; it must also be asserted. APNs must themselves have confidence in the power of their expert knowledge and service and in their right and responsibility to use their skills fully in the public's behalf.

Two milestones in establishing APNs' authority have been recognition of APNs for reimbursement by the government and other payers and the National Council of State Boards of Nursing's (NCSBN, 1993) Position Paper on the Regulation of Advanced Nursing Practice. In this document, the NCSBN encourages state regulatory bodies to recognize APNs by conferring an expanded legal scope of practice. The central thrust is to authorize, through the jurisdiction of states, greater authority in decision making for the highly educated, expert APN (NCSBN, 1993).

Finally, research on patient outcomes and cost-effectiveness that leads to increased knowledge about advanced nursing practice is critical. The worth of any service depends on the extent to which practice meets the needs and priorities of the society, health care systems, and the public policy arena. These needs are, by and large, for appropriate services at a reasonable cost. Critical challenges to APNs are to demonstrate enhanced effectiveness in meeting social needs and to increase the public's awareness of the benefit or desirability of those services. APNs must communicate within the nursing profession, to other health-care providers, and to society as a whole, in clear and powerful language, the difference advanced nursing practice makes. The author has identified principles of knowledge empowerment (Styles, 1990), two of which have implications for this discussion:

- Appropriate paradigms or theoretical frameworks must be used to elicit politically powerful knowledge (i.e., knowledge significant to decisions about the allocation of resources). As Harrington (1988) wrote,

  *The new imperative for nursing is to move beyond its heavy
  reliance on individualist frameworks and to include
  theoretical frameworks that examine health care systems,
  organizations, professionals and the society as a whole.
  Only with a basic understanding of the larger issues drawn
  from the fields of sociology, political science, public policy
  and economics, can nursing become a full-fledged player in
  the political arena (p. 121).*

- To have political impact, knowledge must be packaged and presented in such a manner that its meaning and relevance are unmistakable and widely disseminated.

Naylor and Brooten (1993) reviewed research literature demonstrating the differences that CNSs make in health outcomes. Their work (and the review by Girouard in Chapter 26) could serve as a model for other researchers seeking to strengthen the value attributed to advanced nursing practice. Specifically, Naylor and Brooten recommended that additional studies be done on patient and family outcomes, that the next phase of studies relate to unique functions, and that research be conducted to compare the practice patterns and outcomes of CNSs with those of physicians and other health providers (Naylor & Brooten, 1993). See Chapter 26 for further discussion of strengthening ANP evaluation.

SUMMARY

As noted above, conceptual models serve many purposes for the field they seek to describe. Importantly, they are useful for guiding and evaluating the progress of advanced nursing practice. Such progress is dependent upon the extent to which practice meets the needs and priorities of the society, health-care systems, and the public policy arena. Although a number of conceptual frameworks exist, none are fully developed in terms of advanced nursing practice. Continued model development and testing can enable the realization of the two goals of maximum social contribution of the APN to the health needs of society and the actualization of advanced practitioners.

REFERENCES

American Association of Nurse Anesthetists. (1992). *Guidelines and standards for nurse anesthesia practice.* Park Ridge, IL: Author.

American College of Nurse-Midwives. (1992). *Core competencies for basic nurse-midwifery practice.* Washington, DC: Author.

Benner, P. (1984). *From novice to expert.* Menlo Park, CA: Addison-Wesley.

Benner, P. (1985). The oncology clinical nurse specialist as expert coach. *Oncology Nursing Forum, 12*(2), 40–44.

Brown, S. J. (1983). The clinical nurse specialist in a multidisciplinary partnership. *Nursing Administration Quarterly, 8,* 36–46.

Brykczynski, K. A. (1989). An interpretive study describing the clinical judgment of nurse practitioners. *Scholarly Inquiry for Nursing Practice, 3,* 75–104.

Calkin, J. D. (1984). A model for advanced nursing practice. *Journal of Nursing Administration, 14*(1), 24–30.

Carveth, J. A. (1987). Conceptual models in nurse-midwifery. *Journal of Nurse-Midwifery, 32,* 20–25.

Diers, D. (1985). Preparation of practitioners, clinical specialists, and clinicians. *Journal of Professional Nursing, 1,* 41–47.

Donabedian, A. (1966). Evaluating the quality of medical care. *Milbank Memorial Fund Quarterly, 44,* 166–206.

Fenton, M. V. (1985). Identifying competencies of clinical nurse specialists. *Journal of Nursing Administration, 15*(12), 31–37.

Fenton, M. V., & Brykczynski, K. A. (1993). Qualitative distinctions and similarities in the practice of clinical nurse specialists and nurse practitioners. *Journal of Professional Nursing, 9,* 313–326.

Ford, L. C. (1982). Nurse practitioners: History of a new idea and predictions for the future. In L. H. Aiken & S. R. Gortner (Eds.), *Nursing in the 1980's: Crises, opportunities, challenges* (pp. 231–247). Philadelphia: J. B. Lippincott.

Harrington, C. (1988). The political economy of

health: A new imperative for nursing. *Nursing and Health Care, 9,* 121.

Holt, F. M. (1984). A theoretical model for clinical specialist practice. *Nursing and Health Care, 5,* 445–449.

Mezey, M. D., & McGivern, D. O. (Eds.). (1993). *Nurses, nurse practitioners: Evolution to advanced practice.* New York: Springer Publishing Company.

National Council of State Boards of Nursing. (1993). *Position paper on the regulation of advanced nursing practice.* Chicago: Author.

Naylor, M. D., & Brooten, D. (1993). The roles and functions of clinical nurse specialists. *Image, 25,* 73–78.

Oda, D. (1977). Specialized role development: A three-phase process. *Nursing Outlook, 25,* 374–377.

Price, M. J., Martin, A. C., Newberry, Y. G., Zimmer, P. A., Brykczynski, K. A., & Warren, B. (1992). Developing national guidelines for nurse practitioner education: An overview of the product and the process. *Journal of Nursing Education, 31,* 10–15.

Roy, C., & Martinez, C. (1983). A conceptual framework for CNS practice. In A. B. Hamric & J. A. Spross (Eds.), *The clinical nurse specialist in theory and practice* (pp. 3–20). New York: Grune & Stratton.

Shuler, P. A., & Davis, J. E. (1993). The Shuler nurse practitioner practice model: A theoretical framework for nurse practitioner clinicians, educators, and researchers, part I. *Journal of the American Academy of Nurse Practitioners, 5,* 11–18.

Spross, J. A., & Baggerly, J. (1989). Models of advanced nursing practice. In A. B. Hamric & J. A. Spross (Eds.), *The clinical nurse specialist in theory and practice* (2nd ed., pp. 19–40). Philadelphia: W. B. Saunders Company.

Styles, M. M. (1990). A common sense approach to nursing research. *International Nursing Review, 37,* 203–218.

Thibodeau, J. A., & Hawkins, J. W. (1994). Moving

toward a nursing model in advanced practice. *Western Journal of Nursing Research, 16,* 205–218.

Williams, C. A., & Valdivieso, G. C. (1994). Advanced practice models: A clinical comparison of clinical nurse specialist and nurse practitioner activities. *Clinical Nurse Specialist, 8,* 311–318.

Zimmer, P., Brykczynski, K. A., Martin, A. C., Newberry, Y. G., Price, M. J., & Warren, B. (1990). *Advanced nursing practice: Nurse practitioner curriculum guidelines* (Final Report: NONPF Education Committee). Washington, DC: National Organization of Nurse Practitioner Faculties.

CHAPTER 3

A Definition of Advanced Nursing Practice

Ann B. Hamric

INTRODUCTION

Ideally, all nurses share the same definition and core values of the discipline of nursing, which constitute the foundation of professional practice. In its new Social Policy Statement, the American Nurses' Association (ANA, 1995) defined four essential features of contemporary nursing practice:

1. Inclusion of "the full range of human experiences and responses to health and illness without restriction to a problem-focused orientation";
2. Practice based on the integration of objective and subjective experience;
3. The ability to apply "scientific knowledge to the processes of diagnosis and treatment"; and
4. The ability to provide "a caring relationship that facilitates health and healing."

Core values that guide practice include advocating for patients; respecting patient and family values and informed choices; viewing individuals holistically within their environments and cultural traditions; and maintaining a focus on disease prevention, health restoration, and health promotion (Creasia & Parker, 1991; Leddy & Pepper, 1993).

Advanced nursing practice (ANP) builds upon this foundation. The core professional values noted above also inform the central perspective of advanced practice. As Smith (1995) stated,

> The core of advanced practice nursing lies within nursing's disciplinary perspective on human-environment and caring interrelationships that facilitate health and healing. This core is delineated specifically in the philosophic and theoretic foundations of nursing. True advanced practice nursing is theory-based [and] fully integrated into the nurse's way of being and practicing. (p. 3)

In this chapter, advanced nursing practice is defined, and the various ANP roles are differentiated. Elements of the definition and roles that advanced practice nurses (APNs) assume are described in greater detail in subsequent chapters.

DISTINGUISHING BETWEEN SPECIALIZATION AND ADVANCED NURSING PRACTICE

Before exploring the definitions of advanced nursing practice, it is important to distinguish between specialization in nursing and advanced nursing practice. Specialization involves concentration in a selected clinical area within the field of nursing. All nurses with extensive experience in a particular area of practice (e.g., pediatric nursing or trauma nursing) are specialized in this sense. As the profession has advanced and responded to changes in health care, specialization and the need for specialty knowledge have increased. Thus, there are few nurses who are generalists in the true sense of the word (Kitzman, 1989).

The nursing profession has responded in a variety of ways to the increasing need for specialization in both clinical and clinical support arenas. The creation of specialty organizations, such as the American Association of Critical-Care Nurses and the Oncology Nursing Society (ONS), has been one response. The creation of advanced clinical practice roles—the certified registered nurse anesthetist (CRNA) and certified nurse-midwife (CNM) roles early in nursing's evolution and the clinical nurse specialist (CNS) and nurse practitioner (NP) roles more recently—has been another response. The development of specialized faculty, such as pediatric and obstetric faculty; researchers who focus on particular phenomena, such as nursing ethics or the care of dying patients; and nursing administrators who direct clinical nursing services has been a third response. Nurses in all of these roles can be considered specialists in an area of nursing; some of these roles may involve advanced education in a clinical specialty as well. They are not necessarily ANP roles, however.

Advanced nursing practice includes specialization but goes beyond it. In the definition proposed herein, advanced nursing practice involves specialization, expansion, advancement (ANA, 1995; Cronenwett, 1995), as well as additional characteristics. Before proposing this definition, it is necessary to review the current literature on defining ANP.

DEFINITIONS OF ADVANCED NURSING PRACTICE IN THE NURSING LITERATURE

The concept of advanced nursing practice is defined in various ways in the nursing literature. There is no consensus on the definition of advanced nursing practice, and it is difficult to find a clear definition of the term (Davies & Hughes, 1995). The *Cumulative Index to Nursing and Allied Health Literature* defined advanced practice very broadly as anything beyond the staff nurse role: "Nurses who fulfill roles beyond those that require basic educational preparation are practicing at an advanced level" (1991, p. 40). A definition this broad incorporates many nursing roles, not all of which should be considered advanced practice. For example, some authors have proposed the "health policy analyst" as an advanced practice role (Stimpson & Hanley, 1991). This role contains no direct practice component, focusing as it does on consultation to decision makers regarding health policy. As the ANA (1995) noted in its latest Social Policy Statement, "The term advanced practice is used to refer exclusively to advanced *clinical* practice" (p. 15). In this sense, the health policy analyst is a specialized nursing role but not an advanced practice role.

Other sources have defined advanced practice as practice in one of the four roles of CNS, NP, CNM, and CRNA (ANA, 1992; Donley, 1995; Ray & Hardin, 1995). Numerous authors have used the ANA's (1992) designation of these four roles as the definition of advanced nursing practice, identifying APNs as registered nurses who have completed graduate level education and/or are certified in an area of specialization. The ANA has encouraged lawmakers to expand reimbursement for the services of these APNs as a cost-effective alternative to physician care: "Advanced Practice Nurses can provide 60% to 80% of primary and preventative care traditionally performed by physicians. They are educated at one sixth the expense, to perform many of the procedures traditionally associated with physicians. . . . They are additionally cost-effective because they work to prevent illness and hospitalizations" (ANA, 1992, p. 1).

One problem with defining advanced nursing practice in terms of four practice roles is that there are other roles in addition to these four that can also be considered ANP roles, notably, the case manager, the acute care nurse practitioner

(ACNP), and the blended CNS/NP. As advanced practice continues to evolve, permutations of these roles and others will be created. It thus seems preferable to define advanced nursing practice in a way other than referring to particular roles.

A third definition, proposed by Calkin (1984), takes a more conceptual approach. Rather than define advanced nursing practice as any position other than a staff nurse, or as particular roles, Calkin defined it in terms of the diagnosis of human responses (the definition used in the ANA's 1980 Social Policy Statement). To Calkin "advanced nursing practice is the deliberative diagnosis and treatment of a full range of human responses to actual or potential health problems" (p. 27; see Chapter 2 for a description of her model). Calkin maintained that APNs have higher skill and knowledge levels that make them better able to intervene with patients whose problems represent extremes of the response continuum, whether negative or positive. In addition, they rely on deliberative and conscious reasoning and are able to be articulate about the nature of nursing practice. Calkin explicitly referred to NPs and CNSs as advanced practitioners.

Other authors have identified advanced nursing practice with particular roles. For example, Thibodeau and Hawkins (1994), in a study entitled "Moving Toward a Nursing Model in Advanced Practice," focused exclusively on the NP role. Snyder and Mirr (1995) defined advanced nursing practice as the merged roles of the CNS and NP. These definitions of advanced practice in terms of particular roles limit the concept and deny the reality that nurses practicing in other roles are also APNs.

DEFINITIONS OF ADVANCED NURSING PRACTICE PUT FORTH BY PROFESSIONAL GROUPS

One specialty organization, the ONS (1990) has developed a core definition of advanced practice for its specialty. "Advanced oncology nursing practice is defined as 'expert competency and leadership in the provision of care to individuals with an actual or potential diagnosis of cancer' " (p. 4). The ONS includes CNS, educator, researcher, and administrator roles as advanced nursing practice and requires the minimum of a master's degree for advanced practice. The inclusion of roles that do not have direct clinical practice as their main focus is not consistent with the definition of advanced nursing practice advocated here.

In a Position Paper on the Regulation of Advanced Nursing Practice, the National Council of State Boards of Nursing (NCSBN, 1993) proposed a definition of advanced practice based on registered nurse licensure and basic nursing education in addition to

> *a graduate degree with a major in nursing or a graduate degree with a concentration in an advanced nursing practice category, which includes both didactic and clinical components, advanced knowledge in nursing theory, physical and psychosocial assessment, appropriate interventions, and management of health care.* (p. 2)

The skills and abilities the NCSBN considers essential for the advanced practice registered nurse within a designated area of practice are listed in Table 3–1.

As noted earlier, in 1992 the ANA defined advanced nursing practice in terms

TABLE 3–1. SKILLS AND ABILITIES THAT THE NCSBN CONSIDERS NECESSARY FOR ADVANCED PRACTICE REGISTERED NURSES

- Assessing clients, synthesizing and analyzing data, and understanding and applying nursing principles at an advanced level;
- Providing expert guidance and teaching;
- Working effectively with clients, families, and other members of the health care team;
- Managing clients' physical and psycho-social health-illness status;
- Utilizing research skills;
- Analyzing multiple sources of data, identifying alternative possibilities as to the nature of a health care problem and selecting appropriate treatment;
- Making independent decisions in solving complex client care problems;
- Performing acts of diagnosis and prescribing therapeutic measures consistent with the area of practice; and
- Recognizing limits of knowledge and experience, planning for situations beyond expertise, and consulting with or referring clients to other health care providers as appropriate.

(From National Council of State Boards of Nursing. (1993). *Position paper on the regulation of advanced nursing practice* (pp. 2–3). Chicago: Author. Used with permission.)

of four roles. In a more recent publication, its latest Social Policy Statement, the ANA (1995) described advanced nursing practice as having three components: specialization, expansion, and advancement.

> *Specialization is concentrating or delimiting one's focus to part of the whole field of nursing. Expansion refers to the acquisition of new practice knowledge and skills, including the knowledge and skills that legitimize role autonomy within areas of practice that overlap traditional boundaries of medical practice. Advancement involves both specialization and expansion and is characterized by the integration of a broad range of theoretical, research-based, and practical knowledge that occurs as a part of graduate education in nursing.* (p. 14)

Advanced practice is further characterized by "autonomy to practice at the edges of the expanding boundaries of nursing's scope of practice," a "preponderance of self-initiated treatment regimens as opposed to dependent functions," and greater "complexity of clinical decision making" and "greater skill in managing organizations and environments" than basic nursing practice (ANA, 1995, p. 16).

These definitions of advanced practice from the NCSBN and the ANA go beyond a definition based on core qualifications or practice roles to a definition that includes key skills and competencies integral to ANP.

CORE DEFINITION OF ADVANCED NURSING PRACTICE

As can be seen from this review of recent nursing literature, advanced nursing practice is defined in differing and sometimes contradictory ways. A central and agreed upon definition of advanced nursing practice and clarity regarding how it is enacted in various health-care settings are critical to the continued development of advanced practice and, indeed, the nursing profession itself.

The definition proposed in this chapter and used throughout this book builds on and extends the discussion in the two landmark papers from the ANA (1995) and the NCSBN (1993). In the next section, a core definition of advanced nursing practice is proposed; the differences among the advanced practice roles are described in the following section. Important assertions of this two-phased definition are as follows:

- Advanced nursing practice is a function of educational and practice preparation *and* a constellation of primary criteria and core competencies.
- All APNs share (or ought to share) these same core criteria and competencies.
- Actual practices differ significantly based on the needs of the specialty patient population served and the organizational framework within which the role is performed. Particular ANP roles have different "shapes" and include additional competencies specific to them. Consequently, it is both necessary and preferable to retain varied job titles that reflect these actual practices, rather than reduce all APNs to one title.

In spite of the need to keep job descriptions and job titles distinct in practice settings, it is critical that the public's confusion about advanced practice be decreased and its acceptance of advanced nursing practice be enhanced. As Safriet (1993) noted, nursing's future depends on reaching consensus on titles and consistent preparation for these title holders. The burden is clearly on the nursing profession and its APNs to be clear, concrete, and consistent about ANP titles and their functions with nursing's larger constituencies: consumers, other health-care professionals, health-care administrators, and health-care policymakers.

CONCEPTUAL DEFINITION

Davies and Hughes (1995) noted, "The term advanced nursing practice extends beyond roles. It is a way of thinking and viewing the world based on clinical knowledge, rather than a composition of roles" (p. 157). The conceptual definition of advanced nursing practice used in this book is as follows:

Advanced nursing practice is the application of an expanded range of practical, theoretical, and research-based therapeutics to phenomena experienced by patients within a specialized clinical area of the larger discipline of nursing.[1]

This definition incorporates the features of specialization, expansion, and advancement proposed by the ANA in its latest Social Policy Statement. The term *therapeutics* refers to any of the activities undertaken as part of the nursing process: assessment, diagnosis, planning, intervention, and evaluation. Although many of these activities are also performed by physicians and other health-care professionals, the experiential, theoretical, and philosophical perspectives of nursing make these activites advanced *nursing* practice. The definition recognizes that not all nursing therapeutics are research based at this point in nursing's evolution. It further recognizes the strong experiential component necessary to develop the competencies of advanced nursing practice. Although graduate education in nursing provides a critical foundation for the expanded knowledge and theory base

---

[1]The reader will note that the term *patient* is intended to be used interchangeably with *individual* and *client*.

necessary to support advanced practice, graduate education and clinical practice experience work synergistically to develop the APN. The definition also emphasizes the patient-focused and specialized nature of advanced practice. Finally, the critical importance of ensuring that any type of advanced nursing practice is grounded within the larger discipline of nursing is made explicit.

The defining characteristics of advanced nursing practice include three primary criteria and eight core competencies, which are represented in Figure 3–1 and presented in the next two subsections. This discussion and the chapters in Part II will segregate these core competencies to clarify them. It is important for the reader to recognize that this is only a cognitive device for clarifying the conceptualization of advanced nursing practice used in this book. In reality, these elements weave throughout an APN's practice and are not separate and distinct features. The circle in Figure 3–1 represents the seamless nature of this interweaving of elements. In addition, the APN's skills function synergistically to produce a whole that is greater than the sum of its parts. The essence of advanced nursing practice is found not only in the primary criteria and competencies demonstrated, but also in the synthesis of these elements along with individual nurse characteristics into a unified composite practice (Davies & Hughes, 1995) that conforms to the conceptual definition presented above.

PRIMARY CRITERIA

Certain criteria (or qualifications) must be met before one can be considered an APN. While these baseline criteria are not *sufficient* in and of themselves, they are *necessary* core elements of advanced nursing practice. These criteria include an earned graduate degree with a concentration in an ANP category, professional

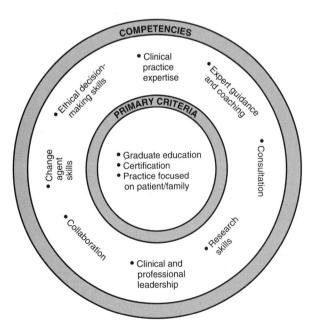

FIGURE 3–1. Defining characteristics of advanced nursing practice.

certification of practice at an advanced level within a given specialty, and a practice that is focused on patients and their families.

First, the APN must possess *an earned graduate (master's or doctorate) degree with a concentration in an ANP category*. Advanced practice students acquire specialized knowledge and skills through study and supervised practice at either the master's or the doctoral level. The content of study includes theories and research findings relevant to the core of the given nursing specialty. The expansion of practice skills is acquired through clinical experience in addition to faculty-supervised practice (ANA, 1995). There is emerging consensus that master's education in nursing should be a requirement for advanced nursing practice. At the National Nursing Summit held in 1993, representatives of 63 out of the 66 organizations attending agreed to this criterion (Cronenwett, 1995).

Why is graduate educational preparation necessary for advanced nursing practice? Some of the differences between basic and advanced nursing practice are apparent in the range and depth of APNs' clinical knowledge; in APNs' ability to anticipate patient responses to health, illness, and nursing interventions; in their ability to analyze clinical situations and produce explicit clinical judgments (Calkin, 1984) and to explain why a phenomenon has occurred or why a particular intervention has been chosen; and in their skill in assessing and addressing nonclinical variables that influence patient care. Because of the interaction and integration of graduate education in nursing and extensive clinical experience, the APN is able to exercise a level of discrimination in clinical judgment that is unavailable to other experienced clinicians (Spross & Baggerly, 1989). Professionally, requiring graduate preparation is important to create parity between all ANP roles, so that all can move forward together in addressing policymaking and regulatory issues. This parity will advance the profession's standards as well as standardize credentialing mechanisms. Creating a normative educational expectation enhances nursing's image and credibility with other disciplines, especially medicine. Finally, the research and theory base required for advanced nursing practice mandates education at the graduate level.

Second, APNs must have *professional certification of practice at an advanced level within a specialty*. The reality of specialization has dramatically increased the amount of knowledge and experience required to practice safely in the modern health care setting. National certification examinations have been developed by specialty organizations and are used to determine whether nurses meet standards for specialty practice in a particular clinical specialty. By and large, these examinations have tested the specialty knowledge of experienced nurses and not ANP knowledge. Two notable exceptions are CNM and CRNA certifying examinations (see Chapter 1). Advanced practice certification examinations have been slow to develop, although they are beginning to appear in some specialties. For example, the ONS began administering an advanced practice certification examination in 1995, and the ANA and AACN have collaborated to offer an ACNP certifying examination by the end of 1995.

If no certification examination exists for the ANP level of a particular specialty, the APN should be certified at the highest level available. As mentioned, the ANA and various specialty organizations are developing and should continue to develop certification for advanced nursing practice based on graduate education. Ultimately, all APN certifications must be at the graduate level.

Third, the APN engages in a *practice focused on patients* and their families. The term *advanced nursing practice* should be used to describe advanced *clinical* practice

(ANA, 1995). As noted earlier, there are certainly other types of specialized roles in the profession, notably, educators, administrators, and researchers, and these roles are vital to the profession's continued development. They are "critical to the preparation of nurses for practice, the provision of environments that are conducive to nursing practice, and the continued development of the knowledge base that nurses use in practice" (ANA, 1995, p. 15). Some of these nurses possess advanced practice knowledge and skills as well. However, if they do not have a patient/family-focused clinical practice, they are not considered APNs by this definition.

There are APNs in community practices who take a community view of their practice and are involved in program development in community health settings. Indeed, the broad perspective of the APN "allows for concerns to encompass not only the care delivery system in which the [APN] practices, but also the community and society in which that care is provided" (Davies & Hughes, 1995, p. 157). However, advanced nursing practice is focused on and realized at the patient/family level. So long as APNs in community health practices maintain a direct clinical practice focused on patients and their families in addition to their programmatic responsibilities, they are APNs in this definition.

Why limit the definition of advanced nursing practice to roles focused on clinical practice? The nurse-patient interface is the core of nursing practice; in the final analysis, the reason the profession exists is to render nursing services to individuals in need of them. Clinical practice expertise in a given specialty develops from these nurse-patient encounters. This expertise brought to the nurse-patient interface is at the heart of advanced nursing practice. Immersion in practice is required to maintain and continue developing the cutting-edge clinical practice expertise found in ANP practices.

The focus of all the ANP roles discussed in this book is the patient/family. Newly emerging roles must be similarly focused on direct clinical practice to be considered advanced practice. If every specialized role in nursing were considered advanced nursing practice, the term would become so broad as to lack meaning and explanatory value (see also Cronenwett, 1995). For example, a nurse administrator functions very differently than does a CNM. Distinguishing between ANP roles and other specialized roles in nursing can help clarify the concept of advanced nursing practice to consumers, to other health-care providers, and even to other nurses. In addition, the monitoring and regulation of advanced nursing practice are increasingly important issues as APNs work toward more authority for their practices (see Chapter 22). If the definition of advanced nursing practice included nurses in nonclinical roles, developing sound regulatory mechanisms would be impossible.

CORE COMPETENCIES

As noted above, the primary criteria are necessary but not sufficient elements of the definition of advanced nursing practice. Advanced practice is further defined by a set of core competencies that are enacted in each ANP role. The term *competency* is used here to refer to a defined area of skilled performance. The following are the core competencies that further define advanced nursing practice:

1. Expert clinical practice;
2. Expert guidance and coaching of patients, families, and other care providers;
3. Consultation;

4. Research skills including utilization, evaluation, and conduct;
5. Clinical and professional leadership;
6. Collaboration;
7. Change agent skills; and
8. Ethical decision-making skills.

These competencies mark advanced practice regardless of role function or setting and have repeatedly been identified as essential ANP features (Davies & Hughes, 1995; O'Rourke, 1989; Patterson & Haddad, 1992; Price et al., 1992; Spross & Baggerly, 1989). The specific content for some of these areas differs significantly by specialty; for example, clinical practice expertise for a CNS dealing with critically ill children differs from the expertise of a NP managing the health maintenance needs of elderly persons or a CRNA administering anesthesia in an outpatient surgical clinic. Other core competencies, such as consultation, collaboration, and ethical decision making, are processes that are similarly learned by all APNs, who then apply them to specific patient populations and settings. Individual ANP roles each have additional competencies that help distinguish between roles. For example, the American College of Nurse-Midwives (ACNM, 1992) and the National Organization of Nurse Practitioner Faculties (NONPF, 1990) have identified additional core competencies for the CNM and NP roles, respectively.

It is important to emphasize that these complex competencies develop over time. No APN emerges from a graduate program fully prepared to enact them all. However, it is critical that all ANP graduate programs provide exposure to each competency in the form of didactic content as well as practical experience, so that new graduates can be tested for initial credentialing and be given a base on which to build their practices. Each of these key competencies is described in detail in subsequent chapters and so is not further elaborated here.

DIFFERENTIATING ADVANCED PRACTICE ROLES: OPERATIONAL DEFINITIONS OF ADVANCED NURSING PRACTICE

As the NCSBN (1993) stated, "The scope of practice in each of the advanced roles of a NP, CRNA, CNM, or CNS is distinguishable from the others. While there is overlapping of activities within these roles, there are activities which are unique to each role" (p. 3). Differentiation between APNs occurs along a number of dimensions: nature of the patient population, additional competencies required, organizational expectations, emphasis given to specific competencies, and practice characteristics unique to each role. It is important to note at the outset of this discussion that these differences between ANP roles are not rigid demarcations. Nursing's scope of practice is dynamic and continually evolving, and this is especially true at the boundaries of the discipline, where advanced practice occurs (ANA, 1995). "Differences among nurses in their scopes of practice can be characterized as intraprofessional intersections across which collegial, collaborative practice occurs" (ANA, 1995, p. 12). These intersections are not rigid lines, but rather are fluid and involve overlapping areas. The intent of this discussion is not to create stereotypical divisions or to deny the dynamic and evolving nature of advanced nursing practice, but rather to describe key differences that are evident in actual practices at this stage in the evolution of advanced practice.

As noted earlier, it is critical to the public's understanding of advanced nursing practice that advanced roles and resulting job titles reflect actual practices. Because actual practices differ, job titles should differ. (The corollary is also true: if the actual practices do not differ, the job titles should not differ.) These differences among roles must be clarified in ways that promote understanding of advanced practice, rather than divide the profession (Davies & Hughes, 1995). It is this spirit of promoting understanding and clarity that informs the ensuing discussion. A key assumption is that *all of these APN roles are valuable* in meeting the needs of patients in current and evolving health care settings.

APN competencies are applied in a variety of roles, some established, some newly emerging. Figure 3–2 illustrates the differing "shapes" of ANP roles. These roles can be considered to be the operational definitions of the conceptual definition of advanced nursing practice. Although each ANP role has the core definition, criteria, and competencies of advanced nursing practice at its center, it has its own distinctive form. Some distinctive features of various ANP roles are listed below. Differences and similarities between roles are further explored in Part III.

The CNS role is distinguished by the expectation of practice in four subroles: clinical expert, consultant, educator, and researcher. CNSs are first and foremost clinical experts, who provide direct clinical practice to patients with complex health problems. CNSs not only learn consultation processes as do other APNs, but also function as formal consultants within their organizations. Their multifocal practice in these different subroles means that CNS practice is fluid and changeable. Managing system change in complex organizations to improve nursing practices, "massaging the system" (Fenton, 1985) to advocate for patients, and developing nursing staff are unique role expectations of the CNS. Expectations regarding research activities have been central to this role since its inception.

NPs, whether in primary care or acute care, possess advanced health assessment, diagnostic, and clinical management skills that include pharmacology management. Their focus is expert primary health care practice in managing the health

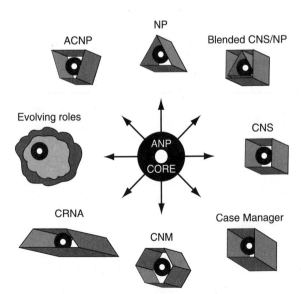

FIGURE 3–2. Different advanced practice roles. ANP = advanced nursing practice; NP = nurse practitioner; CNS = certified nurse specialist; CNM = certified nurse-midwife; CRNA = certified registered nurse anesthetist; ACNP = acute care NP.

needs of individuals and their families. NPs, particularly those in private or small collaborative practices, also use business and marketing principles in practice management. The classic NP role provides primary health care focused on wellness and prevention; NP practice also includes caring for patients with minor, common, acute conditions and stable chronic conditions. The newer ACNP brings this holistic primary prevention focus to a specialized patient population within the acute care setting. The ACNP's focus is the diagnosis and clinical management of acutely or critically ill patient populations in a particular specialized setting.

The blended CNS/NP role combines the CNS's in-depth specialized knowledge of a particular patient population with the NP's primary health care expertise. In addition to the core ANP competencies, education for this role must include functional role preparation for both the CNS and the NP roles. The CNS/NP provides primary and specialty care, including clinical management, to a complex patient population, such as children with diabetes. A unique feature of this role is the provision of primary and specialized care such that the blended CNS/NP crosses setting boundaries to provide continuity of care. This role combines individual patient management with expectations to change complex organizational practices.

The CNM has advanced health assessment and intervention skills focused on women's health and childbearing. CNM practice involves "the independent management of women's health care, focusing particularly on pregnancy, child-birth, the postpartum period, care of the newborn, and the family planning and gynecological needs of women" (ACNM, 1993). The CNM's focus is on direct practice to a select patient population.

CRNA practice is distinguished by advanced procedural and pharmacological management of patients undergoing anesthesia. CRNAs practice independently, in collaboration with physicians, or as employees of a health-care institution. Like CNMs, their focus is on direct practice to a select patient population. Both CNM and CRNA practices are also distinguished by well-established national standards, national examinations, and certification for practice at the advanced specialty level.

APN case managers provide complex patient management of high-risk or resource-intensive patients. They identify patient needs for interdisciplinary care and develop and coordinate an integrated plan of care. In addition to direct clinical practice, APN case managers develop interdisciplinary clinical guidelines that support quality and cost outcomes for individual patients and patient populations. Patient management across delivery networks is an expectation of some of these roles. APN case managers are responsible for patient outcome identification and evaluation and share the risk for accomplishing or not accomplishing outcomes with other team members, and the institution as well.

These differing roles and their similarities and distinctions are explored in detail in subsequent chapters. This brief discussion underscores the rich and varied nature of advanced nursing practice and the necessity for retaining and supporting different ANP roles and titles. At the same time, there is a need for a consistent definition of advanced practice that undergirds each of these roles.

IMPLICATIONS OF THIS DEFINITION OF ADVANCED PRACTICE

Many of the implications of the definition of advanced nursing practice presented here have been noted throughout the chapter, such as the necessity for graduate preparation for ANP roles and the need for an individual nurse to meet the core definition, criteria, and competencies to be considered an APN. There are other implications as well.

It should be clear from this discussion that direct expert clinical practice is the nucleus of all of these ANP roles. It is essential that APNs hold onto and make explicit their direct patient care activities.

ANP roles involve many components and competencies. As a result, APNs require a considerable period of role development to implement fully the varied aspects of their practice (see Chapter 5). Graduate programs should provide anticipatory socialization experiences to prepare students for their chosen ANP role. It is important that graduate experiences include practice in all the competencies of advanced practice, not just clinical practice expertise. For example, students who have no theoretical base or guided practice experiences in consultative skills or clinical leadership will be ill equipped to enact these competencies upon entering a new ANP role. However, even with the most excellent graduate education, no APN new to practice can be expected to perform all the role components and competencies with equal skill.

"Each individual who practices nursing at an advanced level does so with substantial autonomy and independence requiring a high level of accountability" (NCSBN, 1993, p. 3). ANP roles require considerable autonomy and authority to be fully enacted. Practice settings have not always structured ANP roles to allow sufficient autonomy or accountability to achieve the patient and system outcomes that are expected of advanced practice. Federal and state regulations have further limited the potential of ANP roles by not recognizing advanced practice or by placing APNs in dependent positions with respect to their physician colleagues. Both of these barriers are discussed in subsequent chapters. APNs and their advocates must be prepared to work actively for removal of these barriers if advanced nursing practice is to flourish.

It is equally important to emphasize that APNs have direct and expanded responsibilities to patients. Expanded authority for practice requires expanded responsibility for practice. It is crucial for APNs to demonstrate a higher level of responsibility and accountability if they are to be seen as legitimate providers of care and full partners on provider teams responsible for patient populations. This willingness to be accountable for one's practice will also further consumers' and policymakers' perceptions of the APN as a credible provider in line with physicians.

Two key elements of APN leadership involve APNs serving as visible role models and mentors for other nurses (Cronenwett, 1995; also see Chapter 10) and being actively involved in research related to patient care. If research is to be relevant to care delivery and to nursing practice at all levels, APNs must be involved. Differences in level of involvement in research are discussed in Chapter 9. But APNs must recognize the importance of advancing both the profession's and the health care system's knowledge about effective patient care practices. Indeed, APNs are in a key position to uncover the knowledge imbedded in clinical practice (Benner, 1984). Related to this research involvement is the necessity for more research differentiating basic and advanced nursing practice, identifying which patient populations benefit from APN intervention, and linking advanced nursing practice to specific patient outcomes.

Two final implications concern the education of APNs, which is discussed in more detail in Chapter 4. Schools of nursing must not completely homogenize the preparation for advanced practice. Certainly, all students need exposure to the core definition and competencies of advanced practice described here. But APNs enact these competencies in widely varying ways in differentiated positions. It is essential that schools provide sufficient functional role preparation that students are prepared to enter a specific work role. As Price et al. (1992) noted, "Curricula for advanced practice must provide a theoretical and research base specific to the practice area" (p. 12). Programs that prepare only a generic APN who has no preparation for the reality of assuming one of the ANP roles (or more, in the case of the blended CNS/NP) are doing their students, prospective employers of APNs, and the nursing profession a disservice.

It is equally critical that universities (a) develop articulation programs to help certificate-prepared nurses currently functioning in ANP roles obtain master's preparation and (b) begin to transition certificate programs to the master's level. Graduate educators need to support these articulation programs and assist in developing curricula to enable this education. As discussed in Chapter 4, more creative articulation models are needed. Also needed is research on the outcomes of different types of APN master's educational programs in terms of APN graduate experiences and patient outcomes. Such data would be invaluable in continuing to refine ANP education.

CONCLUSION

Today's APNs, future APNs, educators, administrators and other nursing leaders need to be clear and consistent about the definition of advanced nursing practice so that the profession speaks with one voice. For a profession to succeed it must have internal cohesion and external legitimacy, at the same time (Safriet, 1993). Development of a single core definition of advanced nursing practice and recognition of the core criteria and competencies necessary for all APNs will enhance nursing's external legitimacy. At the same time, recognizing the differences among and the legitimacy of different ANP roles will enhance nursing's internal cohesion.

REFERENCES

Advanced nursing practice. (1991). *Cumulative Index to Nursing and Allied Health Literature, 36,* 1599–1600.

American College of Nurse-Midwives. (1992). *Core competencies for basic nurse-midwifery practice.* Washington, DC: Author.

American College of Nurse-Midwives. (1993). *Position statement.* Washington, DC: Author.

American Nurses' Association. (1980). *Nursing: A social policy statement.* Kansas City, MO: Author.

American Nurses' Association. (1992). *Nursing facts.* Washington, DC: Author.

American Nurses' Association. (1995). *Draft: Nursing's social policy statement.* Washington, DC: Author.

Benner, P. (1984). *From novice to expert.* Menlo Park, CA: Addison-Wesley Publishing.

Calkin, J. D. (1984). A model for advanced nursing practice. *Journal of Nursing Administration, 14(1),* 24–30.

Creasia, J. L., & Parker, B. (1991). *Conceptual foundations of professional nursing practice.* St. Louis, MO: Mosby-Year Book.

Cronenwett, L. R. (1995). Modeling the future of advanced practice nursing. *Nursing Outlook, 43,* 112–118.

Davies, B., & Hughes, A. M. (1995). Clarification of advanced nursing practice: Characteristics and competencies. *Clinical Nurse Specialist, 9,* 156–160.

Donley, S. R. (1995). Advanced practice nursing after health care reform. *Nursing Economics, 13(2),* 84–88.

Fenton, M. V. (1985). Identifying competencies of clinical nurse specialists. *Journal of Nursing Administration, 15(12),* 31–37.

Kitzman, H. (1989). The CNS and the nurse practitioner. In A. B. Hamric & J. A. Spross (Eds.), *The clinical nurse specialist in theory and practice* (2nd ed., pp. 379–394). Philadelphia, PA: W. B. Saunders Company.

Leddy, S., & Pepper, J. M. (1993). *Conceptual bases*

of professional nursing (3rd ed.). Philadelphia: J. B. Lippincott.

National Council of State Boards of Nursing. (1993). *Position paper on the regulation of advanced nursing practice.* Chicago: Author.

National Organization of Nurse Practitioner Faculties. (1990). *Advanced nursing practice: Nurse practitioner curriculum guidelines.* Washington, DC: Author.

Oncology Nursing Society. (1990). *Standards of advanced practice in oncology nursing.* Pittsburgh, PA: Oncology Nursing Press.

O'Rourke, M. (1989). Generic professional behaviors: Implications for the clinical nurse specialist role. *Clinical Nurse Specialist, 3,* 128–132.

Patterson, C., & Haddad, B. (1992). The advanced nurse practitioner: Common attributes. *Canadian Journal of Nursing Administration, 5(3),* 18–22.

Price, M. J., Martin, A. C., Newberry, Y. G., Zimmer, P. A., Brykczynski, K. A., & Warren, R. (1992). Developing national guidelines for nurse practitioner education: An overview of the product and the process. *Journal of Nursing Education, 31(1),* 10–15.

Ray, G. L., & Hardin, S. (1995). Advanced practice nursing: Playing a vital role. *Nursing Management, 26(2),* 45–47.

Safriet, B. (1993, February). Keynote Address—One Strong Voice. Paper presented at the National Nurse Practitioner Leadership Summit, Washington, DC.

Smith, M. C. (1995). The core of advanced practice nursing. *Nursing Science Quarterly, 8,* 2–3.

Snyder, M., & Mirr, M. P. (1995). *Advanced practice nursing: A guide to professional development.* New York: Springer Publishing Company.

Spross, J. A., & Baggerly, J. (1989). Models of advanced practice. In A. B. Hamric & J. A. Spross (Eds.), *The clinical nurse specialist in theory and practice* (2nd ed., pp. 19–40). Philadelphia, PA: W. B. Saunders Company.

Stimpson, M., & Hanley, B. (1991). Nurse policy analyst: Advanced practice role. *Nursing and Health Care, 12,* 10–15.

Thibodeau, J. A., & Hawkins, J. W. (1994). Moving toward a nursing model in advanced practice. *Western Journal of Nursing Research, 16,* 205–218.

CHAPTER 4

Education for Advanced Nursing Practice

Doreen Harper

INTRODUCTION

Education for advanced nursing practice (ANP) has received significant attention from the power brokers: health-care corporations, insurance companies, state and federal policymakers, physicians, and other providers. This external recognition has prompted ANP educators to refocus their energies toward increasing access to advanced practice education and refining educational standards in anticipation of the changes in the health-care system and to renew their commitment to prepare competent advanced practice nurses (APNs) for present and future practice.

Graduate educational programs have led the way for the successful development of cutting-edge roles for APNs, providing the foundational components for practice. Graduate nursing educators have been instrumental in shaping the present and future health-care system by designing new fields of learning revolving around ANP roles. In this chapter, the components of graduate level education necessary for the preparation of current APNs are delineated, and conclusions about the clinical practice graduate programs of the future are offered. For the purposes of this chapter, the ANP roles with clearly delineated educational standards and competencies are described. These include the roles of the nurse practitioner (NP), the clinical nurse specialist (CNS), the certified nurse-midwife (CNM), and the certified registered nurse anesthetist (CRNA). Issues relevant to evolving ANP roles in which educational standards and competencies are in early stages of development, such as the case manager and acute care nurse practitioner (ACNP) roles, are also addressed. Finally, issues of ANP education are examined from the perspective of educational standards for ANP programs, interdisciplinary imperatives, and articulated educational models for certificate to graduate level NPs, CRNAs, and CNMs.

DEFINING ANP EDUCATION

The definition proposed by Hamric in Chapter 3 states that the APN "applies an expanded range of practical, theoretical and research-based therapeutics to phenomena experienced by patients within a specialized clinical area of the larger discipline of nursing." As Hamric explains, this definition recognizes the performance-based features of advanced nursing practice as well as the core theoretical and research knowledge and skills needed by APNs to practice in clinical settings.

The core elements incorporate several performance-based features, including: (1) an earned graduate degree in nursing at either the master's or doctoral level, (2) the integration of theory and ANP role function into practice (Smith, 1995), (3) the acquisition of specialized knowledge and skill relevant to the core of the particular nursing specialty, and (4) sufficient faculty-supervised clinical practice. The specialized clinical knowledge and skill base, essential to the provision of care, allows the APN to exercise highly refined clinical judgment in a given specialty within the context of a patient-provider relationship.

The core elements and performance-based features of ANP graduate educational programs are derived from the core values inherent in the nursing profession and the needs of the health-care marketplace. Central among these core values are a holistic perspective, partnerships with patients, clinical reasoning, and diverse management approaches (for a more detailed discussion, see Chapter 6). Because educational programs pertain to society's fundamental needs for health care, the curriculum content, skills, and competencies needed by APNs are constantly evaluated for their practice-based relevance. As such, the health-care market has exerted influence on the educational preparation for the CNS, NP, CRNA, and CNM roles and continues to do so.

ANP educators have defined the specialized knowledge and skills needed in the advanced roles of NP, CNM, CNS, and CRNA. The knowledge and skills can be organized according to domains and competencies derived from qualitative analysis of expert nurses in practice (Benner, 1984; Fenton & Brykczynski, 1993). Benner (1984) defined *domain* as a cluster of competencies with similar intentions, functions, and meanings. Graduate nursing educators have used domains to identify and cluster curriculum knowledge and skills needed for the education of APNs. *Skill* was defined as a practical ability based on the application of knowledge. *Competency* was designated as an interpretively defined area of skilled knowledge, identified and described by its intent, function, and meanings. Benner derived seven domains from her observations of the practice roles developed by hospital-based nurses. These seven domains are described in detail in Chapter 2 and have provided a potential curriculum infrastructure (Fenton & Brykczynski, 1993; National Organization of Nurse Practitioner Faculties [NONPF], 1995) for ANP clinical education, particularly for NPs and CNSs.

The domains and their associated competencies are embedded in the practice-based knowledge and skill components of the ANP roles. The domains and competencies converge in ANP educational programs through curriculum guidelines and the identification of competency behaviors needed for graduation from ANP programs. Curriculum guidelines detail content specific to the ANP roles. Moreover, several ANP roles have proffered program standards to support the development and maintenance of quality programs. For example, NP, CRNA, and CNM groups have identified standards and curriculum guidelines specific to the evaluation of each of these ANP educational programs (ACNM, 1993; Jordan, 1994; NONPF, 1995). Within program standards, selected criteria are addressed, such as organization and administration, faculty, curriculum, students, resources, facilities, and services. These standards define the minimum requirements for the designated roles while simultaneously maintaining a degree of flexibility to accommodate new ANP roles evolving in response to society's changing health-care needs.

Graduate education for these roles enables APNs to provide direct care beyond the basic professional functions. Therefore, preparation for competency-based practice has associated educational and regulatory requirements that extend beyond basic nursing preparation and the registered nurse (RN) license. These educational and regulatory requirements include significant internal and external forces influencing ANP educational programs. Therefore, knowledge of regulatory and educational requirements such as accreditation and preparation of graduates for certification must also be considered by programs seeking to prepare nurses for advanced clinical practice roles. With the maturation of graduate education for advanced practice roles, internal professional requirements and external forces impacting the profession have converged to improve the legitimacy of APNs.

THE EVOLUTION OF ANP EDUCATION

The evolution of ANP education has paralleled the development of ANP roles. As has often been the case, ANP education matured with the growth and development of each of the these respective roles. Because each of the ANP roles originated at different points in time over the past 60 years, the educational programs for NPs, CNSs, CRNAs, and CNMs were formed as separate entities, rather than in one unified educational framework in graduate nursing (see Chapter 1). This section describes the context for the development of the educational programs preparing nurses for each of these roles.

The majority of APNs are prepared at the graduate level in either master's or post-master's educational programs. Typically, these graduate programs are 1 to 2 years of full-time study or 2 to 4 years of part-time study. Clinical practicum training in which students provide direct care is an essential part of the educational program. ANP graduate programs incorporate direct care experiences in required clinical practica, preparing students to function in advanced clinical decision making for both professional nursing functions and in selected roles, for medical functions traditionally performed only by physicians (Safriet, 1992).

Although variation has existed in the level of preparation for the NP, CNM, and CRNA roles, from master's, to post-master's to post-basic (certificate), the nursing profession has now established the graduate degree in nursing as its minimum standard. There are exceptions, however. For example, the American Association of Nurse Anesthetists (see Chapter 19) has mandated that the master's degree will be required as of 1998, but the master's degree will not be required in the nursing discipline. Although this past variation in educational level has been a long-standing issue for graduate nursing education in the past, the vast majority of ANP programs are currently offered in graduate nursing schools (NLN, 1994). The trend toward graduate preparation of ANP roles began in the 1980s as these roles developed external legitimacy.

It is estimated that approximately two-thirds of all currently practicing NPs, CNMs, and CRNAs were prepared in certificate programs, with the remaining third prepared in graduate nursing programs (Aiken, Gwyther, & Whelan, 1994). Although these NPs, CRNAs, and CNMs were originally prepared in certificate level programs, they have contributed significantly toward meeting primary care needs by offering safe, competent care (NONPF, 1995). However, the educational requirements for each of these roles have shifted toward graduate nursing education as the nursing profession has recognized the need for the master's degree to be the educational standard for advanced practice. With the external funding and infrastructure provided through federal and foundation support, the majority of ANP programs have been incorporated into graduate level nursing programs (Bullough, 1992).

In contrast, CNSs have traditionally been graduates of master's level nursing programs. The CNS role has consistently established its roots in and been supported by the nursing education and practice community since its inception. In the past 2 years, a new trend has emerged in response to the perceived demand for ANPs. This trend consists of offering programs to prepare nurses (usually CNSs) with graduate clinical nursing degrees (master's and doctoral) as NPs, CNMs, or CRNAs through post-master's graduate nursing coursework. Likewise, with the merger of the NP and CNS roles, blending and reconfiguration of ANP roles have begun to occur in response to society's need for health care.

One of the most significant influences in developing educational programs for NPs, CNMs, CNSs, and CRNAs in the past twenty years has been the Title VIII funding for advanced education of professional nurses provided by the Division of Nursing of the U.S. Department of Health and Human Services. From the perspective of the federal government, these programs are an innovative way to both prepare new types of advanced nurses with an emphasis on delivering care and to provide access for medically underserved populations. For this reason, some of the Title VIII monies were originally designed to provide line-item funding for CNS, NP, CNM, and CRNA educational programs. This legislation provided the stimulus to support faculty and operational costs for many of the ANP programs in the United States. The legislative mandate primarily supported new ANP programs targeted to vulnerable populations and ANP programs in remote geographic locations.

The Nursing Education Act (Title VIII of the Public Health Service Act) was enacted 30 years ago and is reauthorized every 2 years through the federal legislature. This federal support funds ANP programs in several ways through its annual Congressional appropriations. The fiscal year 1995 programs and APN entitlements were as follows: advanced nursing education program, $12.25 million; NP and CNM program grants, $16.94 million: CRNAs, $2.72 million; and traineeships for advanced education of professional nurses, $15.47 million. Other federal initiatives that support APN preparation are the National Health Service Corps scholarships and the Office of Rural Health (Nurse Education & Practice Improvement Amendment of 1994). As is evident, federal funding for ANP programs has had a significant impact on the maturation of ANP roles through the nursing educational environment.

The ANP roles began at the grassroots level as distinct entities, their educational requirements, including didactic and clinical content, have been divergent even within master's-level programs. Although graduate nursing programs have traditionally been accredited by the National League for Nursing (National League for Nursing, 1992) the purpose of this national accreditation process has been to evaluate the overall master's nursing program, rather than the specialty content of the ANP curriculum. Most ANP programs prepare providers of care who must meet minimal standards for competency-based practice through national credentialing exams and associated state regulatory requirements. In the following section, the data trends in ANP educational programs for the CNS, NP, CNM, and CRNA roles are discussed.

DATA TRENDS IN ANP EDUCATIONAL PROGRAMS AND EMERGING NEW ANP ROLES

The NLN (1994) collected trend data for nursing master's programs for the years 1991 to 1993 in its survey of master's programs. According to the data, the total enrollment in master's programs in 1993 was 30,385. More than 75% of total enrollments were part-time, and the total number of graduates from all types of master's programs was 7,882. Among the ANP master's program enrollments in 1993, the following total enrollments were reported: CNS students, 10,454: NP students, 8,096; nurse anesthetist students, 590; and nurse-midwifery students, 438. Between 1992 and 1993, a significant shift occurred among part-time students. Of the master's graduates in 1993, 5,422 were identified as APN students. Within these clinical graduate programs, the percentage of enrolled NP students increased from 16.2% in 1992 to 22.9% in 1993 and the percentage of CNS students decreased from 46.9% in 1992 to 36.1% in 1993. In addition, there was an upward shift among enrolled part-time NP students and a downward shift among enrolled part-time advanced clinical students.

The most recent data on ANP education programs, based on trends for the 1994–95 academic year, were compiled by the American Association of Colleges of Nursing (AACN, 1995). According to the AACN, enrollment of all types of master's degree students in 257 nursing schools rose by 10.7% in the 1994–95 academic year as compared with the data from 1993–94. Schools that responded to the AACN survey reported a total of 30,718 students enrolled in master's degree nursing programs. Among the enrolled ANP master's students, 10,935 were identified as pursuing study as NPs in a range of specialties; 8,332 were identified as CNSs; 544 were identified as nurse-midwifery students; and 770 were identified as nurse anesthetist students. The number of master's degree graduates reported for the ANP programs totaled 4,989, with 2,648 CNS, 1,867 NP, 216 CNM, and 196 nurse anesthetist graduates, respectively. Neither the NLN nor the AACN reported the trend toward post-master's preparation for APNs. As further evidence of these shifts, the number of institutions offering graduate level programs for NPs grew 63% between 1992 and 1994 (Harper & Johnson, 1995). This program growth parallels the rapid increase in ANP student enrollment.

Throughout these recent years of health-care revolution, other new ANP clinical roles have begun to emerge in response to demands from the health-care marketplace. Among these are the blended NP/CNS role, the case management role, and the acute care NP (ACNP) role. The new ANP roles are in the early stages of developing standards, curricula, and competencies for graduates that will guide graduate program development.

The influence of the marketplace on educational programs is best exemplified by the current trend for CNSs to seek preparation for the NP role or move into new case management roles. By adding the diagnostic and management components common for NP practice to their specialty knowledge and skill repertoire, CNSs are shaping their roles to the needs of the changing marketplace (see Chapter 17 for discussion of the blended role). These newly evolving roles are being accompanied by changes in the educational preparation and standards for these roles.

FORCES INFLUENCING ANP EDUCATION

Graduates from ANP programs have withstood repeated tests for more than 30 years, consistently breaking down national and state barriers to practice and education. This successful outcome attests to the relevance of ANP education and the ability of graduate nursing educators to prepare health-care providers with marketable skills and competencies despite significant resistance from the medical field. With new paradigms for care management systems being mounted, ANP education has become pivotal among the health-care workforce issues, particularly from a supply-and-demand perspective. ANP workforce issues and educational tracks have received attention from policymakers, payers, regulatory agencies, health-care professionals, and foundations. Likewise, the internal professional nursing environment has reexamined issues surrounding ANP education in efforts to clarify and enhance future ANP role development. In this section, the external and internal forces affecting ANP educational programs are discussed.

EXTERNAL FORCES

Driven by external forces, the shift from traditional fee-for-service to managed competition health-care delivery has created not only provider challenges, but also educational challenges for the training and preparation of APNs. Advanced nursing practice has been particularly responsive to society's needs by developing the cutting-edge roles described throughout this book. The general goal of ANP education programs is threefold:

1. To continue to prepare competent APNs as members of the future health-care workforce;
2. To prepare APNs as cost-effective, competent health-care providers, based on supply-and-demand needs; and
3. To maintain flexibility in educating APNs for innovative new roles in the changing health-care system.

Three major foundations have had significant external influence on APN education as part of the future health system. These foundations are the Pew Charitable Trusts, the W. K. Kellogg Foundation, and the Robert Wood Johnson Foundation. For the past 5 years, the Pew Health Professions Commission, funded by the Pew Charitable Trusts, has focused its efforts on restructuring health professions education. Among these efforts, the Commission's report on schools in service to the nation (O'Neil, 1993) has exerted the most direct impact on ANP education. The characteristics of the emerging health-care system are outlined in the report. These characteristics, listed in Table 4–1, are predictive of fundamental changes in the future health-care system and are considered by the Pew Commission to be essential to quality health care. These characteristics of the emerging health-care system are being demonstrated as the trends toward interdisciplinary team care, population-based and outcomes care, information systems, and limited resources have become recurrent themes in health care. In this era of extensive information systems and limited resources, the prevailing emphasis is on providing cost-effective, quality care for all segments of society.

The report on schools in service to the nation also identifies the competencies needed by health professionals to cast the future health-care system. These generic competencies, summarized in Table 4–2, serve as an overall guide for refining the competencies needed by APNs so that they may function effectively in the present and future health-care systems. Another major impetus has been provided by Phase Two of the Pew Health Professions Commission (1995) in its paper "Shifting the Supply of Our Health Care Workforce." In this paper, the Commission proposed that NPs and CNMs could fill the anticipated gap in the primary care workforce created by efforts to control health-care costs.

In concurrent projects, both the W. K. Kellogg Foundation and the Robert Wood Johnson Foundation have focused initiatives on the development and training of interdisciplinary community-based primary care providers. Through its academic-community-based partnership initiatives, the W. K. Kellogg Foundation has helped to craft new community-based, academic-service collaboratives to improve primary care delivery. These partnerships involve schools of medicine, schools of nursing, and communities as equity partners in attempts to shift the graduate and undergraduate education and clinical training of nurses, APNs, and physicians from traditional medical centers to the community. Likewise, the Robert Wood Johnson Foundation has provided significant support to increase the supply and distribution of generalist physicians as well as NPs, physician assistants, and CNMs. Each of these interdisciplinary primary care initiatives designates APNs as bona fide providers and essential members of the health care team. Although these two initiatives are in the early phases of development and implementation, they are potential

TABLE 4–1. CHARACTERISTICS OF THE EMERGING HEALTH-CARE SYSTEM

Orientation Toward Health—Greater emphasis on prevention and wellness and greater expectation of individual responsibility for healthy behaviors.

Population Perspective—New attention to risk factors affecting substantial segments of the community, including inaccessibility and physical and social environments.

Intensive Use of Information—Reliance on information systems to provide complete, easily assimilated patient information, as well as ready access to relevant information on current practice.

Focus on the Consumer—Expectation and encouragement of patient partnerships in decisions related to treatment, facilitated by the availability of complete information on outcomes and partly evaluated by patient satisfaction.

Knowledge of Treatment Outcomes—Empahsis on the determination of the most effective treatment under different conditions and the dissemination of this information to those involved in treatment decisions.

Constrained Resources—A pervasive concern for increasing costs, coupled with expanded use of mechanisms to control or limit available expenditures.

Coordination of Services—Increased integration of providers, with a concomitant emphasis on teams to improve efficiency and effectiveness across all settings.

Reconsideration of Human Values—Careful assessment of the balance between the expanding capability of technology and the need for humane treatment.

Expectations of Accountability—Growing scrutiny by a larger variety of payers, consumers, and regulators, coupled with more formally defined performance expectations.

Growing Interdependence—Further integration of domestic issues of health, education, and public safety, combined with a growing awareness of the importance of U.S. health care in global context.

(Adapted from O'Neil, E. (1993). *Health professions education for the future: Schools in service to the nation.* San Francisco, CA: Pew Health Professions Commission.)

interdisciplinary educational models of learning for nursing and medicine. Common elements of interdisciplinary education for graduate medicine and nursing are discussed later in this chapter.

Another force that has had a significant impact on graduate ANP curricula has been developed through the *Healthy People 2000: National Health Promotion and Disease Prevention Objectives* by the Office of Disease Prevention and Health Promotion (ODPHP) of the U.S. Department of Health and Human Services (U.S. Public Health Service, 1991). With the current health policy emphasis on effective, economical care, ODPHP developed the national Put Prevention into Practice campaign to improve the consistent, systematic delivery of clinical preventive services. As part of this campaign, several resources have been developed, including curriculum materials, practice-based protocols, and research-based tools. Although health promotion and disease prevention activities have historically been the cornerstone of nursing practice, the delivery of preventive services by nurses has often been invisible because of reimbursement constraints. As policymakers have begun to learn the value of preventive services, APNs have been identified as among the essential providers to implement these services VRI-(Vector Research Incorporated, 1995). ANP faculty and students have the opportunity to provide

TABLE 4–2. SUMMARY OF COMPETENCIES FOR 2005

Care for the Community's Health—Understand the determinants of health and work with others in the community to integrate a range of activities that promote, protect, and improve the health of the community. Appreciate the growing diversity of the population, and understand health status and health-care needs in the context of different cultural values.

Provide Contemporary Clinical Care—Acquire and retain up-to-date clinical skills and apply them to meet the public's health-care needs.

Participate in the Emerging System and Accommodate Expanded Accountability—Function in new health-care settings and interdisciplinary team arrangements designed to meet the primary health-care needs of the public, and emphasize high-quality, cost-effective, integrated services. Respond to increasing levels of public, governmental, and third-party participation in, and scrutiny of, the shape and direction of the health-care system.

Ensure Cost-Effective Care and Use Technology Appropriately—Establish cost and quality objectives for the health-care process and understand and apply increasingly complex and often costly technology appropriately.

Practice Prevention and Promote Healthy Lifestyles—Emphasize primary and secondary preventive strategies for all people and help individuals, families, and communities maintain and promote healthy behaviors.

Involve Patients and Families in the Decision-Making Process—Expect patients and their families to participate actively both in decisions regarding their personal health care and in evaluating its quality and acceptability.

Manage Information and Continue to Learn—Manage and continuously use scientific, technological, and patient information to maintain professional competence and relevance throughout practice life.

(Adapted from O'Neil, E. (1993). *Health professions education for the future: Schools in service to the nation.* San Francisco, CA: Pew Health Professions Commission.)

leadership in applying health promotion and disease prevention content and skills for the integration of clinical preventive services throughout the health-care system.

Each of these external forces has created provocative issues for graduate educators, causing them to reevaluate the generic and particular characteristics expected of their APN graduates. Recurrent themes have emerged, which have led to beginning efforts to unify and standardize the core elements of ANP curricula.

INTERNAL PROFESSIONAL FORCES

Beyond the external factors, ANP clinical educators have begun to review the components of ANP education systematically (AACN, 1994; NONPF, 1995). These efforts were stimulated in part by the external forces discussed in the preceding section. Likewise, with health reform, the nursing community has mobilized its efforts to promote ANP roles and education by working to establish consensus among professional organizations (NONPF, 1995). ANP education has been significantly influenced by the three major nursing organizations: the NLN, the ANA, and the AACN. Each of these organizations in conjunction with specialty practice organizations has shaped the ANP roles, steering the direction of ANP education.

Research on ANP Education

A comprehensive study on the state of the art of master's level education within the context of the projected trends in health care was conducted by Burns et al. (1993). They analyzed the curricula of 176 NLN-accredited nursing master's programs using program information usually sent to prospective applicants. Among the variables analyzed descriptively were length of program, credit requirements, academic degree offered, number and area of major and subspecialties, curricular organizing framework, and curricular organization of courses. Results showed that the semester-hour credits varied from 29 to 54, with 36 credits the mode and nine different categories of courses identified. The most commonly cited categories were core courses, ANP courses, research, and theory. Findings showed considerable variation in curriculum, courses, credit structure and titling for majors, subspecialties, and role functions. These findings led Burns et al. to develop recommendations for an "Essentials of Master's Curriculum" document related to the communication and curriculum issues for master's nursing education. With the convergence of the external factors and internal professional forces, this process of systematic review of ANP education has been accelerated in the past 3 years.

The National League for Nursing Accreditation Process

As the major accrediting body for all types of nursing education, the NLN accredits master's level nursing programs. The NLN accreditation process uses 20 outcome-based criteria as essential components for achieving positive graduate and program outcomes. These 20 outcome-based criteria are categorized according to (1) structure and governance, (2) material resources, (3) students, (4) faculty, (5) curriculum, and (6) required outcome criteria for the program. In addition to the outcome-based criteria, other specific areas are required of each educational institution as part of the evaluation for accreditation. These areas include critical thinking, communication, therapeutic nursing interventions, graduation rates, and patterns of employment. This outcome-based approach is particularly relevant for the preparation of ANP providers because graduate nursing educators must validate educational outcomes for the production of skilled competent providers. Hence, the current NLN accreditation process enables graduate educators to move toward this goal.

The American Nurses Association Social Policy Statement

The ANA's (1995b) social policy statement provides a strong philosophical foundation for educating nurses in advanced practice roles. In this newly revised social policy statement, the notion is proposed that APNs must maintain flexible practice boundaries responsive to the needs of society and that these boundaries in turn lay the foundation for further development of cutting-edge roles. Advanced nursing practice is described as the incorporation of specialization, expansion, and advancement in practice. Advancement involves specialization and is characterized by the integration of a broad range of theoretical, research-based, and practical knowledge gained during graduate nursing education. The social policy statement identifies the essential elements of ANP education as (1) the graduate study of nursing, (2) development of specialty knowledge and skills, and (3) faculty supervision of clinical practice. These elements become the cornerstone for the acquisition of knowledge and skills in the preparation of ANPs, according to the social policy statement (ANA, 1995b).

American Association of Colleges of Nursing Essentials Project

Other internal forces are furthering the master's degree in nursing as a basic prerequisite for ANP preparation. The AACN (1994) has recently developed a statement on the essentials of master's education for APNs. The AACN established this project because of the growing debate over the education of ANP clinicians. Through the identification of the core elements of curricula of master's programs for nurses, this project seeks to establish a unifying framework for ANP curricula through the identification of a "common educational core." This important project has been useful in providing leadership among graduate nurse educators to work toward the standardization of a common core curriculum in programs for NPs, CNSs, CNMs, and CRNAs as well as other evolving roles. In addition, this project has been instrumental in distinguishing the common features of ANP graduate education. These features include (1) the graduate core generic to all master's nursing degrees, (2) the advanced practice core generic to all advanced nursing practice, and (3) the specialty role core specific to each ANP role.

The areas identified thus far through consensus among graduate nursing educators include (1) a common graduate core curriculum for all master's degree nursing students and (2) the ANP core curriculum content for APNs. In this project, the graduate core curriculum for all master's students identified the common content areas of research, economics, ethical/legal issues, health policy, professional role development, nursing theory, and cultural diversity. The ANP core curriculum content identified advanced health assessment, pathophysiology, and advanced pharmacology (AACN, 1995) as common core content.

The analysis of core components of ANP education has been a progressive process, building on organizational and individual linkages and contributions. Cronenwett (1995) maintained that all segments of the profession must work toward developing common ground at the graduate level for the education of APNs. The most efficient mechanism for developing consistency in the education of nurses for advanced practice is to identify the common graduate educational requirements for each of these roles and to compare and contrast the differences and similarities in these requirements and specific content among the roles and specialties. Future work needs to be done to analyze the content of specific ANP roles, including their associated competencies. These external and internal professional forces have led to a convergence of opinion among professionals regarding the need for a standardized core ANP curriculum.

CORE ANP CURRICULUM

The external and internal forces that have been influencing graduate nursing education stimulate questions about master's preparation for ANP roles. What is the core curriculum needed to prepare competent APNs? What is the educational process within graduate clinical programs that provides the central core of knowledge and skills needed to develop ANP competencies for all roles? Are the ANP core competencies based on advanced nursing practice, specialty practice, or both?

Resolution of these questions by graduate educators can potentially strengthen and forecast the future of ANP education.

Graduate nurse educators have assumed that the ANP curriculum infrastructure is substantive core content encompassing the essential components of theoretical perspectives, practice-based competencies, and functional role preparation. However, drastic changes in the health-care system have highlighted the reality that ANP education often falls short of this assumption. This is evidenced in the variations cited previously for master's nursing programs in general and for ANP programs specifically (Burns et al., 1993). The substantive core content integrated throughout curricula for all APNs (CNSs, NPs, CNMs, and CRNAs) must be explicit if ANP competencies are to be achieved. However, review of existing ANP standards and competencies (AANA, 1992; ANA, 1995a; ACNM, 1992; NONPF, 1995) reveals inconsistencies among theoretical perspectives, clinical-practice-based competencies, and functional role preparation.

With the bulk of the preparation for ANP roles offered in graduate nursing programs, graduate nursing educators are keenly aware of the need to delineate and standardize the common core of theoretical, practice-based, and functional role content for each of the ANP roles. Graduate nursing content, advanced practice nursing content, and specialty role practice content must be identified to delineate ANP knowledge, skills, and competencies. This process will permit ANP educators to refine the graduate curriculum, resulting in improved educational outcomes for the preparation of APNs.

ANP CURRICULUM FRAMEWORK

The framework that illustrates the components of the ANP core curriculum for the clinical nursing master's degree is analogous to a wheel with concentric circular layers and spokes rotating around an axis (Fig. 4–1). In this three-concentric-layer framework, the three substantive curriculum components are, in order, the graduate nursing core content, the advanced practice core content, and the specialty practice core content. The components of this framework provide the foundation for specialization and expansion of clinical practice competencies at an advanced practice level.

Core Graduate Nursing Content

The commonly occurring core graduate nursing content consists of research, health policy, nursing and health-related theory, organizational/leadership theory, ethical/legal issues, multicultural care, economics, community-based care, managed care, and health-care delivery systems. This content is generic to all master's level nursing programs, be they ANP programs or other types of advanced nursing programs, such as administration or informatics.

Advanced Practice Core Content

The second curriculum layer is the ANP core content. This content is foundational to the development of depth in the clinical specialty and differentiates the advanced clinical nursing roles from other advanced roles, such as administration and education. Among the components common to all ANP curricula are advanced health assessment; pharmacology; physiology; advanced pathophysiology or other related

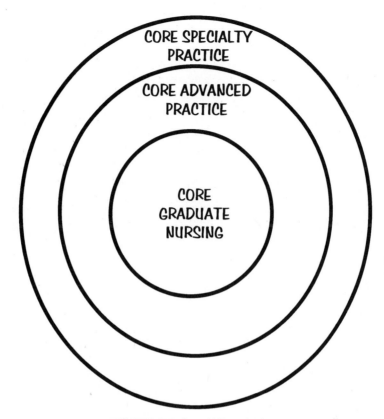

FIGURE 4–1. Core ANP curriculum.

sciences (depending on the ANP specialty); the process of clinical decision making; complex or advanced nursing interventions/therapeutics; health promotion/disease prevention; community-based practice; role differentiation, interpersonal and family theory.

Advanced assessment incorporates health assessment and risk appraisal; physical and mental status assessment; interpretation of diagnostic studies; and psychosocial, family, and/or community assessment. Advanced pathophysiology consists of the study of disease and provides the basis for medical and/or nursing clinical decision making. Advanced nursing therapeutics consists of the study of patient responses and related nursing interventions for special patient populations. It may be instituted as distinct interventions but most often is combined with medical therapeutics. Pharmacology includes pharmacokinetics, pharmacodynamics, drug therapies and their appropriate selection, and particular legal aspects associated with prescriptive authority defined according to regulatory statutes (AACN, 1993). Depending on the specialty role content, other related sciences may be necessary, such as human genetics, which is typically required for nurse-midwifery students; chemistry and physics, required for nurse anesthetist students; and immunology, required for oncology CNS students.

ANP Specialty Core Content

The specialty-related core content is unique to each type of ANP role (NP, CRNA, CNS, or CNM) as well as the health-care needs of the respective specialty population (e.g., oncology, adult health, acute care, women's health, family, or pediatric). The specialty core content frequently must match standards and competencies established by the professional specialty organizations, such as the Oncology Nursing Society, the NONPF's (1995) *Curriculum Guidelines and Program Outcomes,* the ACNM's 1992 *Core Competencies,* and the *Standards and Guidelines for Programs of Nurse Anesthesia* from the AANA's Council on Accreditation (1990). The specialty content core is developed in depth through clinical decision making applied to specialty practice based on the setting and patient population served. Courses in advanced therapeutics include pharmacological and nonpharmacological interventions used in changing health status and frequently combine nursing and medical interventions. Faculty-supervised clinical practice is essential for the expansion of specialty-related content.

ANP Competencies

ANP role content includes the competencies of expert practice, ethical decision making, consultation, expert guidance and coaching, research, leadership, collaboration, and change agent skills (see Chapter 3 and specific chapters). Another competency relates to particular types of functional role, such as the NP, CNM, CRNA, and CNS scope of practice. Content related to these nine competencies is threaded from the axis of graduate nursing core content through each of the concentric layers, much like the spokes of a wheel (Fig. 4–2). This content moves, rotating around the axis from the graduate core. It is this dynamic state that propels learning and the acquisition of knowledge, skills, and competencies essential for advanced nursing practice. Graduate ANP students acquire beginning ability and skills through learning and integrating their knowledge and relevant experiences. The foundation for the acquisition of these competencies is laid in the graduate program, but the ANP competencies continue to develop fully after graduation through practice.

The hallmark of the ANP curriculum model is the rotation of the advanced practice role content on the axis of the graduate nursing advanced practice and specialty practice core content for the development of the critical practice-based competencies (Fig. 4–3). These competencies must be explicitly addressed in all courses if students are to internalize the ANP role. The practice-based competencies are enhanced by each of the concentric core layers as they are integrated with advanced nursing role competencies and conclude with the achievement of ANP competencies. The integration of curriculum content and competency needs to be achieved if nurses are to function as APNs. If the merger of practice and role content fails to occur, nurses educated as CNMs, NPs, CNSs, and CRNAs function in specialty practice roles, rather than ANP roles. Within this ANP curriculum framework, the core graduate nursing content, the core advanced practice content, and the core specialty practice content are foundational to the ANP role content. The major curriculum components of this three-layer concentric framework define the generic educational requisites essential for advanced *clinical* practice, as distinguished from other types of advanced nursing preparation.

The professional challenge is to standardize and unify these core elements of

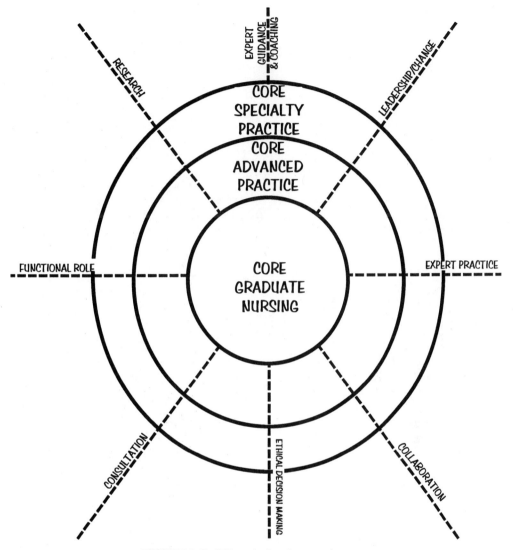

FIGURE 4–2. ANP curriculum framework.

the ANP curriculum and competencies, providing a model for master's level ANP preparation. The integration of curriculum and competencies is foundational to professional growth and positions APNs to be key providers in the emerging health-care system.

A GENERIC ANP CURRICULUM

On the basis of these core curriculum components, a generic curriculum for ANP education may be proposed. It should be noted that this generic curriculum is not proscriptive, but rather serves as a sample to identify the content in each of the

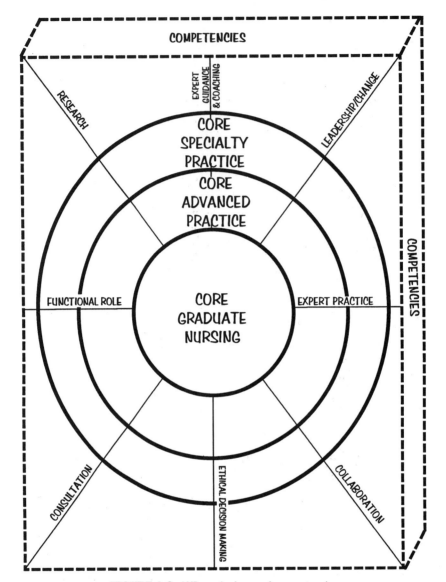

FIGURE 4–3. ANP curriculum and competencies.

core areas. The sample generic curriculum for ANP master's level preparation is presented in Table 4–3.

The sample curriculum and credit structure varies according to the type of ANP specialty being prepared. For example, didactic content and clinical practica for the CNM must integrate perinatal physiology; neonatal, prenatal, intrapartum, and postpartum care; family planning; and well-woman gynecological care. Likewise, the ACNP and the CRNA contents are oriented toward acquisition of the knowledge and competencies needed to care for in-hospital critical care and

TABLE 4–3. SAMPLE GENERIC ANP CURRICULUM FOR GRADUATE LEVEL PREPARATION

CORE NURSING CONTENT
Research—6 credits
Theoretical perspectives—3 credits (nursing and health-related theory, role theory, and ethical decision making)
Organization/policy perspectives—3 credits (organizational/leadership theory, health policy, economics, community-based care, and managed care)

ADVANCED NURSING PRACTICE CORE CONTENT
Pharmacology—3 credits
Advanced health assessment—3 credits
Clinical decision making, advanced therapeutics, health promotion and disease prevention—3 credits
Pathophysiology/genetics/related science—variable credit

SPECIALTY CONTENT
Specialties I, II, and III—12 to 18 credits

surgical patient populations. On the other hand, specialty didactic and clinical practicum content for the family NP incorporates a generalist approach to obstetrical, gynecological, pediatric, adult, and geriatric primary care. Distinguished from these other roles is the CNS. Although most CNS programs do not require the pharmacology and medical clinical management components in the advanced clinical core required by the programs for other established ANP roles, the curriculum for this ANP role substitutes significant content and skill development in formal consultation and educator subroles and in advanced nursing interventions for patients (Hamric & Spross, 1989; Naylor & Brooten, 1993). As is evident from these examples, the specialty content for each of these particular ANP roles is unique to the characteristics of the patient population or clinical environment.

The relatively new development of post-master's graduate nursing programs to prepare nurses with master's degrees in other areas of nursing to become NPs in a designated specialty track (adult NP, family NP, gerontological NP, women's health care NP, and others) also builds on this generic ANP curriculum. Because the post-master's students have taken prior core master's level coursework as part of their original graduate degree, they are not required to repeat this core content as part of their postmaster's certificate. Instead, they take the graduate level coursework in the ANP core and the specialty content, which often leads to a postgraduate certificate with preparation in the specialty areas. This phenomenon demonstrates the utility of having a generic ANP curriculum.

TEACHING/LEARNING STRATEGIES FOR ANP EDUCATION

ANP educators use several strategies in the process of teaching students to integrate the ANP core content, role functions, and competencies. Among them are the processes of clinical decision making, critical thinking, and clinical practicum experiences.

CLINICAL DECISION MAKING

Clinical decision making is a complex process that involves several steps. These include

1. Collection and interpretation of data,
2. Formulation of hypotheses about the continuum of human experiences and responses to health and illness,
3. Hypotheses testing, and
4. Diagnostic reasoning (the application of scientific knowledge to diagnosis and treatment).

Clinical decision making incorporates the knowledge, skills, and competencies needed for assessment, diagnosis, and management of all types of clinical situations. In clinical decision making, the benefits and costs of any nursing/and or medical actions with the identified population are weighed before a decision is made. Graduate educators thread critical-thinking teaching strategies as part of the clinical decision-making process throughout ANP master's programs. Evaluated throughout the didactic and clinical required coursework at each layer of the curriculum model, clinical decision-making outcomes are developed sequentially through the ANP core courses. Finally, clinical decision making is fully developed throughout the specialty coursework and in clinical practicum experiences for each ANP role. The ANP core courses develop clinical decision making through the presentation of content and skills that are logically clustered to enhance diagnostic reasoning in didactic and clinical practice situations. In the specialty core, ANP students expand their specialized clinical decision-making knowledge and skills in classroom settings through the analysis of paradigm clinical cases and in clinical practice supervised by graduate faculty and preceptors. An implicit part of clinical decision making is advanced therapeutics. Advanced therapeutics provides the knowledge and skills needed to prescribe all pharmacological and nonpharmacological therapies/interventions and to assess patients' responses to these therapies. Directed at influencing measurable change in health status and quality of life, advanced therapeutics delineates the end products or measurable outcomes that result from interventions (Buchanan, 1994). Through faculty supervised clinical practice of adequate duration, students integrate and synthesize theory about health and disease, findings of clinical research, and knowledge of advanced therapeutics to meet the health-care needs of patients and their families (AACN, 1993).

CLINICAL PRACTICUM EXPERIENCES

Clinical practicum experiences consist of direct client care to individuals and families and must be a required component of all ANP programs. In addition to giving students practice in the direct caregiver role, the clinical practica allow students to learn particular aspects of the ANP role, to function as members of an interdisciplinary team, and to develop programs targeting system-based needs.

Typically, a faculty-supervised clinical practicum consists of both direct and indirect supervision. In direct supervision, faculty provide on-site clinical supervision for students. Faculty who provide direct supervision usually bring students to ongoing faculty practice sites, where the faculty serve as role models and direct supervisors. Indirect supervision involves faculty supplementation of a preceptor's clinical teaching. It has three components: Faculty serve as students' mentors, act as community liaisons, and evaluate students' progress (NONPF, 1995).

Among the teaching strategies that serve to guide ANP students through the process of clinical decision making in clinical practicum experiences are analysis of case studies; critique of research findings and scholarly literature as applied to the diagnosis and management of conditions or problems for individuals, families, or communities; case presentations; oral presentations; class discussions; seminars; clinical journals; preceptor and self-evaluation; and written and performance examinations. Through these teaching strategies, graduate nursing educators develop criteria to measure ANP core content, role functions, and competencies. These criteria allow students to progress toward increasing clinical expertise and the development of ANP competencies under the direction of faculty guidance and supervision throughout the ANP program.

ISSUES IN ANP EDUCATION

INTERDISCIPLINARY EDUCATION

Interdisciplinary education for health professionals has not been operationalized to its full extent within ANP education over the years. As advanced nursing practice has become established in the health-care system, new educational models of interdisciplinary collaboration have been developed. Yet, interdisciplinary activities have not been a consistent part of the formal educational process of APNs, instead occurring in on-the-job training with little assistance or support from health professional educational programs. It is frequently assumed that interdisciplinary education will occur when different disciplines are placed in proximity to one another. What happens more often is a random event with little strategic planning and minimal attention to outcomes. If collaboration competencies are an expected outcome of ANP programs, educators must attend to the development and improvement of interdisciplinary teaching/learning strategies. The focus on the changing health system has led to an outgrowth of several interdisciplinary initiatives that are funded by foundations and were mentioned earlier in this chapter. Each of these initiatives has sought to include APNs as the common denominator in interdisciplinary team models to restore the failing health-care system.

Senge's (1990) work on learning communities has also played a key role in promoting the notion of interdisciplinary learning. Building on the concepts of shared vision, communication, reflective inquiry, and teams, health-care systems have been challenged to look at new ways of thinking and being. Given the fact that the education of health professional disciplines has occurred independently, with minimal interdisciplinary team learning between faculty and/or students, APN educators need to reflect on the preponderance of discipline-specific content and learning in ANP programs. Interdisciplinary teams have been identified as one unfulfilled resource in the health-care environment (Institute of Medicine [IOM], 1994), with most interdisciplinary teams developed at the grassroots provider level. Educational programs have been slow in improving the function and outcomes of these teams, maintaining their discipline-specific domains as they do.

As an example of the thrust toward interdisciplinary models, the IOM (1994) recently published the preliminary *Report on Defining Primary Care*, which focuses on developing the interdisciplinary team as the provider of care. A new emphasis has also been placed on developing interdisciplinary core content for primary care providers, including primary care physicians, advanced practice nurses, physician assistants, and nurse-midwives. A new initiative entitled "Partners in Training" (Robert Wood Johnson Foundation, 1995) has been funded by the Robert Wood Johnson Foundation to develop interdisciplinary training models for NPs, CNMs, and physician assistants. Among the areas having been identified as core interdisciplinary content are health assessment, pharmacology, pathophysiology, health promotion and disease prevention, and selected aspects of specialty content. Other content areas identified center on team development: collaboration, continuous quality improvement, interdisciplinary team building, and community-oriented primary care.

Interdisciplinary educational models for primary care training have been in existence since the early 1970s. However, it has been only since the Pew Health Professions Commission Report (O'Neil, 1993) that innovative models of interdisciplinary team education and training for primary care professionals have been resurrected as a way of developing more effective service delivery. These foundation initiatives have challenged educators to expand their ways of thinking and being. The challenge inherent in health care interdisciplinary education is to create innovative, cutting-edge models for practice while maintaining equity among the disciplines and the integrity of each discipline's philosophy and practice style. Shared interdisciplinary instruction has multiple benefits. Among them are the conservation of curriculum, instructional resources, and faculty (Johnson-Pawlson & Harper, 1993) and the opportunity to develop and test models of team learning with faculty and students that extend to clinical agencies and other providers.

EDUCATIONAL STANDARDS FOR ANP PROGRAMS

The need to maintain consistent quality standards for ANP educational programs at the graduate level is paramount, given the increased use of APNs in the health-care workforce. During the initial phases of role development, ANP educators were particularly successful in safeguarding the quality of educational programs through careful attention to educational program outcomes. Among the educational strategies used to safeguard the quality of program outcomes were selective admission to ANP programs, limited numbers of ANP students, low faculty-to-student ratios, and systematic evaluation of clinical knowledge and skills.

Quality control was furthered by ensuring that graduates of ANP programs met established competency levels for designated clinical practice areas. For example, the ACNM (1992) delineated the fundamental knowledge, skills, and behaviors expected of new nurse-midwifery graduates in *Core Competencies for Basic Nurse Midwifery Practice.* NONPF (1995) delineated the fundamental knowledge, skills, and behaviors expected of new graduates in *ANP: Curriculum Guidelines and Program Standards for Nurse Practitioner Education.* The NONPF Guidelines include core-competencies for NPs. Because of the distinctive nature of specialty content in ANP programs, professional associations define their own specialty content through standards of practice and competencies. As examples of this, the Oncology Nursing Society, the National Association of Pediatric Nurse Associates and Practitioners, and the National Association of Nurse Practitioners in Reproductive Health all stipulate content, standards, and competencies for graduates of these respective specialty programs.

Quality standards have been met in the majority of ANP education programs, particularly those requiring national and state certification. This credentialing process has promoted the uniform standards and outcomes for certain ANP roles, notably the CNM and the CRNA, withstanding the test of variable educational levels and criteria for national and state certification/credentialing. However, the trend toward rapid expansion of NP programs in the past 3 years (from 201 tracks offered in 73 institutions in 1992 to 372 tracks offered in 158 institutions in 1994; Harper & Johnson, 1995) has led organizations and credentialing centers to reconsider the voluntary nature of establishing standards, particularly for NP programs. Likewise, standards for the CNS role have been highly variable because of the lack of core ANP requirements, with the exception of well-developed specialties such as oncology and acute care nursing. Graduate educators must define the central core of knowledge, skills, and competencies in conjunction with the standards and collaborate on developing a system to administer them if this ANP role is to survive. Whether ANP programs can continue to meet program standards through professional autonomy and accountability is unknown.

CERTIFICATION, CREDENTIALING, AND ACCREDITATION

Given the abilities of educational programs, state regulatory agencies, accrediting bodies, and credentialing centers to independently establish differing standards, it is incumbent upon ANP educators to exercise leadership in promoting the maintenance of quality ANP programs through consistent standards. Certainly, the current wide variation in master's programs (Burns et al., 1993) does not serve the profession well in advocating for stronger roles for APNs in the evolving health-care system. External processes intrinsic to the regulation of advanced nursing practice include national and state certification, credentialing processes, and program approval and accreditation. Each of these external processes supports mechanisms for validating knowledge and competencies for graduates of ANP programs. These external processes have had a major influence on ANP education, linking educational preparation to professional competency and accountability.

Each of the advanced practice roles has its own distinct procedures for obtaining certification, credentialing, and accreditation. These credentialing programs have distinct requirements that influence the development and structure of educational programs. For example, CRNA and CNM programs must receive preaccreditation program approval from their respective accreditation bodies (AANA, 1992; ACNM 1993) before they open their doors. This guarantees that the essential components needed to ensure standards and the core competencies are in place, including program instructional objectives and materials reviewed according to designated criteria. As for NP educational programs, the NONPF (1995) has established minimum standards for NP programs in its *ANP: Curriculum Guidelines and Program Standards for NP Education.* In addition, depending on the NP specialty (i.e., OB/GYN NP, pediatric NP, family NP, adult NP, women's health NP, neonatal NP) several mechanisms for certification and credentialing are available. Each of these respective NP specialties has separate credentialing bodies: the National Certification Center, the American Nurses Credentialing Center, the National Certification Board for Pediatric Nursing Specialties, and the American Academy of Nurse Practitioners. Similarly, each credentialing body has its own distinct criteria to allow graduates of NP programs to sit for their respective national certification exams. Some of these criteria are

- the type of educational degrees or certificates awarded (i.e., graduate nursing credit, post-basic nursing, or continuing education units);

- the number of didactic and faculty-supervised clinical hours in the educational program;
- the type of curriculum offered in the program, including specialty content, and
- whether the curriculum matches the standards of practice for each particular specialty.

Likewise, the ACNM and the AANA allow only those graduates of approved programs to sit for the national certification exams. CNSs are able to receive national certification through the ANA and a variety of other specialty organizations, but frequently certification is not a requirement for CNSs to practice in their role. Through these credentialing centers and certification bodies, the ANP community has established links with educational institutions, accrediting and regulatory bodies, as well as other ANP organizations. However, much work remains to develop common standards among national and state certification, credentialing processes, and mechanisms of accreditation if APNs are to gain widespread public support.

ARTICULATED EDUCATIONAL MODELS

Educational mobility has been a prevailing issue for nurses, including APNs, and continues to be an issue. Considering that an estimated 66% of practicing NPs, CNMs, and CRNAs (Aiken et al., 1994) were not educated in master's nursing programs, there is an apparent need for a process through which individuals practicing in ANP roles progress to higher levels of education with minimal barriers and minimal duplication of knowledge and skills (AACN, 1993). Educational mobility is an issue primarily for three of the ANP roles: NP, CNM, and CRNA. Likewise, the number of students seeking a second degree in nursing has increased with the call to double the number of APNs (Pew, 1995) and parallel shifts in the marketplace. These shifts have been felt by ANP programs nationally as program inquiries, applications, and enrollments have risen, with the exception of CNS tracks (AACN, 1995; Harper & Johnson-Pawlson, 1995; NLN, 1994).

In the past two decades, nursing education has had great success in developing articulated educational models, particularly with RN-to-BSN programs (Rapson, 1987). The principles of educational mobility for RN-to-BSN programs can be applied to nurses needing either undergraduate or graduate coursework for ANP preparation. There are three general types of students who need articulated educational programs:

1. Certificate-prepared NPs, CNMs, and CRNAs;
2. RNs without BSN preparation seeking accelerated master's preparation as an APN; and
3. Students who have a baccalaureate degree other than nursing and are seeking ANP preparation.

These three types of students have different needs based on their personal and educational characteristics. The educational issues and strategies of the students who have the basic preparation and licensure as an RN are somewhat different from those of the students who have no education in nursing. Numerous programs have been tailored to the specific needs of each of these student groups. The common denominators in these programs are flexibility, acceleration and consolidation of content to avoid repetition, identification of a common core of content at either the graduate or undergraduate level, and an established programmatic curriculum model for articulation. These characteristics define the type of articulation model according to the particular needs of the group of students being served.

An articulated curriculum model for RNs seeking master's preparation as an APN frequently includes advanced placement credit for undergraduate nursing coursework through examination, an accelerated curriculum that consolidates core graduate coursework with undergraduate coursework, and specially tailored clinical practice experiences. An articulated curriculum model for a certificate-prepared NP, CNM, or CRNA who does not have a baccalaureate degree often incorporates baccalaureate content for nursing and general education courses. Advanced placement exams are used for advanced placement in both undergraduate and graduate nursing courses, with standard ANP core courses identified to prevent duplication of content. Graduate nursing coursework is tailored to incorporate a stronger emphasis on theory and research application. These programs need to explicitly address the ANP core competencies identified earlier, so that graduates are prepared to function at an advanced level. Generic master's ANP programs are designed for students who have a degree in a field other than nursing. Articulated educational programs usually incorporate accelerated content for undergraduate and graduate knowledge, skills, and competencies. These programs must prepare students for both professional nursing and ANP competencies. They are typically offered over a 2- to 3-year period, with intensive clinical practice incorporating both undergraduate and graduate level ANP clinical experiences. The accelerated programs for students seeking a second degree are relatively expensive, because of the faculty resources needed to prepare these students as competent APNs.

CONCLUSION

APNs must standardize the level of educational preparation to strengthen their internal professional cohesion and extend their external professional validity among health-care providers. Although there has been much debate among members of the nursing community, standardizing the minimum level of preparation for APNs at the master's level in nursing graduate programs is essential in order to establish credibility among nurses, other health-care providers, consumers, and policymakers. In addition, progress toward standardizing graduate nursing programs, including core curricula and competencies for APNs, is necessary to derive credibility for each of these roles in the emerging health-care system. APNs and ANP educators cannot afford to stand still. Instead, they must continually evaluate, refine, and redesign educational programs that are responsive to society's needs and those of the existing and future health-care system.

REFERENCES

Aiken, L., Gwyther, M., & Whelan, E. (1994). *Advanced practice nursing education: Allocation of the proposed graduate nursing education account* (Report submitted under contract to the Office of the Assistant Secretary of Health, U.S. Department of Health and Human Services). Philadelphia, PA: Center for Health Policy Research, University of Pennsylvania School of Nursing.

American Association of Colleges of Nursing. (1993). *Position statement on educational mobility*. Washington, DC: Author.

American Association of Colleges of Nursing. (1994). *Annual report: Unifying the curricula for advanced practice*. Washington, DC. Author.

American Association of Colleges of Nursing. (1995). *1994–1995 Special Report on master's and post master's nurse practitioner programs; faculty clinical practice; faculty age profiles; undergraduate curriculum expansion in baccalaureate & graduate programs in nursing*. Washington, DC: AACN.

American Association of Nurse Anesthetists.

(1992). *Guidelines and standards for nurse anesthesia practice.* Park Ridge, IL: AANA.

American Association of Nurse Anesthetists Council on Accreditation. (1990). *Standards and guidelines for programs of nurse anesthesia.* Park Ridge, IL: AANA.

American College of Nurse Midwives. (1992). *Core competencies in nurse-midwifery.* Washington, DC: Author.

American College of Nurse Midwives. (1993). *Criteria for accreditation of basic certificate, graduate, and pre-certification nurse-midwifery programs.* Washington, DC: Author.

American Nurses' Association. (1995a). *Draft scope and standards of advanced practice nursing.* Washington, DC: Author.

American Nurses' Association. (1995b). *Nursing's social policy statement.* Washington, DC: Author.

Benner, P. (1984). *From novice to expert: Excellence and power in clinical nursing practice.* Menlo Park, CA: Addison Wesley.

Buchanan, L. (1994). Therapeutic nursing intervention knowledge development and outcome measures for advanced practice. *Nursing and Health Care, 15,* 190–195.

Bullough, B, (1992). Alternative models for specialty nursing practice. *Nursing and Health Care, 13,* 254–259.

Burns, P., Nishikawa; H., Weatherby, F., Forni, P., Moran, M., Allen, M., Baker, C., & Booten, D. (1993). Masters degree nursing education: State of the art. *Journal of Professional Nursing, 9,* 267–276.

Cronenwett, L. (1995). Molding the future of advanced practice nursing. *Nursing Outlook, 43*(3), 112–118.

Fenton, M., & Brykczynski, K. (1993). Qualitative distinctions and similarities in the practice of clinical nurse specialists and nurse practitioners. *Journal of Professional Nursing, 9,* 313–326.

Hamric, A., & Spross, J. (1989). *The clinical specialist in theory and practice.* Philadelphia, PA: W. B. Saunders Company.

Harper, D., & Johnson, J. (1995, July). *Interim preliminary report of the workforce policy project: Comparison of the 1992 to 1994 national nurse practitioner program directories.* Paper presented at the annual conference of the National Organization of Nurse Practitioner Faculties National Conference, Denver, CO.

Institute of Medicine. (1994). *Defining primary care: An interim report.* Donaldson, M., Yordy, K., & Vanselow, N. (eds.). Washington, DC: National Academy Press.

Johnson-Pawlson, J., & Harper, D. (1993). An economic paradigm for NP education program development. *Journal of Professional Nursing, 9,* 148–152.

Jordan, L. (1994). Qualifications and capabilities of the certified registered nurse anesthetist. In S. D. Foster & L. Jordan (Eds.), *Professional aspects of nurse anesthesia practice.* Philadelphia, PA: F. A. Davis. pp. 3–10.

National League for Nursing. (1994). *Nursing datasource, 1994: Volume II. Graduate education in nursing, advanced practice nursing* (Pub. No. 19-2643). New York: National League for Nursing.

National League for Nursing Accreditation Committee, Council of Baccalaureate and Higher Degree Programs. (1992). *Criteria and guidelines for evaluation of baccalaureate and higher degree programs in nursing* (Pub. No. 15-2474). New York: National League for Nursing Press.

Naylor, M., & Brooten, D. (1993). The roles and functions of clinical nurse specialists. *Image, 25,* 73–78.

National Organization of Nurse Practitioner Faculties. (1995). *Advanced nursing practice: Curriculum guidelines and program standards for nurse practitioner education.* C. A. Boodley, D. C. Harper, C. M. Hanson, P. Jackson, D. D. Russell, D. Taylor, and P. Zimmer (Eds.). Washington, DC: NONPF.

Nurse Education and Practice Improvement Amendment of 1992. Title II Public Law 103-3331 September 30, 1994.

O'Neil, E. (1993). *Health professions education for the future: Schools in service to the nation.* San Francisco, CA: Pew Health Professions Commission, Pew Charitable Trust Foundation.

Pew Health Professions Commission, Phase Two. (1995). *Shifting the supply of our health care workforce: A guide to redirecting federal subsidy of medical education.* San Francisco, CA: Pew Charitable Trusts Foundation.

Rapson, M. (Ed.). (1987). Collaborating for articulation: RN to BSN. New York: National League for Nursing.

Robert Wood Johnson Foundation. (1995). *Partnerships in training: Regional education systems for nurse practitioners, certified nurse midwives and physician assistants.* Washington, DC: Association of Academic Health Centers.

Safriet, B. (1992) Health care dollars and regulatory sense: The role of advanced practice nursing. *Yale Journal on Regulation, 9,* 417–487.

Senge, P. (1990). *The fifth discipline: The art and practice of the learning organization.* New York: Doubleday.

Smith, M. (1995). The core of advanced practice nursing. *Nursing Science Quarterly, 8,* 2–3.

U.S. Department of Health and Human Services, Public Health Service. (1991). *Healthy People 2000: National health promotion and disease prevention objectives.* (DHHS Publication No. (PHS) 91-50213). Washington, DC: U.S. Government Printing Office.

Vector Research, Incorporated. (1995). *Development of integrated requirements for PAs, NPs, CNMs, and physicians (MDs and DOs)* Final Report (HRSA contract No. 240-94-0033). Arlington, VA: Vector Research Incorporated.

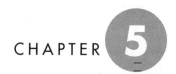

CHAPTER 5

Role Development of the Advanced Practice Nurse

Karen A. Brykczynski

INTRODUCTION

Role development in clinical nursing practice is described here as a process that evolves over time (Hamric & Taylor, 1989; Mauksch, 1981; Oda, 1977; Sparacino & Cooper, 1990). Over the years nurses have taken on many tasks or procedures that were once under the exclusive purview of medicine, but the core of nursing is not defined by the tasks nurses perform. This task-oriented perspective is inadequate and does violence to the complex nature of nursing. Nursing practice is distinguished by an orientation to holistic care, a philosophy of collaboration with patients and their families, a tradition of care and concern, a disciplinary matrix, a rich and varied history, and an ever-growing body of knowledge. Open acknowledgment of the knowledge that develops as nurses expand their scope of practice and incorporate new knowledge and skill into their repertoire is required for advancing understanding of clinical nursing practice (Benner, 1985).

The processes of acquiring and implementing advanced practice roles in nursing are complex, dynamic, and varied. The discussion of role development as presented in this chapter differs from previous literature in several major ways. First, this chapter derives from a holistic perspective characteristic of phenomenological and feminist philosophical perspectives. Secondly, this chapter consolidates literature from all of the advanced practice nurse (APN) roles, including clinical nurse specialists (CNSs), nurse practitioners (NPs), nurse-midwives (CNMs), and nurse anesthetists (CRNAs), to present a generic process relevant to all APN roles. Third, a situational model of the development of expertise is presented to guide understanding of the development of advanced practice roles in nursing.

Reference to general professional role development literature in nursing is followed by discussion of the utility of the generic situational model of expertise for understanding the acquisition of APN skills and knowledge. Next a professional career development model is presented. Exploration of inter-professional and intra-professional role issues follows. Then the discussion is separated into the educational component of APN *role acquisition* and the occupational or work component of *role implementation*. This division in the process of role development is intended to clarify and distinguish between the changes occurring during role transitions experienced during the educational component of learning an APN role (role acquisition) and the changes occurring during the actual performance of the role following program completion (role implementation). Strategies for enhancing APN role development are again divided into role acquisition and implementation sections. The chapter concludes with summary comments and suggestions regarding facilitation of future APN role development.

PERSPECTIVES ON APN ROLE DEVELOPMENT

PROFESSIONAL ROLE DEVELOPMENT LITERATURE

Professional role development literature in nursing is abundant and complex, involving as it does multiple component processes. These include (1) aspects of adult development, (2) development of clinical expertise, (3) modification of self-identity through initial socialization in school, (4) development and integration of professional subrole components, and (5) subsequent resocialization in the work setting. Like socialization for other professional roles such as attorney, teacher, and social worker, the process of becoming a professional nurse involves aspects of adult socialization as well as occupational socialization (Lum, 1988). Leddy and Pepper (1993) adapted the stages, tasks, and goals of Erikson's (1982) developmental life cycle model for depicting role development in nursing. This model may be useful for understanding professional role transition experiences. A broader developmental view that incorporates socialization as a component process but allows for more holistic understanding is advocated here. In discussing development, Benner and Wrubel's (1989) use of the term "life course" rather than "life cycle" conveys the contextual meanings of these life situations and their connection to past experiences and anticipation of future possibilities. Aspects of adult socialization that often occur concurrently with becoming a professional include life transitions such as becoming a spouse or a parent.

SITUATIONAL MODEL OF DEVELOPING EXPERTISE

A phenomenological and interpretive understanding of human expertise is fundamental to the Dreyfus model of skill acquisition (Dreyfus & Dreyfus, 1986). A phenomenological perspective provides data about lived experiences while an interpretive approach takes the situational context into account. The Dreyfus model is a situational model, not a trait model. An expert in one situation is not necessarily an expert in another. When a novel situation is encountered or a situation is grasped erroneously, there is regression to less skilled levels of performance. Expertise, according to this model, differs from predominantly cognitive, rationalist perspectives in that extensive personal experience in actual situations is required for its development (Benner, 1984; Dreyfus & Dreyfus, 1986; Heidegger, 1927/1962; Kuhn, 1970; Polanyi, 1958). Expertise, a hybrid of practical and theoretical knowledge, develops as skills and knowledge become embodied.

Embodied knowledge is knowledge that involves all the senses, not just the rational mind. Mulligan (1976) provided an illustration of embodied knowledge in describing the development and refinement of perceptual knowledge that occurs with learning the skills to become a CNM. She noted that the fingers and hands learn to detect distinctions in shape, size, consistency, and location; the eyes learn to recognize fetal position by observing the shape of the contracting abdomen, and these data are confirmed by touch. The ears learn to detect changes in fetal heart tones, and the nose provides clues that distinguish some common vaginal infections that the eyes and the microscope confirm or refute. This concept of embodied knowledge and skill underlies not only clinical practice but all APN core skills, including expert guidance and coaching, consultation, research, leadership, collaboration, change agency, and ethical decision-making (see Chapter 3).

The Dreyfus model was originally developed with pilot trainers, chess players, and adult learners of second languages (Dreyfus & Dreyfus, 1986). According to this model there is a generic process of skill acquisition through which humans proceed in stages from novice to expert as they acquire new psychomotor, perceptual, and judgment skills. The Dreyfus model has been applied in a variety of disciplines. Benner's (1984) application of it to nursing is particularly relevant here. Expertise, according to this model, develops over time through direct personal encounters that alter preconceptions and prior understanding developed from one's own background of particular experiences. Though personal, such knowledge is not totally idiosyncratic. It can be shared in ways described by Benner (1984), such as identifying maxims, common meanings, assumptions, expectations, sets, exemplars, and paradigm cases that convey the contextual meanings of the embedded knowledge.

This is a situational model, as noted earlier, and the novice-to-expert trajectory has important implications for graduate nursing programs. It might be argued that this model lends substance to graduate program entry requirements of a year or more of clinical practice experience. On the other hand, it might be argued that this model helps explain the success of generic graduate APN programs wherein non-nurse graduates from other fields such as counseling, biology, or sociology have acquired practical and theoretical knowledge in related fields that facilitates their learning of APN roles and functions. Most importantly, this model gives explicit recognition to the fact that even experienced experts perform at less proficient levels when they enter new situations. Thus, it must be acknowledged that new master's APN graduates cannot be expected to perform at expert levels immediately upon graduation. Readers are encouraged to keep these implications of the Dreyfus model in the background as concepts of role development are explored throughout this chapter.

PROFESSIONAL CAREER DEVELOPMENT MODEL

A variety of models have been developed to illustrate the phases of career development in professions. The stages of (1) apprentice, (2) colleague, (3) mentor, and (4) sponsor were described by Dalton and colleagues (1977) from interviews with several hundred professionally trained employees. These stages form the framework for a model (Table 5–1) that offers an alternative to the more traditional pyramidal model by which authority, status, and salary all increase as individuals advance in administrative positions. The relevance of this model for APN role development is that it incorporates advancement in professional roles without necessitating movement into management positions.

A dynamic, situational interpretation of the Dalton and colleagues (1977) model is useful for depicting the multiple simultaneous processes occurring during APN role development. For example, a professional nurse who functions as a mentor for baccalaureate graduates may decide to pursue an advanced degree as an APN. As an APN student this nurse will experience the challenges of acquiring a new role, the anxiety of unfamiliar skills and practices, and the dependency of being a novice and in the apprentice stage of the career model. At the same time, if this nurse continues to work as an RN, his or her functioning in this work role will be at competent, proficient, and expert levels (depending on experience and

TABLE 5–1. FOUR CAREER STAGES

	Stage I	**Stage II**	**Stage III**	**Stage IV**
Central activity	Helping Learning Following directions	Independent contributor	Training Interfacing	Shaping the direction of the organization
Primary relationship	Apprentice	Colleague	Mentor	Sponsor
Major psychological issues	Dependence	Independence	Assuming responsibility for others	Exercising power

(From Dalton, G.W., Thompson, P.H., & Price, R.L. (1977). The four stages of professional careers—A new look at performance by professionals. Reprinted, by permission of publisher, from *Organizational Dynamics*, Summer/1997, © 1977. American Management Association, New York. All rights reserved.)

the situation) in the mentor career stage. Upon graduation and taking a new APN position, this nurse will experience the phases of role implementation, continued movement along the novice-to-expert trajectory, and resumption of the interrupted course of career development. Years later, the APN may decide to pursue yet another APN role after the mentor or sponsor stages of career development have been reached. The processes of role acquisition, role implementation, and novice-to-expert skill development will again be experienced (though altered and informed by previous experiences) as the student again re-enters the apprentice stage of career development. Role development is thus pictured as multiple, dynamic, situational processes, with each new undertaking being characterized by passage through earlier developmental phases with some movement back and forth, and horizontally, as different career options are pursued.

ROLE CONCEPTS AND PROFESSIONAL ROLE ISSUES

The concepts of role stress and strain discussed by Hardy and Hardy (1988) are useful for understanding the dynamics of role transitions. They described role stress as a social structural condition in which role obligations are ambiguous, conflicting, incongruous, excessive, or unpredictable. Role strain is defined as the subjective feeling of frustration, tension, or anxiety experienced in response to role stress. It is believed that role strain can be minimized though certainly not completely prevented by the identification of potential role stressors, the development of strategies to cope with them, and rehearsal of situations designed to apply those strategies. It is acknowledged here that the difficulties experienced by neophytes in new positions can never be eliminated. As noted above, expertise is holistic, involving bodily perceptual skills and shared background knowledge as well as cognitive ability. A school-work, theory-practice, ideal-real gap will remain because of the nature of human skill acquisition.

This discussion of professional role issues will incorporate additional role concepts from Hardy and Hardy (1988) along with the concept that different APN roles represent different cultural groups within the broader nursing culture (Leininger, 1976). APNs can be described as tricultural and trilingual. They share background knowledge, practices, and skills of three cultures: (1) biomedicine, (2) mainstream nursing, and (3) everyday life. They are fluent in the languages of biomedical science, nursing knowledge and skill, and everyday parlance. Some APNs, CNMs for example, are socialized into a fourth culture as well, that of midwifery. Others are also fluent in more than one everyday language. Just as APN roles can be conceptualized as encompassing skills and knowledge from more than one culture, they can be seen as encompassing aspects of both male and female occupational sex roles (Kritek, 1988). Bem (1977) contended that successful adult existence in society requires the ability to blend both the traditionally masculine and the traditionally feminine domains. These insights that APNs are multicultural, multilingual, and androgenous can be helpful for cultivating expertise in an increasingly multicultural world.

Role Ambiguity

Role ambiguity develops when there is a lack of clarity about expectations, a blurring of responsibilities, uncertainty regarding implementation of subroles, and the inherent uncertainty of the existent knowledge base of a discipline. According to Hardy and Hardy (1988), role ambiguity characterizes all professional positions. They pointed out that role ambiguity may be positive in that it offers opportunities for creative possibilities. It can be expected to be more prominent in professions undergoing change such as those in the health care field. Role ambiguity has been widely discussed in relation to the CNS role (see Chapter 14), but it is a relevant issue for other APN roles as well.

Role Incongruity

Role incongruity is an example of intra-role conflict that Hardy and Hardy (1988) described as developing from two sources. Incompatibility between skills and abilities and role obligations is one source of role incongruity. An example might be an APN with excellent history-taking and therapeutic communication skills whose role requires performing invasive procedures that may be experienced as more stressful and less satisfying. Another source of role incongruity is incompatibility between personal values, self-concept, and expected role behaviors. APNs commonly experience this incongruity when they highly value clinical practice, yet their position requires them to assume administrative functions. An example comes from Banda's (1985) study of psychiatric liaison CNSs in acute care hospitals and community health agencies. She reported that they viewed consultation and teaching as their major functions, whereas research and administrative subroles were associated with role strain.

Inter-Professional Role Conflict

Role conflict develops when role expectations are perceived as contradictory or mutually exclusive. APNs may experience intra-role conflict as well as both inter- and intra-professional role conflicts. Conflicts between physicians and APNs constitute the most common situations of inter-professional conflict of interest here. Major sources of conflict for physicians with regard to APNs are the perceived economic threat of competition, limited resources in clinical training sites, and lack of experience working with APNs.

The relationship between anesthesiologists and CRNAs is an exemplar for considering the issues of inter-professional role conflict between physicians and APNs. Historically, anesthesiologists have interpreted their relationship with CRNAs as one of direct competition, thus creating an adversarial stance. Their relationship over the years might be characterized as a cold war with overt offensives mounted periodically by anesthesiologists. Following World War II, anesthesiologists launched a major effort to eliminate nurses from the field of anesthesia (Gunn, 1991). In the mid-1980s, the concept of all-physician anesthesia was again promoted, and many nurse anesthesia programs were closed (DePaolis-Lutzo, 1987). When CRNAs are viewed as direct competitors, it is understandable that some if not most anesthesiologists would be reluctant to be involved in assisting with their education (National Commission on Nurse Anesthesia Education, 1990).

Improved relationships between APNs and physicians will require redefinition of the situation by both groups. Fagin (1992) asserted that collaboration is imperative: "Comprehensive health care today requires the broad spectrum of knowledge that no one practitioner can provide. Costs of health and medical care have been shown to be reduced by the appropriate utilization of nurses working in teams or in consultative relationships with physicians. Nurses and physicians are not in competition for the patient. As physicians' work roles and autonomy change and more of them are salaried employees, the convergence of issues affecting nurses and doctors will benefit from collaboration" (pp. 357–358).

Redefinition of the situation between APNs and physicians can be facilitated by prioritizing public service over self-serving personal and professional interests. Collaboration between nurses and physicians is good for both groups as well as the public. Research data support the contention that collaboration improves patient outcomes (Baggs, 1989) and decreases mortality rates (Knaus, Wagner, & Zimmerman, 1986). In developing collaborative efforts it may be helpful to recognize that individual physicians and APNs often form practice relationships on institutional or individual levels that are satisfactory and mutually beneficial. The conflicts of interest emphasized at organizational levels often exaggerate the issues.

Rooks (1983) noted that "collegiality, cooperation, communication, and complementarity—not competition—should be the characteristics of nurse-midwives' relationships with physicians" (p. 3). King (1990) observed that "the collegial relationship is built on shared knowledge, confidence, and mutual trust in which an egalitarian working situation develops" (p. 172). Inter-professional role conflict results when any of these factors is deficient. Rooks and Haas (1986) discussed this problem in terms of nurse-midwifery and suggested that educating physicians about nurse-midwifery care with emphasis on its complementary relationship to medical care may decrease conflict. They also recommended CNM appointments on medical school faculties to increase awareness of nurse-midwifery and improve inter-professional communication. These recommendations are relevant for all APN groups.

However, the complementary nature of advanced nursing practice to medical care is a foreign concept for many physicians who view all health care as an extension of medical care and APNs as physician extenders. This misunderstanding of advanced nursing practice underlies their opposition to independent roles for nurses because they believe such nurses want to practice medicine without a license. The fact that nursing has its own knowledge and skills is a novel idea for physicians who see nursing as a subset of medicine. Thus, an information campaign on individual, institutional, and national levels may be necessary to change such perceptions held by physicians and the general public.

More mundane matters also contribute to inter-professional role conflicts. Long and Sharp (1982) surveyed CNMs and OB residents and identified factors contributing to conflictual relationships. Factors identified included residents' perceptions of CNMs as having more favorable work schedules, working with a predominately low-risk patient population, and having positions somewhat separate from the OB faculty-resident hierarchy. These factors would be expected to be applicable to other APN/physician situations as well. Long and Sharp (1982) recommended using differences in practice between APNs and physicians as areas of inquiry rather than as targets of criticism. One way to promote positive inter-professional relationships is to structure education and practice experiences between APNs, medical students, and residents to enhance mutual understanding. Developing such interdisciplinary experiences is difficult because of different academic calendars and clinical schedules. Such obstacles can be overcome if these interdisciplinary activities are considered essential for improved health-care delivery.

Intra-Professional Role Conflict

APNs experience intra-professional role conflict with other nurses and within the nursing profession for a variety of reasons. The historical development of APN roles has been fraught with conflict and controversy in nursing education and nursing organizations for CNMs (Varney, 1987), NPs (Ford, 1982), and CRNAs (Gunn, 1991; see also Chapter 1). Relationships between these APN groups and nursing as a discipline have improved markedly in recent years, yet difficulties remain to be surmounted. For example, the necessity of a nursing foundation for midwifery has been challenged (Flanagan, 1986; Rooks, 1983). One would expect current discussions about broadening the scope of midwifery care to encompass primary care management of women's health to promote renewed interest in and commitment to maintaining a nursing foundation (American College of Nurse-Midwives, 1993).

Kimbro (1978) described communication difficulties between CNMs and staff RNs as developing from lack of communication between the two groups in three areas: (1) on an organizational level, (2) during educational programs, and (3) in the literature. She also noted that value differences and structural role differences set up a situation for intra-professional role conflict in that staff RNs were concerned with 24-hour coverage and smooth functioning of the unit as a whole, whereas CNMs were more concerned with direct care of their individual patients.

Hazle's (1985) descriptive study of inter-role conflict between OB nurses and CNMs indicated that they generally viewed one another positively, but that conflicts did arise over intrapartum management. Lack of communication seemed to be a major source of conflict in the critical incidents reported (Hazle, 1985). She commented that when the OB nurse in the hospital setting encounters a CNM, a hierarchical relationship results in which another nurse (the CNM) performs functions usually within the purview of medicine and beyond the usual scope of nursing practice. If OB nurses are not informed and oriented about CNM roles and functions, conflict may ensue. Familiarizing OB nurses with CNM job descriptions was recommended to decrease confusion about CNM role expectations. In developing strategies to manage these conflicts it may be helpful to note that there are marked similarities between physician/APN inter-professional role conflict and CNM/OB nurse intra-professional role conflict.

Hamric and Taylor (1989) pointed out that staff resistance to change, complacency or apathy, and the fact that nurses are generally not accustomed to seeking consultation from other nurses as experts can impede CNS role development. Studies by Lurie (1981) and Brykczynski (1985) reported refusals by staff nurses to perform support functions, such as taking vital signs and drawing blood, for patients assigned to NPs and the absence of negative sanctions by their supervisors for these behaviors. These behaviors suggest the horizontal violence commonly observed within oppressed groups as discussed by Roberts (1983). Framing intra-professional conflict in the context of acting out hostility toward one's own less powerful group instead of toward the more powerful oppressors can be useful for developing strategies to overcome these difficulties. Such a perspective indicates that by providing information and support, nurses can learn to value their own worth and significance, becoming empowered and consequently supportive rather than destructive toward other nurses.

According to Curry (1994), an important component of successfully integrating NP practice in an emergency room setting is thorough orientation of staff nurses about the APN role, including clear guidelines and policies regarding responsibility issues. Another significant strategy for minimizing intra-professional role conflict is for the new APN to spend time with the nursing staff to establish rapport and learn as much as possible about the new setting from those who really know what is going on—the nurses. This affirms the value and significance of the nurses and sets up a positive atmosphere for collegiality and intra-professional role cooperation and collaboration.

REVIEW OF APN ROLE DEVELOPMENT

ROLE TRANSITIONS

Hardy and Hardy (1988) maintained that role strain invariably accompanies major role transitions. They suggested that role strain may be prerequisite to acquiring and implementing a new role and may actually facilitate role transition by increasing awareness of gaps in knowledge and skill. Professional socialization in nursing involves role transitions from layperson to RN (RN to BSN for some), from RN to APN, or from non-RN to APN. These transitions occur over time as the individual nurse pursues additional education and changes roles or positions. Selected literature relating to initial processes of role development in basic nursing education, which can enhance the understanding of APN role transition by providing sociohistorical context, is included in the following discussion of role acquisition and role implementation.

NURSING ROLE ACQUISITION (IN SCHOOL)

Each individual's unique personality, background experiences, repertoire of abilities and skills, and culturally defined values and beliefs affect role development (Thorton & Nardi, 1975), thus contributing to the variability of individual role trajectories. In spite of these individual variations, the intense and extensive processes of socialization into a professional role often involve alteration in the role incumbent's self-identity and self-concept (Hardy & Hardy, 1988). In a review of the role development literature in undergraduate, certificate, and graduate nursing these alterations of self-identity and self-concept emerged as a consistent theme with role acquisition experiences commonly depicted as identity crises (Anderson, Leonard, & Yates, 1974; Elkema & Knutson, 1983; Klaich, 1990; Malkemes, 1974; Oleson & Whittaker, 1968; Russell, 1988).

The contention that the personal upheaval experienced by APN students constitutes an identity crisis early in the program is common to literature inclusive of certificate as well as graduate level programs across APN specialty groups. Anderson and colleagues (1974) observed the crisis within the first 2 to 3 months of all three programs studied (a graduate program, a post-baccalaureate certificate program, and a continuing education program), whereas Malkemes (1974) reported that the role crisis occurred after the first 4 weeks of a year-long certificate program that admitted nurses from ADN to post-master's levels. In 1988, Russell reported a marked decrease in students' perceptions of their learning and their concepts of themselves as NPs during the fourth to the sixth weeks of a master's level program.

Elkema & Knutson (1983) observed that the identity crisis occurred during the middle of their 12-month family NP certificate program. They speculated that the identity crisis apparently facilitated the role change critical to NP role development.

This observation can be understood from the role strain perspective. As noted earlier, the experience of role strain resulting from awareness of the gap between one's current knowledge and ability and that required of the new APN role may energize active involvement in trying to learn the expected role behaviors. Klaich's (1990) qualitative study of 18 CNS graduate students suggested that the multiple changes associated with the transition from generalist BSN nurse to specialist MSN nurse were associated with disruption in self-esteem and self-concept. Thus, APN role transition experiences are reported to be associated with sufficient ego disequilibrium to result in identity transitions of sufficient magnitude to constitute a crisis.

Insights from feminist critiques and further elucidation of developmental phenomena from a feminist perspective (Spross, 1992) allow for a reinterpretation of the transitions associated with APN role development. It is important to note here that these insights from feminist philosophy are intended to be holistic and inclusive of both males and females in APN roles. Grimshaw's (1988) feminine perspective of the development of self-understanding as a dialectic of autonomy in which the search for control and coherence needs to be balanced with realism and tolerance provides useful insight here. Such self-understanding enables one to tolerate contradictions and be more comfortable with ambiguity as opposed to being burdened with anxiety and guilt. The self from the feminist perspective is viewed as a becoming, a process—responsive to experiences and relationships (Spross, 1992). Thus, the crisis of identity associated with APN role transition can be reframed in feminist terms as a reshaping or reconstitution of the self in the context of experience (Spross, 1992).

Spross described how this feminine perspective can sustain integrity or stability in the face of change: "Women trying to make sense of their experiences often face contradictions and ambiguity. These very experiences may underlie the dynamic stability of an individual's self, so that even as one responds to the environment and redefines self and meaning, the authentic self is experienced as whole" (Spross, 1992, p. 20). These feminist ideas are congruent with the phenomenological concepts of the development of expertise and role development over the life course presented earlier. Perhaps by understanding APN role transition experiences holistically as relational and situational, one can develop additional strategies to facilitate role development.

NURSING ROLE IMPLEMENTATION (AT WORK)

Kramer (1974) described a phenomenon of reality shock experienced by baccalaureate graduates as they encountered conflict between academic values, attitudes, and behaviors and the values, attitudes, and behaviors of the work world. This phenomenon was considered analogous to the cultural shock experienced by persons who move into another culture. Kramer's work provides meaningful background for understanding APN role development by virtue of the similarities in the experiences reported for new BSN graduates in the 1970s and those reported and observed for new APN graduates today. For example, Kramer noted that the dominant emphases in initial work experiences were organizational efficiency regarding the numbers of patients cared for and specific role behaviors, such as documentation. Similarly, current APN graduates commonly describe feeling pressured to see large numbers of patients and to keep their charting complete yet concise. These experiences of graduate APNs can also be conceptualized as bureaucratic versus professional role conflict occurring when the realities of the work world conflict with the ideals of academia.

The phases of professional nursing work role implementation with BSN graduates described by Kramer (1974) share many similarities with those described by Oda (1977), Baker (1979), and Hamric and Taylor (1989) with CNS graduates (Table 5–2). There is general agreement that there is significant overlap and fluidity among the phases (Hamric & Taylor, 1989; Kramer, 1974; Oda, 1977). However, for purposes of discussion the phases of role implementation will be considered sequentially, and Hamric and Taylor's (1989) descriptors will be used.

Phase one, orientation (see Table 5–2), is characterized by enthusiasm, optimism, and attention to mastery of clinical skills. The second phase, frustration (see Table 5–2), was not noted by Oda, yet it was commonly observed by the other authors. It is associated with feelings of conflict and inadequacy. The next phase, implementation, is described similarly by all of the authors (see Table 5–2) as one of role modification in response to interactions with others. This phase is associated with a renewed or returning perspective. The models suggest that the fourth phase, integration, is reached only after successful transition through the earlier phases. This phase is characterized by refinement of clinical expertise and integration of role components appropriate for the particular situation. The three additional phases described by Hamric and Taylor (1989) are discussed in the following section.

DEVELOPMENTAL PHASES OF APN ROLE IMPLEMENTATION

Hamric and Taylor's (1989) study of CNS role development warrants further discussion here because it may be useful as a model for understanding implementation of all APN roles. In addition, their research built on Kramer's, Baker's, and Oda's earlier work. Hamric and Taylor's (1989) analysis of questionnaires returned by 100 CNSs indicated that role development experiences were highly variable and complex. These authors described seven phases of CNS role development along with associated characteristics and developmental tasks (Table 5–3). Progression through the first three phases (identical to those identified by Baker, 1979) was commonly experienced by CNSs in their positions for 3 years or less. Data indicated that all but 5% of the 42 CNSs in their first positions for 3 years or less experienced these three phases. The phases were not necessarily experienced sequentially as evidenced by reports of overlapping of the first four phases, presence of some

TABLE 5–2. PHASES OF APN WORK ROLE IMPLEMENTATION

Kramer (1974), BSN Grads Page & Arena (1991), CNSs	Oda (1977), Specialists	Baker (1979), CNSs	Hamric & Taylor (1989), CNSs
Honeymoon	Role identification	Orientation	Orientation
Shock		Frustration	Frustration
Recovery	Role transition	Implementation Reassessment	Implementation
Resolution	Role confirmation		Integration Frozen Reorganization Complacent

TABLE 5–3. PHASES OF APN ROLE DEVELOPMENT

Phase	Characteristics	Developmental Tasks
Orientation	Enthusiasm, optimism, eager to prove self to setting Anxious about ability to meet self- and institutional expectations Expects to make change	Learn formal and informal organizations Learn key players; begin establishing relationships and power base Explore expectations to see if compatible with own Identify and clarify role to self and others
Frustration	Discouragement and questioning due to unrealistic expectations (either self- or employer); difficult and slow-paced change; resistance encountered Feelings of inadequacy in response to the overwhelming problems encountered, pressure to prove worth	Develop more realistic expectations Work on time management and setting priorities Develop short-term goals or projects to get tangible results/feedback Develop support system within and/or outside work setting
Implementation	Returning optimism and enthusiasm as positive feedback received and expectations realigned Organization and reorganization of role tasks, modified in response to feedback Implementing and balancing new subroles Regaining sense of perspective *May* focus on specific project(s)	Enhance visibility and power base within informal and formal organizations; build coalitions and networks Identify tangible accomplishments Complete transition to advanced practice level, if necessary Continue to reassess and refocus direction
Integration	Self-confident and assured in role Rated self at advanced level of practice Activities reflect wide recognition, influence in area of specialty Continuously feels challenged; takes on new projects; expands practice Either moderately or very satisfied with present position Congruence between personal and organizational goals and expectations	Continued role evolution and skill development to strengthen subroles and competencies Share expertise and experience with others through publications, research, professional activities Maintain flexible approach Be alert for signs of complacency or boredom
Frozen	Self-confident, assured in role Rated self at intermediate or advanced practice level Experiencing anger/frustration reflecting experience Conflict between self goals and those of organization/supervisor Report sense of being unable to move forward due to forces outside of self	Obtain feedback from supervisor and peers Re-evaluate self goals in relation to CNS role and organization Objective assessment of organization: Is there potential for compatibility? Attempt to redesign or renegotiate the role If unsuccessful consider change in position/career direction
Reorganization	Reported earlier experiences that represent integration Organization experiencing major changes Pressure to change role in ways that are incongruent with own concept of CNS role and/or self goals	Open discussion with change agents Attempt compromise to preserve integrity of role and still meet needs of organization If unsuccessful, change position/title or negotiate job change
Complacent	Experiences self in role as settled and comfortable Variable job satisfaction Questionable impact on organization	Need to re-energize Reconfigure role to allow growth by identifying new need of client population or institution

(From Hamric, A. B., & Taylor, J. W. (1989). Role development of the CNS. In A. B. Hamric & J. A. Spross (Eds.), *The clinical nurse specialist in theory and practice* (2nd ed., p. 48). Philadelphia: W. B. Saunders. Used with permission.)

elements of all phases together, and being in different phases in different work settings at the same time. Data collected by Hamric and Taylor (1989) did not support Baker's (1979) fourth phase of reassessment. Instead, the implementation phase was interpreted by Hamric and Taylor (1989) as encompassing characteristics Baker categorized as the reassessment phase.

The CNSs with more than 3 years' experience described their role development experiences in terms very different from Baker's (1979) phases. Content analysis of these data led to description of four additional phases (see Table 5–3). The integration phase (a new phase replacing Baker's [1979] reassessment phase) was identified and characterized by "self-confidence and assurance in the role, high job satisfaction, an advanced level of practice, and signs of recognition and respect for expertise within and outside the work setting" (Hamric & Taylor, 1989, p. 56). Only 10% of the CNSs studied with less than 5 years' experience in the role met the criteria for this phase, whereas 50% of those with more than 6 years' experience could be categorized as being in this phase.

Hamric and Taylor's (1989) study was significant in that more than half of the CNSs studied had been in practice for 3 or more years. Study of experienced CNSs allowed for identification of additional phases of role development that were not evident in previous studies. The frozen phase was described as being associated with frustration, anger, and lack of career satisfaction. The reorganization phase was characterized by restructuring of role responsibilities and changing expectations. The complacent phase was characterized by comfort, stability, and maintenance of the status quo. These additional phases share a negative, nonproductive character unlike the integration phase. One might speculate that APNs experiencing these phases would be more vulnerable to position changes in response to health care reform.

The integration phase described by Hamric and Taylor (1989) appears to be a chronological progression from the earlier implementation phase. The additional phases of role development that are described—specifically, frozen, reorganization, and complacent—rather than being separate phases, are proposed here instead as variants of the earlier phases. Hamric and Taylor's speculation that the frozen phase of CNS role development might be analogous to the "lateral arabesquers" described by Kramer (1974) prompted this reinterpretation of these additional phases as alternative lateral categories.

In this reinterpretation, the frozen phase may represent an alternative to integration resulting from lack of resolution of bureaucratic versus professional value conflict. The lateral arabesquers were described by Kramer as having high professional and low bureaucratic role orientations. Job hopping was common in this group. An example of the frozen phase for an APN might be an APN who perceives organizational imperatives to be incompatible with personal and professional goals, resulting in a cessation or halt of role development. This may prevent further career advancement and prompt the APN's resignation and search for a more compatible position.

The reorganization phase may be a variant of the implementation phase reverted to after having reached the integration phase. This reinterpretation is based on Hamric and Taylor's report that this phase was typically experienced by CNSs in settings undergoing major organizational change whose earlier experiences in the same settings were characteristic of the integration phase. Finally, the complacent phase may constitute a lateral variant of the integration phase similar to the "organization woman" and "the rutter" described by Kramer (1974), which also result from less-than-ideal resolution of bureaucratic versus professional value conflict. Kramer's "organization woman" was classified as high on bureaucratic orientation and low on professional orientation, whereas "the rutter" was classified as low in both bureaucratic and professional orientation. The complacent CNS was described by Hamric and Taylor (1989) as "settled into a comfortable position" or "plugging along," descriptions similar to Kramer's "organizational woman" and "rutter" categories, respectively. Hamric and Taylor (1989) noted that the complacent phase is not necessarily negative, especially if it is temporary and allows for energy renewal. However, they noted that when CNSs are in this phase for long periods of time, they are not perceived as change agents.

Additional reinterpretations and adaptations of this framework for APN role development can be anticipated with its application to other APN roles. For example, one might speculate that persons in APN roles that are more focused on clinical practice with less emphasis on other subrole components may not experience the frustration phase with the same intensity and duration as would persons in APN roles with more diffuse role demands. Further research with this framework may indicate that the experience of the frustration phase is inversely related to the degree of realistic role rehearsal experienced during the role acquisition period in school. It is interesting to note here that Oda's (1977) model, which was "developed, tested, and refined in actual work settings through graduate practice and residencies, consultation with staff nurse groups, and as a continuing education course for employed nurses" (p. 377) did not include a frustration phase.

The role trajectory proposed by Sparacino and Cooper (1990) offers another framework for understanding role development for APNs. Their approach integrates the work of Baker (1987), Cooper (1983), Holt (1987), and Oda (1985; note that they referred to Oda's further refinement and development of the 1977 model). This framework complements the work of Hamric and Taylor (1989) by illustrating the gradual implementation of the multiple role components of the CNS role over time. Sparacino and Cooper (1990) identified role markers (described as specific time-phased behaviors and activities) as follows: (1) role identity and visibility, (2) role implementation, (3) incorporation of subrole components of education and research, and (4) expansion of consultant subrole, refinement, and integration of all role components. Following initial emphasis on clinical mastery over the first 2 years, other role components are gradually integrated into practice so that by 5 years post graduation, the multiple role components have been integrated and are being refined and modified. This corresponds to and supports the integration phase described by Hamric and Taylor (1989).

The complexity of role development processes is further demonstrated by preliminary findings of Brown and Olshansky's (1995) grounded theory study of the role transition experiences of 35 novice NPs during their first year of practice. They described a four-phase process occurring during the first year of practice: (1) laying the foundation, (2) launching, (3) meeting the challenge, and (4) broadening the perspective. Analysis of the relationships between these phases and those identified by Hamric and Taylor (1989) is needed to put these findings into the context of current understanding of APN role implementation. Initial comparisons of the descriptions of the four phases identified with CNSs by Hamric and Taylor (1989) and the four phases identified with new NPs by Brown and Olshansky (1995) suggest that they are similar. The implications of Brown and Olshansky are described further in the "Strategies" sections of this chapter. Further refinement of these various frameworks is needed for their incorporation into APN teaching, research, and practice.

ENHANCING APN ROLE DEVELOPMENT

STRATEGIES TO FACILITATE ROLE ACQUISITION (IN SCHOOL)

Anticipatory socialization is analogous to immunization (Kramer, 1974). The overall objective is to expose role incumbents to as many real-life experiences as possible during the educational program to minimize their reality or cultural shock upon graduation and beginning role implementation. Anticipatory socialization is referred to here as role resocialization for APN programs to point out that role incumbents are already socialized into nursing. Role resocialization may be used as the overall framework for designing an APN curriculum (Igoe, 1977; Malkemes, 1974), a specific role course, or role seminars that span an entire curriculum. All APN programs today, regardless of specialty, should have requirements for basic content related to professional roles and issues.

Specific strategies for facilitating role acquisition are presented here from a variety of sources (Table 5–4). Many of the strategies developed by Kramer and associates (1974) for anticipatory socialization of baccalaureate students have relevance and utility for today's APN programs. The basic structure of the anticipatory socialization program was a series of seminars continued throughout the educational program. Appropriate content and experiences used by Kramer (1974) that can be useful for APN programs include information about the cultural phenomenon of reality shock, role negotiation scenarios, change agent skills, conflict resolution strategies, identification with a role model, and development of peer support networks. Kramer's strategy of using taped conflict situations for students to respond to during a role seminar would be appropriate for APN programs. Becoming aware of potential conflict situations and responding to them would help students be more aware of their own feelings and experiences and perhaps help them recognize conflicts they may be unaware of in their own clinical preceptorships.

Igoe (1977) designed interdisciplinary role seminar groups to simulate life-like situations of threat and confrontation to provide NP students with opportunities to practice role negotiation and conflict resolution skills. Another strategy Igoe (1977) used was to refer to NP students as "participants" rather than "students" to reinforce

TABLE 5–4. STRATEGIES TO FACILITATE APN ROLE ACQUISITION (IN SCHOOL)

Life-like role negotiation seminars	Holistic situational perspective
Identify with a role model	Professional marketing portfolio
Establish peer support network	Students as colleagues
Diagram role sets	Share self- and peer evaluations
Competency profiles	Panel discussions
Directly experience all core skills	Critical incident presentations
Realistic clinical immersion experiences	Faculty/student social functions
Clinical logs	Faculty practice
Burning question interviews	

the importance of their pre-student experiences. The overall approach to teaching and learning was designed to provide participants with the opportunity to rehearse new role behaviors and to acquire personal experience with the dynamics of role definition, clarity, conflict, and negotiation.

Russell (1995) suggested having APN students diagram a role set. A typical role set for an APN student would include the multiple roles of student, employee, wife/husband, mother/father, daughter/son, sister/brother, and friend. This exercise helps illustrate why students experience the tension of being pulled in many different directions at the same time. Sharing their role sets with other APN students helps validate that the stresses they are experiencing are normal and expected. The competency profiles described by Callahan and Bruton-Maree (1994; see also Chapter 19) offer a realistic, flexible framework for conceptualizing multiple subroles. They constitute another way for APN students to depict the multiple core skills they will be expected to implement. The role set and competency profile together help clarify the complexity of the multiple roles and core skills expected of APNs.

It is important that APN students experience all aspects of the core skills (see Chapter 3) directly while faculty and fellow students are readily available to help them "process" or debrief these experiences (Hamric & Taylor, 1989). APN students should become aware that other nurses, physicians, and administrators in the work setting may only value clinical expertise and not the other core skills. Strategies for enhancing acquisition of all the core skills include preparation of short- and long-term goals to use as guides in the development of professional portfolios, analysis of existing position descriptions, and development of the ideal position description.

Realistic learning experiences facilitate APN role acquisition. In a study of adult NP students, Knafl (1979) found that students evaluate the realism of their clinical experiences. Students explained that the more realistic a learning experience was in terms of making a contribution to patient care, the more they learned from it. Learning experiences that offer students realistic opportunities for applying assessment, management, and role negotiation skills will enhance APN role acquisition. Clinical immersion experiences were considered essential for CNS students by a group of oncology nursing leaders (Donoghue & Spross, 1985). Identification with a role model is important here. Clinical logs were recommended by Hamric and Taylor (1989) to document experiences during the educational program for CNSs. They can also be used by faculty and students for identifying problem situations and exploring issues. Spross (1995) recommended that beginning APN students conduct "burning question" interviews with experienced APNs to develop a realistic vision and focus for their role acquisition experiences.

Resocialization experiences for APN students should emphasize realism and a holistic situational perspective rather than being compartmentalized, dichotomized, and idealized. In planning these experiences, artificially separating theory from practice in ways such as Hupcey's (1990) categorization of clinical skills as technical (medical) behaviors and designation of all other core skills as master's level behaviors, should be avoided. A more holistic perspective is imperative for recognizing that the complex clinical judgments involved in APN assessment and management of patient situations over time is not simply technical medical knowledge. Teaching and learning experiences for the direct provider role of the APN in a graduate program should integrate elements of research, teaching, nursing theory, personal and professional philosophy, health promotion, illness prevention, epidemiology, economics, ethics, nutrition, family-focused interventions, and community assessment into the clinical management courses and clinical preceptorship experiences. These learning experiences build on the knowledge gained in the traditional graduate core and clinical support courses in the curriculum. This is a critical issue. If the clinical knowledge and skills of APNs are classified only as technical medical skill separate from graduate level nursing knowledge there would be no need for master's level programs in advanced nursing practice. Studies of APN practice demonstrate that advanced practice roles incorporate a holistic approach that blends elements of nursing and medicine (Brykczynski, 1989; Johnson, 1993). *Advanced Nursing Practice: Curriculum Guidelines and Program Standards for Nurse Practitioner Education* (Boodley et al., 1995) is a guide for NP education that utilizes this integrated program planning approach.

An additional tool for facilitating role acquisition is the preparation of a marketing portfolio as recommended by Hawkins and Thibodeau (1993). The marketing portfolio consists of the APN student's personal philosophy of nursing and health care, a resumé targeted for the desired position, a detailed position description, clinical logs, state nurse practice act, rules and regulations for APN practice, malpractice insurance information, salary ranges for similar positions, certification materials, brochures and articles describing the APN role, information about interviewing, and ideas for selecting a suitable position. These materials can be used for learning assignments and seminar discussions by having APN students share drafts of their portfolio components with peers, faculty, and preceptors and then revise them according to the feedback received. These strategies contribute to refinement and modification of definitions and expectations for future APN roles and promote development of students as colleagues and peer evaluators.

A variety of panels can be convened during role seminars to stimulate exploration of issues and promote greater role clarity. For example, a panel composed of various APNs is helpful for students to gain an appreciation of similarities as well as differences in available roles. Another useful panel is one composed of program graduates and potential employers, which helps APN students target their resumés and position descriptions. The impact and significance of seeing successful APN graduates cannot be overstated. An interdisciplinary panel made up of a nurse in an APN role and a physician in a complementary role can help with clarifying perceptions and discussing strategies for minimizing inter-professional role conflict.

Two popular role course activities are a discussion in which students present critical incidents encountered in beginning to develop their roles and a get-together at a faculty member's home specifically focused on describing the APN role in a social setting. Critical incident presentations require students to identify an actual role conflict situation from their nursing practice. Students analyze these situations using the critical incident format developed by Gordon and Benner (1980) and present them for class discussion. As for the second activity, Diers' (1992) brief article serves as a conversation starter at the get-together, which includes faculty, graduates, and students who have completed at least one clinical preceptorship experience.

Finally and perhaps most importantly, an overall strategy for facilitating APN role acquisition is for faculty to maintain competency in clinical practice. This is essential to avoid a wide gap between education and practice and to mediate against intense reality shock experiences for new APN graduates. APN faculty must value clinical practice knowledge and skills equally with knowledge and skills for the other core APN skills (see Chapter 21).

STRATEGIES TO FACILITATE ROLE IMPLEMENTATION (AT WORK)

APN faculty, students, new graduates, and practicing APNs might find review of Kramer's (1974) *Reality Shock* and Kramer and Schmalenberg's (1977) *Path to Biculturalism* beneficial for understanding, facilitating, and implementing role development. Kramer (1977) maintained that the content could be useful not only for nurses at various levels but also for members of other occupational groups who are moving into a new position or setting. *Path to Biculturalism* is composed of five self-instructional programs with activities designed to stimulate thinking about reality shock, interpersonal competence, informal norms, seeking feedback on performance, and conflict resolution. New APN graduates may find completion of the modules useful for promoting the achievement and maintenance of competence in the new work world with minimal reality shock.

The four major developmental phases (orientation, frustration, implementation, and integration) identified by Hamric and Taylor (1989) to describe CNS role development are selected here to structure the discussion of APN role implementation. As noted earlier, these phases of CNS role development may be applicable to implementing all APN roles regardless of specialty. Future application and research using this model is encouraged. Strategies for facilitating APN role implementation are described for each of these developmental phases in the following section (Table 5–5).

Orientation Phase

A strategy to facilitate role implementation for all APNs during the orientation phase is to develop a structured orientation plan. An APN in a new position (whether experienced in the role or not) needs to be aware of the importance of being informed about the organizational structure, philosophy, goals, policies, and proce-

---

TABLE 5–5. STRATEGIES TO ENHANCE APN ROLE IMPLEMENTATION (AT WORK)

Orientation Phase
Structure an orientation plan
Establish mutually agreed upon role expectations
Circulate literature on APN role
Meetings with key individuals
Peer networking
Identify with a role model
Goal-oriented evaluation
Concentrate on clinical mastery
Postpone recommendations for major changes
Join key committees
Recognize transitions as time-limited

Frustration Phase
Schedule debriefing sessions
Practice time management
Maintain professional portfolio
Continue seeking peer support
Maintain communication with administrators
Consult with experts
Recognize that all novices need more time
Organize resources for easy accessibility

Implementation Phase
Reassess demands, priorities, goals
Plan for performance and impact evaluation
Sustain communication with peers, administrators, and others
Recognize that repetition builds competence and confidence
Formulate short-term goals for further development

Integration Phase
Continue debriefing sessions
Plan for role expansion and refinement
Schedule performance and impact evaluations
Develop broader professional interests

Frozen, Reorganization, and Complacent Phases
Self-assessment and early recognition of problems
Conflict resolution and role clarification discussions
Appraisal of APN goals in relation to organizational goals
Renegotiate role expectations
Consider career move/change

dures of the agency. Holt (1984) recommended formulating a role development growth plan and then conducting periodic self-assessment of role implementation according to the plan. The plan should include clearly formulated purposes and goals (Ball, 1990). Other important components of the plan are scheduling meetings with key individuals and the opportunity to mutually share philosophies, expectations, and goals. Peer support, both within and outside the work setting, is important. APNs should be encouraged to join local APN groups. Designating a more experienced APN in the work setting as a preceptor would be a useful support for all APNs new to a position.

Page and Arena (1991) recommended scheduling and fulfilling the major portion of time in direct patient care to substantiate the clinical expert role. They also suggested making appointments with nursing leaders, physicians, and other health professionals during this phase to garner administrative support. They recommended distributing business cards and making the APN job description available for discussion. Strategies suggested for networking within the system include developing peer support groups, being accessible by beeper, and getting involved in interdisciplinary committees. They recommended withholding suggestions for change until the system is more fully assessed. Spross (1995) suggested that when a new APN joins the staff of an organization, the administrator should send a letter describing the APN's background experiences and new position to key people in the organization. Strategies suggested by Brown and Olshansky (1995)—taken from their qualitative study describing the first year of NP practice as one of major transition—are clarification of values, needs, and expectations and recognition that transitional experiences are time-limited. They also pointed out the importance of anticipatory guidance and normalization of transition experiences for new graduates.

Frustration Phase

Hamric and Taylor (1989) observed that the frustration phase may come and go and may overlap other phases. They noted that painful affective responses are typical of this difficult phase. They suggested that monthly sessions for sharing concerns with a group of peers and an administrator may facilitate movement through this phase. Strategies identified as helpful for energizing movement from the frustration phase to the implementation phase included assistance with time management, support groups to ameliorate feelings of inadequacy, conflict resolution and role clarification discussions, reassessing priorities and setting realistic expectations, and focusing on short-term, visible goals. Page and Arena (1991) recommended keeping a work portfolio to document activities so that progress is more readily visible. They noted that seeking peer support continues to be important at this time. Brown and Olshansky 1995) pointed out that organized sources of support, such as phone calls, seminars, planned meetings with mentors, and scheduled time for consultation, can significantly decrease feelings of anxiety. They noted that recognizing that part of the discomfort arises from moving from "expert back to novice" and realizing that previous expertise can be valuable in the new role may help to reduce feelings of inadequacy. They suggested that requesting reasonable time frames for initial patient visits is key to initial adjustment, because novices take longer than experienced practitioners.

Implementation Phase

During the implementation phase it is important for the APN to reassess demands to guard against feeling overwhelmed. Priorities may need to be readjusted, and short-term goals may be reformulated. During the implementation phase, APNs may plan and execute small-scale projects to demonstrate their effectiveness. Feedback about areas of strength and any need for improvement should be sought as part of the evaluation process during this phase. Strategies mentioned as important during this time include seeking administrative support through involvement in meetings, maintaining visibility in clinical areas, and developing inservice programs with input from staff (Page & Arena, 1991). Brown and Olshansky (1995) observed that competence and confidence are fostered through repetition. They pointed out that formulating short-term goals is important to further development, and recommended scheduling a formal evaluation after approximately 6 months.

Integration Phase

Hamric and Taylor's (1989) survey data indicated that CNSs maximize their role potential during the integration phase. They surmised that satisfactory completion of the earlier phases appears to be essential for passage into the integration phase. Strategies for enhancing and maintaining optimal role implementation during this phase include having a trusted colleague who can act as a safe sounding board for "feedback, constructive criticism, and advice" (Hamric & Taylor, 1989, p. 79). During this phase, it is important to have a plan to guide continued role expansion and refinement. Seeking appointment to key committees is important to broaden organizational impact. Competing or conflicting demands may arise during this phase and other phases. Administrative support and constructive feedback from a trusted mentor continues to be important. Development of a promotional system that offers professional advancement in the APN practice role remains a challenge for practitioners and administrators. Page and Arena (1991) observed that less time is required for establishing relationships and assessing the system during this phase so more time can be devoted to areas of scholarly interests.

Frozen, Reorganization, and Complacent Phases

Whether the frozen, reorganization, and complacent phases are distinct developmental phases or variations of the implementation and integration phases, they are clearly negative resolutions for APNs and their organizations. Strategies described by Hamric and Taylor (1989) for enhancing role development in these phases are included in Table 5-5. They pointed out that APNs should engage in periodic self-assessment so that they recognize beginning signs or characteristics associated with these phases, such as feelings of anger or dissatisfaction, conflict between self-goals and those of the organization or supervisor, feeling pressure to change one's APN role in ways that are incongruous with one's concept of the role, or feelings of complacency. Early problem recognition and taking proactive steps to deal with organizational changes can help prevent or ameliorate the negative feelings associated with these phases.

Hamric and Taylor (1989) stated that honest and open discussions with supervisors or individuals with whom the APN is experiencing conflict should be initiated to resolve conflicts and clarify role issues before they become serious problems. In situations of organizational turmoil, which characterize the reorganization phase, APNs should evaluate their goals in relation to the organizational changes and renegotiate role expectations if necessary. Hamric (1995) suggested that, for example, in an organization increasingly concerned with fiscal efficiencies and patient outcomes, CNSs could negotiate to add a component of nurse case management to their practices for complex patients in their specialty. Temporary role realignment may also be negotiated to meet short-term crises, with explicit negotiated agreement that APNs would return to their original role after an agreed-upon time.

Hamric (1995) asserted that APNs should not allow themselves, nor should administrators allow them, to remain in these negative phases. If discussion, compromise, and negotiations are unsuccessful, the APN should consider a career move, either to another position within the organization or to another organization. Career counseling may be a helpful strategy for the seriously disaffected APN.

WORK SETTING FACTORS

Aspects of the work setting exert a major influence on APN role definitions and expectations, thereby affecting role ambiguity, role incongruity, and role conflict. Factors found to facilitate role development for NPs (Lurie, 1981) included being assigned their own caseload of patients and having access to their own examination room. Economic factors such as pressure to manage large numbers of patients impeded role development for the NPs studied. Lurie maintained that requirements to see 22 patients in one 8-hour day and the physician evaluator's emphasis on assessment and management skills over counseling and patient education skills were two major factors that constrained NP teaching and counseling activities.

Lurie (1981) observed that in spite of time pressures some NPs managed to integrate counseling and teaching into the history and physical examination by performing these activities simultaneously. Brykczynski (1985) and Johnson (1993) also reported that NPs incorporated counseling and teaching into the flow of patient visits—capturing the teachable moment without setting aside special time for it. The ability to incorporate teaching and counseling into the patient visit may be a factor of skill development that comes with experience in the role. This observation may be used as rationale for structuring time for longer visits and fewer total patients for new APNs, with gradual increases in caseloads as experience is accrued.

ADMINISTRATIVE STRUCTURE

Administrative factors—including whether APNs are placed in line or staff positions; whether they are unit-based, population-based, or in some other arrangement; who evaluates them; and whether they report to administrative or clinical supervisors—are important to consider. Baird and Prouty (1989) maintained that the organizational design should have enough flexibility to change as the situation changes. Specific individual placements of APN positions may differ even within one setting depending on size, complexity, and distribution of the patient population (Baird & Prouty, 1989; see also Chapter 24).

Issues of professional versus administrative authority underlie the importance of the structural placement of the APN within the organization. Effectiveness of the APN role is enhanced when there is a mutual fit between the goals and expectations of the individual and those of the organization (Cooper & Sparacino, 1990). Clarification of goals and expectations prior to employment and periodic reassessments can minimize conflict and enhance role development and effectiveness. Cooper and Sparacino (1990) suggested that one way to clarify goals and expectations is to share one's position description with peers for critique and revise it according to their feedback before sharing it with one's supervisor or future employer and subsequently other staff and colleagues.

EVALUATION

Evaluation is fundamental to enhancing role implementation. Evaluation of APNs should comprise both performance and impact (process and outcome) components (see Chapter 26). Development of a professional portfolio to document APN accomplishments can be useful with both performance and impact evaluation. Performance evaluation for APNs should include self-evaluation, peer review, and administrative evaluation (Cooper & Sparacino, 1990; Hamric & Taylor, 1989). A competency profile can be helpful for organizing evaluation in a dynamic way that allows for changes in subrole implementation over time as expertise, situations, and priorities change (Callahan & Bruton-Maree, 1994). The competency profile can be employed as an assessment of performance (novice to expert) on each of the core APN skills. Impact evaluation is important to demonstrate the effectiveness of the APN role. Ongoing development of appropriate impact evaluation measures, such as patient outcomes and patient satisfaction, are important. A reward system to provide for career advancement through a clinical ladder program and accrual of additional benefits is particularly important for retaining APNs in clinical roles. In less-structured situations, APNs can negotiate for periodic reassessments and salary increases through options such as profit-sharing.

When APN practice includes hospital privileges, prescriptive privileges, and third-party reimbursement, the evaluation process expands to include interdisciplinary review. This expansion of the evaluation process has both positive and negative aspects. As Lurie (1981) noted, physicians may evaluate performance without recognizing the value of teaching and counseling, whereas a nursing supervisor may be more focused on general system components than individual patient care situations. Advantages to the review process associated with securing and maintaining hospital privileges include the multiple aspects that are considered in the evaluation, the variety of perspectives, and the visibility afforded APNs. To promote APN roles within organizations, it is important that APNs have key positions on hospital review committees. A major difficulty in implementing interdisciplinary peer review is the previously noted lack of interaction between and among the incumbents of the various health professional groups during their formative educational programs (Brykczynski, 1989).

CONCLUSION

A holistic, inclusive perspective is advocated here for advancing APN role development. Role development experiences for APNs encompass role acquisition processes in school and role implementation processes after graduation. The limits of the educational process for preparing graduates for the realities of the work world need to be acknowledged. Students need to be informed about the human skill acquisition process and its stages as well as the processes of adult and professional socialization, identity transformation, role acquisition, role implementation, and overall career development. Knowing about and actually experiencing are different phenomena, but at least students can be forewarned. Anticipatory guidance can be provided through role rehearsal experiences, such as clinical preceptorships and role seminars. Students need to be encouraged to begin networking with practicing APNs through local, state, and national APN groups. This is especially important for APNs who will not be practicing in close proximity to other APNs. Experienced APNs and new APN graduates can form mutually beneficial relationships.

There needs to be open acknowledgment that anticipatory socialization experiences in school can facilitate role acquisition, but they cannot prevent the upheaval that occurs with movement into a new position and actual role implementation. It is essential that APN programs have a firm foundation in the real world. However, an awareness of a certain degree of incongruence or conflict between academic ideals and work world realities must always be fostered to guide and direct planned change and guard against mere maintenance of the status quo. Support for the developmental phases of role implementation in the work setting needs to be ongoing. Support groups in local APN organizations are especially useful for enhancing both role acquisition and role implementation.

APN role development has been described as dynamic, complex, and situational. It is influenced by many factors, such as experience, level of expertise, personal and professional values, setting, specialty, relationships with co-workers, aspects of role transition, and life transitions. Frameworks for understanding role development processes have been discussed. Research applying these frameworks to additional APN specialty groups will further the development of strategies to enhance role development. Strategies for facilitating role acquisition and role implementation that have implications for educators, administrators, and APNs have been presented.

REFERENCES

American College of Nurse-Midwives. (1993). *Certified nurse-midwives as primary care providers.* Washington, D. C.: ACNM.

Anderson, E. M., Leonard, B. J., & Yates, J. A. (1974). Epigenesis of the nurse practitioner role. *American Journal of Nursing, 10*(18), 12-16.

Baggs, J. G. (1989). Intensive care unit and collaboration between nurses and physicians. *Heart & Lung, 18,* 332.

Baird, S. B., & Prouty, M. P. (1989). Administratively enhancing CNS contributions. In A. B. Hamric & J. A. Spross (Eds.), *The clinical nurse specialist in theory and practice* (2nd ed., pp. 261-283). Philadelphia: W. B. Saunders.

Baker, P. O. (1987). Model activities for clinical nurse specialist role development. *Clinical Nurse Specialist, 1*(3), 119-123.

Baker, V. (1979). Retrospective explorations in role development. In G. V. Padilla (Ed.), *The clinical nurse specialist and improvement of nursing practice* (pp. 56-63). Wakefield, MA: Nursing Resources.

Ball, G. B. (1990). Perspectives on developing, marketing, and implementing a new clinical nurse specialist position. *Clinical Nurse Specialist, 4*(1), 33-36.

Banda, E. E. (1985). *Role problems, role strain: Perception and experience of the clinical nurse specialist.* Unpublished master's thesis, Boston University School of Nursing.

Bem, S. L. (1977). On the utility of alternative procedures for assessing psychological androgyny. *Journal of Consulting and Clinical Psychology, 45,* 196-205.

Benner, P. E. (1984). *From novice to expert. Excellence and power in clinical nursing practice.* Menlo Park, CA: Addison-Wesley.

Benner, P. E. (1985). The oncology clinical nurse specialist: An expert coach. *Oncology Nurse Forum, 12*(2), 40-44.

Benner, P. E., & Wrubel, J. (1989). *The primacy of caring.* Menlo Park, CA: Addison-Wesley.

Boodley, C. A., Harper, D. C., Hanson, C., Jackson, P., Russell, D. D., Taylor, D., & Zimmer, P. A. (1995). *Advanced Nursing Practice: Curriculum guidelines and program standards for nurse prac-*

titioner education (2nd ed.). Washington, D. C.: National Organization of Nurse Practitioner Faculties.

Brown, M. A., & Olshansky, E. (1995, July). *Supporting novice nurse practitioners: The experience of the first year of NP practice.* Paper presented at the annual meeting of the National Organization of Nurse Practitioner Faculties, Keystone, CO.

Brykczynski, K. A. (1985). Exploring the clinical practice of nurse practitioners (Doctoral dissertation, University of California San Francisco, School of Nursing). *Dissertation Abstracts International, 46,* 3789B (University Microfilms No. DA8600592).

Brykczynski, K. A. (1989). An interpretive study describing the clinical judgment of nurse practitioners. *Scholarly Inquiry for Nursing Practice: An International Journal, 3*(2), 75-104.

Callahan, L., & Bruton-Maree, N. (1994). Establishing measures of competence. In S. D. Foster & L. M. Jordan (Eds.), *Professional aspects of nurse anesthesia practice* (pp. 275-290). Philadelphia: F. A. Davis.

Cooper, D. (1983). A refined expert: The clinical nurse specialist after five years. *Momentum, 1,* 1-2.

Cooper, D. M., & Sparacino, P. S. A. (1990). Acquiring, implementing, and evaluating the clinical nurse specialist role. In P. S. A. Sparacino, D. M. Cooper, & P. A. Minarik (Eds.), *The clinical nurse specialist implementation and impact* (pp. 41-75). Norwalk, CT: Appleton & Lange.

Curry, J. L. (1994). Nurse practitioners in the emergency department: Current issues. *Journal of Emergency Nursing, 20*(3), 207-215.

Dalton, G. W., Thompson, P. H., & Price, R. L. (1977). The four stages of professional careers—A new look at performance by professionals. *Organizational Dynamics, 6*(1), 19-42.

DePaolis-Lutzo, M. V. (1987). Factors influencing nurse anesthesia educational programs: 1982–1987. Unpublished doctoral dissertation, University of Pittsburgh.

Diers, D. (1992). One-liners. *Image: Journal of Nursing Scholarship, 24*(1), 75-77.

Donoghue, M., & Spross, J. A. (1985). A report from the first national invitational conference: The oncology clinical nurse specialist role analysis and future projections. *Oncology Nursing Forum, 12*(2), 35-73.

Dreyfus, H. L., & Dreyfus, S. E. (1986). *Mind over machine.* New York: Free Press.

Elkema, R. C., & Knutson, M. (1983). Basic principles for new role development: A ten year experience. *Journal of Long-Term Care Administration, 11,* 10-14.

Erikson, E. H. (1982). *The life cycle completed.* New York: Norton.

Fagin, C. M. (1992). Collaboration between nurses and physicians no longer a choice. *Nursing & Health Care, 13*(7), 354-363.

Flanagan, J. (1986). Childbirth in the eighties what next? When alternatives become mainstream. *Journal of Nurse-Midwifery, 31,* 194-199.

Ford, L. C. (1982). Nurse practitioners: History of a new idea and predictions for the future. In L. H. Aiken (Ed.), *Nursing in the 1980s: Crises, opportunities, challenges* (pp. 231-247). Philadelphia: J. B. Lippincott.

Gordon, D., & Benner, P. E. (1980). Guidelines for recording critical incidents. AMICAE Project, University of San Francisco.

Grimshaw, J. (1988). Autonomy and identity in feminist theory. In M. Griffiths & M. Whitford (Eds.), *Feminist perspectives in philosophy.* Bloomington, IN: Indiana University Press.

Gunn, I. P. (1991). The history of nurse anesthesia education: Highlights and influences. Report of the National Commission on Nurse Anesthesia Education. *Journal of the American Association of Nurse Anesthetists, 59*(1), 53-61.

Hamric, A. B. (1995). Personal communication.

Hamric, A. B., & Taylor, J. W. (1989). Role development of the CNS. In A. B. Hamric & J. A. Spross (Eds.), *The clinical nurse specialist in theory and practice* (2nd ed., pp. 41-82). Philadelphia: W. B. Saunders.

Hardy, M. E., & Hardy, W. L. (1988). Role stress and role strain. In M. E. Hardy & M. E. Conway (Eds.), *Role theory. Perspectives for health professionals* (2nd ed., pp. 159-239). Norwalk, CT: Appleton & Lange.

Hawkins, J. W., & Thibodeau, J. A. (1993). Negotiating an employment contract. In J. W. Hawkins & J. A. Thibodeau (Eds.), *The practitioner* (3rd ed., pp. 130-140). New York: Tiresias Press.

Hazle, N. R. (1985). Perceptions of role conflict between obstetric nurses and nurse-midwives. *Journal of Nurse-Midwifery, 30*(3), 166-173.

Heidegger, M. (1962). *Being and time.* New York: Harper & Row. (Originally published in German, 1927).

Holt, F. M. (1984). A theoretical model for clinical specialist practice. *Nursing and Health Care, 5*(8), 445-449.

Holt, F. M. (1987). Executive practice role. Editorial. *Clinical Nurse Specialist, 1*(3), 116-118.

Hupcey, J. E. (1990). The socialization process of master's level nurse practitioner students. *Journal of Nursing Education, 29*(5), 196-201.

Igoe, J. (1977). One experience in the preparation of nurse practitioners. In J. E. Hall & B. Weaver (Eds.), *Distributive nursing practice. A systems approach to community health* (pp. 309-319). Philadelphia: J. B. Lippincott.

Johnson, R. (1993). Nurse practitioner-patient discourse: Uncovering the voice of nursing in primary care practice. *Scholarly Inquiry for Nursing Practice: An International Journal, 7*(3), 143-157.

Kimbro, C. D. (1978). The relationship between nurses and nurse-midwives. *Journal of Nurse-Midwifery, 22*(4), 28-31.

King, M. B. (1990). Clinical nurse specialist collaboration with physicians. *Clinical Nurse Specialist, 4*(4), 172-177.

Klaich, K. (1990). Transitions in professional identity of nurses enrolled in graduate educational programs. *Holistic Nursing Practice, 4*(3), 17-24.

Knafl, K. A. (1979). How real is the practicum for nurse practitioner students? *Nursing Outlook, 27,* 131-135.

Knaus, W. A., Wagner, D. P., & Zimmerman, J. E. (1986). An evaluation of outcome from Intensive Care in major medical centers. *Annals of Internal Medicine, 104,* 410-418.

Kramer, M. (1974). *Reality shock.* St. Louis: Mosby.

Kramer, M., & Schmalenberg, C. (1977). *Path to biculturalism.* Wakefield, MA: Contemporary Publishing.

Kritek, P. (1988). Gender roles and the professional. In M. E. Hardy & M. E. Conway (Eds.), *Role theory perspectives for health professionals* (2nd ed., pp. 309-341). Norwalk, CT: Appleton & Lange.

Kuhn, T. (1970). *The structure of scientific revolutions* (2nd ed.). Chicago: University of Chicago Press.

Leddy, S., & Pepper, J. M. (1993). Socialization for professional practice. In S. Leddy & J. M. Pepper (Eds.), *Conceptual bases of professional nursing* (3rd ed., pp. 43-59). Philadelphia: J. B. Lippincott.

Leininger, M. A. (1976). Two strange health tribes: The Ginsrun and Enicidem in the United States. *Human Organization. Journal of the Society for Applied Anthropology, 35*(3), 253-261.

Long, W. N., & Sharp, E. S. (1982). Relationships between professions: From the viewpoint of the physician and nurse-midwife in a tertiary center. *Journal of Nurse-Midwifery, 27*(4), 14-24.

Lum, J. L. J. (1988). Reference groups and professional socialization. In M. E. Hardy & M. E. Conway (Eds.), *Role theory. Perspectives for health professionals* (2nd ed., pp. 257-272). Norwalk, CT: Appleton & Lange.

Lurie, E. E. (1981). Nurse practitioners: Issues in professional socialization. *Journal of Health and Social Behavior, 22,* 31-48.

Malkemes, L. C. (1974). Resocialization: A model for nurse practitioner preparation. *Nursing Outlook, 22*(2), 90-94.

Mauksch, I. G. (1981). Introduction. In I. G. Mauksch (Ed.), *Primary care. A contemporary perspective* (pp. 1-11). New York: Grune & Stratton.

Mulligan, J. E. (1976). Professional transition: Nurse to nurse-midwife. *Nursing Outlook, 24*(4), 228-233.

National Commission on Nurse Anesthesia Education. (1990). Summary of Commission findings: Issues and review of supporting documents. *Journal of the American Association of Nurse Anesthetists, 58*(5), 394-398.

Oda, D. (1977). Specialized role development: A three phase process. *Nursing Outlook, 25,* 374-377.

Oda, D. S. (1985). Community health nursing in innovative school health roles and programs. In S. E. Archer & R. P. Fleshman (Eds.), *Community health nursing* (pp. 368-393). Monterey, CA: Wadsworth Health Sciences.

Oleson, V., & Whittaker, E. (1968). *The silent dialogue.* San Francisco: Jossey-Bass.

Page, N. E., & Arena, D. M. (1991). Practical strategies for CNS role implementation. *Clinical Nurse Specialist, 5*(1), 43-38.

Polanyi, M. (1958). *Personal knowledge.* Chicago: University of Chicago Press.

Roberts, S. J. (1983). Oppressed group behavior: Implications for nursing. *Advances in Nursing Science, 5,* 21-30.

Rooks, J. P. (1983). The context of nurse-midwifery in the 1980s: Our relationships with medicine, nursing, lay-midwives, consumers and health care economists. *Journal of Nurse-Midwifery, 26*(5), 3-8.

Rooks, J. P., & Haas, J. E. (Eds.). (1986). *Nurse-Midwifery in America.* Washington, D. C.: American College of Nurse-Midwives Foundation.

Russell, D. (1988, April). *Role theory: Role development of nurse practitioners.* Paper presented at the annual meeting of the National Organization of Nurse Practitioner Faculties, Minneapolis, MN.

Russell, D. (1995). Personal communication.

Sparacino, P. S. A., & Cooper, D. M. (1990). The role components. In P. S. A. Sparacino, D. M. Cooper, & P. A. Minarik (Eds.), *The clinical nurse specialist implementation and impact* (pp. 11-40). Norwalk, CT: Appleton & Lange.

Spross, J. (1992). Feminist theory: Implications for the epistemology of nursing. Unpublished paper.

Spross, J. (1995). Personal communication.

Thornton, R., & Nardi, P. M. (1975). The dynamics of role acquisition. *American Journal of Sociology, 80*(4), 870-885.

Varney, H. (1987). *Nurse-midwifery* (2nd ed.). Boston: Blackwell Scientific.

PART II

COMPETENCIES OF ADVANCED NURSING PRACTICE

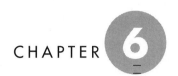

CHAPTER 6

Direct Clinical Practice

Sarah Jo Brown

INTRODUCTION

Today people are asking that health-care professionals respect them as individuals, focus on their concerns, consider their physical comfort and emotional distress, provide them with information, and coordinate care within and across settings (Gerteis, Edgman-Levitan, Daley, & Delbanco, 1993). In fact, these are the very aspects of health care in which advanced practice nurses (APNs) excel and the aspects they have been working to improve. It is important that members of the nursing profession be able to describe advanced direct care practice to the public, who, once they become aware of it, may choose to use APNs' services. It is also important to be able to convey clearly the nature and outcomes of direct patient care by APNs to policymakers, who have the power to sanction advanced nursing practice (ANP) through legislation, regulations, and funding.

FOUR CHARACTERISTICS OF THE DIRECT CARE OF ADVANCED PRACTICE NURSES

This chapter is offered in the spirit of creating a dialogue regarding the essential characteristics of ANP care and to help the profession, policymakers, and the public appreciate the uniqueness and value of APN direct care. It is proposed that the direct care competency of advanced nursing practice has four characteristics: the use of a holistic perspective, the formation of partnerships with patients, the use of expert clinical reasoning, and the use of diverse health and illness management approaches. These characteristics are widely present in APN practice, have some research support, and are the themes one hears when APNs describe what they do. The strategies APNs use to enact the four practice characteristics are also examined (see Table 6–1). In this chapter, it is assumed that a majority of APNs are expert nurses; this assumption has research support (Fenton & Brykczynski, 1993), but to pursue it would divert from the present focus, which is to describe advanced direct care practice.

ACKNOWLEDGMENT: The author wishes to recognize the contributions of Carol Williams-Suich, MSN, to this chapter. Carol is a family nurse practitioner employed by the Family Health Center in Lebanon, New Hampshire.

TABLE 6–1. CHARACTERISTICS OF ADVANCED DIRECT CARE PRACTICE AND STRATEGIES FOR ENACTING THEM

Use of a Holistic Framework
- Take into account the complexity of human life
- Recognize and address person-context interactions and their effects on health and illness
- Consider the multiple effects of illness, aging, and stress
- Focus on functional abilities and needs
- Consider quality-of-life effects of symptoms and therapies

Formation of Partnerships with Patients
- Interact in an egalitarian manner
- Use a conversational style
- Encourage active participation in decision making
- Give mute patients a voice
- Advocate patient's perspective and concerns to others

Use of Expert Clinical Reasoning
- Acquire specialized knowledge
- Generate and test hypotheses
- Use base rate information
- Use associative and integrative thinking
- Avoid common thinking errors
- Consider multiple factors when deciding how to treat
- Develop a strategy for documenting patients' problems

Use of Diverse Management Approaches
- Use interpersonal interventions
- Use multiple and diverse types of interventions
- Actively manage complex situations
- Help patients maintain or regain health
- Help patients manage chronic illness
- Coordinate services

ORIGINS OF THE CHARACTERISTICS

The four characteristics of advanced direct care practice have their roots in the traditional values of the nursing profession. Nurses have always been person centered, holistic, and committed to patient self-determination; since the inception of the profession, nurses have taken into account the numerous, intricately related factors that shape individual responses and patterns of health, illness, recovery, and aging. Although basic nursing education is built on these values, the ability to enact them is developed during post-basic work experiences and graduate education. Full enactment of these values is realized when the nurse assumes an advanced practice role and is able to practice within the context of an expanded scope of practice and greater role autonomy than is afforded in basic practice.

Specialization is essential to advanced direct care practice, because it deepens knowledge and understandings in a particular domain, which in turn enables the APN to deal competently with a greater range of problems and with more complex problems. In advanced practice, the domain refers to extensive knowledge of the experiences, issues, and problems that occur frequently in a particular clinical population. APNs know the usual illness and developmental trajectories that occur within their specialties and can help patients and families anticipate problems they might encounter. Specialized knowledge also requires a deep understanding of the processes that underlie problems, an appreciation of the wide variety of ways in which persons respond to problems, and knowledge of the circumstances under which particular therapeutic approaches work.

An APN's specialized knowledge may have begun to develop during work experiences before graduate school, but graduate coursework and practica expand and deepen that knowledge. Experience with a population of patients develops the APN's abilities to analyze ambiguous situations, discriminate between similar conditions, and anticipate problems. With experience, the APN becomes open to a broader range of explanations for common events and experiences and synthesizes experiential knowledge with knowledge from other sources. Experience also confers increased comfort with uncertainty in clinical situations and helps the APN realize that the so-called experts, i.e., specialists, often don't have better answers or approaches than those the APN has selected. One APN described his hesitancy in digitalizing patients until he realized that the cardiologist to whom he was referring patients did exactly what he would have done. Thus, with experience, the APN becomes confident in managing a broad range of problems.

ANP specialization frequently involves knowledge, skills, and services that overlap with those traditionally viewed as within the medical domain. The success of certified nurse-midwives (CNMs), nurse practitioners (NPs), and certified registered nurse anesthetists (CRNAs) in expanded practice domains has established that a wide range of health-care services can be safely and effectively provided by APNs. More recently, clinical nurse specialists (CNSs) have expanded or focused their practices to manage health-care problems and conditions hitherto managed by physicians and are treating patients across health-care settings. The increasingly flexible boundaries between nursing and medicine and the trend toward providing care across in-patient and out-patient clinical settings should enable APNs to use their holistic clinical expertise more effectively to influence patients' experiences of care and improve health outcomes. The four characteristics of direct care provided by APNs set forth in this chapter can provide a basis for research questions about the differences between advanced nursing practice (ANP) and medical care and the impact of those differences on patient outcomes.

Lastly, the specialized knowledge of advanced practice includes familiarity with theoretical models and research findings relevant to the clinical area of practice. Midrange theories, in particular, provide models for thinking about clinical situations and help organize substantive clinical knowledge.[1] The ability to critique and evaluate the clinical applicability of research promotes practice that is based on scientifically validated knowledge. Thus, APNs' knowledge goes beyond basic practice knowledge in that it is more conceptually organized and distinguishes research-based knowledge from other ways of knowing used in nursing practice.

USE OF A HOLISTIC PERSPECTIVE

HOLISM DESCRIBED

Holism is a greatly abused term, but there is general agreement that it involves:

1. Viewing the patient as an integral part of larger social, physical, and energy environments;

---

[1]Midrange theories address specific kinds of situations, as opposed to the full range of nursing situations, like conceptual models do. As a result, midrange theories are more directly applicable to practice, albeit only to those situations that they address. Examples of evolving midrange theories include theories of the experience of dyspnea (Carrieri & Janson-Bjerklie, 1986; Gift, 1993; Steele & Shaver, 1992), childbearing fatigue (Pugh & Milligan, 1993), and care-seeking behavior (Lauver, 1992).

2. Assuming that the mind, body, and spirit are closely related, so that one dimension should not be considered in isolation from the other;
3. Centering on the meanings patients assign to health, illness experiences, and health-care choices; and
4. Viewing patients' current behaviors and responses as contiguous with their life-span patterns of response and choice (Hall & Allan, 1994; Kinney & Erickson, 1990).

This kind of comprehensive and integrated view of human life and health is evident in the issues experts address when caring for persons with chronic illness. These include

- Physical issues, including functional status, symptom distress, symptom meaning, and symptom management;
- Psychosocial issues, such as the search for meaning, quality of life, personal control, changing human relationships, and the need for self-enhancement;
- Sociocultural issues, such as the significance of social support, cultural values, and interpretations;
- Spiritual issues pertaining to the meaning of life and suffering;
- Economic impact issues; and
- Ethical issues related to matters such as the sanctity of life, the right to self-determination, and concern for others' well-being (Johnson-Taylor, Jones, & Burns, 1995).

A powerful case example of the importance of recognizing how chronic illness affects a patient's life was reported by a CNS in a rheumatology screening clinic (Benner & Wrubel, 1989). While examining the patient's joints, the CNS commented on her findings in ways that indicated that she understood that it must be difficult to do everyday activities with the amount of pain, stiffness, and deformity this woman had. At the end of the examination, the CNS said something like, "Rheumatoid arthritis really has not been very nice to you." The patient burst into tears, eventually explaining, "You know, no one has ever talked about it as a personal thing, no one's ever talked to me as if this were a thing that mattered, a personal event" (Benner & Wrubel, 1989, p. 9).

NURSING AND MEDICINE: CONTRASTING VIEWS OF THE PATIENT

Although many APNs provide services that once were provided only by physicians, they do not approach their practice from within a traditional medical model (Thibodeau & Hawkins, 1994). APNs typically elicit considerable psychosocial information and use that information to individualize care (Brown, 1994; Johnson, 1993; Thibodeau & Hawkins, 1994). Underlying the obtaining of psychosocial information, there appears to be a deep commitment to understanding the patient's lived health and illness experiences, as well as an interpersonal competence that enables experts to interpret accurately the information the patient puts forth (Kasch, 1984). Experts are able to "escape the confines of personal perspective and to assume or construct the viewpoint of the other person" (Kasch, 1984, p. 78). To achieve this kind of connectedness with patients, expert nurses (including APNs) convey interest and concern in their patients as valued and unique individuals (Brown, 1994). They provide opportunities for patients to tell their stories in their own words and to explain how they see their situations. In short, APNs focus on persons, their experiences, their worries, their aspirations, and the contexts of their lives.

Lynaugh (1988) contrasted the questions nurses and physicians attempt to answer in clinical encounters that apparently have the same purpose. Nurses asked, "What are this patient's problems, how is he or she coping with them, what help is needed, and what should be left up to the patient?" The physicians' question was likely to be, "What is this patient's diagnosis and what treatment does he or she need?" (Lynaugh, 1988). Despite acknowledged changes in medical curricula aimed at improving physician-patient communication and humanizing medical care, this emphasis on the diagnostic process and therapeutics was recently reaffirmed (Siegler & Whitney, 1994). The persistence of these differences may be attributed as much to the socialization of the two disciplines as to substantive differences in curricular content.

HOLISM AND ANP HEALTH ASSESSMENT

Because assessment serves multiple purposes (i.e., gathering data, coming to know the patient as an individual, and putting the patient at ease in the clinical relationship), a holistic approach is essential. One way to gain a holistic understanding of patients and their health is to prompt patients to talk about how they conduct various aspects of daily living. Functional-abilities assessment is one strategy for acquiring a comprehensive knowledge base regarding the patient's daily living experiences. Most functional-abilities formats focus on (1) how patients view their health or quality of life; (2) how they accomplish self-care and household or job management; (3) the social, physical, financial, and environmental resources that augment or tax their abilities; and (4) the strategies they and their families use to cope with the problems in their lives. The ability to function in daily activities and relationships is an important consideration for patients when they evaluate their health (Herth, 1989; Loomis & Conco, 1991), so it is an appropriate and essential focus for a holistic, patient-focused assessment of individuals.

In a text on history taking and physical examination (Bates, 1987) commonly used in APN programs, the comprehensive history described has a holistic focus and elicits data on functional abilities (pp. 3–9). Although this text was written by a physician, it is unusual in that it is informed by suggestions, critiques, and contributions provided by APNs acknowledged by the author. Use of this guide to comprehensive history taking is one way to address the challenge of combining holistic assessment with more traditional symptom-based assessment.

Functional health patterns (FHP) assessment (Gordon, 1994) is a functional-abilities format that has wide applicability. Although developed from a nursing perspective, FHP has been used in expanded role practice and in a variety of care settings. It is particularly valuable for establishing a person-centered baseline of health status. FHP may seem like an unfamiliar or unworkable idea to some APN students and APNs who may practice in settings (especially those primary care settings) in which a traditional medical approach to interviewing, diagnosing, treating, and documentation prevails. Although data regarding the chief complaint, history of illnesses, past health history, patient profile/lifestyle, family health history, and review of systems are important, they are only one type of information; the APN also needs to assess how the patient is experiencing everyday life (Gordon, 1994).[2]

A screening FHP assessment that can be used for out-patients or in-patients is presented in Table 6–2. This form includes questions that allow the APN to identify problem areas efficiently. The questions can be asked conversationally in interviews with patients to ensure that all functional areas have been considered. Alternatively, patients can complete the questionnaire while waiting to be seen, or support staff can administer it before the interview with the APN. The questions allow patients to indicate the areas of their life in which they have problems or concerns without requiring a series of specific, symptom-focused questions. The APN can use the answers to focus the visit/interview on problems and potential illness areas that need to be explored. The screening questions provide a time-efficient way of zeroing in on health issues that are of concern to patients, which may or may not be the issue that brought the patient to the APN.

When APNs initially try a functional-abilities assessment approach, such as Gordon's (1994) FHP assessment or the screening FHP questionnaire presented herein, they are often surprised at the kinds of information and insights they acquire. One NP student who used Gordon's FHP assessment for the first time said, "I feel like I got to know this patient and her problems better, and faster, than I do using my usual clinical interview questions." As advanced nursing practice evolves and as APNs from different specialties collaborate among themselves and with other disciplines, the profession is likely to learn more about what constitutes holistic, efficient, and effective assessments that address the concerns of patients seeking care.

FORMATION OF PARTNERSHIPS WITH PATIENTS

APNs' person-centered, holistic perspective is the foundation for the kinds of relationships they co-create with patients. The following quote describes how one NP thought about her relationships with patients:

> Rather than going in with the professional mind set of "I know the goal. I want to take you there," it becomes a much more equal kind of action. . . . You can't teach people things they don't want to know. You can't solve problems that aren't seen as problems. And I've thrown a lot of my health goals [for patients] out the window in terms of universalizing them. I finally came to realize that it doesn't matter what my health goals are unless they're the patient's goals too. The whole mutual goal setting concept is real central to how I feel about what I do. (Brown, 1990, p. 138)

This APN recognized that effective relationships with clients require that providers not control or dominate what is talked about in the health-care encounter.

---

[2]The author is not suggesting that an FHP format, or any other cognitive framework the provider uses to organize thinking about clinical problems, be used to structure the clinical interview interpersonally. Instead, the patient's story and concerns should provide the interpersonal framework for the interview.

TABLE 6–2. HEALTH SCREENING QUESTIONS

Your answers will help the advanced practice nurse in talking with you about your health and health problems.

1. How has your health been recently?

    Very good _____   Good _____   Fair _____   Poor _____

2. What "new" health problems do you have?

3. What "old" health problems still bother you?

4. Are you physically able to do the activities you would like to be able to do?

    Yes _____   No _____

5. Do you have pain, aches, or discomfort of any type?

    Yes _____   No _____   Not sure _____

6. Do you believe you eat well?   Yes _____   No _____   Not sure _____

    Are you satisfied with your weight?   Yes _____   No _____

7. Do you have any problems with your bowels or bladder?

    Yes _____   No _____   Maybe _____

8. Are you satisfied with the amount of sleep and rest you get?

    Yes _____   No _____   Not sure _____

9. Do you notice any problems with your vision, hearing, or feeling in your hands or feet?

    Yes _____   No _____   Maybe _____

10. Are you satisfied with how you handle the problems of daily life and with the decisions you make?

    Yes _____   No _____   Not sure _____

11. Do you generally feel good about yourself?

    Yes _____   No _____   Not sure _____

12. Are you generally satisfied with your relationships with others?

    Yes _____   No _____   Not sure _____

13. Are you satisfied with your sexuality and sexual relations?

    Yes _____   No _____   Not sure _____

14. Do you have beliefs about life that are very important to you and that you think we need to know to provide health care for you?

    Yes _____   No _____   Not sure _____

APNS' INTERPERSONAL STYLES

Descriptions of APNs' interpersonal styles have documented the use of informal and egalitarian interpersonal styles (Brown, 1994; Johnson, 1993; Morten, Kohl, O'Mahoney, & Pelosi, 1991). APNs engage in social story exchanges, express regard for patients, and ask about patients' home lives, all the while discussing the clinical issue. This less structured and less dominating style of interviewing has been called "conversational interviewing" (Brown, 1995) and offers a contrast to the interrogative style of the prototypic medically focused interview. The interrogative style is dominated by the questions and clinical reasoning of the health-care provider and is oriented more toward information gathering and problem solving than toward understanding the patient's experiences and life contexts. Conversational health-care interviewing serves several purposes: (1) It breaks down whatever social barriers may exist between the patient and the provider; (2) it establishes concern for the patient; (3) it helps the provider acquire a sense of the patient as a person; and (4) it provides the patient with multiple opportunities to express his or her concerns, beliefs, preferences, and expectations. The use of the conversational style may also influence the extent to which patients reveal what is going on in their lives and affect whether they take the provider's advice or follow recommendations (Rodin & Janis, 1982; Squier, 1990).

ESTABLISHING PARTNERSHIPS WITH PATIENTS

In a partnership, individuals complement one another; different areas of expertise are joined to accomplish a shared goal. Just as it takes collaboration between a score writer and a lyricist to write a musical play, so collaboration between patient and provider is needed to shape health care that is meaningful and helpful. Patients have knowledge about themselves, whereas the APN has expertise in helping people think about their lives, in identifying what may be going on that is causing them health problems, and in suggesting ways for dealing with the underlying issues or processes. *Together* they can usually identify the problems that need to be addressed, figure out what is causing or contributing to the problems, and decide what can be done to alleviate them. At the outset, this collaboration may also require negotiation about each participant's priorities and responsibilities.

Patients and families who are faced with treatment decisions that will influence their lives in important ways often need a provider partner who will take the time to describe the scenarios that could accompany each option; help them examine their own values, priorities, and preferences; and weigh these values, priorities, and preferences vis-à-vis the options available. The parents' decision whether to continue aggressive treatment in a seriously injured and unresponsive adolescent or not, an elderly woman's decision to place her husband, who is cognitively deteriorating, in a nursing home or have him stay at home, a menopausal woman's decision regarding hormone replacement therapy—these are the kinds of decisions that APNs can help patients make. They are ideal persons to help patients with these kinds of decisions, because they possess the technical knowledge, the knowledge of human responses, the ethical commitment to self-determination, and the interpersonal skills to illuminate the choices.

A nursing strategy to provide decisional support for patients with cancer who want to participate in medical treatment decisions has been developed by Neufeld, Degner, and Dick (1993). Patients are first assisted to identify exactly how they want to participate in decisions and then are helped to formulate and voice their questions and preferences to their physicians.

Not all patients want to participate actively in their health-care decisions and plans, however. Older persons in particular may prefer a more passive role (Greene, Adelman, Friedmann, & Charon, 1994), whereas others may feel ambivalent about taking an active role in decision making. For example, a 34-year-old woman related to her family NP that she appreciated the recent telephone conversation regarding her mammogram, but that she wished the NP would just tell her what to do, like in the "good old days" with her physician. She went on to acknowledge that she sought care from NPs because they gave her more information and considered her as a person when developing a plan of care. Nevertheless, when faced with a decision and asked to share responsibility for developing a plan of care, she had an inclination to revert to a more passive role. Often, APNs must socialize patients to a more active role, by discussing the notion and assuring them that they will be given information and be helped to think through the ramifications of each option, not just presented with options and asked for a decision.

PARTNERSHIPS WITH NONCOMMUNICATIVE PATIENTS

Some patients are not able to enter fully into partnership with APNs because they are too young, have compromised cognitive capacity, or are unconscious. Clinical populations who may be unable to participate fully in the therapeutic partnership are listed in Table 6–3. Although these patients may be limited in their abilities to speak for themselves, they are not entirely without voice. Several strategies can be used to give such patients a voice. APNs can often anticipate situations during which patients will experience temporary alterations in cognition or verbal abilities, such as the intense pain of labor or elective procedures and surgeries for which the patient is anesthetized, and can collaborate with these patients prior to their incapacity, to develop plans for handling certain contingencies.

In the absence of this kind of prior dialogue, the APN draws on other knowledge and skills. Many noncommunicative patients have very basic ways of expressing discomfort and preference (Smith, 1988). Experts who work with these patients learn to pay close attention to how patients respond to what happens to them and to discern fine levels of response in their facial expressions, body movements, physiological parameters (Tanner, Benner, Chesla, & Gordon, 1993), types of cries or vocalizations, and other behaviors. Because of their knowledge of patients' underlying physiological conditions and the psychological aspects of their conditions, their experience with previous patients with similar conditions, and their attentiveness to what family members say about the patient, APNs are often able to interpret the meaning of patient behaviors that are obscure to other providers. Undergirding the attempt to figure out what the patient's behavior means is a deep commitment to the belief that all behavior is an expression of need or the desire to stay connected with other human beings, and APNs try to respect that expression, regardless of how rudimentary it may be.

TABLE 6–3. PATIENT POPULATIONS UNABLE TO PARTICIPATE FULLY IN PARTNERSHIP

Infants and preverbal children
Anesthetized patients
Unconscious/comatose patients
Persons in severe pain
Patients receiving medications that impair cognition
Persons with dementia
Persons with psychiatric conditions that seriously impair rational thought
Persons with conditions that render them incapable of speech and conversation

The importance of identifying alternative sources of data in patients who are unable to respond physically or to communicate was illustrated in a study of persons who had experienced and recovered from unconsciousness (Lawrence, 1995). In this study, 27% of the patients were able to hear, understand, and respond emotionally while unconscious. Lawrence cited evidence that some patients under anesthesia have some level of awareness (1995). These findings suggest that nurses should communicate with unconscious patients by providing them with interventions such as reassurance, explanations, and comforting touch.

Several scenarios illustrate this ability to intervene effectively when the patient's ability to communicate is compromised. The CNM reminds the woman in intense labor of the strategies they developed to deal with the woman's desire to avoid pharmacological intervention as part of her birth plan. When the ability to participate in the partnership is temporarily but fully compromised, such as in the anesthetized patient, APNs rely on the data collected when the patient was conscious, including specific requests and concerns. The CRNA makes sure that for a patient who had had negative experiences with patient-controlled analgesia (PCA) and specifically requested that PCA not be used that the postoperative prescriptions include intravenous analgesics that will be administered by the staff nurse.

There are yet more ways to determine what patients want. One strategy is to talk with family members or those legally authorized to make health-care decisions for the patient. Most parents and families are eager to give accounts of the person's life and health and illness experiences before he or she became incapacitated. Through these accounts, the nurse can come to know the patient as a person who lived life in a particular way. These insights may provide links that explain the patient's current behavior pattern or may suggest ways to approach the patient who has been rendered silent by disease or injury.

Other forms of the patient's voice are advance care directives, health-care proxy documents, and organ donation cards the patient may have completed prior to the present illness. These documents all represent the patient's thinking and should be respected in times of crisis and when difficult decisions regarding treatment must be made. APNs are often in situations in which they can remind the health-care team that the patient has spoken through these documents and thus can give patients a voice at a time when they are physically mute.

Whether patients are able to participate fully in a therapeutic partnership or not, the partnership approach is used to establish a relationship with them and their agents. The nature of the partnership is such that the APN is an advocate for patients and gives voice to their discomforts, concerns, and desire for dignity. For the conscious, communicative patient, the APN's voice joins that of the patient; for unconscious, non-communicative, or powerless patients, the APN's voice is raised on their behalf.

USE OF EXPERT CLINICAL REASONING

KNOWLEDGE

Specialized knowledge and accrued experience working with a population of patients lay the foundation for the expert clinical reasoning that is associated with advanced direct care practice.[3] Graduate education launches APNs in the acquisition and organization of an in-depth body of clinical knowledge relevant to understanding, diagnosing, and treating problems that they will encounter in practice. As experience accumulates, the distinguishing and common features of particular conditions are noted and imprinted in memory. Illness trajectories and presentations of particular patients make an impression and come to mind when a patient with a similar problem is seen later (Benner, 1984). Eventually, the expert's clinical knowledge consists of a complex network of memorable cases, prototypic images, maxims, probabilities, associations, theories, conceptual categories, research findings, and therapeutic information.

All of this information is stored in memory, somewhat like files on various topics, that can be accessed or activated with the aid of a cue, or signal, from the current clinical situation (Carnevali & Thomas, 1993). There probably are "symptom files," "problem files," "diagnosis files," "situation files," and "treatment files," all intricately linked. The various types of files ensure that the expert is flexible in analyzing a situation; that is, the APN can approach it from more than one perspective and recognize the connections between the various aspects of the situation. Over time, the files are enriched, refined, and cross-referenced with other files that may be connected in some situations. Thus, experts have extensive, varied, and intricately connected knowledge about the clinical problems they encounter.

THINKING PROCESSES

Expertise involves more than accumulated stores of knowledge, however. Experts also process information differently than less experienced practitioners do (Benner, 1984). Very early in the patient's telling of his or her story, expert clinicians generate hypotheses (diagnoses) that could explain the patient's experiences (Gordon, 1994). Over the course of the interview, experts listen for, ask about, and look for information that increases or decreases the likelihood of a hypothesis, so as to narrow the field of viable hypotheses. The goal, of course, is to arrive at a working diagnosis, which is the diagnostic hypothesis with the best fit between the presenting data and the mental images stored in memory. However, experts do not pursue this goal in a linear manner; they do not let this goal dominate their conversations with patients. For example, several studies have shown that NPs' interactions with patients are not highly hypothesis driven; rather, client-centered questions and hypothesis-driven questions are interspersed throughout encounters (Brown, 1992; White, Nativio, Kobert, & Engberg, 1992).

Experts use several types of thinking processes to narrow the field of hypotheses and eventually select the best one. They look for patterns in the data that match, or have a good fit with, the mental pictures of each diagnosis that are stored in memory (Benner & Tanner, 1987). They are skilled in recognizing patterns in the presenting information, despite confusing presentations and marked differ-

---

[3]Unfortunately, there are few studies of APNs' clinical reasoning. Therefore, the information presented in this section is based on findings regarding how health-care providers with experience are different from those with minimal experience. The information has been assembled from studies of nurses, physicians, and occupational therapists. Where information was specifically obtained regarding APNs, this will be explicitly stated. Otherwise, the assumption that most APNs are experts is invoked throughout this section.

ences between past and present presentations. Often, pattern-matching thinking occurs with great rapidity and a great deal of it takes place below the level of conscious awareness—much like riding a bicycle once one has mastered the skill. Yet, some situations do not declare themselves clearly or quickly and require the expert to be more deliberate. In these situations, experts methodically and logically try to rule out hypotheses in the process of determining the one that best matches the clinical data. Often, nonfitting data suggest to experts that they need to generate new hypotheses, because none of the ones being considered account for the nonfitting piece or pieces. Recognition that there are nonfitting data can be particularly important in figuring out what is going on in complex and problematic situations. It can be the clue that initiates the search for a better-fitting explanation of the situation.

Knowing the patient as a particular person with certain patterns of response enables experienced nurses to detect subtle changes in patients' conditions (Tanner et al., 1993). In one study, experienced acute care nurses reported that they often sensed nonspecific changes in patients and experienced a gut feeling that the patient was somehow different before they were able to detect significant objective changes (Smith, 1988). These subjective feelings led to "close searching" for confirming evidence, which gradually led to detection and recognition of an objective pattern indicating deterioration in condition. Premonitory feelings were also reported by an NP in primary care. The NP reported attending to her "feelings of lack of closure, of uneasiness, incompleteness or discomfort" (Brykczynski, 1989, p. 83) because they often indicated that something important was going to come up in the conversation. Thus, knowing patients well and attending to their own subjective responses inform and complement experts' deliberative assessment and reasoning, adding to the data available for solving problems.

BASE RATE INFORMATION

The accuracy of diagnosis also depends on whether the practitioner uses base rate data (O'Neill, 1994). The base rate is the incidence of the condition in a relevant population and can be based on either objective or subjective estimates of the frequency with which the condition occurs in the practitioner's population. There is evidence that some practitioners rely too much on matching the clinical picture to mental images of a diagnosis and forget to consider the base rate of the problem in the population (O'Neill, 1994). Keeping in mind the maxim "When you hear hoofbeats in Kansas, think horses, not zebras" is one way clinicians remind themselves, and each other, to consider base rate data when making a diagnosis.

ASSOCIATIVE AND INTEGRATIVE THINKING

APNs typically go beyond diagnosing patients' conditions to develop a deep understanding of how patients view their life or life situation, given their current health state, be it illness, wellness, surgery, childbearing, or aging. The dual objective of understanding patients' views of their situations and diagnosing underlying processes and conditions requires APNs to work with tremendous amounts of information; this involves putting together a meaningful interpretation of the situation from what patients say: their stories about their experiences, which relate sequences of events and provide descriptions of their daily life, home environment, and social relationships; their opinions; and their expressed and implied concerns. The APN is also aware that patients' nonverbal behaviors offer important insights into what is meant. In addition, physical observations, findings from the physical examination, and diagnostic tests must be interpreted within the context of patients' stories. Thus, APNs are constantly developing associations between data bits and comparing the patterns and partial patterns with information stored in memory to understand and interpret the data coming from the encounter (see Figure 6–1).

Arriving at accurate and meaningful understandings of human responses is infinitely more complicated than trying to understand diseases, because diseases to a great extent follow deterministic paths, whereas human responses are shaped by multiple layers of influence, values, interactions between personal tendencies and circumstances, and are expressed in a diversity of forms. Thus APNs must make connections between pieces of seemingly unrelated data and be flexible in their thinking to construct accurate understandings and explanations of what is going on.

A form of integrative clinical reasoning was identified in a study of occupational therapists. Experienced therapists were found to "imagine how the [patient's] condition could change" (Mattingly & Fleming, 1994, p. 133). This way of thinking involved "imagining and integrating images of the past, present and possible futures" of the person (Mattingly & Fleming, 1994, p. 135). Although envisioning patients' possible futures has not been studied in nursing, it is likely that APNs use this method, given nursing's tradition of incorporating outcomes into care planning and the contextual way in which APNs work with patients. Simon (1969) went so far as to call actions involved in "changing existing situations into preferred ones" the central concern of *all* professions.

THINKING ERRORS

The clinical acumen of APNs and the hypotheses they generate are highly dependable. However, as practice becomes repetitive, APNs may develop routine responses and they run the risk of making certain types of thinking errors (Schön, 1983). Errors of expectancy occur when the correct diagnosis is not generated as a hypothesis because there is a set of circumstances, in either the clinician's experience or the patient's circumstances, that predisposes the clinician to disregard it. For example, the NP who over several years has seen an elderly woman for

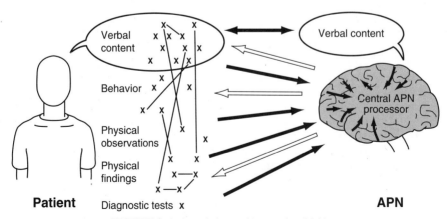

FIGURE 6–1. Associative and integrative thinking.

problems associated with chronic pulmonary disease may fail to consider that the most recent onset of shortness of breath and fatigue could be related to worsening aortic stenosis; the NP has come to expect pulmonary pathology, not cardiac pathology.

Erroneous conclusions are also more likely when the situation is ambiguous, that is, when the meaning or reliability of the data is unclear, the interpretation of the data is not clear-cut, the best approach to treatment is debatable, or one cannot say for sure whether the patient is responding well to treatment (Brykczynski, 1991). To avoid errors in these kinds of situations, experts often revert to the use of maxims to guide their thinking (Brykczynski, 1989). One of the maxims that NPs use to deal with uncertain diagnoses is "Real disease will declare itself" (Brykczynski, 1989). This maxim recognizes that with the passage of time, amorphous signs and symptoms may become more distinct, so that suspending judgment and monitoring the situation may be preferable to accepting a diagnosis that has a less than good fit with the data. This way of proceeding in circumstances of ambiguity is different from Scheff's (1963) observation that an implicit guideline in medicine is "When in doubt, diagnose disease." A leaning toward either the monitor-and-wait approach or the when-in-doubt-treat approach is not an issue of right and wrong. Each approach has its consequences, requiring that benefit/risk ratios, probabilities, and clients' values must be considered when deciding how to proceed. In these situations, clinicians should explain the uncertainty to the patient and reach a joint decision about how to proceed.

TREATMENT DECISIONS

The decision whether to treat or not can be complex, because the practitioner is faced with a string of probabilities that do not all point to the same decision. APNs consider four types of information when deciding whether and how to treat:

1. The degree of certainty about the diagnosis/condition,
2. What is known about the effectiveness of the various treatment alternatives,
3. What is known about the risks of the treatment alternatives, and
4. The clinician's comfort with a particular treatment or intervention.

The most clear-cut situation is when the condition is assuredly present, a particular treatment is known to be highly effective, the treatment can be expected to be low in risk for the particular patient, and the clinician is comfortable with the treatment. Unfortunately, many (probably most) therapeutic decisions are not so clear-cut. Instead, the weight of factors in support of a particular treatment and the weight of those against treatment, or in support of another treatment, are close to equivalent. The goal is to choose from among several possible courses of action the one that will have the highest probability of achieving the outcome the patient most desires. However, outcomes are not the only elements that need to be considered. The final decision should also factor in the acceptability of the treatment to the patient, his or her motivation and ability to use or follow the treatment, the likelihood that the patient will continue to use the treatment even if side effects are experienced, and the financial burden of the treatment.

The relative suitability of the various options to the patient can be analyzed using the quantitative method of decision analysis (Pauker & McNeill, 1981). This adjunct to treatment decision making requires structuring all the initial choices and their possible outcomes (or sets of outcomes) into a decision tree. Then the value to the patient of each outcome and the probabilities of various events are added to the tree. Calculations are done that result in numerical values for each choice that reflect a combination of patient values and the likelihood the outcomes will occur as a result of that choice. The choice with the highest expected value is the one recommended by the decision analysis. Corcoran (1986) applied the method to treatment choices for pain control in a patient admitted to a hospice program. In the near future, computer applications of this kind of analysis may serve as guides for clinical decision making. Even with this kind of computer assistance, however, each treatment decision ultimately should be made interpersonally between the provider and the patient, just as it now is.

Clinical reasoning is very complex when dissected and analyzed, yet experts are sound and efficient clinical problem solvers. The experienced APN trusts the almost instantaneous, apparently nonanalytical reasoning that produces a working diagnosis and a treatment choice. Nevertheless, vigilance requires that APNs make deliberate efforts to maintain a body of current knowledge, pay close attention to what patients say, avoid the most common sources of error in clinical thinking, and evaluate their clinical decision making in light of patients' progress and attainment of desirable outcomes.

NAMING PATIENTS' HEALTH CONCERNS AND PROBLEMS

At some point during health assessment and documentation, APNs are faced with decisions regarding how to describe, name, or otherwise characterize the patient's health status and problems. Most NPs use a medical diagnosis only and subsume the patient's other problems under it (Elder & Bullough, 1990; Fenton & Brykczynski, 1993). This does not imply that they do not attend to patients' illness experiences, but only that they use medical diagnosis terminology to organize their documentation. In contrast, CNSs are more likely to use nursing diagnoses or a combination of nursing and medical diagnoses in their documentation. These differences in practice reflect in part the practice settings in which these APN roles evolved. Most NPs practiced primarily with physicians in settings where reimbursement was determined by medical diagnosis. Even now, reimbursement mechanisms are based on diagnostic codes that do not take into account the full range of conditions that APNs treat, manage, and address. Most CNSs practiced primarily with nurses within nursing departments, many of which had adopted nursing diagnosis terminology as the basis for documentation of nursing care. The adoption of a nursing diagnosis framework was not driven by existing financial incentives.

APNs who are committed to explicitly naming the patient's health-related concerns, functional problems, and lifestyle risks are faced with the dilemma of what terminology to use. Consider the case of an elderly woman who has been seen in a clinic on a regular basis for chronic congestive heart failure (CHF). Over the last year, in spite of maximal drug therapy, she has been experiencing gradually increasing shortness of breath and fatigue. The APN could view the woman's problems as all related to the CHF and make this the only problem on the problem list, or the APN could list (1) CHF, (2) shortness of breath with modest activity, (3) decreased social activity related to fatigue or fear, and (4) difficulty with home maintenance related to fatigue and shortness of breath.

There are several advantages to explicitly recognizing the patient's problems as discrete issues in documentation. First, the patient's experiences are kept in the foreground and are not buried beneath what is implicitly deemed to be a more important category of problem—the medical diagnosis. Second, the longer, more definitive list more accurately conveys the holistic nature of the APN's assessment. Third, in our outcome-driven health-care system, the explicit documentation of each problem *actually* identified by the APN enables the APN, collaborating physicians, and payers to track the processes that enable the patient to cope with and compensate for the CHF-related problems. Tracking processes that minimize complications and hospitalizations enables APNs and health-care organizations to provide cost-effective clinical services. A fourth advantage is that the APN's practice becomes more visible within the practice setting.

Disadvantages can be identified for any type of diagnostic nomenclature that is used exclusively. By using only medical diagnosis, the risk is that the problems that are of concern to patients will not be given the attention they deserve and the impression is given that treating the disease condition is the most important service provided. Advanced nursing practice is rendered invisible at a time when its characteristics and contributions need to be most explicit. The use of *only* nursing-derived nomenclature obscures the contributions APNs make to managing symptoms and diseases, which could lead administrators and payers to question APNs' value, since symptoms and disease are often the overt reasons for which people seek health care. In short, if only one profession's nomenclature is used, the talents and contributions of the other disciplines are masked, undermining the potential for mature, interdisciplinary collaboration. Integration of the nomenclatures of all the health-care disciplines is needed.

An altogether different approach is to use nonstandardized, close-to-the-patient (emic) terminology to describe patients' responses to illness and their functional difficulties. Such an approach might capture individual situations better but creates difficulties in developing nursing science and in storing and retrieving clinical data of interest to nurses and health-care systems.

Because APNs are often involved in health promotion as well as illness management, any system of naming the conditions addressed by health care should recognize patient responses that are adaptive and helpful. Advocates of wellness diagnoses point out that healthy responses and strengths often coexist with adversity, transition, and illness (Popkess-Vawter, 1991). Thus, APNs need a comprehensive lexicon that provides names for the issues, conditions, and states that are addressed in giving care. Such a lexicon is not available at present, and as a result many of the health problems that patients experience remain invisible in documentation and reimbursement systems. As advanced nursing practice and health care evolve, the issue of naming problems will be debated within the nursing profession, among APNs, between APNs and physicians, and within policy circles. The nursing profession will pursue standardized, integrated nomenclatures as one way of developing health policies that support basic and advanced nursing practice. APNs should critically evaluate their problem-naming strategies and participate in efforts to shape a lexicon that captures patients' experiences and responses, makes advanced nursing practice visible, and promotes collaboration.

USE OF DIVERSE MANAGEMENT APPROACHES

APNs' holistic approach to care shapes how they help patients. Generally, they use a variety of interventions to effect change in the health status or quality of life of an individual and/or family, including interpersonal interventions and discrete actions. Interpersonal interventions are frequently referred to as "support," whereas discrete actions are those nonpharmacological and pharmacological interventions used to alleviate, prevent, or manage a specific physical symptom, condition, or problem.

INTERPERSONAL INTERVENTIONS

Support is not a discrete intervention; it is a composite of interpersonal interventions that is based on the patient's unique psychological and informational needs. Supportive interpersonal interventions include providing reassurance, giving information, affirming, providing anticipatory guidance, guiding decision making, listening actively, expressing understanding, and being available. Each of these interventions can be described in terms of the circumstances under which it is indicated; for example, reassurance is indicated when clients are experiencing uncertainty, distress, or lack of confidence (Boyd & Munhall, 1989), and active listening is indicated when patients have a strong need to tell their story. The actions that constitute these interventions are not mutually exclusive. Giving factual information can be reassuring, instructional, guiding, or all of these things at the same time. In practice, these interpersonal interventions blend together, and APNs are not consciously aware of when they are doing one and when another. And that's as it should be. There is no need to think "Now I'm doing active listening, now I'm going to do anticipatory guidance." Instead, APNs interact with patients in ways that intermingle the conceptually separate interventions. This crafting of support evolves as the APN talks with patients; infers their worries, fears, and concerns; and, without a great deal of conscious thought, acts to alleviate their distress. The patient may experience the interaction as just a good talk with the APN or as a feeling of being understood. However, support is a complex nursing intervention that is strategically crafted and purposefully administered and often makes a difference in how the patient feels and acts. Thus it is an intervention in the finest nursing tradition. Chapter 7 elaborates on the interpersonal interventions APNs use to teach and coach patients.

DISCRETE INTERVENTIONS

Even the discrete interventions that APNs use are diverse in nature, incorporating nonpharmacological and pharmacological therapies. In a study of 501 physicians and 298 NPs who were asked to describe how they would treat simulated cases involving patients with epigastric pain, the NPs were more likely than the physicians to recommend stopping aspirin; changing diet; reducing alcohol, caffeine, and tobacco intake; and obtaining counseling for stress (Avorn, Everitt, & Baker, 1991). They were also far less likely to recommend a prescription drug. APNs in oncology settings reported that recommending nonpharmacological interventions for symptom management to physicians or nurses was one of their most frequently performed direct care activities (McMillan, Heusinkveld, & Spray, 1995). Similarly, CNMs use significantly less analgesia and anesthesia; perform less fetal monitoring, episiotomies, forceps deliveries, and amniotomies; use less intravenous fluids; and induce labor less frequently than do physicians (Brown & Grimes, 1993). In a study of APNs' use of *Current Procedural Terminology (CPT)* codes, family NPs and nurse-midwives used, on average, 30 to 33% of the codes, a relatively broad usage

(Griffith & Robinson, 1993). Thus, there is evidence that APNs use a broad range of interventions, with substantial reliance on interpersonal and low-technology interventions.

The work of the Nursing Interventions Classification Project (Iowa Intervention Project, 1993) has begun to capture the range of treatments nurses use and should enable identification of interventions used by APNs in particular. This classification system has the potential to recognize nursing interventions that currently are not recognized as contributing to patients' outcomes. If the system were linked with the *CPT* classification system, a complete profile of the interventions patients receive from APNs in various roles and settings would be available.

APNs who prescribe medications report considering many factors when they prescribe: the patient's financial status, the patient's previous experience with similar medications, the ease of taking the medication and how often it must be taken, the side effect profiles of the drugs being considered, and potential drug and disease interactions (Brown & Grimes, 1993). One CNM described prescriptive authority as the "great freedom," because it allowed her to truly integrate drug therapy into the plan of care, rather than having to negotiate pharmacological management with another provider.

The repertoire of interventions used by individual APNs clearly depends on the problems experienced by the population of patients with whom they work and how the health-care agency defines provider roles, but it also depends on the effort they have made to extend and refine their repertoire beyond the interventions they learned during basic and graduate education.

MANAGEMENT OF COMPLEX SITUATIONS

APNs' direct care often involves management and/or coordination of complex situations; many illustrations of this ANP characteristic may be found in the chapters on specific ANP roles (see Chapters 14 through 20). In some settings, APNs have been designated the providers responsible for coordinating discharge for patients with complex follow-up care or for conducting patient education with high-risk patients (Damato et al., 1993; Naylor & Brooten, 1993). In other settings, APNs are assuming management responsibilities for discrete and complex aspects of care, such as care of the elderly who become confused during hospitalization, pain management in patients who are chronically or terminally ill, skin care for patients at risk for skin breakdown or delayed healing, and care coordination for certain kinds of neurological defects. Daleiden (1993) described the role of the CNS as trauma case manager. The CNS assesses each patient daily, rounds with the medical director, does clinical nursing rounds on all trauma patients in the hospital, and meets regularly with families. This coordination of care has resulted in early identification of changes in patients' conditions and smooth transition of patients from unit to unit.

Many CNSs have had the experience of being called in on consultation and finding that there is a need for skilled communication, advocacy, care planning, or—as is often the case—all three. The patient may not be progressing because wound care, pain management, and physical therapy have not been well thought out and coordinated. Or the family may be angry because plans keep changing and they are receiving conflicting information from various providers. Typically, the CNS talks with the patient and family, becomes familiar with the patient's problems and the care required, and then brokers a new plan of care that reflects the patient's and family's needs and preferences and coordinates the objectives of the various providers (and third-party payers) (Steele & Fenton, 1988). This brokering requires broad clinical knowledge regarding the objectives of various providers, interpersonal skill in calming the results of misunderstandings, diplomacy to get the stakeholders to see each other's points of view, and a commitment to keeping the patient's needs and experiences the center of attention.

HELPING PATIENTS MANAGE CHRONIC ILLNESSES

Another type of complex situation that APNs manage effectively is chronic illness. Chronic diseases such as multiple sclerosis, arthritis, cognitive degeneration, psoriasis, cancer, AIDS, and organ failure with subsequent transplantation affect individuals and families in profound ways. The extent to which the disease can be altered significantly by treatment is often unknown. Individuals and their family members, however, develop perceptions about how the illness may unfold over time for them. The term *trajectory* has been used to describe the perceived illness course, because it conveys a sense of phases that unfold over time, each with different illness management issues and ways of intruding on life (Corbin & Strauss, 1992). Individual illness, however, is characterized by a great deal of uncertainty— uncertainty about the future life course, the effectiveness of treatment, the chances of leading a happy life, bodily functions, medical bills, and intimate relationships. APNs often realize that uncertainty is the single most stressful aspect of the illness experience (Mast, 1995) and take steps to help the patient and family overcome their powerlessness by helping them acquire a sense of control over their lives (Miller, 1992).

A study of families coping with breast cancer showed that the issues, problems, and challenges the families dealt with changed as the families moved through the year after diagnosis (Hilton, 1993). Facing the diagnosis, experiencing family communication problems, and dealing with the effects of tests and treatment were more prevalent during the diagnosis and treatment phases, whereas disruption of plans, household organization, and the health of other family members became issues later. However, for most of the families uncertainty remained a major issue throughout the course of the illness.

The spouses and significant others of persons with chronic illness often bear considerable emotional and workload burdens (Gaynor, 1990; Laizner, Yost, Barg, & McCorkle, 1993; Northouse & Peters-Golden, 1993). One intervention approach is to enhance the couple's ability to work together. A study of 60 couples over a 2-year period showed that couples who worked together well (1) had come to terms with the illness and the reality that it would have major effects on their lives; (2) were committed to the relationship and to the work that had to be done to manage the illness; (3) were sensitive to cues indicating each other's moods, needs, and wants; (4) recognized the need for self-renewal activities; (5) were willing to negotiate and compromise; (6) knew how to use resources; and (7) trusted that each was doing everything possible to make their shared and separate lives good (Corbin & Strauss, 1984).

A final issue related to the care of persons with chronic illness is that the APN who sees patients either in a primary care setting or in a follow-up specialty setting can assist greatly by coordinating the services these people receive from a variety of providers. Because many chronic illnesses affect several body systems or have numerous sequelae, persons who are chronically ill are often receiving care from a primary care provider, one or several specialty providers, and adjunct providers such as a physical therapist or dietitian. Some are also receiving home care, and family members, particularly children, may be receiving adaptive supportive services of some kind. Insurance providers and health maintenance organizations are also powerful players in the situation, having the authority to allow or disallow services and stipulate providers. As a result, families with chronic illness can find themselves in an "agency maze" (Burton, 1995). This vivid phrase captures the confusing experiences that ensue when the various providers and payers don't communicate with one another. Many families use a trial-and-error approach to getting what they need and suffer the negative effects of conflicting approaches and unsolved problems. Getting needed services can be a nightmare. Families dealing with chronic illness often receive erroneous information about available services, have difficulty locating services for which they qualify, and spend a great deal of time describing their situation to various intake workers. A resource-savvy APN can often pull together these kinds of situations in a way that results in tremendous benefit to patients and families. By contacting other providers to develop a coordinated plan of management and by linking patients with suitable agencies, the APN can do much to relieve the burdens of chronic illness on a family.

CONDITIONS CONDUCIVE TO THE APN'S PRACTICE

SCOPE-OF-PRACTICE AGREEMENTS AND PRACTICE PRIVILEGES

Scope-of-practice agreements are usually worked out before employment. Typically, these agreements spell out the types of patients for whom APNs will render services and the activities APNs may perform and for which they will be accountable. In effect, these agreements are job descriptions or contracts outlining responsibilities and expectations. Scope-of-practice agreements must be consistent with the jurisdiction's requirements, and all APNs are responsible for knowing and abiding by the laws and regulations governing advanced practice in the jurisdiction in which they practice.

The process of credentialing in the practice setting is a very important determinant of success for some APNs (Smith, 1991). *Credentialing* refers to the licensure, certification, and experience requirements needed to obtain privileges to practice in an organization in which the APN is not an employee. For example, CNMs in private practice must obtain privileges at their local hospitals in order to attend their clients' deliveries. The process of credentialing establishes acceptance of the ANP role, defines the APN's practice privileges, and promotes credibility within the medical and health-care communities. Inability to obtain practice privileges particularly affects APNs in primary care and can be a barrier to the full expression of the APN's direct care competency.

ORGANIZATIONAL SUPPORT

The direct care of APNs who practice in in-patient settings is interdependent with that of other providers of nursing and medical care and must be integrated with their care. Organizational factors can either lend support to their direct care activities or impede them (see Chapters 10 through 12). Therefore, it is very important that these APNs' scopes of practice be specifically defined and explicitly authorized by the organization (Smith, 1991). Clarification of the scope of responsibility and accountability is particularly important since the APN's responsibilities may be a source of conflict if other providers perceive that the APN is impinging on staff nurses', physicians', or another professional's job.

Organizational support is important for any APN role, but it is especially critical for CNSs. For a variety of reasons, the direct care competencies have not been consistently viewed as vital, as have the competencies of the other ANP roles (Koetters, 1989). For other APNs, their direct accountability for panels of patients often secures their positions. For CNSs, the absence of such links is a factor that has made their position vulnerable to budget cuts. Therefore, the success of CNSs in establishing a direct care practice has depended on the extent to which nursing administrators support them in doing so (Baird & Prouty, 1989). In the current climate, such support should take the form of explicit accountability for patient care, documented in the job description. CNSs must maintain a direct care practice to continue to acquire and refine their experiential knowledge and skill and develop as clinical experts. They must do this while still fulfilling other CNS responsibilities valued by the organization. This may require considerable planning by CNSs and nursing administrators. Eventually, if the full benefit of CNSs' expertise is to be realized by patients, statutory, reimbursement, and organizational constraints on CNSs' scope of practice must be removed, particularly in the areas of independent prescribing of medications and devices, ordering and interpreting of diagnostic tests, and ordering of therapies. Safreit (1992) has addressed the issue of constraints as they pertain to NP and CNM practice, but her recommendations apply equally well to CNS and CRNA practice.

APPOINTMENT SCHEDULING

APNs who practice on an appointment basis are being pressured by third-party payers to reduce the length and frequency of patients' visits. The main concern expressed is that restrictions on the length of visits and the number of visits a patient may make have the potential to erode holistic health care. A brief visit is expected to last 15 to 20 minutes; 45 to 60 minutes may be allotted for an initial visit. This time pressure is acutely felt by student and novice APNs, who are still trying to master and apply a large body of knowledge. Often, all that can be accomplished in one 15-minute visit is direct treatment of the patient's explicit concern, and that may be all that is needed. Fifteen minutes is insufficient for a thorough assessment of issues contributing to that concern or for the teaching and counseling that might be needed.

Several strategies can be used to deal with this issue. One strategy used by NPs to deal with short appointments is to address the problem that is of most concern to the patient and then schedule a return visit in a week or two to address other issues. Another way to counter the effects of short appointments is to employ a basic practice nurse to obtain health screening information, teach patients about upcoming diagnostic tests, call to obtain medical equipment, and make contact with community agencies that the APN and patient have agreed the patient should use.

Experienced APNs can also identify the kinds of recurring concerns in their particular populations that can be effectively addressed in a brief visit or a telephone call. Some occur so commonly that protocols developed by the APN can be implemented by assistive personnel. With experience, the APN learns which brief visits must be extended, which scheduled longer visits can be shortened, and what aspects of a visit can be delegated.

CONSULTATION, COLLABORATION, AND REFERRAL

In describing how they manage patient care, APNs often mention that they refer the patient to another provider for either consultation or specialized management (see Chapters 8 and 11). There is no sense that managing patient situations by themselves is a point of honor for APNs. A family NP was told by a patient that the fact that she called a dermatologist for advice on how to handle a persistent rash was one of the reasons he trusted her so much. He said, "You know what you know, and you know what you don't know. I like that." One gets the same sense from talking to patients who have received care from CNMs; one woman said, "She didn't take any chances with me or my baby. She just got on the phone and called the obstetrician—and she was right." CNMs and CRNAs have worked closely with physicians for years and are quite clear regarding what they can manage independently and when they need to consult, comanage, or refer.

Experienced APNs who are in joint practices with physicians find them an important source of affirmation for the nursing perspective that APNs bring to care. APNs report that consultation is just as likely to consist of the physician's seeking the APN's opinion as it is the APN's seeking the physician's opinion. For the new APN, a carefully chosen joint practice provides ready consultation as well as opportunities for case review and discussions. Joint practice can make available to patients the benefits of different perspectives on care and can result in patients' being linked with the provider who has the interests and skills that correspond with their needs.

APNs who work in settings with APN peers report that relationships within the group are important sources of support and professional growth (Winch, 1989). Although many APNs work in geographical areas where peers are a considerable distance away, electronic communication has the potential to increase opportunities for dialogue and mutual support.

EDUCATIONAL STRATEGIES

The education of APNs should consider the health-care problems and needs of the population the graduates of the program will serve, the expressed preferences of the public, the health-care policy of the state and the nation, and the competencies set forth by professional nursing organizations and national commissions. In this brief discussion, selected issues that pertain directly to the four characteristics of APN practice discussed in this chapter are addressed.

HOLISTIC PERSPECTIVE

When student APNs begin to have learning experiences in the expanded domain of advanced practice (i.e., assessment and management of medical problems), they often experience a deterioration in their comfort level, motor skills, interviewing competency, and clinical problem-solving ability. As they become more competent in the new domain, they eventually emerge and recognize that they want to retain the holistic perspective from their basic nursing education and career experiences. They don't want to simply diagnose and treat disease; they want to continue to attend to how patients are responding to disease and to the effects patients' social and physical environments have on their illness, and they want to continue to be responsive to the health problems patients experience in their daily lives. Part of the solution may be to address the continued importance of a holistic perspective up front and to encourage students to evaluate the different perspectives they observe in their clinical placements.

Unfortunately, the theoretical, empirical, and educational literatures are rather silent on how the medical and nursing perspectives can be brought together. A first thought may be that what is needed is to learn how to unite cognitively the purposes of diagnosing and treating patients' disease-based problems with the purposes of helping patients adjust to and cope with their experiences of development, parenting, aging, and illness. But union of the two perspectives on health and health care may not be possible, or even desirable, because the two perspectives have very different philosophical assumptions, traditions, and assessment interests that inform the design of medical and nursing curricula and affect role socialization. Each perspective has something unique to contribute to health care. Perhaps what should be pursued is facility with both perspectives and awareness of when to use one rather than the other. Although one cannot take the nursing perspective out of the APN, some issues patients raise during health-care encounters may be better addressed by emphasizing the diagnostic processes and therapeutic approaches characteristic of the medical perspective. Other issues are likely to be better addressed by the holistic, functional perspective characterized by the nursing view of the patient. Until the blending of the two perspectives is better understood, the most effective strategy is to approach and think about patient care within a holistic framework but recognize that when disease-related issues surface, it is necessary to think in a more causal way. The holistic framework is the most helpful for seeing issues from patients' perspectives and for seeing the relationship between disease and illness, but the linear cause-and-effect perspective may be necessary when underlying disease processes need to be considered. Dialogue on interdisciplinary education and demonstration projects that evaluate effects of interdisciplinary education of APNs and physicians is likely to illuminate this discussion (Larson, 1995).

Allan and Hall (1988) contrasted the technocratic framework of health care (i.e., the medical model) with the ecological framework of health care. The ecological model focuses on the interaction between the person and the environment and quality-of-life issues. The three major concepts that distinguish the ecological viewpoint are environment, holism, and process. Newman's (1994) conceptual model of health as expanding consciousness is one of several ecological theories in nursing. It provides a useful way of thinking about patients' experiences, about how people develop lifestyle patterns that affect their well-being, and about how people's choices can bring about expanding consciousness; it also suggests new ways of helping patients. However, this author does not find Newman's model particularly helpful for deliberating on how to join the medical and the holistic perspectives, because it places considerable emphasis on refraining from fixing things and letting go of personal control. It doesn't take into account the reality that many diseases are highly treatable using technological interventions. Yet, the ecological paradigm has generated ideas that could eventually result in the evolution of a new holistic framework that brings together person-environment interaction care and disease-focused care.

PARTNERSHIPS WITH PATIENTS

Creating partnerships with patients, refraining from dominating patients, and helping patients be self-determining are values that are taught in basic education, yet student APNs need opportunities to revisit these values and strategize about how they can enact them in their busy day. After a discussion of person-centered communication and conversational interviewing in one of this author's classes, students reflected on taped interviews they had had with patients, and several realized how controlling they had been. The assignment moved them to alter drastically their approaches to assessment interviewing.

CLINICAL REASONING

There are learning strategies that can be used to assist students in becoming good clinical thinkers. First, it is important to recognize that expert clinical reasoning is more than arriving at a correct diagnosis, even though that is an important objective. Expert clinical reasoning also requires that the practitioner use communication competency as a medium of practice and be sensitive to the broader contexts in which disease, illness, and individual responses occur. To produce broad-based, discriminating, and proficient clinical thinkers, some combination of the following learning experiences is most likely needed: substantive clinical content, top-down sensitizing concepts and theories,[4] bottom-up case analysis, experiential learning assignments, self-directed study, practice in evaluating clinical research, and mentored clinical experiences in actual practice.

One approach to bottom-up case analysis is problem-based learning (PBL), in which the student is guided through standardized cases by the tutor-teacher (Barrows & Pickell, 1991). The tutor is responsible for the process of learning, not for content. In PBL, the tutor guides students through analysis and synthesis by pushing them to identify what they know, what they do not know, and what resources they will have to use to acquire the information they need to manage a case. During the ensuing week, the students are expected to acquire the needed information so that they can continue analysis and synthesis at a more informed level. Evaluations of PBL indicate that it produces more self-motivated learners than do traditional learning methods and that students prefer it to traditional methods (Vernon & Blake, 1993). The evidence regarding its effect on clinical performance suggests that PBL does result in a higher level of clinical functioning, although this is not a consistent finding across all applications of PBL (Moore, Block, Style, & Mitchell, 1994; Vernon & Blake, 1993).

Like PBL, experiential learning requires students to be active learners, and it is also particularly useful in helping students approach care from an entirely new perspective. In this learning method, assignments require students to try an ap-

---

[4]Definition of the situation, adaptation, and culture-sensitive care are examples of concepts that can be used to think about how to design education for particular patients. Irritable infant syndrome theory (Keefe, 1988), the theory of passage through infertility treatment (Blenner, 1990), and the interaction model of client health behavior (Cox, 1982) are examples of midrange theories that can be used to plan care.

proach to care or intervention that they haven't previously used and then to reflect on whether the approach has advantages over the method they are currently using (Jarvis, 1987). For example, an assignment might require students to conduct several health assessments to try out different interview formats—conversational assessment interviewing, functional health assessment, and a comprehensive health history. The reflection phase of experiential learning is crucial in helping students evaluate whether (and how) they should incorporate the method into their practices.

DIVERSE APPROACHES TO MANAGEMENT

Graduate school should be a time when APN students expand their repertoire of interventions. They learn new skills and therapies and refine and expand existing ones. In a course taught by this author, students are required to use several interventions that are not in their current repertoire. They are also required to evaluate the research base regarding the intervention and to report back to the class on their experiences in learning and using the new intervention. One student tried foot reflexology, another used a transcutaneous nerve stimulation unit for a certain kind of pain, and another used guided imagery with adolescents in a psychiatric unit who were experiencing difficulty settling for sleep at bedtime. Students frequently expressed that the assignment forced them to try a new intervention and that the learning experience made them recognize the importance of continuing to expand their repertoire of interventions. In summary, if graduate APN students are to begin to demonstrate the four qualities of direct care described in this chapter, they need a broad range of learning experiences (see Table 6–4).

EVALUATION STRATEGIES

Evaluation of APNs' direct care competencies can be conducted at the individual practitioner level, at the multidisciplinary or group practice level, or at one of several health-care systems levels. Regardless of the level, the task of evaluating direct care practice is extremely complicated in terms of both criteria (or standard) setting and methodology. Hamric (1989) and Koetters (1989) have described evaluation strategies that APNs may find useful.

At the individual practitioner level, site-based peer review (Winch, 1989) on a daily, informal basis as well as on a more formal basis and periodic assessment of patient satisfaction with services would seem to be the most efficacious approaches. Case review by peers can be a helpful learning experience as well as a check on

TABLE 6–4. LEARNING EXPERIENCES TO DEVELOP CLINICAL REASONING

Exposure to substantive clinical content
Practice using concepts and theories as thinking tools
Tutored bottom-up case analysis
Experiential learning assignments
Self-directed study
Discussion and debriefing of clinical decision making
Research critique and integrative review practice
Mentored clinical practice

quality, but it should be included in the structure of the practice, not left to individual initiative. Assessment of patient satisfaction, in the form of either periodic questionnaires or focus groups, can help individual practitioners and group practices stay in touch with the populations they serve as well as provide information about whether patients' needs are being met.

At the organization level, the Pew Health Professions Commission (1993) recognized continuous quality improvement (CQI) as a model that evaluates past performance yet emphasizes a continuous striving for future quality. One advantage of the model is that it recognizes the shared responsibilities of the whole organization (i.e., top management, middle management, support departments, and direct care providers) in determining the quality of care provided by an organization. Participation in CQI gives APNs an opportunity to voice their views of health care and ensure that humanistic care is one objective of the organization's decision making, planning, and activities.

Rigorous, scientific evaluation of the quality of the direct care provided by APNs is particularly difficult (Brown & Grimes, 1993). Studies that link the processes of care provided by APNs to desired outcomes are needed to establish that the unique aspects of advanced nursing practice have positive effects on clients' well-being. In addition, patient outcomes such as functional status, quality of life, and avoidance of illness need to be examined (Crosby, Ventura, & Feldman, 1987).

CONCLUSION

APNs are currently providing direct health-care services that

1. Are qualitatively different from those provided by other health-care professionals,
2. Positively affect patient health-care outcomes,
3. Achieve equal or superior health outcomes when compared with similar services provided by physicians, and
4. Are cost-effective.

In spite of research and anecdotal evidence supporting these claims, health maintenance organizations, hospitals, long-term care facilities, and home care agencies rarely feature APN providers in marketing strategies. This neglect is financially unwise, because many people who have experienced ANP health care value it as an alternative, or complement, to traditional medical care and are quick to recommend it to others. Thus, the demand often grows once ANP services are introduced. The CNM role is the major exception to facilities' disregard of marketing of advanced nursing practice, in that the availability of CNMs within a hospital-based obstetrical service is often presented as an asset in local media advertisements and hospital promotional literature. One reason for this is that the childbearing public values holistic, humanistic care, so there is demand for the service. Unfortunately, in the same care systems that promote CNM services, there are often CNSs, NPs, and CRNAs whose presence and services are neither promoted nor used to solicit patients. Perhaps these APNs need to push for greater promotion of their services by the organizations for whom they work, rather than relying on patients discovering them incidentally.

Despite the invisibility of APNs and ANP practice, there is sufficient evidence to warrant the nursing profession's confidence that its commitment to advanced practice roles is well founded. APNs need to continue to base their direct care on the holistic perspective, partnerships with patients, expert clinical reasoning, and the use of diverse management approaches. Together, these qualities provide a solid foundation for providing high-quality, humanistic health care.

REFERENCES

Allan, J. D., & Hall, B. A. (1988). Challenging the focus on technology: A critique of the medical model in a changing health care system. *Advances in Nursing Science, 10*(3), 22–34.

Avorn, J., Everitt, D. E., & Baker, M. W. (1991). The neglected medical history and therapeutic choices for abdominal pain. *Archives of Internal Medicine, 151,* 694–698.

Baird, S. B., & Prouty, M. P. (1989). Administratively enhancing CNS contributions. In A. B. Hamric & J. A. Spross (Eds.), *The clinical nurse specialist in theory and practice* (2nd ed., pp. 261–284). Philadelphia, PA: W. B. Saunders Company.

Barrows, H. S., & Pickell, G. C. (1991). *Developing clinical problem-solving skills.* New York: Norton.

Bates, B. (1987). *A guide to physical examination and history taking.* Philadelphia, PA: J. B. Lippincott.

Benner, P. (1984). *From novice to expert: Excellence and power in clinical practice.* Menlo Park, CA: Addison-Wesley.

Benner, P., & Tanner, C. (1987). Clinical judgment: How expert nurses use intuition. *American Journal of Nursing, 87,* 23–31.

Benner, P., & Wrubel, J. (1989). *The primacy of caring: Stress and coping in health and illness.* Menlo Park, CA: Addison-Wesley.

Blenner, J. L. (1990). Passage through infertility treatment: A stage theory. *Image: The Journal of Nursing Scholarship, 22,* 153–158.

Boyd, C. O., & Munhall, P. L. (1989). A qualitative investigation of reassurance. *Holistic Nursing Practice, 4*(1), 61–69.

Brown, S. A., & Grimes, D. E. (1993). *Nurse practitioners and certified nurse-midwives: A meta-analysis of studies on nurses in primary care roles.* Washington, DC: American Nurses Publishing.

Brown, S. J. (1990). Tailoring nursing care to the individual client: An analysis of client-nurse dialogue. *Dissertation Abstracts International, 51*(10), 4774B. (University Microfilms No. 9106506)

Brown, S. J. (1992). Tailoring nursing care to the individual client: Empirical challenge of a theoretical concept. *Research in Nursing & Health, 15,* 39–46.

Brown, S. J. (1994). Communication strategies used by an expert nurse. *Clinical Nursing Research, 3*(1), 43–56.

Brown, S. J. (1995). An interviewing style for nursing assessment. *Journal of Advanced Nursing, 21,* 340–343.

Brykczynski, K. A. (1989). An interpretive study describing the clinical judgment of nurse practitioners. *Scholarly Inquiry for Nursing Practice: An International Journal, 3,* 75–104.

Brykczynski, K. A. (1991). Judgment strategies for coping with ambiguous clinical situations encountered in primary family care. *Journal of the American Academy of Nurse Practitioners, 3*(2), 79–84.

Burton, D. (1995). Agency maze. In I. M. Lubkin (Ed.), *Chronic illness: Impact and interventions* (3rd ed., pp. 457–480). Boston: Jones & Bartlett.

Carnevali, D. L., & Thomas, M. D. (1993). *Diagnostic reasoning and treatment decision making in nursing.* Philadelphia, PA: J. B. Lippincott.

Carrieri, V. K., & Janson-Bjerklie, S. (1986). Strategies patients use to manage the sensation of dyspnea. *Western Journal of Nursing Research, 8,* 284–305.

Corbin, J. M., & Strauss, A. L. (1984). Collaboration: Couples working together to manage chronic illness. *Image: The Journal of Nursing Scholarship, 16,* 109–115.

Corbin, J. M., & Strauss, A. (1992). A nursing model for chronic illness management based upon the trajectory framework. In P. Woog (Ed.), *The chronic illness trajectory framework: The Corbin and Strauss nursing model* (pp. 9–28). New York: Springer Publishing Company.

Corcoran, S. (1986). Decisional analysis: A step-by-step guide for making clinical decisions. *Nursing & Health Care, 7,* 149–154.

Cox, C. L. (1982). An interaction model of client health behavior: Theoretical prescription for nursing. *Advances in Nursing Science, 5*(1), 41–56.

Crosby, F., Ventura, M. R., & Feldman, M. J. (1987). Future research recommendations for establishing NP effectiveness. *Nurse Practitioner, 12,* 75–79.

Daleiden, A. L. (1993). The CNS as trauma case manager: A new frontier. *Clinical Nurse Specialist, 7,* 295–298.

Damato, E. G., Dill, P. Z., Gennaro, S., Brown, L. P., York, R., & Brooten, D. (1993). The association between CNS direct care time and total time and very low birth weight infant outcomes. *Clinical Nurse Specialist, 7,* 75–79.

Elder, R. G., & Bullough, B. (1990). Nurse practitioners and clinical nurse specialists: Are the roles merging? *Clinical Nurse Specialist, 4,* 78–84.

Fenton, M. V., & Brykczynski, K. A. (1993). Qualitative distinctions and similarities in the practice of clinical nurse specialists and nurse practitioners. *Journal of Professional Nursing, 9,* 313–326.

Gaynor, S. E. (1990). The long haul: The effect of home care on the caregiver. *Image: The Journal of Nursing Scholarship, 22,* 208–212.

Gerteis, M., Edgman-Levitan, S., Daley, J., & Delbanco, T. L. (1993). *Through the patient's eyes: Understanding and promoting patient-centered care.* San Francisco: Jossey-Bass.

Gift, A. G. (1993). Dyspnea. *Nursing Clinics of North America, 25,* 955–965.

Gordon, M. (1994). *Nursing diagnosis: Process and application* (3rd ed.). St. Louis, MO: Mosby.

Greene, M. G., Adelman, R. D., Friedmann, E., & Charon, R. (1994). Older patient satisfaction with communication during an initial medical encounter. *Social Science and Medicine, 38,* 1279–1288.

Griffith, H. M., & Robinson, K. R. (1993). Current procedural terminology (CPT) coded services provided by nurse specialists. *Image: The Journal of Nursing Scholarship, 25,* 178–186.

Hall, B. A., & Allan, J. D. (1994). Self in relation: A prolegomenon for holistic nursing. *Nursing Outlook, 2,* 162–170.

Hamric, A. B. (1989). A model for CNS evaluation. In A. B. Hamric & J. A. Spross (Eds.), *The clinical nurse specialist in theory and practice* (2nd ed., pp. 83–196). Philadelphia, PA: W. B. Saunders Company.

Herth, K. A. (1989). The relationship between level of hope and level of coping response and other variables in patients with cancer. *Oncology Nursing Forum, 16,* 67–72.

Hilton, B. A. (1993). Issues, problems, and challenges for families coping with breast cancer. *Seminars in Oncology Nursing, 9,* 88–100.

Iowa Intervention Project. (1993). The NIC taxonomy structure. *Image: The Journal of Nursing Scholarship, 25,* 187–192.

Jarvis, P. (1987). Meaningful and meaningless experience: Towards an analysis of learning from life. *Adult Education Quarterly, 37,* 164–172.

Johnson, R. (1993). Nurse practitioner-patient discourse: Uncovering the voice of nursing in primary care practice. *Scholarly Inquiry for Nursing Practice: An International Journal, 7,* 143–163.

Johnston-Taylor, E., Jones, P., & Burns, M. (1995). In I. M. Lubkin (Ed.), *Chronic illness: Impact and interventions* (3rd ed., pp. 193–212). Boston: Jones & Bartlett.

Kasch, C. R. (1984). Interpersonal competence and communication in the delivery of nursing care. *Advances in Nursing Science, 6*(2), 71–88.

Keefe, M. R. (1988). Irritable infant syndrome. *Advances in Nursing Science, 10*(3), 70–78.

Kinney, C. K., & Erickson, H. C. (1990). Modeling the client's world: A way to holistic care. *Issues in Mental Health Nursing, 11,* 93–108.

Koetters, T. L. (1989). Clinical practice and direct patient care. In A. B. Hamric & J. A. Spross (Eds.), *The clinical nurse specialist in theory and practice* (2nd ed., pp. 107–124). Philadelphia, PA: W. B. Saunders Company.

Laizner, A. M., Yost, L. M., Barg, F. K., & McCorkle, R. (1993). Needs of family caregivers of persons with cancer: A review. *Seminars in Oncology Nursing, 9,* 114–120.

Larson, E. L. (1995). New rules for the game: Interdisciplinary education for health professionals. *Nursing Outlook, 43,* 180–185.

Lauver, D. (1992). A theory of care-seeking behavior. *Image: The Journal of Nursing Scholarship, 24,* 281–287.

Lawrence, M. (1995). The unconscious experience. *American Journal of Critical Care, 4,* 227–232.

Loomis, M. E., & Conco, D. (1991). Patients' perceptions of health, chronic illness, and nursing diagnoses. *Nursing Diagnosis, 2,* 162–170.

Lynaugh, J. E. (1988). Narrow passageways: Nurses and physicians in conflict and concert since 1875. In N. H. P. King, L. R. Churchill, & A. C. Cross (Eds.), *The physician as captain of the ship: A critical reappraisal* (pp. 23–37). Boston: D. Reidel.

Mast, M. E. (1995). Adult uncertainty in illness: A critical review of research. *Scholarly Inquiry for Nursing Practice: An International Journal, 9,* 3–24.

Mattingly, C., & Fleming, M. H. (1994). *Clinical reasoning: Forms of inquiry in a therapeutic practice.* Philadelphia, PA: F. A. Davis.

McMillan, S. C., Heusinkveld, K. B., & Spray, J. (1995). Advanced practice in oncology nursing: A role delineation study. *Oncology Nursing Forum, 22,* 41–50.

Miller, J. F. (1992). *Coping with chronic illness* (2nd ed.). Philadelphia, PA: F. A. Davis.

Moore, G. T., Block, S. D., Style, C. B., & Mitchell, R. (1994). The influence of the new pathway curriculum on Harvard medical students. *Academic Medicine, 69,* 983–989.

Morten, A., Kohl, D., O'Mahoney, P., & Pelosi, K. (1991). Certified nurse-midwifery care of the postpartum client: A descriptive study. *Journal of Nurse-Midwifery, 36,* 276–288.

Naylor, M. D., & Brooten, D. (1993). State of the science: The roles and function of clinical nurse specialists. *Image: The Journal of Nursing Scholarship, 25,* 73–78.

Neufeld, K. R., Degner, L. F., & Dick, J. A. (1993). A nursing intervention strategy to foster patient involvement in treatment decisions. *Oncology Nursing Forum, 20,* 631–635.

Newman, M. A. (1994). *Health as expanding con-*

sciousness (2nd ed., Publication No. 14-2626). New York: National League for Nursing.

Northouse, L. L., & Peters-Golden, H. (1993). Cancer and the family: Strategies to assist spouses. *Seminars in Oncology Nursing, 9,* 74–82.

O'Neill, E. S. (1994). Home health nurses' use of base rate information in diagnostic reasoning. *Advances in Nursing Science, 17*(2), 77–85.

Pauker, S. G., & McNeill, B. J. (1981). Impact of patient preference on the selection of therapy. *Journal of Chronic Disease, 34,* 77–86.

Pew Health Professions Commission. (1993). *Resource book for health professions education strategic planning and policy development.* San Francisco: University of California, San Francisco, Center for the Health Professions.

Popkess-Vawter, S. (1991). Wellness nursing diagnosis: To be or not to be? *Nursing Diagnosis, 2,* 19–25.

Pugh, L. C., & Milligan, R. (1993). A framework for the study of childbearing fatigue. *Advances in Nursing Science, 15*(4), 60–70.

Rodin, J., & Janis, I. L. (1982). The social influence of physicians and other health care practitioners as agents of change. In H. S. Friedman & M. R. DiMatteo (Eds.), *Interpersonal issues in health care* (pp. 33–49). New York: Academic Press.

Safreit, B. J. (1992). Health care dollars and regulatory sense: The roles of advanced practice nursing. *Yale Journal of Regulation, 9,* 417–488.

Scheff, T. J. (1963). Decision rules, types of error, and their consequences in medical diagnosis. *Behavioral Science, 8,* 97–108.

Schön, D. A. (1983). *The reflective practitioner: How professionals think in action.* New York: Basic Books.

Siegler, E. L., & Whitney, F. W. (1994). Education of physicians and nurses. In E. L. Siegler & F. W. Whitney (Eds.), *Nurse-physician collaboration: Care of adults and elderly* (pp. 11–20). New York: Springer Publishing Company.

Simon, H. (1969). *The science of the artificial.* Cambridge, MA: MIT Press.

Smith, S. (1988). An analysis of the phenomenon of deterioration in the critically ill. *Image: The Journal of Nursing Scholarship, 20,* 12–15.

Smith, T. C. (1991). A structured process to credential nurses with advanced practice skills. *Journal of Nursing Quality Assurance, 5*(3), 40–51.

Squier, R. W. (1990). A model of empathic understanding and adherence to treatment regimens in practitioner-patient relationships. *Social Science and Medicine, 30,* 325–339.

Steele, B., & Shaver, J. (1992). The dyspnea experience: Nocioceptive properties and a model for research and practice. *Advances in Nursing Science, 15*(1), 64–76.

Steele, S., & Fenton, M. V. (1988). Expert practice of clinical nurse specialists. *Clinical Nurse Specialist, 2,* 45–52.

Tanner, C. A., Benner, P., Chesla, C., & Gordon, D. R. (1993). The phenomenology of knowing the patient. *Image: The Journal of Nursing Scholarship, 25,* 273–280.

Thibodeau, J. A., & Hawkins, J. W. (1994). Moving toward a nursing model in advanced practice. *Western Journal of Nursing Research, 16,* 205–218.

Vernon, D. T., & Blake, R. L. (1993). Does problem-based learning work? A meta-analysis of evaluative research. *Academic Medicine, 68,* 550–563.

White, J. E., Nativio, D. G., Kobert, S. N., & Engberg, S. J. (1992). Content and process in clinical decision-making by nurse practitioners. *Image: The Journal of Nursing Scholarship, 24,* 153–158.

Winch, A. E. (1989). Peer support and peer review. In A. B. Hamric & J. A. Spross (Eds.), *The clinical nurse specialist in theory and practice* (pp. 299–321). Philadelphia, PA: W. B. Saunders Company.

CHAPTER **7**

Expert Coaching and Guidance

Ellen B. Clarke
Judith A. Spross

INTRODUCTION

Patient education is a central and well-documented function of all nurses. Patient and other types of education provided by advanced practice nurses (APNs) are best conceptualized as interpersonal processes of coaching through transition. In this chapter the use of the terms *coach* and *coaching,* rather than *patient education,* is deliberate, because these terms imply the existence of a relationship that is fundamental to effective teaching. Coaching people through transitions is a relatively invisible, intangible, but complex process that must be made more explicit if APNs are to be seen by consumers and policy-makers as a solution to health policy concerns such as access to and continuity of care and if they are to secure reimbursement for their care. Because numerous resources exist to help APNs develop and implement educational programs for individuals and groups, this chapter describes the coaching competence of APNs and strategies for acquiring and using the skills needed to coach effectively. The authors synthesize their own advanced practice and teaching experiences with theoretical, research, and clinical literature to develop a picture of coaching through transitions as the complex, interpersonal process APNs use to enlist clients' active and effective participation in their care. Although the focus is on coaching of patients and families, the processes of coaching can also be applied to student and staff education.

PATIENT EDUCATION: SELECTED LITERATURE REVIEW

Research has demonstrated that effective patient education is associated with improved patient outcomes in diverse populations, including persons with diabetes or hypertension, people undergoing surgery and procedures, and women preparing for childbirth. Research and anecdotal reports indicate that teaching is a core function and clinical activity of advanced nursing practice (ANP) (Brooten et al., 1991; Brown & Waybrant, 1988; Mezey, Dougherty, Wade, Mersmann, 1994; Priest, 1989). According to a number of studies, one outcome of care provided by APNs is increased patient knowledge (Alexander, Younger, Cohen, & Crawford, 1988; Brooten et al., 1988; Brooten et al., 1986; Lipman, 1986; Office of Technology Assessment, 1986; Pozen et al., 1977). These and other studies (Brown & Waybrant, 1988; Brykczynski, 1989; Davis, Sawin, & Dunn, 1993; Fenton, 1984, 1985; Fenton & Brykczynski, 1993) suggest that APNs build on and extend the teaching/coaching functions that Benner (1984) identified as characteristic of the practice of experts by experience.

Redman (1988) described patient education as a complex set of interactions that include a diversity of subtasks and approaches. What and how to teach patients and how to help them cope with or master their health concerns have long been concerns of nurses in basic and advanced practice. Studies on client education were among the earliest types of clinical research performed by nurses. Much of what is considered standard practice in nursing, such as preparing patients for procedures and surgery by providing sensory, procedural, and other information, is based on a program of research initiated by Johnson and her colleagues (e.g., Johnson, Rice, Fuller, & Endress, 1978; Leventhal & Johnson, 1983) and replicated and extended by subsequent investigators.

Sufficient research on patient education exists to indicate how teaching should be done and that it influences outcomes. In an integrative review of research on patient education, Lindemann (1988) found that most teaching strategies—booklet, programmed instruction, modeling, lecture, and discussion—are effective. Although this may be an artifact of various research designs, it may also underscore the strength of patient education as an intervention. A meta-analysis of patient teaching strategies revealed that nine strategies had small to moderate effect sizes (Theis & Johnson, 1995). The largest effect sizes were associated with structured approaches, reinforcement, independent study, and multiple strategies. Regardless of a strategy's effect size, all subjects in experimental groups had better outcomes than did those in control groups. In a meta-analysis of 84 experimental studies, Heater, Becker, and Olson (1988) evaluated the effectiveness of patient education for 4,000 subjects, including neonates, preterm infants, preschool children, grade school children, adolescents, new parents, parents and infants, adults, and elderly. They concluded that the average subject in an experimental group had a better outcome than did 72% of the subjects in comparison groups. Improved outcomes occurred in the cognitive (knowledge), behavioral, physiological, and psychosocial areas.

Many studies document the content and amount of time APNs spend in teaching and counseling as well as the outcomes of these interventions (see Chapter 26 for more detail on outcome studies). Studies of nurse practitioners (NPs) indicate that they spend a significant proportion of their direct care time in teaching and counseling (Brown, 1995; Brown & Waybrant, 1988; Draye & Pesznecker, 1980; Mezey, Dougherty, Wade, & Mersmann, 1994). Health promotion topics covered by NPs include diet, exercise, smoking cessation, family planning, and stress management (Brown & Waybrant, 1988). Teaching and counseling are significant clinical activities in nurse-midwifery practice (Scupholme, Paine, Lang, Kumar, & DeJoseph, 1994; Scupholme & Walsh, 1994). In the Quality-Cost Model of Early Discharge and Nurse Specialist Transitional Care, teaching and counseling are provided during face-to-face contacts in the home as well as through regular telephone contact; these services are regarded as critical (Brooten, Kumar, Brown, et al., 1986). Analysis of clinical nurse specialists' (CNSs') interventions revealed that 68% could be categorized as teaching; other types of interventions were liaison, consultation, and referral; encouragement of self-care and infant care; and reassurance and reinforcement of client actions (Brooten, Gennaro, Knapp et al., 1991).

Smith (1989) believed that managed care and cost containment were likely to increase the focus on patient education as a means of improving effectiveness and efficiency and achieving cost and quality outcomes. If patient education is this effective, as the above reports suggest, and if efficient patient education is one of the solutions to reducing the costs of health care, more needs to be understood about the process of patient teaching used by APNs and how it promotes adherence to therapies and self-care. Given the research-based evidence of the effectiveness of nurses' and APNs' patient education, some investigators have questioned why the nature, process, and characteristics of nurse-client interactions have rarely been the focus of research on patient teaching and patient adherence to therapies (Kasch, 1983; Schwartz-Barcott, Fortin, & Kim, 1994; Squier, 1990).

The foregoing review, though not exhaustive, supports the authors' premise that expert guidance and coaching are key foci of the APN's direct care role. APNs' coaching of clients as it is described in this chapter assumes an understanding of basic principles of education and an awareness of the research on which patient education is based. APNs are responsible for knowing the theoretical and scientific bases for patient teaching in their specialties and practice settings. For many specialties, this literature is substantial. Examples of the APN's integration of specialty knowledge with principles of patient education to operationalize the coaching competency are incorporated into the chapters on the different ANP roles in Part III.

COACHING THROUGH TRANSITIONS: A SYNTHESIS OF THEORETICAL PERSPECTIVES

COACHING: AN INTERDISCIPLINARY PERSPECTIVE

The word *coach* is derived from the Middle English word, *coche,* meaning "wagon or carriage, a means of conveyance from one destination to another." The advent of horse-drawn carriages made journeys less arduous for travelers, who no longer had to travel by foot or on horseback. The coach also offered protection from the elements and a modicum of safety and security. Other advantages of travel by coach might have included the comfort of having fellow travelers and being driven by a knowledgeable guide who knew the route well enough to ensure timely arrival at one's destination. Modern usage of *coach* to mean a teacher is apt—a coach facilitates the safe passage of a person in transition from one situation to another. Coaching is complex interpersonal work that helps people who are facing equally complex personal transitions or journeys. These meanings of coaching can be applied to nurse-patient, faculty-student, preceptor-student, and mentor-protégé relationships.

Coaching has been used by several disciplines to describe interactions between experts and learners that focus on developing the learner's knowledge and skill in an area that is within the coach's expertise (Spross, 1994). The following literature summary is based on a more extensive review (Spross, 1994). The review supports the use of *coach* and *coaching* as terms that describe the teaching functions of APNs better than the term *patient education*. The fact that *coach* and *coaching* are common terms may also make it easier for APNs to communicate with consumers and policy-makers about what it is they do.

In cognitive psychology, social skills tutoring (Frisch, Elliott, Atsaides, Salva, & Denny, 1982) and interpersonal cognitive problem solving (Hops, 1983) are coaching techniques that have been used to improve individuals' social skills, language skills, and problem-solving abilities. Both techniques include direct verbal instructions in problem-solving principles. Interpersonal cognitive problem solving also emphasizes thinking processes such as identifying problems, generating alternative solutions, and anticipating the consequences of solutions (Pelligrini & Urbain, 1985).

Adler's (1985) description of the art of coaching in music conveyed the depth of human connection needed between coach and singer:

> *The specific art of coaching lies in the ability to deeply feel the singer's intentions and artistry . . . to attune oneself to [her style]; to recognize the singer's shortcomings and to make up for them by extending a helping hand to lead [her], giving her a sense of . . . mastery and matching it by following [her]. . . . Coaching is a continuous give and take, a molding of two personalities into one. . . . A coach must try to search for and understand where the*

> *roots of [the singer's individuality and being] lie. Faith . . . is one of the strongest roots; faith in oneself is part of it; another root is [the ability to compensate] for shortcomings in one's makeup . . . [another root is] sensitivity. . . . Without sensitivity, the ability to feel influences from without and within and to [transform them], there can be no becoming.* (p. 82)

Participation in sports affects an athlete's personal development physically, cognitively, psychologically, and affectively (Lombardo, 1987). The coach creates and presents complex challenges for athletes to develop these capacities while simultaneously providing support and motivation (Sullivan & Wilson, 1991). Coaches are expected to have technical competence, interpersonal skills, and leadership skills. Lombardo (1987) described humanistic coaches as those who are not only competent but also secure in their self-concepts and self-accepting, so that they are able to focus on strengthening the athlete's performance and self-concept. Such coaches help athletes believe in themselves; through coaching, athletes learn that they are trustworthy, responsible, capable of self-direction, and able to identify relevant goals.

Heifetz' (1994) work on leadership illuminates Lombardo's (1987) description of humanistic coaching. According to Heifetz, leadership is "mobilizing people to tackle tough problems" (p. 15). Situations that require leadership or expert coaching are those in which the problems are complex—a technical solution is unavailable, and would be inadequate anyway, and the problem demands adaptive work (Heifetz, 1994). Leaders identify the adaptive task (see Chapter 10). Leadership, as a type of coaching, can be viewed as helping people uncover opportunities for personal growth through transitions by helping them clarify their goals, decide what matters most to them, acknowledge tradeoffs and losses, and develop coping strategies. Becoming a parent, losing a job, adjusting to and living with a chronic illness, and facing impending death are examples of transitions requiring complex, adaptive work that can be facilitated by APNs. APNs prepare the way or help clients break a trail in making the adjustments needed to facilitate transitions.

In a qualitative study of nurses' clinical experiences, Benner (1984) identified the teaching-coaching role as one of seven domains of nursing practice. Subsequent studies, based on Benner's work, have confirmed that APNs demonstrate this role as part of their practice (Fenton, 1984; Fenton & Brykczynski, 1993; Steele & Fenton, 1988). Benner (1985) elaborated on the teaching-coaching role of APNs who work with patients with chronic illness: "Coaches learn what the illness means to the individual, what the adaptive demands, tasks, and resources are for the patient at different stages in the illness" (p. 43). APNs use their knowledge of a patient as well as knowledge from past experiences with similar patients to craft patient-specific coaching interventions. Benner's description of coaching by nurses is consistent with the concepts of coaching from other disciplines discussed above.

Several studies of patient education done by nurses in basic and advanced practice indicate that the nurse-patient relationship is the basis for successful educational interventions (Benner, 1984; Fenton, 1984; Lamb & Stempel, 1994; Morgan, 1994; Steele & Fenton, 1988). A patient who happened to be a communications expert also believed that interpersonal competence was the major determinant of a nurse's effectiveness (Kasch & Lisnek, 1984). He further believed that this competence explained NPs' effectiveness.

In a phenomenological study of nurses, nurse-patient interaction and the development of rapport were foundational in accomplishing patient education (Morgan, 1994). In a study of public health nurses, de la Cuesta (1994) affirmed that relationships or therapeutic alliances with patients had an important enabling function—the relationship was seen as "a medium or vehicle for achieving goals" (p. 452) and as having a mediating function that allowed the nurse to adopt conflicting roles (e.g., being able to point out the patient's self-neglect behaviors while supporting the patient as a person or intervening to help the patient accomplish self-care goals).

Lamb and Stempel's (1994) qualitative study of patients' experiences with nurse case management offers additional insight. The basic social process that emerged was that patients became "their own insider-experts" (Lamb & Stempel, p. 9). This process consisted of three intrapersonal and interpersonal phases: bonding, working, and changing. Lamb and Stempel noted that "the demonstration of concern appears to be a key factor in triggering cognitive change" (p. 10). Once the nurse was seen as both expert and insider, the working phase could begin. Patients were willing to examine relationships among their attitudes, behaviors, illness exacerbations, and use of health-care resources. Affective and cognitive changes occurred that enabled patients to see themselves and their situations differently. Patients reported that changes in self-image, changes in meaning, and mastery occurred throughout the process. As mentioned, many patients became their own insider-experts, skilled at identifying changes in illness patterns, selecting self-care interventions that were likely to work, and using the health-care system in a timely and appropriate way.

In describing coaching as the interpersonal process nurses use to help those who suffer, Spross (1996) summarized the elements of the nurse-patient relationship connoted by the term *coaching:*

> *Coaching captures the essence of the relationships nurses create with patients on which their effectiveness depends. . . . It is a term that permits the experience of intense emotions on both sides; it captures the temporal nature of the relationship (which may be brief or extended); it suggests both the one-sided aspect (the coach has information and expertise needed by the patient) and the mutuality (opportunities for personal growth) in the relationship; and it conveys the contractual or voluntary nature of the relationship (if the relationship is not working despite the best efforts of both, another coach may need to be found). (pp. 294–295)*

From the literature on coaching, then, one can clearly see that it is a multidimensional process for the coach and the learner and involves the many aspects of being human—cognitive, affective, behavioral, physical, social, and spiritual.

If the goals of health care are preventing future illness, decreasing chronicity, limiting relapses or exacerbations of illnesses, alleviating suffering, and responding to crises, why is the quality of provider-patient relationships not given more priority, at least as much as is given to technological treatments? This compelling question led Squier (1990) to analyze existing literature from a variety of disciplines (which included studies of APNs) and propose a model linking a clinician's empathic understanding with a patient's adherence to therapeutic regimens. Squier proposed that empathic understanding has two components: cognitive and affective. Clinicians' cognitive ability to take accurately the perspective of the patient, even in situations where it is not obvious, enables them to communicate effectively, reflecting this understanding back to the patient. Patients are then more likely to elaborate their experiences of the concern that brought them to the clinician. Clinicians' emotional sensitivity to the patient's emotions and underlying concerns helps reduce the anxiety and stress that often affect the presenting health problem. Clinicians' cognitive and affective processes occur in parallel but influence each other. Squier further described phases of the clinician-patient consultation and the client outcomes associated with each phase, the ultimate outcome being improved adherence to preventive and therapeutic strategies (self-care) and beneficial health outcomes. Although Squier did not use the terms *coach* and *coaching,* his model is congruent with the ideas proposed herein. Squier sufficiently explicated his model that the concepts of coaching proposed in this chapter could be tested using it.

TRANSITIONS

The word *transition* comes from the Latin *transitus,* meaning "to go across, to pass over or go through." Transition is further defined in the dictionary as "the process or instance of changing from one form, state, activity, or place to another." In music, a transition is a modulation or a passage connecting two themes. The musical connotations of transition are interesting and relevant to the authors' use of transition. As the concept of coaching through transitions is further described, APNs' efforts to make connections and to modulate (adjust, adapt, and shape) individuals' experiences of health and illness will become clear.

Transitions—physiological, developmental, situational, and organizational—make up the natural course of human lives. Throughout life, personal growth involves periodic accelerations, modulations, and transformations (Bridges, 1980). Transitions are paradigms for life and living—"dangerous opportunities" in Chinese culture. Like life, they may be predictable or unpredictable, joyous or painful, obvious or barely perceptible, chosen and welcomed or unexpected and feared. Bridges (1980) described three phases of transition: an ending or leaving; a period of chaos, confusion, and distress; and a new beginning. Bridges indicated that for some, "transitionality" may be a semipermanent state (see Chapter 12 for further discussion of Bridges's work).

Schumacher and Meleis (1994) asserted that transition is a central concept in nursing, and Chick and Meleis (1986) offered a clinically useful definition of it:

> Transition is a passage from one life phase, condition, or status to another. . . . Transition refers to both the process and outcome of complex person-environment interactions. It may involve more than one person and is embedded in the context and the situation. (pp. 239–240)

Like Bridges (1980), Chick and Meleis (1986) characterized the process of transition as having phases during which individuals experience (1) a disconnectedness from their usual social supports, (2) a loss of familiar reference points, (3) old needs that remain unmet, (4) new needs, and (5) old expectations that are no longer congruent with the changing situation. Thus, transition is a passage or movement from one state, condition, or place to another. Many of the clinical phenomena addressed by nurses can be considered transitions. Becoming a parent, giving up cigarettes, learning how to cope with chronic illness, and dying in comfort and dignity are just a few examples. Transitions can also be characterized according to type, conditions, and universal properties. Schumacher and Meleis (1994) identified nursing therapeutics that support or facilitate transitions, and education was one of them.

Other models also inform the present conceptualization of APN coaching through transition. Corbin and Strauss's (1992) *chronic illness trajectory framework* is a model derived from qualitative research on chronic illnesses. A chronic illness has a course that varies and changes over time. Nurses collaborate with patients and families in "shaping and managing" illness trajectories through nursing interventions such as teaching. Braden's (1990, 1993) *self-help model* emerged from several quantitative studies that tested hypotheses from three different learning theories. Braden's program of research led to the elucidation of five stages of response to chronic illness and the testing of interventions to facilitate the acquisition of self-help behaviors. Connelly's (1993) *self-care in chronic illness model* is a research-based adaptation and extension of the health belief model, which identified variables that influence self-care. Lamm, Dungan, and Hiromoto (1991) described processes that would ease the transition from entry into the health-care system for an acute problem to home. These processes included counseling, social support, and teaching/learning. Common to all of these models are teaching and mobilizing social support to accomplish health- and illness-related outcomes. Thus, this discussion of APN coaching draws on and extends the theoretical work and research of Meleis and her colleagues and others to support the idea of coaching through transitions as a practice focus.

A Typology of Transitions

On the basis of their review of the literature, Schumacher and Meleis (1994) proposed that there are four categories of transitions in which nurses are involved: developmental, health/illness, situational, and organizational. *Developmental* transitions are those that reflect life cycle transitions, such as adolescence, parenthood, and aging. For the purposes of discussing APN coaching, the authors consider developmental transitions to include any intrapersonally focused transition, including changes in life cycle, self-perception, motivation, expectations, or meanings. *Health/illness* transitions were described by Schumacher and Meleis (1994) primarily as illness related, ranging from adapting to a chronic illness to being discharged from the hospital to home. In this chapter, health/illness transitions are defined as transitions that are driven by an individual's experience of the body in a holistic sense. Such transitions can include modifying risk factors, adapting to a chronic illness, adapting to the physiological and psychological demands of pregnancy, and numerous other clinical phenomena. Some health/illness changes are self-limiting (e.g., the physiological changes of pregnancy), whereas others are long-term or chronic, reversible or irreversible. Although Schumacher and Meleis excluded acute self-limiting illnesses (e.g., a cold) from the notion of transition, other variables are likely to influence whether a transition occurs in illnesses that are usually self-limited (e.g., if the cold prevents the person from attending an important event). Changes in educational, professional, or family roles were given as examples of *situational* transitions by Schumacher and Meleis (1994). The authors also include situational transitions occurring as a result of changes in intangible or tangible structures or resources (e.g., role changes and financial reversals) that are specific to individuals and their relationships. *Organizational* transitions were defined as those that occur in the environment—within agencies, between agencies, or in society. Organizational transitions reflect changes in structures and resources but at a system level. The first three types of transitions are the ones most likely to lead to clinical encounters between APNs and patients in which expert coaching is required. However, APNs must also be skilled at dealing with organizational transitions, which tend to affect structural and contextual aspects of providing care (see Chapter 12). Wise APNs pay attention to all four types of transitions in their personal and professional lives, because transitions can affect the development and effectiveness of APNs' expert coaching.

The APN is also aware of the possibility of multiple transitions occurring as a result of one salient transition. While eliciting information on the primary transition that led the client to seek care, the APN is attending to verbal, nonverbal, and intuitive cues to identify other transitions and meanings associated with the primary one. Attending to the possibility of multiple transitions enables the APN to tailor coaching to the individual's particular needs and concerns. Table 7–1 lists some situations, based on this typology, that require APN coaching.

Characteristics, Conditions, and Outcomes of Transitions

Transitions can be characterized along the dimensions of time, the nature of the process that occurs, and the type of change that occurs (Schumacher & Meleis, 1994). All transitions seem to have a temporal nature; that is, they unfold over time, as opposed to being a one-time event. A single event may precipitate the transition, but the transition is experienced over some period of time. The process that occurs is directional, entailing movement from one state to another, and is often described as occurring in stages. The third characteristic is the type of change that occurs. The change tends to be substantive and internal, rather than incidental or superficial; transitions affect personal identities, roles, relationships, functional status, and behaviors (Schumacher & Meleis, 1994). The experience of transition can vary considerably from one individual, group, or organization to the next as a result of conditions affecting the transition (Corbin & Strauss, 1992; Schumacher & Meleis, 1994). Regardless of the type of change that occurs, similar conditions seem to

TABLE 7–1. TRANSITION SITUATIONS THAT REQUIRE COACHING

Health/Illness	Developmental	Situational	Organizational
Pregnancy/labor	Parenting	Job loss or change	Mergers
Hospitalization	Puberty	Divorce	Policy changes
Risk reduction	Suffering	Natural disasters	Change in leadership
Lifestyle changes	Loss of significant others	Quality of life	Change in organizational
Chronic illness	Caregiving for elderly	Change in social supports	structure
Disability	relatives	Social isolation	
Weight loss or gain	Changes in sexual function	Financial reversals or	
Symptoms	or activity	windfalls	
Violence		Change in living situations	

Note. The situations are categorized according to the initiating change. Many of these transitions have reciprocal impacts across categories.

influence transitions. These conditions include meanings, expectations, motivation, level of knowledge and skill, the environment, level of planning, and well-being.

Outcomes of transitions proposed by Schumacher and Meleis (1994) included subjective well-being, role mastery, and well-being of relationships. Quality-of-care outcomes could also be used as indicators of successful transitions. When one considers the direct, individual effects of APN coaching, the most relevant outcomes are those that are patient-related. These could be traditional or emerging clinical outcomes, such as morbidity; mortality; medical complications; comfort; functional, physiological, or mental status; stress level; coping strategies; quality of life; patient satisfaction; and caregiver burden (Kolcaba, 1992; Lang & Marek, 1992; Naylor, Munro, & Brooten, 1991; Peplau, 1994). Other outcomes might examine effective self-care related to health promotion, health maintenance, illness prevention and management, and chronic illness management. Although some researchers are beginning to study intrapersonal phenomena that might be considered outcomes of coaching, such as meaning (e.g., Steeves & Kahn, 1987) and self-transcendence (Reed, 1991), more work is needed on how to assess such outcomes. Organizational or cost outcomes that might be affected by coaching processes include lengths of stay, costs of care, proportion of services that receive reimbursement, and use of health-care services (Lang & Marek, 1992; Naylor, Munro, & Brooten, 1991).

This description of transitions as a focus for APN coaching underscores the need for, and the importance of, a holistic orientation when helping individuals address their health and illness concerns. This conceptualization of transition together with the principles of change discussed in Chapter 10 can also transform APNs' approaches to teaching their patients, staff, and students.

THE FOUNDATIONS OF COACHING THROUGH TRANSITIONS

A MODEL OF APNS' EXPERT COACHING AND GUIDANCE

On the basis of the patient education literature and the theoretical perspectives on coaching and transition presented earlier, a definition of APN coaching can be offered. APN coaching may be defined as a complex, dynamic, collaborative, and holistic interpersonal process that is mediated by the APN-patient relationship and the APN's self-reflective skills. APNs integrate self-reflection and the technical, clinical, and interpersonal competencies they have acquired through graduate education and experience with patients' understandings, experiences, and goals in order to shape transitional experiences and accomplish therapeutic and educational goals.

Expert coaching by APNs depends on the interaction of four factors: clinical competence, technical competence, interpersonal competence, and self-reflection (Fig. 1). (Graduate education is assumed.) It is the interaction of self-reflection with these three areas of competence that drives the ongoing expansion and refinement of expertise in advanced nursing practice.

TECHNICAL COMPETENCE AND CLINICAL COMPETENCE

Several assumptions that underlie this model of APNs' coaching and guiding must be made explicit. First, the entire discussion of coaching assumes the integration

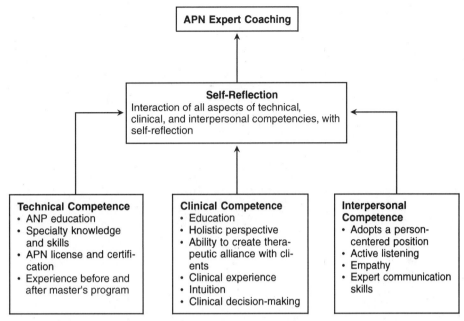

FIGURE 7–1. The coaching competency of an advanced practice nurse (APN).

of the client's significant other or the client's proxy as appropriate. Second, although technical competence and clinical competence may be sufficient to teach a task, they are insufficient to coach patients through transitions. For example, diabetic persons may be taught how to monitor their blood sugar and administer insulin with technical accuracy, but if the impact of the transition from health to chronic illness that requires major lifestyle changes is not evaluated, then coaching and guidance cannot occur.

The third assumption is that the APN's skill as an expert coach and guide depends on a combination of clinical experience with a particular population and graduate education (see also Chapter 3). Although the expert by experience is able to coach effectively, the clinical and didactic content of graduate education extends the APN's repertoire of assessment skills, technical skills, interpersonal behaviors, and self-reflection abilities, enabling the APN to coach in situations that are broader in scope or more complex in nature. APNs are also able to be more explicit about the processes and outcomes of coaching.

The final assumption is that the basis for expert APN coaching is the interaction of interpersonal, technical, and clinical competence with self-reflection. Expert coaching requires that APNs be self-aware and be able to self-reflect *as an interpersonal transaction is unfolding,* so that they can shape communications and behaviors to maximize the therapeutic and educational goals of the clinical encounter. Being able to self-reflect and focus on the process of coaching as it is occurring implies that APNs are also capable of the simultaneous execution of other physical, cognitive, and intuitive skills, such as assessment, physical examination, interpretation, and attendance to both their own noncognitive reactions and those of the client. One might compare the process to a speech's being translated into several languages as it is being given; the difference is that the multiple simultaneous translations are being carried out by one APN, not several translators. De la Cuesta (1994) characterized this as the " 'product' [or outcome] taking shape or being 'manufactured' in the very process of the interaction" (p. 457). This aspect of APNs' practice is not particularly visible, but it accounts for their effectiveness.

The importance of technical and clinical competence to coaching cannot be overestimated. However, these two factors are not addressed in detail in this chapter. The evolution of specialties in advanced nursing practice has focused on defining and describing the technical and clinical skills required for advanced practice with particular populations. Chapter 1 documents this aspect of the evolutions of various ANP roles. In addition, chapters on specific ANP roles (e.g., Part III) illustrate the specificity of technical and clinical skills APNs are expected to acquire through their educational programs. The need for technical and clinical competence is an explicit and often well-defined aspect of established ANP roles.

An important part of clinical competence is clinical experience with the populations that are the APN's focus. Pre-graduate school experiences, experiences within the clinical practica of graduate programs, and post-master's clinical experiences provide the grist for analyzing, developing, and making explicit the coaching competency of APNs. Ongoing development of the APN's coaching competency depends on applying self-reflection to clinical experiences in order to acquire new coaching knowledge and skills that cannot be found in any textbook. Benner (1991) defined experience from a phenomenological perspective as "the turning around, the adding of nuance, the amending or changing of preconceived notions or perceptions of the situation" (p. 2). Over the course of caring for patients, nurses learn the many ways people experience and manage health, birth, illness, pain, suffering, and death (Benner, 1985). These clinical experiences help them identify coaching alternatives that help other patients understand, learn, change, modulate, and control experiences of transitions.

INTERPERSONAL COMPETENCE

Nurse theorists have described the importance of the nurse-patient relationship to effective nursing care (e.g., Peplau, 1952, 1994; Travelbee, 1971). Graduate education should extend and refine interpersonal skills acquired in basic nursing education. Interpersonal interactions can be characterized as position centered or person centered (Bernstein, 1974; Kasch & Knutson, 1985; Kasch & Dine, 1988). Position-centered interpersonal interactions are characterized by dependence on roles and rules and the use of power and authority. A person-centered encounter is characterized by an appreciation for the uniqueness of the individuals involved (the nurse and the patient) and attention to the patient's concerns. Person-centered clinicians are able to bridge the differences between themselves and their clients through communication (Kasch & Dine, 1988). It is their adoption of a person-centered style of interaction that enables APNs to be effective coaches.

Behavioral, cognitive, and affective processes are essential to the person-centered approach to coaching. APNs using a person-centered approach are highly skilled at eliciting information from clients, encouraging self-disclosure, and responding empathetically (Kasch & Dine, 1988). The APN is "fully present" to another person (Davis, 1981). Such presencing transcends role obligations inherent in position-centered approaches; nurses reveal themselves and are attentive with their eyes, tone of voice, affect, body language, and silences. Younger (1995) described such presencing as "being in tune with the patient's messages" so that the patient's alienation begins to dissolve as she or he experiences being heard. Being present in this way is a confirmation of a person's existence and is an expression of concern and caring (Drew, 1986).

In interacting with clients, APNs adopt an open, flexible, nonhierarchical stance and communicate this verbally and behaviorally. Brown (1995) characterized this style of interacting as "conversational interviewing." Other verbal and nonverbal skills that characterize a person-centered approach to interviewing have been identified by Quirk and Casey (1995). Verbal skills include the use of open-ended questions and paraphrasing to convey the APN's inferences regarding the thoughts and feelings underlying the patient's actions and communications and to validate the APN's perception of the patient's message. APNs summarize, recap, and interpret as they coach. They collaborate with the patient to maintain the direction of the interview while listening patiently. Nonverbal skills identified by Quirk and Casey include a tone of voice and pace of speech appropriate to the topic being discussed; the use of eye contact; and a relaxed, forward-leaning posture. Nonverbal behaviors and the sharing of power are the primary means by which APNs convey respect for their clients. Throughout interactions, APNs convey an attitude of openness, elicit and respond to feelings, express concern, confirm the patient's experience, and provide positive reinforcement (Quirk & Casey, 1995).

This approach to interactions enables APNs to bridge the differences between themselves and their clients, and to accurately take the patient's perspective and respond empathically (Squier, 1990). Through effective communication with and assessment of the patient, APNs can see the situation from the patient's point of view (Kasch, 1983; Kasch & Dine, 1988; Squier, 1990). They do not assume they understand the patient's perspective; they validate their understanding with the patient. Once validated with the patient, the APN's ability to understand the patient's perspective comes from a holistic view of human functioning (body, mind, spirit). This view is informed by the APN's education in the biopsychosocial sciences and experiences with patients with similar problems or concerns (Benner, 1985). Most nurses, when taught about interpersonal communication, learn to maintain a professional distance. A person-centered approach challenges this idea. Rather than keep the nurse-as-person out of the interaction, coaching demands that the nurse not be distant but emotionally responsive. Martocchio (1987) emphasized the importance of the nurse's competence as both a professional and a person; the nurse and patient enter the relationship as whole persons, complete with talents, goals, needs, and wishes, but the focus of the interpersonal process is on addressing the patient's potentials and goals. APNs who rely only on the scientific/technical (cognitive) competencies in their relationships with patients are unlikely to enable patients to express themselves holistically. The APN "who withholds parts of herself [or himself] is unlikely to allow the patient to emerge as a whole, or to comprehend that wholeness if it does emerge" (Gadow, 1980, p. 87). In a position-centered interpersonal interaction, patients become discouraged and are less likely to disclose relevant information; they may lose their motivation and be less likely to follow the APN's recommendations. If patients are to be coached effectively in making transitions that are genuinely their own, both the nurse and the patient must enter the relationship as whole persons. A person-centered approach demands an involved, current, individualized, contextual understanding of the patient (Tanner, Benner, Chesla, & Gordon, 1993).

SELF-REFLECTION

Self-reflection is the deliberate, internal examination of experience in order to learn from it. The APN uses self-reflection during interactions with patients as well as retrospectively. Schön (1983) described these as "reflection-in-action" and "reflection-on-action." Reflection-in-action is the ability to pay attention to phenomena as they are occurring, giving free rein to one's intuitive understanding of the situation as it is unfolding. This type of reflection requires skill and courage and involves three functions: exploration, more testing, and hypothesis testing. It is not a mindset that follows only familiar patterns of thought. It is more like the flexible and inventive mind of a jazz musician, who can attend to what is happening in the moment and respond with a varied repertoire of exploratory and transforming actions. The heart of reflective practice is action and paradox, not generalized scripts and certainty (Grimmett, 1988). In the APN-client relationship, it is simultaneously doing and learning and coming to know. Reflection-in-action can be compared to the Zen concept of mindfulness (Tremmel, 1993). *Mindfulness* means paying attention to "right here, right now" and investing the present moment with full concentration. Reflection-in-action, or mindfulness, involves awareness of the world, awareness of the self acting in the world, and awareness of being aware.

Looking within involves listening to one's own thinking processes; it is part of preparing for and enacting reflective practice (Pugach & Johnson, 1990). Extending the work done by Jackson (1986) on expert teaching, APN coaches might be characterized as those who "see more" than nonexperts do. "Seeing more" refers to the practice of "paying attention" (Jackson, 1986). APNs are alive to possibilities—within patients, within the processes of the clinical encounter, and within themselves. They anticipate what might happen during the encounter or after the patient leaves. They are sensitive to incipient difficulty: "Their senses are fully tuned to what is going on around them. They are not easily rattled" (Jackson, 1986, p. 87). APNs' sensibilities, processes (including reflection), and skills interact to shape their interactions with patients, to support patients, and to enable patients to navigate transitions to achieve mutually determined goals. Action without reflection becomes automatic; there can be no transformation in the absence of action with reflection (Freire, 1970).

The capacity to reflect mindfully in action and on action is not readily mastered and requires continuous practice (Tremmel, 1993). However, certain qualities and characteristics can be developed to facilitate self-reflection. These include motivation, commitment, open-mindedness, self-awareness, the ability to describe phenomena or situations, critical analysis, and the ability to synthesize and evaluate (Atkins & Murphy, 1994). It is important to pay attention to both positive and negative experiences. What made this effective? Why didn't this work? APNs may be more likely to reflect on negative experiences than to reflect on positive experiences, because the feeling of failure is more uncomfortable than the feeling of satisfaction or success. However, reflecting on satisfying, successful experiences can provide clues to interventions that will be effective in future interactions. One of the key aspects of self-reflection is paying attention to feelings. Experienced nurses and APNs are more likely than inexperienced ones to pay attention to feelings or intuitions. However, novice APNs need to be taught to recognize that their affective responses to situations are clues to developing their expertise as clinicians and coaches.

COACHING ASSESSMENT, PROCESSES, AND OUTCOMES

ASSESSMENT

Patient assessment is the basis for determining which coaching interventions will be used. APNs use whatever physical and psychological assessment procedures, skills, or tools they need to evaluate the patient's presenting concerns. They understand that assessments have two purposes: (1) establishing and building a relationship and (2) collecting data. They make conscious efforts to build a relationship that will work by conveying caring and concern, being honest and dependable, and displaying professional knowledge and self-confidence. The person-centered approach adopted by nurses has been described by several researchers as *"knowing the patient"* (Jenny & Logan, 1992; Tanner, Benner, Chesla, & Gordon, 1993). This entails getting to know the patient as a person and learning the patient's pattern of responses, including habits, practices, preferences, usual demeanor, and self-presentation (Jenny & Logan, 1992).

The person-centered approach must be extended beyond the individuals to consider the communities and social milieu in which clients live and in which health care is provided, since social and contextual variables often influence the APN's ability to provide effective care. Thus, a vital aspect of knowing the patient and one neglected in previous models of the nurse-patient relationship (Carper, 1978; Jacobs-Kramer & Chinn, 1988) as well as in graduate education is what White (1995) calls "sociopolitical knowing." Past models of the nurse-patient relationship focused on the intimacy of the nurse-patient interaction (e.g., Peplau, 1952; Travelbee, 1971). Sociopolitical knowing includes an understanding of the social and political context of the patient as well as the broader context in which nursing and health care take place. Both the APN's and the patient's cultural and political location powerfully influence their understandings of health, illness, language, identity, social roles, and historical issues. For example, domestic violence, child abuse, malnutrition, substance abuse, and stress-induced illnesses are responses to political, social, and personal problems. Both Steven (1989) and Chopoorian (1986) emphasize the need for nurses to provide a vocal critique of how domination, alienation, poverty, homelessness, and unemployment affect the health of persons and communities. APNs may find that coaching their clients requires that they expose, provoke, and problematize social and political inequities that affect people's health (Hagedorn, 1995; Kendall, 1992). Otherwise the core issues in many patients' transitions will be invisible and unidentified and the coaching strategies employed will be superficial, unfocused, and ineffective.

In addition to getting to know the patient and using strategic communication, APNs use their observations of themselves, the patients, and the interactive process to decode patients' behaviors and the content of their communications for significance (Kasch & Dine, 1988). They need to grasp the patient's perspective, including salient aspects of the patient's self-definition (Olesen, Schatzman, Droes, Hatton, & Chico, 1990). This understanding is critical for selecting coaching behaviors to use with people who need to make lifestyle changes to reduce risk or manage chronic illness.

Several conditions influence the experience of transition and its unfolding (Corbin & Strauss, 1992; Schumacher & Meleis, 1994). Meaning and expectations are subjective phenomena that affect the anticipation and experience of transition (Schumacher & Meleis, 1994). While many transition conditions can be affected by prior experience, meanings and expectations may be the ones most colored by memories and past experiences. Meanings may be positive, negative, or neutral. Regardless of whether the meaning is positive or negative, patients may experience uncertainty, grief, guilt, stress, or other emotional responses. Expectations may be accurate and realistic, or they may be unrealistic, even fantastic. Cognitive variables such as knowledge, self-care skills, motivation, coping style, habitual stressors, and personal preferences for control affect people's experience of and ability to accept, adjust to, or adapt to transitional experiences (Brooten, Gennaro, Knapp, et al., 1991; Corbin & Strauss, 1993; Jenny & Logan, 1992; Kasch & Dine, 1988; Schumacher & Meleis, 1994). The environment, including resources, relationships, social support, setting of care, and contextual variables can mediate transitions (Brooten, Gennaro, Knapp, et al., 1991; Corbin & Strauss, 1992; Schumacher & Meleis, 1994). Role demands and responsibilities that may interfere with therapeutic self-care need to be identified (Connelly, 1993). Level of planning, including problem and need identification; organization of phase-related interventions; and communication influence the success of the transition. Physical and emotional well-being also determine how the transition process is experienced (Schumacher & Meleis, 1994). The nature of the health concern; the degree of symptomatology, perceived vulnerability, and seriousness; and the degree of predictability or certainty about one's experience of the body can make for smooth or chaotic transitions.

APNs identify missing information that they might need for coaching and variables that might enhance or hinder coaching. Throughout the interaction, they try to regulate distress (Heifetz, 1994), respond to patients' needs for information, and create a physically and interpersonally comforting environment (Kasch & Lisnek, 1984). For example, the APN might observe that a patient is becoming fatigued during an examination. In addition to providing for rest and changing the pace of the examination, the causes, duration, and significance of the fatigue will be explored.

Several points can be made about the assessment aspects of coaching through transitions. First, not every encounter will involve a transition; many encounters will be self-limiting. Even in these more routine situations, the APN's coaching competence can result in efficient care delivery, improved patient satisfaction, and return business, all valued outcomes in managed care environments. Second, not every individual immersed in a transitional situation is interested in moving or adjusting; a person can become stuck or immobilized by the demands of the transition. APNs can often help patients who are immobilized. Indeed, these are often the patients for whom the help of an experienced APN is sought by physicians, staff nurses, or novice APNs. By working effectively with difficult cases, APNs expand their repertoire of coaching interventions. Some patients who are stuck simply need a new coach—someone with a different approach or personality. A smaller population may be help rejectors; in this case, coaching is unlikely to be effective and patients can only be "maintained." Third, whereas some conscious patients may reject help, noncommunicative patients can often be coached effectively. For example, the APN who is providing palliative care to a person who is dying talks to the person about letting go, reviews aspects of the patient's life, and provides comforting touch interventions. The APN observes responses that indicate relaxation and peace (e.g., less restlessness and moaning).

PROCESSES AND OUTCOMES

Coaching processes used by APNs focus on fostering involvement, choice, and independence. One study of patient education suggested that a continuum of nurse-patient interactions exists, from simple interactions to decrease anxiety to complex ones such as counseling to enhance problem-solving skills (Morgan, 1994). Benner (1985) elaborated on APNs' coaching behaviors. In coaching a patient, APNs have four main tasks: interpreting unfamiliar diagnostic and treatment demands, coaching the patient through alienated stances (e.g., anger and hopelessness), identifying changing relevance as demands or symptoms of the illness change, and ensuring that cure is enhanced by care. These tasks can be accomplished through coaching processes. Both processes and outcomes can be categorized by focus: bodily or physical, affective/interpersonal/spiritual, cognitive/behavioral, and social. Processes and outcomes derived from the literature review presented earlier and references found in Spross (1996) are listed in Table 7–2. This categorization is merely a device to illustrate the range of coaching behaviors and related outcomes. In reality, coaching is a holistic process, and although there is a primary focus or target, coaching behaviors often have effects across all dimensions of the patient's experience.

APNs attend to issues of timing and sequencing in teaching and counseling patients. Thus, they may need to coach the patient to become motivated before beginning to teach the patient a particular task. APNs integrate coaching into processes of consultation, collaboration, and referral. They use their knowing the patient to mobilize resources and interpret the patient's needs to team members, consultants, and family caregivers. Knowing the patient enables APNs to take risks, adopt stances that are unusual or unpopular, and make the system work in order to shape patients' transitional experiences, a quality of APN direct care that has been described as "fearlessness" (Koetters, 1989).

DEVELOPMENT OF APNS' COACHING COMPETENCE

As noted, becoming an expert coach requires a rich combination of education, experience, interpersonal competence, and self-reflection on one's practice. It is not a technical skill; technical skill is insufficient "in the swampy lowland [of clinical practice] where situations are confusing 'messes' " (Schön, 1983, p. 42). Although scientific and technical knowledge are essential for effective coaching, it is in the coaching of clients that the art of advanced nursing practice is fully expressed. APNs need a highly nuanced range of interpersonal skills to coach people through multifaceted transitions. The strategies used to develop coaching expertise are designed to groom reflective practice and a person-oriented interactive style. These are foundational abilities that APNs must develop to become skilled coaches.

TABLE 7–2. ADVANCED PRACTICE NURSES' COACHING PROCESSES AND POSSIBLE OUTCOMES

Dominant Focus	Coaching Processes	Possible Outcomes*
Physical	Using comforting touch Demonstrating self-care or self-monitoring skills Describing the likely physical trajectory of the health or illness concern, including physical and psychological demands, tasks, and resources Describing the possibilities inherent in the physical transitions experienced Interpreting the person's experiences of the body Offering alternative (e.g., more hopeful) interpretations of bodily sensations/functions Implementing pain and symptom management Providing hygiene and toileting and conducting invasive procedures and other physical interventions while preserving dignity Identifying risk factors Offering strategies to modify risk factors	Effective self-care (e.g., fewer symptoms) Improved functional status Improved mental status (e.g., as a result of decreased pain or normalized blood sugars)
Affective, interpersonal, spiritual	Accepting the person as he or she is Acknowledging the person's courage, strength, or other personal qualities Acknowledging both expressed and possible fears and concerns Attuning oneself to client's needs and goals Being available/presencing Being honest Bonding, establishing a therapeutic alliance Comforting through touch, behavior, and interactions Counseling Eliciting expectations, fears, meanings, and values Enabling Encouraging, praising Ensuring safe passage Expressing confidence in clients and their abilities Inspiring/inspiriting Listening Keeping a vigil Making a commitment to help Offering hope Reassuring Supporting Validating	Acceptance of help from others Decreased anxiety, stress, or uncertainty Hope Improved quality of life Increased ability to initiate self-care Increased comfort, decreased suffering Revised future agendas Self-acceptance Self-report of satisfaction with decision making Self-transcendence

TABLE 7–2. ADVANCED PRACTICE NURSES' COACHING PROCESSES AND POSSIBLE OUTCOMES *Continued*

Dominant Focus	Coaching Processes	Possible Outcomes*
Cognitive, behavioral	Challenging Coaching in communication and technical skills Communicating strategically Confronting and identifying contradictions Dealing with conflict Demonstrating and role-modeling Explaining Guiding, offering a map Identifying adaptive tasks Identifying the goals of interventions Improving problem-solving skills Mediating Monitoring Motivating Negotiating Offering options Organizing goals Presenting challenges Providing cognitive strategies to alter negative thought patterns Providing feedback Reframing expectations, goals, and meanings Setting tasks Using a variety of teaching strategies Using humor	Behavior change Decreased stress Effective self-care and problem solving related to clinical issues Effective use of cognitive coping strategies Improved functional status Improved quality of life
Social	Advocating Bonding Collaborating with the client and with other providers Facilitating important relationships Interpreting patients' behaviors, needs, and goals to members of the health-care team and patients' families Keeping tradition Mobilizing community, financial, and social resources Strengthening social supports through teaching, consultation, and referral	Affection Comfort Coordinated care Decreased caregiver burden Decreased costs of care Improved satisfaction with care Improved self-care Satisfaction with social support

From Spross, J.A. (1996). Coaching and suffering: The role of the nurse in helping people face illness. In B.R. Ferrell (Ed.), *The human dimensions of suffering* (Table 8.3, pp. 198–199). Boston: Jones & Bartlett. The reader is encouraged to refer to that publication for additional references from which the coaching processes were derived.
*Although most outcomes are client/family related, some systems outcomes are included to help readers connect the individual coaching by advanced practice nurses with organization-level outcomes.

GRADUATE NURSING EDUCATION: THE INFLUENCE OF FACULTY AND PRECEPTORS

Graduate faculty and clinical preceptors are highly influential models for APN students seeking to develop coaching skills. A key step in assisting APN students to develop as coaches is for faculty to be reflective and assess their own educational experiences. In particular, faculty need to name and evaluate the processes and pedagogies to which they were exposed, distinguishing between effective, respectful experiences of being taught/coached and ineffective, disrespectful ones. Students who have been effectively coached by teachers and preceptors will know experientially what respectful coaching "feels like." They will be more likely to reproduce these behaviors with patients. Schön (1987) calls this the "Hall of Mirrors" effect—the teacher, in the very process of supervising and coaching the student, exemplifies the coaching repertoire that the student is attempting to acquire. If ineffective, disrespectful teaching is recognized for what it is—a position-centered style—then students also learn how not to coach.

Clinical preceptors play a particularly salient role with APN students. In effect, there is a "double exposure" to coaching: the student experiences being coached and observes how patients are coached by the preceptor. Similarly, preceptors need to be able to coach students while coaching patients. The authors believe that a person-centered style of interaction on the part of the preceptor is just as important to developing the APN student's coaching skills as it is to helping clients accomplish their health goals. It is possible to have preceptors who use a person-centered style of interaction with clients, yet because of their own student experiences, adopt a position-centered style of interacting with students. Very experienced APNs can be novice preceptors (Meng & Morris, 1995), so that preceptors themselves may need coaching by faculty to develop in their preceptor roles. Davis, Sawin, and Dunn (1993) identified strategies preceptors should employ to create the best conditions for learning: using orientation strategies; managing the clinical environment to decrease student anxiety; and optimizing patient, student, and preceptor interactions. Just as APNs tailor their coaching to meet individual client needs, so APN preceptors need to tailor their coaching of students to the level of the student and the situation (Davis, Sawin, & Dunn, 1993).

Faculty and APN preceptors need to be explicit with students in articulating the range of coaching strategies used in the classroom and the clinical area. In this way, the student learns the components of coaching. What was ineffable and undervalued in the process of coaching becomes defined, contextualized, reproducible, and valued (McKinnon & Erickson, 1988). Developing coaching competence requires attention to all ways of knowing, including personal knowing (Diemert Moch, 1990). Therefore, faculty and APN preceptors need to encourage students to pay close attention to their experiences. APN students should reflect on their past educational experiences, identifying and evaluating effective and ineffective coaching that they experienced. Bringing these educational moments to full consciousness and naming them is a key first step to envisioning coaching processes the students want to emulate or discard.

STRATEGIES FOR DEVELOPING COACHING COMPETENCE

Coaching activities can be conceptualized along two dimensions: the degree of structure and the focus. Activities may be very structured (e.g., a lecture) or unstructured (e.g., storytelling). The focus of the APN's coaching may be individuals or groups. Table 7–3 organizes teaching activities and strategies along these dimensions. These strategies can be used to foster the development of coaching processes and can also be used to evaluate the APN's competence at coaching.

Less traditional teaching strategies must be used if one is to enlarge the APN student's interpersonal repertoire and self-reflective abilities. Expressive writing (Fulwiler, 1987; Sorrell, 1994; Van Manen, 1989) enables the student to recapture important experiences in nursing and reflect on them to arrive at new insights and interpretations. Keeping a journal and poetry writing are examples of expressive writing. Storytelling is another expressive strategy in which stories, the products of reflection, are relayed orally. Storytelling can build community and mutual respect among nurses (Lindesmith & McWeeny, 1994). Sharing stories from practice enables APN students to establish a shared history, and provides a means of offering and receiving support. The process promotes critical thinking, strengthens collegiality, and builds self-esteem and rapport (Lindesmith & McWeeny, 1994). One author (Spross) included journal writing as a teaching strategy in courses on role development. The journals were not graded. Through the students' writings and the instructor's responses, salient experiences were debriefed, a process described by Davies (1995). Sometimes debriefing consisted of the instructor's written response to the student's reflections. Other times, with the student's permission, the journal entries became the focus of a seminar discussion. Students' reflections on the

TABLE 7–3. EDUCATIONAL STRATEGIES TO DEVELOP THE COACHING SKILLS OF THE ADVANCED PRACTICE NURSE

Individual	Group
Unstructured	
Coaching	Discussion group
Debriefing	Grand rounds
Discovery	Online communication
Experiential learning	Storytelling
Expressive writing (e.g., poetry)	Support groups
Use of humor	Use of movies/media with a health-care theme
Individual clinical supervision	Walking rounds
Journal keeping	
Mentoring	
Peer coaching	
Reading about others' health-care experiences	
Support for risk taking	
Structured	
Chart review	Continuing education programs
Critical incidents/exemplars	Group patient education
Demonstrations	In-services
Clear, immediate feedback on strengths *and* areas for growth	Lecture
Competency-based instruction	Orientation
Computer-assisted learning	Staff development
Individualized media (e.g., patient education booklets and self-study programs)	Standardized curricula
Objective tests	Standardized patient teaching plans
Practice laboratories	
Precepting	
Self-learning modules	

experience of being new or uncertain of their skills led to discussions of developmental tasks such as embracing novicehood or learning to trust one's hands, heart, gut, and observations. Through journals and storytelling, cues and strategies for coaching used by different APN students and preceptors became available to a larger group of learners.

Aesthetic approaches to developing interpersonal competence can also develop APNs' coaching skills. The intense insights that can come from reading poetry and literature or watching a movie are often unexplored ways of knowing. Some of the most profound aesthetic experiences in which nurses are involved can never be known through the limitations imposed by scientific and transactional writing. The acutely personal, reflective nature of poetry especially captures for nurses the person-oriented stance of interpersonal interaction that is required in APN coaching. Introducing students to relevant poetry and literature have been potent triggers for reflective practice. For example, one of the authors (Clarke) had the experience of being invited to bring a short piece of prose, a poem, or a song that was meaningful to her. Students could volunteer to share the piece with the class. When a student volunteered, the teacher coached the student in the process of delivering the piece effectively by focusing and calming the student, demonstrating the process, standing close to the student, and offering encouragement. Similarly, movies with plots revolving around illness or disability, such as *Heart Sounds* and *Regarding Henry*, can help APN students evaluate ineffective and effective interpersonal styles and articulate the gaps in care that might have been met by an APN.

One of the authors (Clarke) integrated aesthetic approaches into a 3-credit graduate course on pathophysiology. The basic sciences and clinical features of various pathologies were presented to teach students "what disease is." Poetry and literature were used to help students understand the lived experience of illness—"What it is like for a person to have this disease." These educational experiences and take-home tests that incorporated patient stories (cases) enabled students to acquire the hybrid of knowledge *and* clinical experience that Benner (1985) described as essential for APN coaching. Other uses of art can be considered to explicate coaching.

Additional strategies and resources are available to APNs interested in refining their coaching skills: peer coaching (Robbins, 1991), thinking aloud (Corcoran & Moreland, 1988), and mentoring (Daloz, 1986).

CONCLUSIONS

APNs coach patients through transitions. In the APN, graduate education and technical, clinical, and interpersonal competence interact with self-reflection to produce a diverse set of coaching skills and the ability to invent new coaching processes in the midst of novel clinical encounters. This is an extremely complex skill that relies on APNs' human and professional qualities. Although coaching processes occur simultaneously, they are not automatic. APNs can usually describe the intent of coaching interventions and explain their selection of one approach over another. What may seem automatic is actually very deliberate; the APN has learned what has worked in similar encounters and uses it over and over. In using a person-centered style with a patient, the APN remains open to cues that the approach may not work in this particular encounter, thereby remaining flexible and aware of alternatives. An observer seeing the APN in action may think these processes are automatic because of how natural they seem. That such interactions appear to occur naturally arises from the APN's mindfulness of the encounter and the patient's and the APN's own responses.

In many arts and sports, coaches no longer perform the skill they coach and yet are still able to coach effectively. The nature of the health-care environment and the delivery of clinical services are dynamic and complex—they could be considered to be in a semipermanent state of "transitionality" (Bridges, 1980). A nurse's coaching expertise can still develop when the nurse's primary responsibility shifts from direct care to another area within nursing, such as teaching or administration. However, the coaching processes that are developed will be related to the learners—students or staff. The ability to coach patients *depends* on direct care experiences in which new human responses, possibilities for growth, and new coaching strategies are revealed through APNs' encounters with patients and families as they experience health and illness and new technologies and therapies.

REFERENCES

Adler, K. (1985). *The art of accompanying and coaching*. Chicago: Dacapo Publishers.

Alexander, J., Younger, R., Cohen, R., & Crawford, L. (1988). Effectiveness of a nurse managed program for children with chronic asthma. *Journal of Pediatric Nursing, 3*, 312–317.

Atkins, S., & Murphy, K. (1994). Reflective practice. *Nursing Standard, 8*, 39, 49–54.

Benner, P. (1984). *From novice to expert: Excellence and power in clinical nursing practice*. Menlo Park, CA: Addison Wesley.

Benner, P. (1985). The oncology clinical nurse specialist as expert coach. *Oncology Nursing Forum, 12* (2), 40–44.

Benner, P. (1991). The role of experience, narrative, and community in skilled ethical comportment. *Advances in Nursing Science, 14* (2), 1–21.

Bernstein, B. (1974). *Class, codes, and control: Theoretical studies towards a sociology of language*. New York: Schocken Books.

Braden, C. (1990). Learned self-help response to chronic illness experience: A test of three alternative learning theories. *Scholarly Inquiry for Nursing Practice, 4* (1), 23–41.

Braden, C. (1993). Research program on learned response to chronic illness experience: Self-help model. *Holistic Nursing Practice, 8* (1), 38–44.

Bridges, W. (1980). *Transitions: Making sense of life's changes*. Reading: Addison Wesley Publishing.

Brooten, D., Brown, L., Hazard Munro, B., York, R., Cohen, S., Roncoli, M., & Hollingsworth, A. (1988). Early discharge and specialist transitional care. *Image—The Journal of Nursing Scholarship, 20* (2), 64–68.

Brooten, D., Gennaro, S., Knapp, H., Jovene, N., Brown, L., & York, R. (1991). Functions of the CNS in early discharge and home followup of very low birthweight infants. *Clinical Nurse Specialist, 5* (4), 196–201.

Brooten, D., Kumar, S., Brown, L., Butts, P., Finkler, S., Bakewell-Sachs, S., Gibbons, A., & Delivoria-Papadopoulos, M. (1986). A randomized clinical trial of early hospital discharge and home followup of very low birthweight infants. *New England Journal of Medicine, 315*, 934–939.

Brown, M., & Waybrant, K. (1988). Health promotion, education, counseling, and coordination in primary health care nursing. *Public Health Nursing, 5* (1), 16–23.

Brown, S. (1995). An interviewing style for nursing assessment. *Journal of Advanced Nursing, 21*, 340–343.

Brykczynski, K. (1989). An interpretive study describing the clinical judgment of nurse practitioners. *Scholarly Inquiry for Nursing Practice, 3* (2), 75–112.

Carper, B. (1978). Fundamental patterns of knowing in nursing. *Advances in Nursing Science, 1* (1), 13–23.

Chick, N., & Meleis, A. (1986). Transitions: A nursing concern. In P. Chinn (Ed.), *Nursing research methodology: Issues and implementation* (pp. 237–258). Rockville, MD: Aspen Publishers.

Chopoorian, T. (1986). Reconceptualizing the environment. In P. Moccia (Ed.), *New approaches to theory development*. New York: National League for Nursing.

Connelly, C. (1993). An empirical model of self-care in chronic illness. *Clinical Nurse Specialist, 7*, 247–253.

Corbin, J., & Strauss, A. (1992). A nursing model for chronic illness management based upon the trajectory framework. In P. Woog (Ed.), *The chronic illness trajectory framework: The Corbin and Strauss model* (pp. 9–28). New York: Springer Publishing.

Corcoran, S., & Moreland, H. (1988). "Thinking aloud" as a strategy to improve clinical decision making. *Heart & Lung, 17*, 463–468.

Daloz, L. (1986). *Effective teaching and mentoring: Realizing the transformational power of adult learning experiences.* San Francisco: Jossey Bass Publishers.

Davies, E. (1995). Reflective practice: A focus for caring. *Journal of Nursing Education, 34,* 167–174.

Davis, A. (1981). Compassion, suffering, morality: Ethical dilemmas in caring. *Nursing Law & Ethics, 2,* 2.

Davis, M., Sawin, K., & Dunn, M. (1993). Teaching strategies used by expert nurse practitioner preceptors: A qualitative study. *Journal of the American Academy of Nurse Practitioners, 5,* 27–33.

de La Cuesta, C. (1994). Relationships in health visiting: Enabling and mediating. *International Journal of Nursing Studies, 31,* 451–459.

Diemert Moch, S. (1990). Personal knowing: Evolving research and practice. *Scholarly Inquiry for Nursing Practice, 4,* 155–170.

Draye, M., & Pesznecker, B. (1980). Teaching activities of nurse practitioners. *Nurse Practitioner, 5,* 28–33.

Drew, N. (1986). Exclusion and confirmation: A phenomenology of patients' experiences with caregivers. *Image—The Journal of Nursing Scholarship, 18* (2), 39–43.

Fenton, M. (1984). Identification of the skilled performance of master's prepared nurses as a method of curriculum planning and evaluation. In P. Benner (Ed.), *From novice to expert* (pp. 262–274). Menlo Park, CA: Addison Wesley Publishers.

Fenton, M. (1985). Identifying competencies of clinical nurse specialists. *Journal of Nursing Administration, 15* (12), 31–37.

Fenton, M., & Brykczynski, K. (1993). Qualitative distinctions and similarities in the practice of clinical nurse specialists and nurse practitioners. *Journal of Professional Nursing, 9,* 313–326.

Freire, P. (1970). *Pedagogy of the oppressed.* New York: Continuum Publishing.

Frisch, M., Elliott, C., Atsaides, J., Salva, D., & Denney, D. (1982). Social skills and stress management training to enhance patients' interpersonal competencies. *Psychotherapy Theory, Research and Practice, 19,* 349–358.

Fulwiler, T. (1987). *Teaching with writing.* Upper Montclair, NJ: Boynton/Cook.

Gadow, S. (1980). Existential advocacy: Philosophical foundations of nursing. In S. Spicker & S. Gadow (Eds.), *Nursing: images and ideas* (pp. 79–101). New York: Springer Publishing.

Grimmett, P. (1988). The nature of reflection and Schön's conception in perspective. In P. Grimmett & G. Erickson (Eds.), *Reflection in teacher education* (pp. 5–15). New York: Teacher's College Press.

Hagedorn, S. (1995). The politics of caring: The role of activism in primary care. *Advances in Nursing Science, 17* (4), 1–11.

Hathway, D. (1986). Effect of preoperative instruction on postoperative outcomes: A meta-analysis. *Nursing Research, 35,* 260–275.

Heater, B., Becker, A., & Olson, R. (1988). Nursing interventions and patient outcomes: A meta-analysis of studies. *Nursing Research, 37,* 303–307.

Heifetz, R. (1994). *Leadership without easy answers.* Cambridge, MA: The Belknap Press of Harvard University Press.

Hops, H. (1983). Children's social competence and skill: Current research, practices, and future directions. *Behavioral Therapy, 14,* 3–18.

Jackson, P. (1986). *The practice of teaching.* New York: Teacher's College Press.

Jacobs-Kramer, M., & Chinn, P. (1988). Perspectives on knowing: A model of nursing knowledge. *Scholarly Inquiry for Nursing Practice, 2,* 129–139.

Jenny, J., & Logan, J. (1992). Knowing the patient: One aspect of clinical knowledge. *Image—The Journal of Nursing Scholarship, 24,* 254–258.

Johnson, J., Rice, V., Fuller, S., & Endress, M. (1978). Sensory information about a threatening procedure on patients' expectations and emotional distress. *Nursing Research, 1,* 4–17.

Kasch, C. (1983). Interpersonal competence and communication in the delivery of nursing care. *Advances in Nursing Science, 5* (1), 71–88.

Kasch, C., & Dine, J. (1988). Person-centered communication and social perspective taking. *Western Journal of Nursing Research, 10,* 317–326.

Kasch, C., & Knutson, K. (1985). Patient compliance and interpersonal style: Implications for practice and research. *Nurse Practitioner, 10* (3), 52–64.

Kasch, C., & Lisnek, P. (1984). Role of strategic communication in nursing theory and research. *Advances in Nursing Science, 6* (1), 56–71.

Kendall, J. (1992). Fighting back: Promoting emancipatory nursing actions. *Advances in Nursing Science, 15* (2), 1–15.

Koetters, T. L. (1989). Clinical practice and direct patient care. In A. B. Hamric & J. A. Spross (Eds.), *The clinical nurse specialist in theory and practice* (2nd ed.) (pp. 107–124). Philadelphia: W. B. Saunders.

Kolcaba, K. (1992). Holistic comfort: Operationalizing the construct as a nurse-sensitive outcome. *Advances in Nursing Science, 15* (1), 1–10.

Lamb, G., & Stempel, J. (1994). Nurse case management from the client's view: Growing as insider-expert. *Nursing Outlook, 42* (1), 7–13.

Lamm, B., Dungan, J., & Hiromoto, B. (1991). Long-term lifestyle management. *Clinical Nurse Specialist, 5* (4), 182–188.

Lang, N., & Marek, K. (1992). Outcomes that reflect clinical practice. In U.S. Department of Health and Human Services (Ed.). *Patient outcomes research: Examining the effectiveness of nursing practice* (pp. 27–38). Rockville, MD: U.S. Department of Health and Human Services, Public Health Service, National Institutes of Health. NIH Publication No. 93-3411.

Leventhal, H., & Johnson, J. (1983). Laboratory and field experimentation: Development of a theory of self-regulation. In P. Woolridge, M. Schmitt, J. Skipper, & P. Leonard (Eds.), *Behavioral science and nursing theory* (pp. 189–262). St. Louis: C. V. Mosby.

Lindemann, C. (1988). Nursing research in patient education. *Annual Review of Nursing Research, 6,* 29–60.

Lindesmith, K., & McWeeny, M. (1994). The power of storytelling. *Journal of Continuing Education in Nursing, 25,* 186–187.

Lipman, T. (1986). Length of hospitalization of children with diabetes: Effect of a clinical nurse specialist. *The Diabetes Educator, 14* (1), 41–43.

Lombardo, B. (1987). *The humanistic coach: From theory to practice.* Springfield, IL: Charles C Thomas, Publisher.

McKinnon, A., & Erickson, G. (1988). Taking Schön's ideas to a science teaching practicum. In P. Grimmett & G. Erickson (Eds.), *Reflection in teacher education* (pp. 113–137). New York: Teacher's College Press.

Martocchio, B. (1987). Authenticity, belonging, emotional closeness, and self representation. *Oncology Nursing Forum, 14* (4), 23–27.

Meng, A., & Morris, D. (1995). Continuing education for advanced nurse practitioners: Preparing nurse-midwives as clinical preceptors. *Journal of Continuing Education in Nursing, 26,* 180–184.

Mezey, M., Dougherty, M., Wade, P., & Mersmann, C. (1994). Nurse practitioners, certified nurse-midwives, and nurse anesthetists: Changing care in acute care hospitals in New York City. *Journal of the NY State Nurses' Association, 25* (4), 13–17.

Morgan, A. (1994). Client education experiences in professional nursing practice—a phenomenological perspective. *Journal of Advanced Nursing, 19,* 792–801.

Naylor, M., Munro, B., & Brooten, D. (1991). Measuring the effectiveness of nursing practice. *Clinical Nurse Specialist, 5,* 210–215.

Office of Technology Assessment, U.S. Congress (1986). *Nurse practitioners, physician assistants, and certified nurse-midwives: A policy analysis* (Health Technology Case Study 37, No. OTA-HCS-37). Washington, DC: U.S. Government Printing Office.

Olesen, V., Schatzman, L., Droes, N., Hatton, D., & Chico, N. (1990). The mundane ailment and the physical self: Analysis of the social psychology of health and illness. *Social Science and Medicine, 30,* 449–455.

Pelligrini, D., & Urbain, E. (1985). An evaluation of interpersonal cognitive problem solving training with children. *Journal of Psychology and Psychiatry, 26,* 17–41.

Peplau, H. (1952). *Interpersonal relations in nursing: A conceptual frame of reference.* New York: G.P. Putnam.

Peplau, H. (1994). Quality of life: An interpersonal perspective. *Nursing Science Quarterly, 7* (1), 10–15.

Pozen, M., Stechmiller, J., Harris, W., Smith, S., Fred, D., & Voight, G. (1977). A nurse rehabilitator's impact on patients with myocardial infarction. *Medical Care, 15,* 830–837.

Priest, A. R. (1989). The CNS as educator. In A. B. Hamric & J. A. Spross (Eds.), *The clinical nurse specialist in theory and practice* (2nd ed.) (pp. 147–168). Philadelphia: W.B. Saunders.

Pugach, M., & Johnson, L. (1990). Developing reflective practice through structured dialogue. In R. Clift, W. Houston, & M. Pugach (Eds.), *Encouraging reflective practice in teacher education* (pp. 186–207). New York: Teacher's College Press.

Quirk, M., & Casey, L. (1995). Primary care for women: The art of interviewing. *Journal of Nurse-Midwifery, 40* (2), 97–103.

Redman, B. (1988). *The process of patient education.* St. Louis: Mosby-Year Book.

Reed, P. (1991). Toward a nursing theory of self-transcendence: Deductive reformulation using developmental theories. *Advances in Nursing Science, 13* (4), 64–77.

Robbins, P. (1991). *How to plan and implement a peer coaching program.* Alexandria, VA: Association for Supervision and Curriculum Development.

Schön, D. (1983). *The reflective practitioner: How professionals think in action.* New York: Basic Books.

Schön, D. (1987). *Educating the reflective practitioner: Toward a new design for teaching and learning in the professions.* San Francisco: Jossey Bass.

Schumacher, K., & Meleis, A. (1994). Transitions: A central concept in nursing. *Image—The Journal of Nursing Scholarship, 26,* 119–127.

Schwartz-Barcott, D., Fortin, J., & Kim, H. (1994). Client-nurse interaction: Testing for its impact in preoperative instruction. *International Journal of Nursing Studies, 31* (1), 23–35.

Scupholme, A., Paine, L., Lang, J., Kumar, S., & DeJoseph, J. (1994). Time associated with components of clinical services rendered by nurse-midwives: Sample data from Phase II of nurse-midwifery care to vulnerable populations in the United States. *Journal of Nurse-Midwifery, 39,* 5–12.

Scupholme, A., & Walsh, L. (1994). Home-based services by nurse-midwives: Sample data from Phase II of nurse-midwifery care to vulnerable populations in the United States. *Journal of Nurse-Midwifery, 39,* 358–362.

Smith, C. (1989). Overview of patient education: Opportunities and challenges for the twenty-first century. *Nursing Clinics of North America, 24,* 583–587.

Sorrell, J. (1994). Remembrance of things past through writing: Esthetic patterns of knowing in nursing. *Advances in Nursing Science, 17* (1), 60–70.

Spross, J. (1994). Coaching: An interdisciplinary perspective. Unpublished manuscript. Boston College, Doctoral Program in Nursing, Chestnut Hill, MA.

Spross, J. (1996). Coaching and suffering: The role of the nurse in helping people face illness. In B. Ferrell (Ed.), *Suffering* (pp. 173–208). Boston: Jones & Bartlett.

Squier, R. (1990). A model of empathic understanding and adherence to treatment regimens in practitioner-patient relationships. *Social Science and Medicine, 30,* 325–339.

Steele, S., & Fenton, M. (1988). Expert practice of clinical nurse specialists. *Clinical Nurse Specialist, 2* (1), 45–52.

Steeves, R., & Kahn, D. (1987). Experience of meaning in suffering. *Image—The Journal of Nursing Scholarship, 19,* 114–116.

Steven, P. (1989). A critical social reconstruction of environment in nursing: Implications for methodology. *Advances in Nursing Science, 11* (4), 55–68.

Sullivan, P., & Wilson, D. (1991). The coach's role. In G. Cohen (Ed.), *Women in sport: Issues and controversies* (pp. 230–237). Newbury Park, CA: Sage.

Tanner, C., Benner, P., Chesla, C., & Gordon, D. (1993). The phenomenology of knowing the patient. *Image—The Journal of Nursing Scholarship, 25,* 273–280.

Theis, S., & Johnson, J. (1995). Strategies for teaching patients: A meta-analysis. *Clinical Nurse Specialist, 9,* 100–105, 120.

Travelbee, J. (1971). *Interpersonal aspects of nursing.* Philadelphia: F. A. Davis.

Tremmel, R. (1993). Zen and the art of reflective practice in teacher education. *Harvard Educational Review, 63,* 434–458.

Van Manen, M. (1989). By the light of anecdote. *Phenomenological Pedagogy, 7,* 232–253.

White, J. (1995). Patterns of knowing: Review, critique, and update. *Advances in Nursing Science, 17* (4), 73–86.

Younger, J. (1995). The alienation of the sufferer. *Advances in Nursing Science, 17* (4), 53–72.

CHAPTER 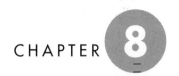 8

Consultation

Anne-Marie Barron
Patricia White

Consultation is an important aspect of advanced nursing practice. The nursing literature on consultation is largely focused on the clinical nurse specialist (CNS) role. Historically, CNS practice in the acute care setting has emphasized consultation as a critical role component while other advanced practice nurses (APNs) have emphasized the direct care role. As the profession of nursing considers the educational and practice issues relevant to all advanced practice, it is important that consultation be considered an essential core competency of all advanced practice roles. Although CNSs have developed this aspect of their practice more completely, all APNs offer and receive consultation.

The authors are a psychiatric CNS with a background in psychiatric liaison nursing and a primary care nurse practitioner (NP) with a gerontology emphasis. Both are currently nursing faculty members. The synergy that developed from their collaboration and the sharing of experiences and perspectives was enriching and energizing and perhaps underscores the most fundamental points of this book—that there is much common ground across roles, that APNs have much to offer one another, and that together they can effect important changes.

This chapter has several goals. First, consultation is defined, and the purposes and processes of consultation are discussed. Current realities of practice are considered, and future possibilities are explored. Second, consultation is distinguished from supervision, collaboration, and referral. The assumption of direct patient care responsibilities is considered in some detail. Third, the authors describe their model of consultation in advanced practice and outline issues in developing the consultative role. Finally, the value of consultation as a means of increasing practice knowledge and skill, enhancing nursing care, and fostering professional development is underscored.

The goals of consultation are relevant to the current health-care debate. APNs can help to bring about the national goal of high-quality, cost-effective health care for every American. Through consultation APNs create networks with other APNs, physicians, and other colleagues, offering and receiving advice and information that can improve patient care and one's clinical knowledge and skills. Interacting with colleagues in other disciplines can enhance interdisciplinary collaboration (see Chapter 11). Consultation can also help to shape and develop the practices of nurse consultees and proteges, thereby indirectly but significantly improving the quality, depth, and comprehensiveness of nursing care available to populations of patients and families. Consultation offers APNs the opportunity to positively influence health-care outcomes beyond the direct patient care encounter.

DEFINING CONSULTATION

The term consultation is used in many ways. It is sometimes used to describe direct care: the practitioner is in consultation with the patient. It is also used interchangeably with referral or collaboration. For example, a staff nurse requested consultation with the oncology CNS so that the CNS could assume management of the patient's pain. It is also used when there is a hierarchical relationship and the person without decision-making authority presents an issue to the person with such authority for a decision. For example, a psychiatric CNS might consult with the psychiatrist regarding in-patient admission for a patient. Some consultants always see the patient being considered, and some consultants never see the patient being considered. It can be confusing, indeed, to know how the term is being used in any given situation and to therefore know exactly what is being requested and what is expected. The more precisely consultation is defined, the more likely consultation will be utilized well for its intended purposes. Because consultation is a core competency of advanced nursing practice, such precision is needed for communication within and outside the profession regarding APN roles and patient care. In addition to enhancing patient care, consultative interactions can promote collegiality and teamwork and foster the development of mature collaborative relationships.

CAPLAN'S CONSULTATION MODEL

Gerald Caplan is considered the father of mental health consultation theory (Simmons, 1985). He recognized that there were many more mental health needs to be addressed in the Israeli community in which he worked than could possibly be met by available mental health professionals and developed his consultation model in response to these pressing needs (Caplan & Caplan, 1993). In the late 1940s, Caplan and a small team of psychologists and social workers were expected to meet the mental health needs of 16,000 new immigrant children in Jerusalem. By consulting with other health-care professionals and community resources, such as teachers and counselors, he found that they (the recipients of consultation) could effectively meet many of the mental health needs of the children. Both the need that gave rise to this model and the model itself are relevant to APNs, who must consider strategies that enable patients and families, beyond their direct practice reach, to benefit from APN knowledge and skills. Although the model was developed for application in mental health, the authors believe it is useful for APNs to know, regardless of specialty.

Consultation is an interaction between two professionals (Caplan, 1970; Caplan & Caplan, 1993). The consultant is recognized as having specialized expertise. The consultee requests the assistance of that expert in the handling of a work-related difficulty that he or she recognizes as falling within the expertise of the consultant. Caplan (1970) described four types of consultation. *Client-centered case consultation* is the most common type of consultation offered. The primary goal of this type of consultation is assisting the consultee to develop an effective plan of care for a patient who has a particularly difficult or complex problem. In *consultee-centered case consultation,* improving patient care is also important, but the emphasis is focused directly on the consultee's problem in handling the situation, and the primary goal is to assist the consultee to overcome the deficits involved. The deficit may be related to lack of knowledge, skill, confidence, or objectivity. In addition to client-centered case consultation, this type of consultation has been an important focus of traditional CNS practice. *Program-centered administrative consultation* focuses on the planning and administration of clinical services. *Consultee-centered administrative consultation* focuses on the consultee's (or group of consultees') difficulties as they interfere with the organization's objectives. APNs may be involved in all four types of consultation at various times. This chapter specifically considers client-centered case consultation and consultee-centered case consultation, because the focus of this chapter is the process of interacting with other professionals regarding the care of individual patients.

In client-centered case consultation, the consultant often sees the patient directly to complete an assessment of the patient and to make recommendations to the consultee for the consultee's management of the case. This is often a one-time evaluation. Follow-up by the consultant sometimes is needed. The primary goal is to assist the consultee in helping the patient. A positive experience with handling that specific case will enhance the consultee's ability so that future patients with similar problems can be managed more effectively.

In consultee-centered case consultation the task for the consultant is to understand and remedy the problems of the consultee in managing a particular case. Usual problems, as noted earlier, are lack of knowledge, skill, confidence, or objectivity. Thus, the consultant may educate the consultee further on the issues presented by the patient or may suggest alternative strategies for dealing with the problem. This is probably the most common type of consultation sought by APNs. The consultant may seek to bolster the confidence of the consultee in handling the problem, if in the opinion of the consultant the consultee has the ability and potential to do so. If the problem presented by the consultee is a lack of professional objectivity, the consultant can help the consultee to identify the factors interfering with the consultee's ability to see the patient realistically. It may be that the consultee holds a stereotyped view of the patient. Or, perhaps, the patient's difficulties in some way mirror or symbolize the consultee's personal difficulties and cloud the consultee's ability to see the reality of the situation.

Lipowski (1981) developed a model of consultation in the general hospital setting. He stressed the perspective that the consultant's appreciation for the context of the consultation situation is essential. Although this is an acute care model, it has relevance for community-based care as well. Lipowski incorporated both client-centered and consultee-centered principles into his model. He described this type of consultation as including an evaluation of the patient, the patient's interaction with the staff, and the specific needs of the consultee. The family and social supports are considered as well. The consultant carefully communicates with the staff and provides regular follow-up of the patient for the course of the hospitalization.

THE NATURE OF ADVANCED NURSING PRACTICE CONSULTATION

Although consultation is part of every APN's practice, the CNS and certified nurse-midwife (CNM) roles appear to address the competency most specifically (American College of Nurse Midwives [ACNM], 1992; Barron, 1983; Barron, 1989). In CNS roles, consultation was primarily directed toward staff nurses as a way of directly or indirectly influencing patient care. Although CNSs might serve as consultants to physicians and other clinicians, staff nurses and their patients are the primary focus. The ACNM identifies consultation with physicians as one of several communicative/interactive processes used in providing well-woman care (ACNM, 1992). For other Advanced Nursing Practice (ANP) roles, consultation seems to have been less formally described. State laws and regulations may mandate a consulting physician as a requirement for advanced practice and prescriptive privileges. The wording of such mandates often directly states or implies a hierarchical relationship between APN and MD, which is contrary to the description being put forth here. As advanced nursing practice evolves, the nature of the consultation competency of APNs will evolve.

APN-Staff Nurse Consultation

As CNSs implemented their consultative roles, it became apparent that the culture of nursing had not adopted consultation as an important strategy in providing patient care (Barron, 1983). Staff nurses were expected to take care of the patients themselves. A novice might consult a head nurse or more senior nurse, but staff were expected to know how to solve problems and use the policy and procedure manual. Part of implementing consultation meant teaching staff how and when to consult. In the early days, CNSs often engaged in active case-finding to identify the patients who needed the knowledge and skills they had, because CNSs were not "assigned" to patients and staff nurses. By building this kind of clinical caseload they demonstrated to staff how consultation might be helpful. Of note, CNSs tended to do both direct consultation and to identify and enlist other professional resources to assist the staff with problem-solving and enhancing patient care. For example, the staff nurses might call the medical-surgical CNS regarding a patient with Guillain-Barré syndrome because they had had no previous experience caring for patients with this disorder. The CNS may have had little or no experience as well but would mobilize the resources needed, such as arranging in-services by the neuroscience or rehabilitation CNS, providing articles, being available to staff on all shifts as they implement unfamiliar assessments, and assisting with care plan development. The CNS would initiate processes (including additional consultation) and provide knowledge directly.

APN-APN Consultation

Within one's specialty or agency, APNs may take for granted the available ANP consulting resources. They may not think of their interactions about patient care as consultation because they occur in the hallway or over coffee. Consultation among APNs may be more or less formal depending on the culture of the unit or clinic, the relationships among the APNs, and the specialty populations seen in the agency. Consultations are likely to involve specific patient issues. For example: "Could you look at this rash, I've never seen one quite like this before." Or, "I've done everything I can think of to try to make sure this pregnant teen comes to her prenatal visits and she still misses them. Here's what I've done . . . can you think of anything else before I get the City Department of Social Services involved?" In many settings, APNs may have some clinical as well as supervisory responsibilities. For example, a senior NP may supervise other APNs and staff as well as have a patient caseload. The supervisory relationship may constrain the consultation process as it is described here. An NP seeking consultation from a supervisor may worry that such a request reflects poorly on clinical competency. It is important to be aware that the nature of the relationship (i.e., whether it is with a colleague or a supervisor) can affect the consultation relationship. Given the authors' belief that a nonhierarchical relationship is essential for true consultation, it may be more accurate to refer to interactions with a supervisor as problem solving. Regardless of what the interaction is called, these types of interactions are important for professional development and optimal patient care. As APNs integrate consultation more explicitly into their practices and reflect on the process and outcomes of consultation, future discussions might illuminate this consultation dilemma.

APN-Physician Consultation

When consulting with other APNs or physicians, an APN is likely to be fairly far along in the problem-solving process. The need for consultation is often related to the consultee's level of diagnostic uncertainty (Colman, 1992). Experienced APNs often have a clear definition of the problem and a preliminary plan to address the problem that they wish to validate or reformulate, depending on the consultant's advice. One might say that APN-APN or APN-physician consultation is sophisticated and high-level.

Unfortunately, APN-physician consultative relationships have often been structured by laws and regulations that mandate or imply a supervisory relationship, which can reinforce stereotypical nurse-physician relationships and the doctor-nurse game. Perhaps to address some of these social/societal aspects of APN/MD relationships, the ACNM (1992) was deliberate in describing the various kinds of interactions CNMs have (primarily with physicians). Many organizational cultures reinforce traditional nurse-physician relationships and the behavioral norms associated with them. One of the major challenges facing ANP educators is to explicitly address socialization to nurse-physician relationships that may undermine full expression of autonomous APN practice. When a hierarchical relationship exists between an APN and a physician, the APN who consults with a physician may defer to the physician's decisions, downplaying or ignoring first-hand knowledge of the patient. APN-physician consultation is further discussed later. On the other hand, numerous descriptions of successful collaborative practices between physicians and APNs exist. Such practices embrace the nonhierarchical relationship we believe is key to effective consultation (see Chapter 11).

A MODEL OF NURSING CONSULTATION

KEY CHARACTERISTICS OF CONSULTATION

Four principles are viewed as essential to consultation (Caplan, 1970; Caplan & Caplan, 1993). The problem is always identified by the consultee, who recognizes the potential helpfulness of the consultant. The relationship between the consultant and the consultee is nonhierarchical. That is, the consultant has no administrative authority over the consultee and is not responsible for the consultee's work. The professional responsibility for the patient remains with the consultee. The consultee is free to accept or reject the ideas and recommendations of the consultant.

Caplan and Caplan (1993) stressed understanding the ecological field of the consultation. This involves an appreciation for the interconnection and interrelatedness of systems and contexts involved in the consultation problem. APNs tend to have a holistic orientation and an understanding of systems theory and apply this knowledge to consultation. Consultation also fosters orderly reflection and widens frames of reference for the consultee (Caplan & Caplan, 1993).

Barron (1989) proposed a nursing model of consultation for CNSs that incorporated principles from Caplan's (1970; Caplan & Caplan, 1993) and Lipowski's (1974, 1981, 1983) work. This model (Table 8–1) for APN consultation extends Barron's work. Each step is explicitly described. With experience and expertise, the process may occur fairly rapidly so that the expert consultant may not be aware of using these steps consciously. In addition, there are situations in which the problem for which help is sought is clear-cut and the consultation is brief. These are discussed later.

PHASES OF CONSULTATION

Assessment of the consultation problem begins with consideration of the request itself. The consultant clarifies the nonhierarchical nature of the relationship between the consultant and consultee and confirms that the problem has been accurately identified and falls within the realm of the consultant's expertise. The consultant also confirms that the consultee will remain clinically responsible for the patient who is the focus of the consultation. In addition, the consultee is ultimately free to accept or reject the recommendations of the consultant. Once the request itself has been considered the consultant gathers information from the consultee about the specific nature of the problem. The consultant tries to determine whether the patient has unusually difficult and complex problems and whether the problem results from the consultee's lack of knowledge, skill, confidence, or objectivity. An important task of this phase of the process is to confirm with the consultee that consultation is, in fact, the appropriate strategy for addressing the problem (rather than a referral, for example). Once the request, the nature of the relationship, and appropriateness of consultation have been established, the consultant focuses on completing the assessment of the consultation problem. This may include direct assessment of the patient. The consultant considers the ecological field of the consultation, which includes the systems and contexts that may influence the patient and family, consultee and staff, and the setting in which the consultation takes place.

The consultant then *identifies the exact problem* or problems that are to be the focus of consultation. This may or may not be the one for which help was sought. The consultant shares the identified problem with the consultee. If the problem includes lack of expertise of the consultee, the consultant will want to use tact as the problem is identified and discussed. Interpersonal qualities of the consultant are crucial and are discussed later in this chapter.

Once the specific problem or problems have been identified the consultant and consultee *consider interventions* that will address the problems. The consultant may intervene directly with the consultee using an educational approach if the problem is the consultee's lack of experience with the consultation problem. If the problem results from a particularly difficult patient situation, the consultant may assist with the process of clinical decision-making and may recommend interventions specific to the problem. If the consultee accepts the recommendations of the consultant, together they negotiate how the interventions will be carried out and by whom. If the consultant is to intervene directly with the patient, the consultee must understand his or her ongoing responsibility for the patient and agree to the consultant's interventions.

Following the intervention, the consultant and consultee engage in *evaluation*. Evaluating the success or lack of success of the interventions and the overall consultation is essential to the consultation process. If problems remain, evaluation offers the consultant and consultee another opportunity for problem-solving. If the problems are resolved, evaluation offers an opportunity for review, confirmation of the enhanced effectiveness of the consultee in managing the problem (underscoring the new skills and abilities or understanding of the situation by the consultee), and closure. Table 8–1 summarizes the components of this consultation model.

FORMAL AND INFORMAL CONSULTATION

The process of consultation described above is comprehensive and formal. The consultant brings clinical expertise as well as an understanding and appreciation of the process of consultation to the problem presented. According to the model, the consultant considers all elements of the nursing process in relation to the

TABLE 8–1. COMPONENTS OF THE MODEL OF CONSULTATION IN ADVANCED NURSING PRACTICE

Characteristics of the Consultant
Clinical expertise in an area of advanced nursing practice
Interpersonal skills
Demonstrated skill and competence in the consultative process
Accepts request from consultee

Characteristics of the Consultee
Identifies clinical situation in which increased knowledge and assistance with clinical decision-making would enhance practice
Initiates request for consultation
Continues to assume clinical responsibility for the patient who is the focus of the consultation
Is free to accept or reject the recommendations of the consultant

Characteristics of the APN as Consultee
Identifies and articulates the nature of the problem for which help is being sought
Clarifies the collegial, nonhierarchical nature of request, if necessary
Proposes alternative plans that are being considered or have been tried
Clarifies accountability for further assessment and intervention

Phases of Consultation
  Assessment
Considers the request
Clarifies the relationship, responsibilities, and accountability
Confirms that consultation is the appropriate problem-solving strategy
Completes the assessment of the problem

  Problem Identification
Identifies the specific problems involved
Validates problems defined for consultation with consultee

  Interventions (may include):
Assists the consultee with clinical decision-making:
• Asks the consultee to gather more data
• Provides alternative perspectives on problem
• Consultant gathers more data from patient because of nature of problem or to further analyze the situation
• Initiates educational strategies
• Consultant and consultee develop a plan and clarify who will do what, but patient care remains consultee's responsibility
• Consultant and consultee decide that an alternative process is needed (e.g., co-management or referral)

Follow-Up, Evaluation, and Closure
Is problem solved? If not, why and what next?
If problem is solved, review why, confirm new skills and abilities
Review overall process of consultation

consultation problem. What about the quick questions to the consultant, when what is needed is a piece of information and a quick description of how to apply the information? Are these brief interactions around a circumscribed problem true consultation? Absolutely, but the consultant needs to make a conscious decision about responding in a brief and simple way to the request and needs to consider with the consultee whether or not the quick response addresses the problem. There are times when the problem presented oversimplifies a complex concern requiring a more comprehensive approach. If the consultant and consultee consider the problem together, they can determine if the quick response is adequate. On the other hand, there are times when what is truly needed is a short answer to a clinical question or validation that the approach to the problem is appropriate. Staff nurses, at times, equate this brief type of consultation with consultation in general because they have experienced only this type of consultation with physicians, who quickly impart information and are then off to the next patient. The idea of the roving clinical expert dropping by with tidbits of expert advice is indeed the notion non-APNs can have of a consultant. That is another reason why it is important to make a conscious decision about responding in a brief way to the consultation request. In the informal situation the consultee may not realize that a more comprehensive and thorough investigation of the problem and solutions with the consultant is possible. Also, there are clinical situations that require a more formal approach to the consultation problem. The authors suggest that APNs consider the kinds of problems in practice that require a formal approach and develop a system for integrating nurse-nurse and interdisciplinary consultations that make APN skills more visible and extend their knowledge and skills.

DISTINGUISHING CONSULTATION FROM CLINICAL AND ADMINISTRATIVE SUPERVISION

Caplan and Caplan (1993), Critchley (1985), and Lewis and Levy (1982) described clinical supervision in mental health practice. The process of supervision can be helpful for enhancing the practice of clinicians, especially novice clinicians, regardless of specialty area. APNs can be competent supervisors. But there are some important distinguishing characteristics of supervision, and it is important that the supervisor and supervisee understand that supervision is different from consultation. The term *clinical supervision,* as used in mental health, describes an ongoing supportive and educational process between a more senior and expert clinician and a less senior, more novice clinician. The goals of clinical supervision are to develop the knowledge, skills, self-esteem, and autonomy of the supervisee (Caplan & Caplan, 1993). Unlike the consultant, the supervisor generally is responsible for safeguarding the care of the supervisee's patients and is accountable in that respect for the work of the supervisee (Caplan & Caplan, 1993). Also unlike the consultant, who is often an outsider to the organization or unit where the consultation occurs, the supervisor and supervisee commonly are employed by the same organization and work together in the same clinical area. The supervisor and supervisee generally are in hierarchical positions, with the supervisor being in a higher position (Caplan & Caplan, 1993). Although the ultimate goal of supervision and consultation are the same, namely, assisting another professional to enhance knowledge, skills and abilities as they care for patients and families and the processes, relationships, and responsibilities are different. Administrative supervision (e.g., vice president for nursing of APNs) has much in common with clinical supervision (e.g., hierarchical relationship, responsibility for professional development of APNs). In administrative supervision, however, interactions are likely to focus on operations and the APN's ability to meet job responsibilities rather than the day-to-day clinical management of patients.

DISTINGUISHING CONSULTATION FROM CO-MANAGEMENT, COLLABORATION, AND REFERRAL

Expert clinical practice is a hallmark of all advanced practice roles. Providing direct care services is the usual activity of NPs, CNMs, and CRNAs. CNSs provide direct care as well, but their involvement in the indirect care activities of consultation, education, and research has been more explicit than for other ANP roles. Providing direct care involves a variety of interactions with colleagues. APNs who assume responsibility for managing aspects of care that fall within their particular expertise and who coordinate that care with the direct care of other professionals are co-managing a patient's care and collaborating with those professionals. The term co-management may be used when describing the process of managing some aspects of care while another professional manages other aspects of the same patient's care. Often, co-management takes place between professionals who consider themselves part of the same interdisciplinary team. Referral is another frequently encountered term. Referral, however, often results in the APN relinquishing responsibility for care (or aspects of care), either temporarily or permanently. The core concept in collaboration, co-management, and referral is the assumption of responsibility for direct care, which falls within one's specialty area. Consultation, collaboration, co-management, and referral are, at times, used interchangeably but should not be. Lack of clarity about the specific process being used for clinical problem-solving leads to confusion about roles and clinical accountability. Caplan and Caplan (1993), Spross (1989), and Hanson and Spross (see Chapter 11) discuss collaboration in some depth. Collaboration is raised as an issue for consideration in relation to consultation because it has been the authors' experience that APNs are confused about the differences between collaboration and consultation. Collaboration and consultation can be similar, but it is important to understand the different responsibilities inherent in each. To further complicate the discussion there are times when the APN may engage in both activities with the same professional. Consultation can occur in what is usually a collaborative relationship, and collaboration can develop from the consultative relationship. What is essential when the relationship (and, hence, responsibilities) change is that everyone involved understands and agrees to that shift.

The issue of responsibility for the outcome of care separates collaboration from consultation. In consultation, the responsibility for care remains with the consultee. Retaining that responsibility, the consultee is free to accept or reject the ideas and recommendations of the consultant. In collaboration, the responsibility for outcomes of care is shared. With managed care and case management systems the need for clarity regarding responsibility for care and outcomes is critical. The nature of clinical problems demands shared responsibility for outcomes. Most often, one provider oversees or directs these various processes (see discussion of nurse case managers' responsibilities for outcomes, Chapter 20). Whether a consultant or consultee, the APN must recognize the issue of responsibility for outcomes and be clear about what responsibilities are being assumed by which professional.

APNs may recognize that the patient's needs could be better met by having the consultant become more involved in the direct care of the patient. For example, the primary care NP caring for a patient with AIDS may consult with an NP colleague with a specialized expertise with that population early in the patient's care. Later, as the disease progresses, the primary care NP may ask that the NP consultant become involved directly in the ongoing clinical care as a co-manager of care. It is critical when such a shift in roles occurs that the resulting changes in responsibilities be clear to all involved, including patients. Consultation may provide the foundation for co-management or collaborative relationships. Successful consultation experiences can lead APNs into new ways of relating and collaborating with one another and other professionals. Consultation can become a stepping stone into these types of relationships, but use of consultation alone offers APNs additional expertise to enhance the direct care they provide to patients.

MECHANISMS TO FACILITATE CONSULTATION

Mechanisms to facilitate consultation need to be considered by all APNs regardless of setting. Traditionally, CNSs have offered consultation as part of their role for institutions in which they are salaried employees. These services are rarely costed-out or considered as directly reimbursable activities. As health care becomes more community-focused and as APNs provide care to increasingly diverse and vulnerable populations, the need for consultation by and for APNs becomes imperative. Current reimbursement mechanisms do not reimburse indirect patient care activities, as much as those activities may improve outcomes for patient care (Sebus, 1994). To the extent that APNs and other disciplines can demonstrate the benefits of consultation, this shortcoming of the current payment system for health-care services can be addressed as part of reform efforts. With the current focus on reimbursement for direct care activities and capitation-based reimbursement, it seems unlikely that additional, specific funds will be available in the near future for consultative activities. Creative strategies for funding consultation need to be developed. For example, incorporating APN consultation into critical pathways for selected populations can be one strategy for ensuring the cost-effectiveness of capitation-based reimbursement and building in bottom-line consideration of consultation services.

Boyd and co-workers (1991) described CNS revenue-generating activities at their hospital in Columbia, South Carolina. They described relevant strategies for APNs as they creatively consider sources of funding for consultation services. They obtained third-party reimbursement for education and direct patient care. Funding was obtained by selling instructional and informational tapes and books written and produced by CNSs. And, notably, they received substantial funding from grants.

Another strategy is bartering of services among APN colleagues. Members of the Sara Beth Harris Clinical Nurse Specialist Group (A. Spang, personal communication, fall, 1994) described exchanging consultative services with a network of other providers. There was an informal understanding that consultation could be sought with reciprocal availability as consultant when the need arose in the future. APNs may also need to look to professional organizations for assistance in developing mechanisms to market and facilitate nursing consultation. Until the issues of financing and reimbursement in the health-care delivery system are resolved and include mechanisms to reimburse consultative activities, creative strategies for this activity will be the responsibility of the profession.

In addition to funding considerations, it is important to consider new settings and potential beneficiaries of APN consultation (see Doughty, Chapter 23). When the APN is involved in collaborative relationships, clarification of the possibilities for consultation could be discussed and negotiated. The consultant's services could be made available to interdisciplinary teams—even teams of which the APN is a member. Interdisciplinary teams exist in many settings. In addition to working collaboratively on such teams, APNs can offer valuable consultative services. When APNs are the primary providers of care, such as in nursing homes and community health centers, opportunities for consultation may be missed because the most common interactions are collaborative or co-managerial or because of time constraints. Yet, in these settings the outcome of consultation often results in improved patient care. Staff nurses in these settings may be without the benefit of abundant resources to enhance practice and professional development. APNs could offer such opportunities through consultation.

As APNs move into innovative practices, they should determine what consultative services they will market and what types of APN and other consultants are available and will be needed. Consultation between APNs offers the additional benefit of collegial networking. CRNAs are establishing private independent practices (see Chapter 19). As independent practitioners they are offering their services in home health (particularly to assist in the respiratory care of ventilator patients), in pain clinics, and in obstetrical care settings (M. Callahan, personal communication, June 14, 1995). Consultation with other APNs in those settings, in addition to the direct care they offer, has the potential to enhance the knowledge and practice of the APNs and creates co-management and collaborative possibilities for all of the APNs involved.

ISSUES IN DEVELOPING SKILL IN CONSULTATION

EDUCATIONAL ISSUES

To learn the theoretical and practical issues involved with developing the abilities of the APN as consultant, it is important to include relevant content in graduate education curricula. Focusing on the theoretical issues in a seminar and engaging in a project as a clinical consultant was helpful for Barron in her graduate program and has been a strategy that some of her mental health CNS colleagues have described as part of their graduate programs. It is ideal to consider developing consultative skill during the educational process as role identity is beginning to be formed. Although this aspect of skill development may be more commonly part of CNS education, it is relevant for all APN graduate programs if the consultation competency is to be truly integrated into APN practice. Considering how the process of consultation differs from the direct care role and discussing the process and methods is easily accomplished in a professional seminar. The students complete assigned readings ahead of time and engage in a faculty-led discussion of the process and issues. Course requirements should include a clinical consultation project. Students could approach individuals or organizations that might benefit in some way from the sharing of their area of expertise. They would negotiate a consultation issue to focus on and engage in a consultation. In Barron's experience with this model, students were surprised by how well they were received and had a positive experience trying out these skills in a practical and real way. The entire focus on consultation was limited to two seminar discussions and the project, yet it was influential later in terms of position choice and role preparation. Spross (personal communication, May 19, 1995) recommended having graduate APN students from different specialty areas consult one another. She devoted the first 20 minutes of the role seminar she facilitated for graduate APN students to consult with one another.

Graduate educators and APNs could collaborate on much-needed research to evaluate the effects of consultative activities on patient outcomes. Documentation of the value and cost-effectiveness of consultation could help to inform curricular decisions. It could also be presented by APNs to insurers and policymakers who determine policy and payment for health-care services. Gurka (1991) suggested that some research questions could emerge from analyzing one's consultation. In an analysis of her own practice, there were three major outcomes of CNS consultation. The first was prevention of complications. The CNS was able to identify high-risk situations and intervene to prevent complications. The second was the maintenance of standards of care and the development of new standards. The CNS's consultation activities assured that high-quality standards of care were consistently maintained. The third outcome she identified was improvement in staff nurses' clinical judgment skills.

APNs are generally the most knowledgeable and skillful nurses in their settings. It is easy to consider how influential they could be with other practitioners and nurses (in their settings and beyond) if they were equipped with knowledge, skill, and confidence in the consultation process. CNS positions are clearly more often structured to facilitate the formal consultative role, but with creative restructuring and confidence in the process, it is easy to imagine how all APNs could positively affect patient care outcomes through the process of consultation.

DOCUMENTATION AND LEGAL CONSIDERATIONS

Although it has been stressed that the consultee remains clinically responsible for the patient who is the focus of the consultation, it is also critical to appreciate that APN consultants are also accountable for their practices relative to the consultation problem. Marie Snyder, R.N., M.S., J.D. (personal communication, June 14, 1995), described the overall responsibilities of the consultant as gathering accurate data about the consultation problem (or letting the consultee know that the data are incomplete), making reasonable recommendations, and giving good advice. She stressed that APN consultants who are working within the same organization as the consultees have a higher degree of accountability in relation to the patient care situations for which they are consulted than do consultants who come from outside the organization. APNs consulting within their own organizations would be expected to identify and follow through on urgent concerns and particularly problematic situations in ways that outside consultants would not be. APNs who are consulting should, therefore, know the organizational structure well and be certain that the APN consultation responsibilities are consistent with the overall job description of the APN. That is, if the job description required that APNs be in a line position of authority for a unit or a clinic (thereby, being ultimately responsible for clinical care), for example, responsibility would constrain their ability to function as consultants as defined here. The hierarchical/supervisory relationship could interfere with the consultation process.

When the APN consultant sees the patient directly, documentation of the consultation in the patient's record is appropriate and important. The consultant's assessment of the problem and recommendations for clinical problem-solving should be clearly articulated in the documentation. When the patient is not seen directly the consultant will want to decide whether or not it is appropriate to document the consultation in the patient's record. If the primary focus of the consultation is on education of the consultee in relation to the consultation problem, documentation in the patient's chart is not necessary. However, consultants should document all consultations in their own records, outlining the issues, the assessment data, and the recommendations (M. Snyder, personal communication, June 14, 1995). Such records provide important data. They enable APNs to make consultation visible and to analyze the nature, volume, and effects of consultation on patient care outcomes.

Snyder recommends documenting informal consultations (see Formal and Informal Consultation, earlier in this chapter) only if they seem to raise particularly problematic situations (personal communication, June 14, 1995). The APN should keep in mind that an informal consultation may be inadequate in relation to the problem described. For example, there may not be enough assessment data to clearly identify the problem for the consultant, or the problem may be particularly complex or urgent. When that is the case, it is important to acknowledge the lack of sufficient information with the person seeking the informal consultation and recommend that a formal consultation be sought to comprehensively consider the problem. If the situation seems to be potentially urgent or emergent, the consultant should recommend the immediate initiation of an emergency consultation.

The increased responsibilities inherent in ANP expose APNs to increased liability (Poteet, 1989; Survillo & Levine, 1993). Specialists may be held to a higher standard than generalists (Survillo & Levine, 1993). Thus, APNs should be cognizant of legal issues in all areas of ANP, including consultation.

SELF-VALUING

For a model of consultative practice to be implemented it is critical that APNs first value the specialized expertise they have developed. One must appreciate one's skills and knowledge before the possibilities for consultation can be envisioned (see Chapter 3). Direct care providers may need to expand their view of what is possible within their practices in order to make room for consultation. APNs have developed specialized expertise in the direct care of under-served populations, such as the homeless, the frail elderly, the chronically mentally ill, the home-bound, the institutionalized, and patients with HIV. The knowledge and skill developed by these APNs could serve to inform and expand the practices of staff nurses, other APNs, and health-care professionals of various disciplines involved in the care of these populations of patients. The APNs must first appreciate that they have valuable understanding and knowledge to share, however.

SELF-AWARENESS AND INTERPERSONAL SKILL

A theoretical appreciation of consultation is essential, as has been discussed. In addition to theoretical understanding, self-awareness and interpersonal skills are essential for the consultant (Barron, 1989). Consultants ideally know themselves, their personal issues, and motives well. A good consultant must be able to suspend judgment and avoid stereotyping. When consultation is sought, often what is needed is a fresh perspective. Self-understanding allows the consultant to see consultation issues realistically and without prejudice. It is not uncommon for a consultant to step into a highly emotionally charged situation—self-awareness, understanding, and being able to remain centered and self-possessed are key to remaining objective and clear. It can be meaningful and helpful for the consultant to have a trusted colleague or supervisor with whom to share and review consultation situations. Such discussions can offer support and enhance one's understanding of personal and interpersonal responses to the consultation material.

It is also important that the consultant be able to establish warm, respectful, and accepting relationships with consultees. The initiation of a consultation request often is associated with a sense of vulnerability on the part of the consultee, who recognizes that assistance is required to help manage the situation at hand. The consultant must communicate (and sincerely believe) that the problem and the consultee are important and worthy of consideration. The consultant must also communicate confidence in the consultee's ability to overcome the difficulties resulting in the consultation request. When the consultant creates a climate of trust and acceptance, the consultee can then be willing to risk vulnerability and genuineness with the consultant. When a respectful, trusting connection is made between the consultant and consultee, a deep examination of the problem, implications, and solutions is possible.

STEPPING OUT OF THE CONSULTATION PROCESS

The APN must recognize that unusual circumstances could necessitate abandoning the consultation process and assuming the stance of clinically responsible expert (Barron, 1983, 1989). If the APN became aware that the patient being considered during the consultation was in a dangerous situation and the consultee was unable or unwilling to intervene on behalf of the patient, the consultant would then assume direct responsibility for assuring that safety needs were addressed. It is unusual that consultees, once aware of safety concerns, are unable or unwilling to address them, but it does happen. Barron described such a circumstance (1989). She was consulted by the coronary care unit (CCU) nursing staff because of a patient's unwillingness to adhere to the safety guidelines of his care protocol. The patient had had a myocardial infarction two days earlier. It became apparent during the consultant's psychosocial assessment of the patient that he was delirious. Recognizing the potentially dangerous implications of the delirium, the consultant went directly to the intern (having discussed her plan with the consultee, who fully supported her direct action) to share her concern and to recommend that the cause of the delirium be evaluated. The intern and then the resident minimized the delirium and attributed the patient's symptoms to psychological distress. The consultant then initiated a psychiatric consultation by discussing her concerns with one of the psychiatrists on the Consultation and Liaison Service and asked that he contact the attending CCU physician and offer psychiatric consultation. The psychiatrist consultant agreed with the liaison nurse consultant, and an investigation into the causes of the delirium revealed that the patient's digitalis level exceeded the therapeutic range. A potentially dangerous and correctable problem was identified.

DEVELOPING THE PRACTICE OF OTHER NURSES

An outcome of nursing consultation, especially consultation over time, is to enhance the professional development and practice of nurse consultees. Consultation can clearly enhance the clinical knowledge and practice of nurses requesting consultation. One of the most satisfying aspects of the consultaive process is to watch consultees master new skills and become more clinically expert. A goal for consultation is to enable the consultee to manage future similar situations effectively. When the consultant and consultee evaluate the effectiveness of the consultation, they can recognize and reinforce helpful problem-solving strategies, which then can be applied in the future. Evaluation of the consultation itself with the consultee is enormously important. It can enhance the learning and skill of both the consultee and the consultant. APNs can contribute to the development of other APNs in a meaningful way through the consultation process. APNs can also enhance their own professional development and practices by receiving nursing consultation.

MORE ON APN-PHYSICIAN CONSULTATION

APNs and physicians can offer helpful consultation to one another. Nurses commonly request consultation from physicians. Because of the history of nursing and medicine, the APN must safeguard against seeing the physician as being in a position of authority relative to the consultation problem. Indeed, physicians may resist the relinquishing of authority. There may, in fact, be some areas in which the physician is in a position of higher status in relation to the APN who is requesting consultation. Nurse Practice Acts and institutional policy may dictate supervisory relationships between APNs and physicians in relation to aspects of APN practice (Reifsteck, 1990; Lamb, 1991). Such statutory and regulatory barriers to ANP have been analyzed (Safriet, 1992). The need for statutory language that delineates the independent nature of ANP has been addressed (Safriet, 1992; Birkholz & Walker, 1994). If the APN and the physician cannot agree to suspend the hierarchical aspect of their relationship in relation to the consultation problem, however, consultation cannot take place. APNs may establish consultative relationships with certain physicians and be unable to establish consultative relationships with others. Independent CRNAs, for example, may establish relationships with cardiologists, who agree to be available as consultants in the event of cardiac emergencies in the operating room, but may not be able to establish consultative relationships with anesthesiologists, who are unwilling to give up their supervisory stances in relation to CRNAs (M. Callahan, personal communication, June 14, 1995).

Let it be stressed again that communication about what is being specifically requested is essential. When there is clarity and agreement, consultation between nurses and physicians can be successful. APNs may consult with physicians in their specialty regarding complex diagnostic issues while maintaining responsibility for the care of the patient; physicians may consult with APNs regarding the patient's or family's response to a challenging illness. The ultimate outcome of APN-physician consultation can be enhanced practice, collaboration, knowledge, and skill for both and improved patient care. Nursing often intersects with other professions. Ideally, there is an exchange of knowledge, techniques, and ideas between professionals that promotes the health of patients. Even though physician consultation with APNs may often relate to the APN's clinical (nursing and medical) knowledge, the consultation should emphasize the nursing domain. Such consultations are an opportunity to demonstrate and interpret the APN's holistic understanding of human experiences of and responses to health and illness, developmental milestones and crises, adaptation, optimal well-being, and practices that are restorative, supportive, and promotive in nature (American Nursing Association, 1995).

CONSULTATION PRACTICE OVER TIME

Initially, consultants must market their services to potential consultees. Setting, niche identification, workload, and experience are all issues that contribute to the time and focus an APN may have for consultation efforts. Describing the role and potential value of the consultative process can be a hallmark feature of the beginning consultant's practice. Over time, the consultant may find the need to develop strategies to deal with large numbers of requests. Setting priorities and identifying alternative resources when the consultant's caseload is full are important activities as the consultation practice becomes more and more recognized and valued. Clarifying availability and the timing of responses to requests is essential if consultees are to continue to consider consultation as a helpful, timely option for assistance with complex clinical situations. Negotiating directly with the consultee at the time of the request (or shortly thereafter) allows the consultant to express to the consultee the importance and worth of the request, even if the consultant can not meet the need directly. It also provides the opportunity to consider appropriate alternative resources to assist the consultee in addressing the clinical problem. The consultant must have established backup resources who are available to handle emergencies when the consultant is not available. (Establishing such resources at the beginning of the consultant's practice is essential. Consultees should always know who to contact in the event of a clinical emergency.)

Over time the number of consultee-centered requests may increase. After trust has been established with the consultant, the consultee may feel more comfortable and able to focus on specific problems in handling the clinical situation. It may be more comfortable for the consultee, as the relationship is beginning with the consultant, to focus on the needs of the patient. Over time the consultee may be willing to examine lack of understanding, skill, or objectivity. Wonderful professional development can result from that level of self-examination, but trust usually needs to be firmly developed before such self-examination can take place with the consultant.

The consultant may find that the consultees' requests become more sophisticated over time. The consultee who often requested basic assistance with care may develop skill, understanding, and confidence with basic issues and move on to more expert levels of practice. Requests for consultation may reflect more expert levels of concern and understanding. Such requests can be catalysts for the consultant's ongoing professional growth! Experiencing the development of the consultee's professional practice is exciting.

On the other hand, boredom with requests may be an issue for the established consultant. Particularly where there is high turnover of staff, the consultant may focus time and time again on the same clinical concerns. Seeking support from a trusted colleague may help the consultant cope with frustration and avoid sharing it with consultees. Communicating a lack of interest with concerns presented by consultees is a sure way to derail both the specific consultation and the use of consultation as a means to address clinical problems. The consultant may also consider developing an educational program to address, in a different way, the needs commonly being expressed in consultation requests. If the problem is common, the consultant may also want to develop written guidelines, protocols, or care plans to share with consultees.

As the APN's consultation skills become widely appreciated in the system and in the community, the nature and types of consultation requests may change. It can be stimulating to move into different types of consultation such as programmatic or administrative consultation, and indeed APN consultants have much to contribute in these areas. APNs should be careful to consider the impact of such shifts, however, because such requests move them away from their original purposes. Such requests can lead to new positions or job restructuring, which may or may not be advanced practice roles. Initially, the request to move into new professional areas can be seductive. Furthermore, the shifts can also be time- and energy-consuming, leading the APN away from practice and ultimately creating job dissatisfaction.

The message that skills and perspectives are valued and that new avenues are available for exploration is gratifying. Developing new ideas and plans also can be helpful to both the institution and the consultant. Recognizing the meaning that new directions have for consultees who have grown to rely on the consultant is critical. Planning with the consultees when such shifts occur can assure consultees that their concerns will continue to be considered even if the resource person changes temporarily or the response from the consultant is not going to be immediate.

EVALUATION

APNs evaluate individual consultations as the final step of the consultation process. Overall evaluation of the consultative process and skills is also important. Barron (1989) discussed both aspects of evaluation. APNs should consider strategies that will help them to determine their overall effectiveness (see Chapter 26) and their specific effectiveness in relation to consultation. Data may be obtained from consultees, peers, administrators, review of the APN's documentation of consults, and the APN's self-evaluation.

APN practices will vary considerably as to what questions and criteria are considered relevant to evaluation of consultation skills. (See Chapter 26 for a comprehensive discussion of evaluation of APN practice.) Some questions that may be useful in eliciting data regarding consultation have been suggested by Lewis and Levy (1982) and Barron (1989). Is the consultant recontacted after the initial consultation? Are consultation requests becoming more sophisticated over time (Lewis & Levy, 1982)? Was the APN able to respond to all requests for consultation? Do glaring issues or needs seem to be going unaddressed? Do there seem to be patterns in terms of either the theme, number, or the location of consultations (Barron, 1989)?

The subjective experiences of the consultant are also important (Barron, 1989). Sensing openness and enthusiasm on the part of consultees can provide the APN with data. On the other hand, sensing resistance or unwillingness to implement consultation recommendations also can provide data. One would not want to rely solely on subjective data, but the feelings of the consultant can yield important information.

Clinical competency, competency in applying the consultation process, interpersonal skills, and professionalism are all areas to be considered in the evaluation process. Identifying the appropriate people to be involved in the evaluation and developing a systematic approach to data collection regarding the consultation aspects of an APN's practice are important. Evaluation can guide the APN's individual professional growth and can ultimately validate the need for the APN's service and skill in the specific work setting and beyond.

SUMMARY

APNs have had a long tradition in various aspects of direct and indirect patient care activities, including consultation. Consultation has the potential to influence patient care both directly and beyond the direct care encounter. The power of consultative activities to inform and advance practice compels all APNs to consider consultation as an integral aspect of role performance. Consultation offers APNs the opportunity to both share and receive the clinical expertise necessary to meet the increasingly challenging and diverse demands of patient care. This chapter has defined consultation, identified various types of consultation, and distinguished it from collaboration and supervision. The authors have offered a model of consultation for advanced nursing practice and have highlighted issues related to implementation of the consultative process. It is the authors' belief that consultation by and for APNs in all settings can enhance and extend quality nursing care, making specialty knowledge available to all patients who might need it, and that consultation should be an expected and integral aspect of APN role performance.

REFERENCES

American College of Nurse-Midwives (1992). Clinical Practice Statement: *Collaborative management in nurse-midwifery practice for medical, gynecological and obstetrical conditions.* Washington, D.C.: ACNM.

American Nursing Association (1995). *Nursing's Social Policy Statement.* Washington, D.C.: ANA.

Barron, A. M. (1983). The clinical nurse specialist as consultant. In A. B. Hamric & J. A. Spross (Eds.), *The clinical nurse specialist in theory and practice* (pp. 91–113). New York: Grune & Stratton.

Barron A. M. (1989). The clinical nurse specialist as consultant. In A. B. Hamric & J. A. Spross (Eds.), *The clinical nurse specialist in theory and practice* (2nd ed., pp. 125–146). Philadelphia: W. B. Saunders Company.

Birkholz, G., & Walker, D. (1994). Strategies for state statutory language changes granting fully independent nurse practitioner practice. *Nurse Practitioner, 19* (1), 54–58.

Boyd, J. N., Stasiowski, S. A., Catoe, P. T., Wells, P. R., Stahl, B. M., Judson, E., Hartman, A. L., & Lander, J. H. (1991). The merit and significance of clinical nurse specialists. *Journal of Nursing Administration, 21* (9), 35–43.

Caplan, G. (1970). *The theory and practice of mental health consultation.* New York: Basic Books.

Caplan, G., & Caplan, R. (1993). *Mental health consultation and collaboration.* San Francisco: Jossey-Bass.

Colman, N. S. (1992). Variability in consultation rates and practitioner level of diagnostic certainty. *Journal of Family Practice, 35* (1), 31–38.

Critchley, D. L. (1985). Clinical supervision. In D. L. Critchley & J. T. Maurin (Eds.), *The clinical specialist in psychiatric mental health nursing* (pp. 495–510). New York: John Wiley & Sons.

Gurka, A. M. (1991). Process and outcome components of clinical nurse specialist consultation. *Dimensions of Critical Care Nursing, 10* (3), 169–175.

Lamb, G. (1991). Two explanations of nurse practitioner interactions and participatory decision-making with physicians. *Research in Nursing and Health, 14,* 379–386.

Lewis, A., & Levy, J. (1982). *Psychiatric liaison nursing: The theory and clinical practice.* Reston, VA.: Reston Publishing Co.

Lipowski, Z. J. (1974). Consultation—Liaison psychiatry: An overview. *American Journal of Psychiatry, 131,* 623–630.

Lipowski, Z. J. (1981). Liaison psychiatry, liaison nursing and behavioral medicine. *Comprehensive Psychiatry, 22,* 554–561.

Lipowski, Z. J. (1983). Current trends in consultation-liaison psychiatry. *Canadian Journal of Psychiatry, 28,* 329–338.

Poteet, G. W. (1989). Consultation. *Clinical Nurse Specialist, 3* (1), 41.

Reifsteck, S. W. (1990). Physician-nurse relationships. *Topics in Health Care Financing, 16* (3), 12–21.

Safriet, B. J. (1992). Health care dollars and regulatory sense: The role of advanced practice nursing. (Special Issue). *Yale Journal on Regulation, 9* (2), 417–488.

Sebus, M. (1994). Developing a collaborative practice agreement for the primary care setting. *Nurse Practitioner, 19* (3), 44–51.

Simmons, M. K. (1985). Psychiatric consultation and liaison. In D. L. Critchley & J. T. Maurin (Eds.), *The clinical specialist in psychiatric mental health nursing* (pp. 362–381). New York: John Wiley & Sons.

Spross, J. A. (1989). The clinical nurse specialist as collaborator. In A. B. Hamric & J. A. Spross (Eds.), *The clinical nurse specialist in theory and practice* (2nd ed., pp. 205–226). Philadelphia: W. B. Saunders Co.

Survillo, A. I., and Levine, A. T. (1993). Strategies to limit CNS malpractice liability exposure. *Clinical Nurse Specialist, 7* (4), 215–220.

CHAPTER **9**

Research Interpretation, Utilization, and Conduct

Deborah B. McGuire
Kerry V. Harwood

HISTORICAL ANTECEDENTS AND CURRENT TRENDS

RESEARCH COMPETENCIES OF ADVANCED PRACTICE
    NURSES: OVERVIEW OF LEVELS OF RESEARCH
    INVOLVEMENT
Interpretation and Use of Research
Evaluation of Practice
Conducting Research

ACQUIRING AND DEVELOPING RESEARCH
    COMPETENCIES
Graduate Education
Postgraduate Research Development

SUMMARY AND CONCLUSION

The role of "Researcher" has long been considered integral to the practice of clinical nurse specialists (CNSs) (Hodgman, 1983; McGuire & Harwood, 1989) and reflects the critical contribution they have made to nursing knowledge and to scientifically based practice. Research roles of other advanced practice nurses (APNs) (e.g., midwives or anesthetists) typically have not been a major focus of attention in education and practice, nor have they been addressed to any great extent in the professional literature.

With the current movement toward professional consensus on the definition, preparation, and practice of the APN (Cronenwett, 1995) (see Chapter 3), it is essential that the traditional *research role* be reformulated as *research competencies* that are flexible enough to meet the needs of all types of APNs. The academic and experiential preparation required for these competencies must also be defined so that schools of nursing and individual nurses understand their respective responsibilities.

The purpose of this chapter is to describe a set of research competencies for APNs ranging from basic activities that should be evident at graduation from a master's degree program to advanced activities that are developed through experience and individual initiative. Recommendations for academic curriculum content are presented, as are suggestions for how APNs may continue to expand their research competencies following graduate school. An extremely important consideration in the formulation of research competencies, and the preparation of nurses for them, is the wide range of research activities in which APNs may choose or be required to participate following their graduate preparation.

In the health-care environment of today and tomorrow, it is critical that research competencies of the APN, historically acknowledged as important yet never consistently embraced or enacted, now move to the forefront of advanced nursing practice. As Kachoyeanos stated (1995, p. 111),

> Nurses can no longer rely on experience in making policy and patient care decisions. Accreditation bodies, such as the Joint Commission on Accreditation of Healthcare Organizations (JCAHO), want confirmation that patient care is based on research. Administrators and payers want evidence that the care delivery system will substantially affect patient care and contain cost.

Thus, research competencies are now essential for the APN. These competencies must become a major focus in academic programs, individual APN practice, and administrative planning and implementation of APN positions across clinical settings. Further, advanced nursing practice research will guide the future utilization and scope of practice of APNs, as well as support standards of nursing practice that appropriately consider both cost and quality outcomes of care. In this chapter, historical antecedents and current trends affecting research competencies are discussed, a flexible set of competencies, including specific knowledge and skills, is explicated, and recommendations for the responsibilities of both academic institutions and individual practitioners in preparing APNs for these research competencies are given.

HISTORICAL ANTECEDENTS AND CURRENT TRENDS

The research role for nurses with master's degree preparation initially focused on the conduct of research, exemplified by numerous graduate programs that taught the research process and required formal, original research theses for graduation. As doctoral education developed and the American Nurses' Association (ANA) recommended specific research roles (1981), the research role of the master's prepared nurse began to focus on the use of research findings in practice (McGuire & Harwood, 1989), commonly referred to as research utilization (Stetler, 1985). This evolution is demonstrated in part by the inclusion of research utilization content in research courses and elimination of the thesis requirement for graduation. In some schools, students are still required to conduct a research or scholarly project but may elect the thesis as an option, whereas in other schools all research-related requirements are met through coursework alone.

In schools that incorporate research utilization content into formal coursework, the breadth and depth of its presentation and its general integration into the graduate curriculum may be less than optimal (McGuire, 1992). One survey demonstrated that although many schools included this content, few had specific readings on the topic or taught specific research utilization models (Firlit, Walsh, & Kemp, 1987). Thus, the disparity in definitions of and preparation for research competencies is still considerable across APN graduate programs.

Current trends in health-care delivery have dramatically affected how and where APNs practice, as well as the demands placed on them. In the health-care environment of the 1990s, learning to provide care using new techniques, equipment, assistive personnel, and documentation systems has become essential to survival. The external demands placed on the health-care system by the effects of managed competition are rapidly escalating the rate of change. In early managed care efforts, changes in the health-care system were primarily driven by cost (i.e., reducing hospital stays, avoiding unnecessary tests). There is now a clear trend toward more emphasis on quality (albeit within the context of controlling costs) as managed care evolves into capitated care. These changes affect the research competencies needed by the APN, who plays a significant role in defining research-based standards of care for specific patient populations, in evaluating the outcomes achieved by APNs in individuals and groups of patients, and in conducting research to establish appropriate health-care practices.

Primary cost containment tools are differentiated practice and standardization of health care. Differentiated practice is a philosophy that structures roles and functions according to education, experience, and competence (American Organization of Nurse Executives, 1990). This trend is manifested both by APNs' performance of activities previously done by physicians and by unlicensed personnel's increasing performance of activities typically associated with licensed nurses. Many positions are now being restructured, and the innovative use of APNs as care providers is increasing (e.g., acute care nurse practitioners, blended role APNs). This increased utilization of APNs could develop in two ways. The first is that APNs could function in strictly physician surrogate roles, providing equivalent care at a lower cost. This direction might leave the APN vulnerable to displacement by physicians who prefer working for a salary similar to that of APNs over not working at all. The second is that APNs could develop practices that combine both medical and nursing responsibilities to create clinical practices that meet cost and quality objectives. Beginning research indicates that there are many areas in which health care provided by APNs may result in *better* outcomes at lower cost than care provided by physicians (see Chapter 26). The future of this latter, preferred practice style hinges on research in all its manifestations—that is, utilization, evaluation, and knowledge building.

The future of advanced nursing practice roles depends not only on demonstration of positive cost and quality outcomes for patients managed by APNs but on a definition of the specific components of nursing practice that lead to positive outcomes. Current pressures to manage larger clinical caseloads may substantially decrease administrative support for research activities of the APN. APNs are expected to integrate clinical expertise and specific research competencies to improve the care provided directly to patients by them and to provide clinical leadership for other nurses (Cronenwett, 1995). Given the critical need for further studies of the short- and long-term outcomes of APN, RN, and specialty nursing care, a lack of administrative support for involvement in such research activities could adversely affect the future of APN roles and perhaps the nursing profession itself (see Chapter 24).

The trend toward differentiated practice within nursing, using unlicensed personnel under the direction of registered nurses, further supports the need for clearly articulated standards of care, with more attention given to the translation/application component of the research utilization process (Stetler, 1994) and careful evaluation of the outcomes of research-based practice (McGuire et al., 1994). Clarifying both the rationale for and the details of differentiated practices for both licensed and unlicensed personnel is essential to achieve successful and appropriate practice changes. Such changes will also enhance the evaluation of nonfiscal outcomes, such as clinical variables and patient satisfaction.

The question, then, is who will establish the standards in delivering care? Several health maintenance organizations use guidelines such as the Milliman and Roberts publication (Doyle & Feren, 1992), which focus on care provided by physicians, to determine standards of care for specific patient groups. It is estimated that 30 different commissions and 80 professional societies are currently involved in the development of practice standards and guidelines (Sandrick, 1993)! Reimbursement for services will be based on such standards and guidelines; thus, APNs must take an active role in their development. The development of appropriate clinical practice guidelines depends on the research utilization process, clearly within the scope of APNs' current practice, skills, and qualifications (McGuire & Harwood, 1989; Stetler & DiMaggio, 1991; Stetler, Bautista, Vernale-Hannon, & Foster, in press).

An increasing emphasis on interdisciplinary approaches to care is also driving efforts to provide research-based care. Tools used to manage patients include critical pathways. These interdisciplinary plans of care incorporate mechanisms for care documentation and for tracking and analyzing outcome data. APNs often provide leadership in the development of critical pathways, particularly when they function as case managers (see Chapter 20). These activities provide opportunities to use nursing research, to incorporate the services and interventions of APNs into care-delivery systems, and to advocate for holistic care of patients and families.

Both research utilization (RU) and other research processes can be used in the development and evaluation of advanced nursing practice. The use and application of research can enhance the credibility of APNs and their interventions, because the research bases for advanced nursing practice are usually less familiar to physicians and interdisciplinary colleagues. For example, an APN may recommend the incorporation of structured decision support for a woman newly diagnosed with cancer. Through the RU process, data from a review of relevant studies indicates that this intervention can decrease depression at 6 and 12 months after surgery, regardless of the surgical option selected (Fallowfield, Hall, Maguire, &

Baum, 1990). Similarly, an APN may recommend a structured support group intervention for newly diagnosed cancer patients based on data indicating that specific interventions for specific groups of patients are likely to be beneficial with regard to quantity and quality of life (Fawzy, Fawzy, Hyun, et al., 1993; Spiegel, Bloom, Kraemer, & Gottheil, 1989). In addition to using research findings, there is a need to demonstrate through the research process that positive patient outcomes result from APNs' interventions (Brooten & Naylor, 1995). The RU process helps determine whether the application of research findings makes a difference in the care of patients. When APNs' interventions are judged effective through this process, they should be included in interdisciplinary and nursing standards of care.

Another critical factor underlying many of the changes in the health-care system is access to information. The explosion in information technology demands that APNs be skilled in using it. Health-care administrators are demanding not only clinical outcome data but "real-time" data access (that is, immediate information that enables decision-making for clinical problems as they occur, rather than monthly or quarterly reports that allow retrospective analyses and problem-solving). As these information systems are developed, it is important that outcome parameters relevant to APN practice are incorporated into databases. In many instances, these parameters will be common variables such as length of stay, readmission rates, or morbidity and mortality, but it will be important to ensure that outcome variables typifying contributions of APN practice (e.g., patient satisfaction, functional status, symptom management) are included. Additionally, APNs should identify population-specific variables (for individuals, families, or communities) that will reflect the APN's integration of specialty knowledge with a holistic nursing perspective. The challenges inherent in interpreting outcome data and attributing changes to specific variables within complex health-care systems can be mitigated somewhat by knowledge of, and experience with, the research process.

Access to health and medical information is improving, not only within health-care institutions or systems but in general. The capacity for biomedical literature searching is widely available, and abstracts or even full texts can often be printed out if journals are not immediately accessible. Multiple sources on the Internet and World Wide Web contain both peer-reviewed and non-peer-reviewed biomedical information. Information overload can be minimized through the use of literature reviews completed by professional organizations and government agencies. These groups have already applied the RU process by analyzing existing knowledge to develop or validate practice standards (Mitchell, Armstrong, Simpson, & Lentz, 1989) as a means of supporting an organization's members or the health-care and public community at large. Perhaps the most well-known efforts are those of the Agency for Health Care Policy and Research (AHCPR), responsible for developing clinical practice guidelines* to assist practitioners in prevention, diagnosis, treatment, and management of clinical conditions (Carter, Moorhead, McCloskey, & Bulechek, 1995). Among AHCPR guidelines that have been released are acute pain management, urinary incontinence in adults, pressure ulcers in adults, sickle cell disease, early human immunodeficiency virus (HIV) infection, unstable angina, and cancer pain management.

Nursing specialty organizations are also involved in efforts to promote practice standards. For example, the Association of Women's Health, Obstetric, and Neona-

---

*The AHCPR guidelines may be requested by writing to: AHCPR Clearinghouse, P.O. Box 8547, Silver Spring, MD 20907.

tal Nurses (AWHONN) recently published results of a research utilization project that tested a clinical protocol for the transition of the preterm infant to an open crib (Meier, 1994). In some cases, published practice standards are subsequently used to define and provide care in the managed environment. For example, one managed care company in Pennsylvania is linking reimbursement for radiologists and diagnostic facilities to compliance with guidelines on fetal monitoring from the American Institute of Ultrasound in Medicine (Sandrick, 1993).

In summary, the historical development of the traditional CNS research role and the demands imposed by the current and future health-care environment have direct implications for the new research competencies of APNs. It is clear that three areas of research competency will be exceedingly important in defining, implementing, refining, validating, and evaluating advanced nursing practice. There must be (1) use of the research utilization process to interpret and incorporate clinical research findings into practice, (2) evaluation studies to examine broad outcomes of nursing and interdisciplinary standards of care as well as more specific outcomes of the practice of individual APNs, and (3) research studies to generate knowledge that defines optimal nursing interventions for particular populations and specific clinical problems (Brooten & Naylor, 1995). These three areas form the core of the APN's research competencies.

RESEARCH COMPETENCIES OF ADVANCED PRACTICE NURSES: OVERVIEW OF LEVELS OF RESEARCH INVOLVEMENT

The authors (McGuire & Harwood, 1989) previously described a *research role* for CNSs, developed from historical antecedents and the clinical and scientific perspectives of the time. To understand the derivation of the new *research competencies* for APNs, it is essential to briefly review the original research role of CNSs and link it directly with the three competencies proposed here. The research role of the CNS was conceptualized as consisting of three levels of research involvement, each level with specific expectations and functions (Table 9–1). Although at least one level would be commensurate with an individual CNS's personal and institutional characteristics, Level 1 was considered the *minimal* research expectation. Furthermore, the levels were not viewed as mutually exclusive; thus, a CNS could function at one or more levels of research involvement simultaneously.

The three essential research competencies for APNs defined here clearly emanate from the levels of research involvement articulated for CNSs (see Table 9–1). Level 1's activities for CNSs were aimed at facilitating relevant clinical research and using research as a foundation for practice. In the new research competencies for APNs, the major focus is the *interpretation and use of research in practice through the research utilization process*. Level 2's activities for CNSs were focused on evaluating practice and extending nursing knowledge through use of simple research designs and replication activities. The new focus is on the *evaluation of practice* using a range of evaluative methodologies to examine a variety of relevant clinical outcomes. Finally, Level 3's activities focused on the generation of new knowledge through mentoring and through collaborative and independent research. In the new research competencies, the major focus is the *generation of*

TABLE 9–1. LEVELS OF RESEARCH INVOLVEMENT FOR THE CLINICAL NURSE SPECIALIST

LEVEL 1
1. Identifies nursing practice problems and translates them into research questions.
2. Enhances the clinical relevance and quality of research through collaboration with researchers.
3. Facilitates the research of nurses and others in the clinical setting.
4. Helps others to apply scientific knowledge in practice.

LEVEL 2
1. Conducts investigations to monitor or assess the quality of nursing practice in the clinical setting.
2. Conducts virtual replication studies of others' research.
3. Tests the research findings of others in the clinical setting and applies the findings when appropriate.
4. Participates in collaborative research, assuming responsibility for minor aspects of the research process.
5. Conducts single-subject (case study) research.
6. Conducts research using secondary analysis.

LEVEL 3
1. Conducts independent nursing research.
2. Conducts constructive replication research.
3. Participates in collaborative research, assuming responsibility for major aspects of the research process.
4. Serves as a research preceptor or advisor for student or other researchers.
5. Seeks out sources of financial support for research and writes grant applications for such funds.

From McGuire, D. B., & Harwood, K. V. (1989). In A. B. Hamric & J. A. Spross (Eds.), *The clinical nurse specialist in theory and practice* (2nd ed., pp. 169–203). Philadelphia: W. B. Saunders.

knowledge that defines optimal nursing practice, which includes not only advanced nursing practice but also the APN's examination of practices that become standards of care, carried out by staff nurses. Thus, in this chapter, the term "levels of research involvement" is not used; instead, three major areas of "research competency" are discussed. In the old "level" approach, Level 1 was the minimal expectation. The authors conceptualize the three research competencies as consisting of basic and advanced activities (Table 9–2). In this new "competency" approach, one is expected to perform basic activities in all three competencies upon completion of graduate school. In the sections that follow, the necessary knowledge and skills for each competency at the basic level of activity (see Table 9–2) are detailed. The advanced level of activity for each competency (see Table 9–2) develops following graduation and is discussed briefly later in this chapter.

Before describing the research competencies, the authors wish to acknowledge Stetler and Grady (in press), who have described research utilization competencies at three levels: beginner, competent, and proficient. The proficient utilizer of research is characterized by in-depth knowledge of a specialty area and its related literature, familiarity with theories of planned change, and advanced coursework in research conduct, utilization, and statistics. Although Stetler and Grady do not link specific educational preparation with competency level, the proficient individual is likely to be an APN. These authors discuss five categories of utilization: (1) focused inquiry (focused reviews of literature), (2) exploration (search and critique), (3) application (conversion of findings into a usable form), (4) evaluation (use of research as a process and assessment of effectiveness of use of research), and (5) diffusion (dissemination and extension of findings or of research utilization itself). For each of these categories, specific competencies and expectations are defined for each level of user (beginner, competent, and proficient). Although it is not the purpose of this chapter to review Stetler and Grady's (in press) research

TABLE 9–2. OVERVIEW OF RESEARCH COMPETENCIES AND LEVELS OF ACTIVITY

Competency	Basic Level	Advanced Level
I. Interpreting and using research	■ Incorporate relevant research findings appropriately into own practice ■ Assist others to incorporate research into individual or unit practice	■ Develop programmatic and/or departmental research utilization process
II. Evaluating practice	■ Use existing data to evaluate nursing practice, individual and/or aggregate ■ Collaborate in conduct of evaluation studies	■ Identify and/or develop practice-specific package of outcome criteria ■ Lead the conduct of evaluation studies
III. Conducting research	■ Participate in collaborative research	■ Participate in independent research

utilization competencies and expectations, it is noteworthy that many of them are similar to the knowledge and skills for the APN research competencies put forth in this chapter. Interested readers are referred to Stetler and Grady's (in press) excellent work for further detail.

I. INTERPRETATION AND USE OF RESEARCH

Interpreting and using existing research constitute the foundation of research utilization (RU), which is the focal point of this first research competency. Simply defined, research utilization is the use of research findings in practice (Stetler, 1985). In an extensive review of research utilization literature, McGuire (1992) described research utilization as a complex process consisting of five essential components: (1) *dissemination/acquisition* of research findings to and by appropriate individuals and agencies, (2) *evaluation of merit and clinical applicability* of research findings, (3) *incorporation of research findings* into practice through various mechanisms, (4) *evaluation of research-based practice* through assessment of predetermined outcome parameters, and (5) *socialization* of nurses into the belief that research-based practice is not only desirable but necessary. This view of research utilization provides a useful conceptual framework for this competency and is used to organize the specific knowledge and skills that are required (Table 9–2).

In order to begin developing this research competency, the APN must first become knowledgeable about several broad areas related to both the conduct and the utilization of research. It is essential to understand what the National League for Nursing (1987) called nursing's circle of knowledge, which consists of a continuous interaction of theory, research, science, and practice. In this circle, nursing practice is driven by a substantive and cumulative body of theoretical knowledge (nursing science), which is generated by research. Nursing science in turn guides not only practice but also additional theory development and research. These four entities—theory, research, science, and practice—support each other in a continuous process that is widely viewed as the means through which nursing fulfills its societal mission and advances itself as a profession. A general understanding of nursing's circle of knowledge then allows the individual APN student to focus attention on the specific theories, practices, research, and science of clinical specialty areas (e.g., anesthesia, nurse-midwifery, family nursing).

With a general understanding of how research drives practice, how practice drives research, and how theory is related to both, the APN can then focus on the concept of research utilization and its relationship to nursing science. Research utilization is one outcome, in a sense, of nursing research. Why? Because research utilization provides the means through which nursing science (the foundation of practice) is solidified, expanded, and actually used to guide or drive practice. That is, nurses read, evaluate, and use relevant research findings in order to improve the scope, content, and quality of their practice. These improved practices are then evaluated, and if outcomes are positive, the value of the research they are based on is substantiated, and the scientific foundation (science) of nursing practice is strengthened.

Research utilization must, however, be understood within the broader field of study called knowledge utilization, which was defined by Larsen (1980) as "a complex process involving political, organizational, socioeconomic, and attitudinal components in addition to the specific information or knowledge" that is used. Using research information within this broader context is appropriate for nurses, who rarely base their practice on research alone but tend to blend research-based information with information from clinical experience, expert judgment, professional standards, and other sources (Stetler, 1994). Although research-based information is recognized as the "first source of substantiation" in confirming research findings of a given study (Stetler, 1994, p. 21), the pressures of real clinical problems and the need for rapid decisions and solutions also necessitate the use of non–research-based information—hence "knowledge utilization"—to deal with these problems (Stetler, 1994).

Once APN students understand this notion, they can explore ways to understand and apply the process of research utilization. It is essential that they learn about research utilization approaches in nursing, including the original models developed during the 1970s (Horsley, Crane, Crabtree, & Wood, 1983; King, Barnard, & Hoehn, 1981; Krueger, Nelson, & Wolanin, 1978; Stetler & Marram, 1976), their more current refinements (Rutledge & Donaldson, 1995; Stetler, 1994), and some new approaches (Funk, Tornquist, & Champagne, 1989a, 1989b; Mitchell et al., 1989; Titler et al., 1994). It will be particularly informative to study the specific methods used by these approaches and their advantages and disadvantages (Nolan, Larson, McGuire, Hill, & Haller, 1994). Additionally, careful examination of real clinical application of some of these research utilization approaches will assist APNs in evaluating potential usefulness in their own clinical settings (McGuire et al., 1994; Titler et al., 1994). Once the APN clearly understands the concept of research utilization and the available approaches, the idea of research utilization as a complex process can be explored in more depth, and the actual activities and responsibilities of the APN in this process can be characterized.

In addition to the generic knowledge just described, APNs must have some specific areas of knowledge and skills to meet this RU competency. The five components of the RU process described by McGuire (1992) are used to organize the components of RU and the knowledge and skills needed. In Table 9–3, each component is briefly defined: knowledge needed is in the middle column, and skills specific to the particular RU component are in the third column. For example, dissemination/acquisition requires that the APN understand not only theories of communication (as they relate to research findings), barriers, resources, and re-

TABLE 9–3. COMPETENCY I: INTERPRETING AND USING RESEARCH

Component of RU Process*	Knowledge	Skills

Dissemination/Acquisition
Communication of research findings *and* research utilization outcomes to others
	■ Theories of communication
	■ Barriers to RU
	■ Resources:
	   Media
	   Personnel
	   Institutions
		■ Identification of relevant databases, literature, resources, and consultants
		■ Literature searching and retrieval techniques
		■ Computer skills
		■ Interpersonal and group process skills
		■ Effective written and oral presentation techniques
		■ Audiovisual skills

Evaluation of Merit and Clinical Applicability Determination of scientific merit of research studies and their potential for clinical application	■ Basic understanding of research paradigms, designs, sampling, instrumentation, procedures, analysis, and ethical aspects ■ Goals and process of a traditional research critique for scientific merit ■ Goals and process of a utilization critique for clinical applicability ■ Critique for use in practice ■ Awareness of specific critique tools ■ Relationship between type of research and potential type of use in practice	■ Oral and written research critique ■ Oral and written utilization critique based on specific criteria defined by formal RU approaches (e.g., Stetler Model: Conduct and Utilization of Research in Nursing Model) ■ Ability to teach, guide, and mentor other nurses in research and utilization critiques
Incorporation of Findings into Practice Translation of research findings into practice through feasible and relevant application mechanisms that are commensurate with the clinical setting	■ Goals, methods, and strategies of published approaches to RU ■ Clinical relevance of research-based practices to a given setting ■ Barriers and facilitators to RU ■ Goals, process, and outcomes of institutional quality management programs	■ Assessment of institutions and individuals for readiness and receptivity to research-based practice ■ Development of policies, procedures, standards of care, and nursing protocols ■ Ability to identify and appropriately incorporate non–research-based knowledge ■ Negotiation with individuals and groups ■ Ability to teach, guide, and mentor other nurses

Table continued on following page

TABLE 9–3. COMPETENCY I: INTERPRETING AND USING RESEARCH *Continued*

Component of RU Process*	Knowledge	Skills
Evaluation of Research-Based Practice Determination of the value, efficacy, and cost-effectiveness of research-based practice	■ Conceptual approaches to outcome evaluation ■ Relevant clinical and administrative outcomes ■ Methodologic approaches to outcome evaluation that are based on selected outcomes ■ Evaluation strategies of published RU approaches	■ Design and conduct evaluation projects ■ Identification and development of tools to measure outcomes ■ Data collection procedures ■ Analysis techniques ■ Oral and written reports of evaluations
Socialization Integration of the value and necessity of research utilization into the philosophy and practice of nursing at all levels	■ Nursing's circle of knowledge ■ Contribution of RU to nursing knowledge ■ Roles of nurses in RU ■ Approaches for socializing nurses and changing the "research culture"	■ Function as an RU role model for APNs and nursing staff ■ Teach, guide, and mentor other nurses in their RU roles ■ Provide leadership in RU-related activities ■ Negotiation with administrative and clinical leaders regarding incorporation of RU into institutional policy and practice

*The components of the RU process are from McGuire, D. B. (1992). The process of implementing research into practice. *Proceedings of the Second National Conference on Cancer Nursing Research* (92-50m-no.3320.00-PE). Atlanta: American Cancer Society.

search utilization and the relationships among these factors. This knowledge is critical in order for the APN to understand why nurses may or may not use research, how the use of research might be increased, and what their own roles might be.

Skills needed for dissemination/acquisition include being able to identify literature databases and other resources and to find and retrieve literature. Of particular importance to APNs in all specialty areas is the ability to identify existing clinical guidelines based on research, such as those developed by the AHCPR that were mentioned earlier. The authors of such guidelines have already undertaken the task of identifying, retrieving, reviewing, and synthesizing available research and clinical information in order to apply it to practice. Additionally, dissemination and acquisition require that the APN have the ability to use a computer in order to identify and retrieve relevant literature, possess interpersonal and group process skills, write and speak effectively, and use appropriate audiovisual materials. Although some of these skills may seem only peripherally relevant to research utilization, on closer examination, they are important in both finding and communicating research results and thus are critical to this competency.

In summary, this research interpretation and utilization depends highly on both generic and specific knowledge and a set of specific skills that encompass literature retrieval, use of computer technology, evaluation of research merit and clinical applicability, interpersonal communication, proficiency in group process, and understanding of political and organizational systems. Three examples of research utilization projects that exemplify how APNs might use this knowledge and skills to carry out this competency follow. These examples reflect the fact that the majority of published research utilization reports were conducted by CNSs. Any group of APNs, however, can engage in similar projects by using these and other examples as models.

Example 1: Prevention of Patient Falls

Two CNSs, Whedon and Shedd (1989), reviewed the research literature on the prediction and prevention of falls. Studies that identified risk profiles and their specific components, tested the outcomes of fall risk profiles, and tested interventions to prevent or reduce falls were included. The authors concluded that patients should be assessed for characteristics that place an individual at high risk for falling, that more study was needed to evaluate the effects of common fall interventions such as alteration of environment and staff/patient ratios, and that studies also were needed to measure the effects of increasing nursing staff's awareness of the problem. In a subsequent publication, additional CNSs from the same institution (Kilpack, Boehm, Smith, & Mudge, 1991) built on this initial work by publishing a report of their study designed to decrease patient falls through use of relevant interventions from the nursing literature. These clinician investigators implemented a falls prevention program on oncology and neuroscience in-patient units and, after 1 year, calculated a fall rate on these nursing units. They demonstrated that during the project, the overall fall rate decreased, even as patient acuity increased. This two-part research utilization project, although conducted by CNSs in an in-patient setting, is extremely relevant for APNs practicing in all types of settings. For example, a gerontology NP in a primary care setting might use this research-based literature to develop and evaluate a home falls prevention program, or a family NP whose practice includes a significant number of elders could conduct a similar project.

Example 2: Transition of Preterm Infants to Open Cribs

In a series of articles, a group of clinical experts and researchers reported on their research utilization project entitled "Transition of the Preterm Infant to an Open Crib," conducted through the AWHONN (Gelhar, Kobler-Miserendino, & O'Sullivan, 1994; Medoff-Cooper, 1994; Meier, 1994). In this project, nurses used a research literature base to develop and test the effect and feasibility of a protocol for safely moving very-low-birthweight infants from thermoregulated incubators to open cribs in preparation for discharge (Meier, 1994). The protocol spelled out three important components: insulating the infant, decreasing incubator temperature, and making the actual transition to the crib. The project was implemented in 10 test sites and demonstrated that a standardized protocol for weaning preterm infants to an open crib was possible and that it was possible to move preterm infants at lower birth weights than previously published research had indicated (Medoff-Cooper, 1994). Many of the participating institutions adopted the protocol as their standard of care following the project. The importance of this sophisticated, large-scale project is that it used research literature to develop a clear-cut clinical protocol with measurable outcomes (infant temperature, needs for extra layers of blankets or quilts, weight at which infant could be moved to crib). A similar approach might be used on a smaller scale (for example, in a single institution) by perinatal/neonatal NPs to address the same clinical problem in their own institutions. Similarly, CNMs involved in postpartum care could use this approach to develop and test a variety of protocols for infant and mother care, such as effectiveness at breast feeding. Such research-based protocols would be extremely important in today's practice of early discharge following delivery.

Example 3: CNS and NP Participation in Research Utilization

Two groups of CNSs and NPs participated in research utilization projects that helped them learn the process of research utilization and delineate their roles in the process. In the first project, CNSs and NPs in a comprehensive cancer center (Hanson & Ashley, 1994) used the Stetler model for research utilization (Stetler, 1994) to review published articles on bereavement care and make recommendations for clinical practice changes at the programmatic and departmental levels. This paper focused on describing the role that APNs could take in research utilization and the process they went through to identify, review and critique literature and to disseminate it to relevant individuals. Important factors in their success were that use of a specific research utilization model helped APNs feel more secure and confident in fulfilling their research utilization role both individually and organizationally, and that assistance from those more knowledgeable about research utilization, research design, and statistics (e.g., a doctorally prepared nurse researcher) was helpful. In the second paper, the process used by a group of CNSs in two acute care hospitals to enhance their knowledge of research utilization and to increase their systematic use of research findings was described (Stetler et al., in press). Through a voluntary research utilization forum, held monthly and facilitated by a doctorally prepared researcher and expert on research utilization, CNSs learned how to use the Stetler model, applied it to their respective clinical areas, and participated in an evaluation of their ability to engage in specific research utilization behaviors as a result of the forums. Although time was consistently cited as a barrier to participating, factors that enhanced the process included the presence of a "champion" to keep the process going, availability of an expert, and the participants' high levels of clinical knowledge and confidence about their specialty areas. Both of these process examples demonstrate that when working in groups with experienced facilitators, even APNs who are novices at the research utilization process can achieve successful outcomes.

II. EVALUATION OF PRACTICE

The critical importance of evaluating advanced nursing practice was addressed earlier. To this end, APNs can use a variety of research methods and approaches to evaluate outcomes of nursing practice. These activities may involve evaluating specific outcome measures related to general patient management by an APN, specific APN interventions, or general nursing practice standards or norms. Research techniques, although generally used to evaluate outcomes in aggregate, may also be used to assess efficacy of interventions in individual patients. The specific knowledge and skills that are essential for the APN who is evaluating nursing practice are summarized in Table 9–4.

The first component of practice evaluation involves selection of appropriate criteria and outcome measures, which are highly specific to the practice being

TABLE 9–4. COMPETENCY II: EVALUATING PRACTICE

Practice Evaluation Component	Knowledge/Skill
Definition of appropriate outcome criteria	■ Familiarity with nursing practice outcome measures ■ Ability to assess outcome measurement tools ■ Knowledge of existing databases
Selection of appropriate evaluation research study design	■ Knowledge of alternative study designs
Implementation	■ Differentiation of research and quality improvement activities and requirements ■ Data collection and storage techniques
Data analysis/interpretation	■ Selection/application of appropriate statistical techniques ■ Consideration of bias and generalizability of findings
Dissemination	■ Interpersonal and group process skills ■ Effective written and oral presentation techniques ■ Audiovisual skills

evaluated. Multiple studies have examined outcomes in groups of patients receiving care from an APN (see also Chapter 26). For example, Brooten et al. (1986) described the impact of discharge planning and home follow-up of very-low-birthweight infants by a perinatal CNS. Neidlinger, Scroggins, and Kennedy (1987) evaluated the impact of the gerontological CNS on discharge planning for the hospitalized elderly.

Others have compared outcomes of APN care versus that of other care providers. For example, Lombness (1994) used length of stay as the outcome criterion for a retrospective chart audit comparing patients undergoing elective coronary artery bypass surgery co-managed by a CNS and a cardiac surgeon with historical controls co-managed by a physician assistant and cardiac surgeon. Lydon-Rochelle, Albers, and Teaf (1995) used status of the perineum after birth as an outcome measure in an observational cohort study to describe general outcomes of nurse-midwifery care, as well as outcomes with specific types of patients and specific interventions. They compared their results to published reports regarding perineal outcomes in births attended by physicians. Similarly, Ramsay and colleagues (1982) examined physiological parameters of weight and blood pressure in adults with hypertension managed by NPs and compared them with those of patients cared for by a physician.

Although such studies have been critical to establishing the cost-effectiveness of various APN specialties, they leave many questions unanswered regarding the specific APN interventions contributing to favorable outcomes, as well as the "dose" of intervention needed (Brooten & Naylor, 1995). Specific APN interventions require evaluation, as do nursing interventions that serve as nursing practice standards or norms. A variety of general outcome criteria can be selected, such as length of stay, number of clinic visits, readmission rates, overall cost of care, patient satisfaction, and many others. Selection of specific parameters relevant to the individual APN's practice may be more appropriate. Brooten and Naylor (1995) suggested using outcome measures more sensitive to nursing interventions, such as functional status, mental status, stress level, and caregiver burden. In describing outcomes that reflected the impact of nursing practice, Lang and Marek (1992) offered several general categories in addition to those previously described, including knowledge, symptom control, quality of life, goal attainment, utilization of services, and safety. Girouard (see Chapter 26) provides further discussion of relevant outcome measures for advanced nursing practice.

The APN must be able to determine how to measure the desired outcome and, in some cases, assess alternative measures for the same criteria. This process may include selection of (1) equipment, e.g., equipment for monitoring blood pressure; (2) procedures, e.g., techniques for taking central venous pressure measurements, techniques for telephone interviews; and (3) instruments, e.g., those for measuring quality of life or functional status or for scoring subjective physical phenomena. Validity, reliability, sensitivity, and relevance must all be considered in defining appropriate outcome measures. Cost and feasibility of collecting the data must also be considered. It is essential that the APN know of the data available through existing resources and databases when selecting outcome measures.

The second component of practice evaluation involves selection of an appropriate evaluation research study design. The purpose of the study design is to minimize the bias inherent in the research process. Nonexperimental designs and methods are often used for evaluation research, because they describe "what is." Variables are not deliberately manipulated, and the setting is not controlled (Brockopp & Hastings-Tolsma, 1995). It is important to remember that nonexperimental designs may suggest relationships but are not strong enough to allow one to attribute causation. Often, the APN will want to examine relationships among nursing interventions and patient care variables, such as "What is the relationship between perineal support, hot compresses, alternative positions, and rate of episiotomy and lacerations?" Or "What is the relationship between telephone support interventions and self-care efficacy in cancer patients receiving treatment at home?" Or "What is the relationship between implementation of a chest pain management protocol and the timing of the first dose of nitroglycerin?"

APN practice often includes components of primary prevention and health promotion. Evaluating outcomes of these practice components requires the use of nontraditional research designs. The overall goal of prevention and health promotion studies is to measure things that do not happen (i.e., illness). Because the final outcomes may be the absence of specific events over several decades, the selection of interim outcomes may be based on the rationale that they are predictive of the ultimate prevention outcomes. Interim outcome measures may include parameters such as changes in knowledge, attitudes, and behavior; functional status or self-care ability; physiological measurements such as blood pressure, cholesterol, or blood sugar; or other outcomes specific to the goal of health promotion. APNs may use interim outcome measures in descriptive studies to describe the outcomes of their prevention and health promotion efforts, such as monitoring client weight changes, smoking cessation rates, and adherence to recommended cancer-screening evaluations in clients participating in a wellness clinic. These approaches may be used to track trends over time, to detect changes following nursing practice innovations, to compare results with published outcomes, or to participate in more formal research studies. In such studies, the study sample consists of a community, in which some participants receive the interventions and are compared with others who do not. For example, a parallel group randomized trial may be used for evaluating outcomes of APN prevention and health promotion efforts.

In addition to evaluating efficacy of nursing interventions within groups of patients, the APN needs to use an organized approach to evaluate individual responses to interventions and subsequent treatment modifications. Although some components of this process are identical to the evaluation of aggregate data, other components differ. In both situations, the parameters for evaluation should be predefined, the interventions and responses carefully documented, and variables that could potentially confound results considered in decision-making. However, when evaluating the effectiveness of interventions within groups of patients, the data are generally reviewed retrospectively, with outcomes used to make treatment decisions for future patients. For clinical decision-making, data are reviewed in real time, with outcomes affecting the care of a particular patient or group of patients. More data recording is generally required for retrospective analysis, because potentially confounding variables may not be as apparent as in clinical decision-making with individual patients.

Issues in the selection of appropriate outcome measures are similar for individual and aggregate decisions. For example, in the Transition of the Preterm Infant to the Open Crib project previously described (Medoff-Cooper, 1994), research outcome criteria were weight gain, maintenance of body temperature, and absence of medical complications such as sepsis, hypoglycemia, and failure to thrive. These same parameters would be useful for effective clinical decision-making on an individual basis.

In some situations, the "*n* of 1" randomized controlled trial can be used to systematically determine whether an intervention benefits a specific patient. A patient alternately receives an intervention and a placebo. Response is recorded by the patient and health-care professional, each one unaware of which cycles consisted of the active intervention versus the placebo. This approach is useful when response to intervention can be defined through measurable outcomes and bias can be controlled through the use of a placebo treatment. Bruera, Schoeller, and MacEachern (1992) described an *n* of 1 double-blind cross-over trial of the benefit of oxygen versus room air in an individual patient. The patient recorded severity of breathlessness during each alternating cycle and both the patient and a blinded investigator chose which of the two gases better relieved dyspnea during each cycle. An unblinded investigator controlled the intervention while monitoring arterial oxygen saturation using a finger oximeter. Although research has demonstrated that oxygen does not benefit most patients with dyspnea, indicators of who will benefit are not clearly defined. This *n* of 1 methodology allows an APN to use interventions helpful to the individual in the absence of research data that clearly guide practice, yet not waste resources on a treatment ineffective for that individual. Similar methodology, used in a large sample of patients, could help define predictors of benefit from oxygen therapy and could certainly be used to study numerous additional clinical problems.

The third component of evaluating practice involves implementation of the study or evaluation activity. In developing the implementation plan, the APN must differentiate between research and evaluative or quality-improvement activities. This decision-making is linked to the rights and responsibilities of patients and hospitals, respectively. Evaluation data are generally collected to confirm the effectiveness of current standards of care. Patients usually enter the health-care arena expecting the quality of their care to be evaluated. Health-care administrators expect providers to demonstrate the effectiveness of the care they provide. Although research skills may be used in the process of evaluation, the patient is not exposed to some of the potential risks inherent in traditional research conducted to expand existing knowledge or generate new knowledge. Research studies are often conducted to test new outcomes or examine alternative interventions. Participating patients have a right to expect protection from undue risk and information relevant to decision-making. The health-care professions have a responsibility to conduct research to improve health-care outcomes within the context of patients' rights. Thurston, Watson, and Reimer (1993) provided guidelines for differentiating between these two activities and thus determining the appropriate approval process, i.e., departmental review versus institutional review board or another approving body responsible for scientific and ethical review (Table 9–5).

Data collection and storage techniques, as well as data analysis strategies, will vary depending on the type of data being collected. Knowledge and skills related to the handling of data are similar regardless of whether the data are collected for evaluation or for the generation of knowledge. Such techniques are included among the knowledge and skills necessary for the third research competency, conducting research (see next section).

The APN needs a variety of skills in order to use research designs and approaches for evaluating practice. Also needed is an understanding of databases, including the types of data that are stored and retrievable within one's institution, as well as how to plan for the development of additional databases (Wu, Crosby, Ventura, & Finnick, 1994). Such databases can be invaluable in the evaluation of practice. For example, various databases at the Duke University Medical Center include data items related to patient satisfaction following hospitalizations and clinic visits, patients' perception of the adequacy of education provided, and assessments of level of pain and functional status. The potential exists for using these data items in evaluating the effects of APN practice over time. Aggregate data

TABLE 9–5. GUIDELINES DIFFERENTIATING RESEARCH FROM QUALITY IMPROVEMENT

Section A
1. Is a risk involved for subjects?
2. Is the intent to ask a new question that will improve or expand knowledge with some generalizability?
3. Is a new therapy, program, or practice to be compared with standard approaches to determine which is better?
4. Are new technologies, interventions, or assessment tools to be compared with those used in providing standard care?
5. Does the patients' involvement change their relationship with the care giver in terms of patient care?

If the answer is yes to one or more of these questions, the project may require ethical and scientific review as a research proposal.

Section B
1. Is a change in therapy, program, or practice an extension of standard care? (Could include a deviation from normal care where good rationale for the change is readily available.)
2. Is patient/staff satisfaction to be evaluated relative to existing practices?
3. Is a measurement tool for evaluation regularly used in clinical practice?
4. Is data gathering intended to confirm existing standards?
5. Is this development of a new program or refinement of an existing program, with formative or summative evaluation?
6. Is a new technology, intervention, or measurement tool supported by good rationale in the literature, experiences of other professionals, etc.?

Affirmation of these questions suggests a quality improvement project.

Adapted from Thurston, N. E., Watson, L. A., & Reimer, M. A. (1993). Research or quality improvement? Making the decision. *Journal of Nursing Administration, 23*(7/8), 46-49.

could be used to track trends related to APN availability or time spent in a specific unit or clinic. A database set up to record APN consults and follow-ups could be linked to existing databases to track the parameters relative to APN interaction.

The APN also needs an adequate understanding of research methodology to interpret data appropriately and to recognize the potential for confounding variables. For example, in correlating pain and functional status with APN interactions with patients, it would be important to also consider disease status over time. Decreasing functional status in the patient with stable disease has different implications than it would in the context of progressive cancer. The knowledge and skills necessary to interpret data appropriately are also necessary to use research in practice, as discussed earlier and shown in Table 9–2.

In summary, a variety of research skills is essential in order to evaluate practice. Some of these skills are developed in learning the previous research competency—interpreting and using research—whereas others must be learned in order to select appropriate outcome criteria, develop an appropriate evaluation study design, and implement evaluation within one's practice. Finally, additional skills in the research process that may be needed to evaluate practice are addressed in the next section on conducting research.

III. CONDUCTING RESEARCH

This third research competency involves participation in research studies conducted to generate knowledge that defines optimal nursing interventions for particular populations and specific clinical problems (Brooten & Naylor, 1995). In keeping with the National League for Nursing's (1987) circle of knowledge, this research should also advance nursing science and further develop the theoretical underpinnings of nursing practice. In an earlier publication (McGuire & Harwood, 1989), Level 3 research involvement focused on the actual conduct of research in clinical settings (see Table 9–1). Although conduct remains the focus of this reformulated research competency, the emphasis at the basic level of activity is on participating in collaborative nursing and interdisciplinary research. Why collaborative research? As Martin (1995) wrote, most nurses can find the time for research if they really want to be involved. She emphasized the need to make research a priority, *to collaborate with others,* to break projects into manageable parts, to structure work for multiple outcomes, and to garner the necessary resources. Collaborative research is a more realistic goal than is independent research in today's health-care environment. With more experience and the development of additional skills, APNs may eventually also conduct their own individual research, thus moving to the advanced level of activity in this competency.

The APN, regardless of type of practice or setting, is the most likely individual to understand the clinical issues and questions in a given patient population. This individual can identify nursing practice problems and translate them into research questions and can significantly enhance the clinical relevance and quality of research through collaboration with researchers (McGuire & Harwood, 1989). Thus, clinical and academic collaboration in knowledge-building research benefits patients, clinicians, and researchers.

As with the preceding two research competencies, a certain set of knowledge and skills is needed for this third competency. Polit and Hungler (1991) presented a useful description of the major steps in the research process, grouped by phases. Table 9–6 lists each phase, its respective steps, and the knowledge and skills that

TABLE 9–6. COMPETENCY III: CONDUCTING RESEARCH

Major Phases and Steps in the Research Process*	Knowledge	Skills
Phase I: Conceptual Phase		
Step 1 Formulating and delimiting the problem	■ Importance of a good research problem ■ Understanding of research problems, purposes, and questions ■ Understanding of ethical and practical aspects of research problems	■ Identification and documentation of clinical practice problems ■ Ability to articulate researchable problems, purposes, and questions
Step 2 Reviewing literature	■ Basic understanding of purposes of literature review ■ Generating and building of knowledge	■ Identification of relevant databases, literature, resources, and consultants ■ Literature searching and retrieval techniques ■ Computer skills ■ Research critique ■ Synthesis of research ■ Integrative literature review
Step 3 Developing a theoretical framework	■ Understanding of relationship between theory, research, practice, and science (National League for Nursing, 1987)	■ Ability to assess theories for appropriate "fit" with clinical questions
Step 4 Formulating hypotheses (if appropriate for the research problem)	■ Understanding relationships between research problems, questions, and hypotheses ■ Understanding of quantitative, hypothesis-testing research designs	■ Ability to articulate hypotheses in clear, measurable terms
Phase 2: Design and Planning Phase (Developing the Methods)		
Step 5 Selecting a research design	■ Basic understanding of research paradigms, designs, and approaches ■ Distinction between purposes and functions of qualitative and quantitative approaches	■ Selection of an appropriate design or approach that matches research problems and questions ■ Determination of feasibility in a given clinical environment
Step 6 Identifying the population	■ Understand basic concepts and principles of population selection in relation to sample selection ■ Recognize issues related to external validity when selecting sample(s) from population(s)	■ Select an appropriate population ■ Help delineate eligibility and exclusion criteria for sample
Step 7 Selecting measures for the research variables	■ Understanding of principles of measure ■ Psychometric properties of measures ■ Distinction between biophysiologic, self-report, and observational measures	■ Determination of appropriateness of measures in a given sample ■ Determination of feasibility of measures in a given setting
Step 8 Designing the sampling plan	■ Understand probability and nonprobability sampling ■ Understand issues and methods in determining sample size	■ Select an appropriate sample ■ Help determine procedures for identifying and recruiting sample

TABLE 9–6. COMPETENCY III: CONDUCTING RESEARCH *Continued*

Major Phases and Steps in the Research Process*	Knowledge	Skills
Step 9 Finalizing and reviewing the research plan	■ Understand the rationale for developing a full written proposal of the research project: —protection of human subjects —other institutional approvals —submission for funding —methodologic, feasibility, or conceptual critique	■ Participate in drafting full proposal ■ Identify relevant institutional approval mechanisms and assist with applications ■ Make clinical or administrative arrangements necessary for the project
Step 10 Conducting the pilot study and making revisions	■ Understand need for and purposes of a pilot study	■ Help with implementation in clinical setting ■ Identify problematic areas (e.g., procedures, measures) ■ Participate in revising research methods if needed
Phase 3: Empirical Phase		
Step 11 Collecting data	■ Understand the various time frames required ■ Understand the need for standardization and quality control	■ Help develop a feasible data collection protocol ■ Monitor data collection and problem-solve when needed
Step 12 Preparing data for analysis	■ Understand data preparation and entry procedures ■ Understand use of computers in data analysis	■ Assist with preparing data for entry (e.g., checking, coding, cleaning) ■ Assist with actual data entry if appropriate
Phase 4: Analytic Phase		
Step 13 Analyzing data	■ Understand purposes of analysis ■ Distinguish between qualitative and quantitative (statistical) analyses	■ Assist in determining appropriate analyses
Step 14 Interpreting results	■ Understand the process of making sense of results and for examining implications	■ Participate in interpretations and implications of data
Phase 5: Dissemination Phase		
Step 15 Communicating findings	■ Understand importance of disseminating research results ■ Discuss various methods for dissemination	■ Participate in decisions regarding when and where to disseminate results ■ Participate in presentations and publications of results
Step 16 Utilizing findings	■ Understand the use of research findings in relation to nursing practice, theory, and science (see Table 9–2)	■ See Competency I, Table 9–2

*The major phases and steps in the research process are from Polit, D. F., & Hungler, B. P. (1991). *Nursing research: Principles and practice* (4th ed.). Philadelphia: J. B. Lippincott.

should enable an APN to function at the basic level of activity in collaborative research. Many of the knowledge areas and skills listed in Table 9–6 could be applied to both qualitative and quantitative research. However, the table does tend to be more oriented toward quantitative research, which reflects the research backgrounds of the authors. For specific research studies, the design selected (qualitative, quantitative, or a combined approach) will determine the research process. Useful research texts for graduate APN students include Polit and Hungler (1991), Burns and Grove (1993), and Streubert and Carpenter (1995). The first two address both quantitative and qualitative research with an emphasis on the former; the third focuses on qualitative approaches. The emphasis for the APN is on two phases in particular—the conceptual phase and the design and planning phase. It is in these phases that APNs' clinical expertise, identification of problems, knowledge of current research, and contributions to methods, especially in clinical feasibility and implementation, are most critical to the formulation of high-quality clinical research. The expert researchers with whom APNs collaborate (usually doctorally prepared) will assume more of a leadership role in the actual conduct and perhaps analysis of a given study. Certainly all co-investigators, including the APN, should be significantly involved in the interpretation step and dissemination phase.

The range of studies in which an APN might collaborate is broad. Some research questions may emanate from the APN's own practice. For example, Harwood (personal communication, 1995) employed the research utilization process to determine appropriate institutional standards for management of extravasation of a common cancer chemotherapy drug, doxorubicin. Through this process, she determined that current research was inadequate to define effective secondary prevention interventions. Following a series of studies using animal models to evaluate potential antidotes (Harwood & Bachur, 1987; VanSloten, Gee, Bachur, & Wiernik, 1982), Harwood proposed and conducted a study within a national cancer cooperative research group to evaluate the most effective intervention defined through the animal studies (Harwood, Strauman, & Gonin, 1994). This collaborative effort provided access to a larger sample, expert statistical consultation, and data management support through the cooperative group and clearly demonstrated this third research competency.

Research questions may arise directly from nursing care issues on an in-patient unit. For example, Shivnan and colleagues (1991) compared two types of dressings for long-term central catheters in patients receiving bone marrow transplantation. The data supported the use of a controversial dressing in this high-risk population, demonstrating that it was safe, comfortable, and cost-effective. The study also advanced the state of knowledge related to catheter care, dressings, and nursing interventions.

Research questions may also arise when nurses consider predictive models for common clinical problems; such models may be used to institute preventive interventions. Hendrich, Nyhuis, Kippenbrock, and Soja (1995) developed a predictive model for hospital falls, using a retrospective case-control study design. In their recommendations for further research, they emphasized the need to replicate and prospectively evaluate their model and prospectively test recommended fall prevention interventions, among other things. Such research again expands the nursing science knowledge base and provides groundwork for much future work.

Participation in collaborative research is an important competency for APNs. In addition to the preparation for the basic level of activity provided by graduate school (see next section), many resources are available to help with the knowledge and skills necessary for this competency. In addition to APNs' own clinical practices, there are sources of important and relevant research questions. Examples include numerous research priority surveys conducted by specialty organizations (e.g., Stetz, Haberman, Holcombe, & Jones, 1995), federal documents on patient outcomes (National Center for Nursing Research, 1991), and state-of-the-science papers on clinical topics (e.g., National Institute for Nursing Research Priority Expert Panel on Symptom Management: Acute Pain, 1994). Comprehensive research textbooks can help the APN fulfill various aspects of this research competency (Burns & Grove, 1993; Mateo & Kirchhoff, 1991; Polit & Hungler, 1991). Specific research texts on topics such as case-study methodology (Stake, 1995), data collection and management (Stouthamer-Loeber & Van Kammen, 1995), evaluation research (Rossi & Freeman, 1993), focus groups (Krueger, 1994), statistics (Sirkin, 1994), survey research methods (Fowler, 1993), and others will provide valuable assistance to APNs as they fulfill this competency as well as the second competency, evaluation of practice.

ACQUIRING AND DEVELOPING RESEARCH COMPETENCIES

This final section discusses the important roles that graduate education and postgraduate research development play in APNs' achievement of meaningful and realistic research competencies that meet the demands placed on them as practitioners. It is unrealistic to expect that any graduate program can, with its temporal and structural constraints, prepare APNs for the full spectrum of possible research competency activities—that is, both basic and advanced levels of activity (see Table 9–2). Thus, it is important to realize that APNs will develop their research competencies *beginning* in graduate school and *continuing* throughout their careers. Upon graduation, APNs should be able to perform at the basic level of activity shown in Table 9–2. With additional experience, continuing education, and mentorship, they may achieve the advanced level of activity shown in Table 9–2.

GRADUATE EDUCATION

Graduate programs bear the primary responsibility for teaching necessary knowledge and skills for the basic level of activity in each competency (see Table 9–2). It is assumed that faculty are role models for all three competencies consistent with their respective didactic and clinical areas. A discussion of this assumption is beyond the scope of this chapter, but such role-modeling is critical to the successful teaching of research competencies. Adoption of this set of research competencies for APNs will require, for many schools, a rethinking of how "research" is conceptualized and taught at the master's degree level. In essence, it may require an overhaul of all curricula in a given program, as research competencies can—and should—be integrated throughout the entire curriculum, not just isolated in the "research" courses. A hypothetical curriculum is shown in Table 9–7 in order to demonstrate how the three research competencies can be integrated throughout an ANP curriculum. In some courses, the specific areas of knowledge listed in Tables 9–3, 9–4, and 9–6 can be used to develop and organize course content as

TABLE 9–7. INTEGRATING RESEARCH COMPETENCIES INTO AN ADVANCED PRACTICE
NURSING GRADUATE CURRICULUM

Courses	Competency*†	Assignments‡
(Core)§		
Theory/knowledge generation	I. Interpreting/Using Research	■ Integrative review of literature supporting a given theory
Research/statistics	I. Interpreting/Using Research	■ Research-based policy, procedure, or protocol
	II. Evaluating Practice	■ Short-term individual or group project evaluating a specific intervention and its effects on selected outcomes
	III. Conducting Research	■ Carry out specific components of the research process (see Table 9–5) such as preparation of an institutional review board application, design of a data collection protocol, development of testable hypotheses
Health policy/professional issues	I. Interpreting/Using Research	■ Write research-based clinical guidelines for a selected problem and make recommendations for implementation at a policy level
	II. Evaluating Practice	■ Develop an evaluation plan for a set of clinical guidelines
Ethics	I. Interpreting/Using Research	■ Write a research-based paper exploring dimensions of a selected ethical issue (e.g., advance directives)
Pharmacology	I. Interpreting/Using Research	■ Case reports describing selection and use of selected pharmacologic agents based on existing research
	II. Evaluating Practice	■ Written evaluation plan for use of specific pharmacologic agents in treating selected clinical problems (e.g., nonopioid and opioid analgesics for cancer pain)
(Clinical)¶		
Advanced Nursing Practice/ Nurse Practitioner I, II, III, etc. (includes didactic sessions and clinical practice)	I. Interpreting/Using Research	■ Description of comprehensive assessment and intervention plan for individual cases or groups derived from current research; can include critical pathways, care maps, algorithms, protocols, etc.
	II. Evaluating Practice	■ Design and implement an evaluation "study" of a specific intervention; include APN-relevant outcomes; make recommendations for practice based on findings
	III. Conducting Research	■ Carry out specific components of the research process (see Table 9–5) such as problem identification, selection of research design or sample, development of data collection procedures, data entry and analysis

*Refer to Tables 9–3, 9–4, and 9–6 for the specific *knowledge* and *skills* required for each competency.
†Note that the specific *knowledge* shown in Tables 9–3, 9–4, and 9–6 can serve as a foundation for course content in selected courses (e.g., research/statistics).
‡Note that the specific *skills* shown in Tables 9–3, 9–4, and 9–6 can be used to design and organize assignments; the examples in this table are more integrative, requiring various combinations of *skills* and building on *knowledge*.
§It is acknowledged that all ANP programs may not have all of these courses; they are hypothetical only.
¶These hypothetical courses are assumed to exist in some form in any type of ANP program (e.g, CNA, CNM, CNS, NP).

well as assignments (e.g., research). In other courses, it may be more appropriate to use the specific skills shown in Tables 9–3, 9–4, and 9–6 to design and implement student assignments. Table 9–7 also gives examples of integrative types of assignments that operationalize the competencies and provide mechanisms for evaluating students' proficiency in the knowledge and skills needed for the competencies.

POSTGRADUATE RESEARCH DEVELOPMENT

Much of graduate education is geared toward providing broad knowledge and skills that support future learning and development. Postgraduate research development is highly individualized to the APN's practice setting and specialty and serves to move the APN toward the advanced level of activity in the three research competencies (see Table 9–2).

Broad areas of postgraduate research development include (1) expanding knowledge of appropriate clinical research literature, (2) expanding knowledge of appropriate outcome measurement techniques, (3) expanding knowledge of research methodologies, (4) developing and maintaining competency in computer applications related to information access and database management, and (5) honing personal skills as a change agent in complex, fluid environments (see also Chapters 10 and 12). There are numerous ways in which an APN can seek further development in these areas, including academic study, mentoring, and self-study.

Formal coursework offers opportunities for development in each of these areas. Relevant courses may be found within graduate programs in nursing, public health, epidemiology, basic sciences (e.g., physiology), social sciences (e.g., psychology), computer sciences, business management, and others. Appropriate courses may also be offered for professional development within one's work environment or by private companies specializing in professional development. APNs can gain needed skills through selection of individual courses to meet their current development needs or pursuit of an additional academic degree to enhance their research and other competencies.

Pursuing a doctoral degree in nursing or a related field is one means by which an APN can acquire additional research knowledge and skills. Subsequent research roles (not competencies) assumed by APNs who obtain doctoral education must be distinguished. Some APNs will choose to obtain a doctoral degree in order to provide themselves with a more advanced level of research skills that they can apply directly in their clinical practice, providing more research-based care, evaluating their practice, and conducting independent or collaborative research within their specialty areas (Spross, personal communication, October 1995). Other APNs will choose to obtain a doctoral degree with its attendant advanced research skills so that they can become clinical researchers, not practicing themselves but collaborating with active clinicians such as APNs to address important clinical problems and research questions (Haller, 1990; Kirchhoff, 1993).

The mentor-protégé relationship offers another opportunity for development of advanced research skills. These relationships occur on a continuum, ranging from passive role-modeling or active precepting of the APN new in a role or new in an institution, to the classic mentoring relationship, the professional and personal nurturing of a less experienced person (Kinsey, 1990; Vance & Olson, 1991). APNs can seek out role models both within their organizations and within their practice specialties.

Watching and reading about how others have incorporated research findings into their practice, evaluated their practice, or conducted research can be both instructive and motivating. The APN may thus be able to identify a preceptor to assist in the development of a specific skill or group of skills related to any of the research competencies described earlier. For example, an APN may request guidance and feedback from an experienced individual when developing a research proposal for submission to a funding agency or research review board, when selecting or incorporating a new outcome measurement technique, or when designing a database for the collection of outcome data.

Within the mentoring continuum, the classic mentor-protégé relationship offers the maximum opportunity for developing advanced research skills. These relationships are typically initiated by the nurse identifying an individual to be emulated and then approaching the individual with a request for mentorship. If the mentor agrees, he or she then provides teaching, guidance, and feedback in broad areas relative to the protégé's development. The protégé sustains the relationship by providing feedback on how the guidance has been used and by giving status or outcome reports on activities undertaken in this mentoring process. These relationships often provide an opportunity for collaborative research, using the APN's clinical expertise and the mentor's research expertise. APNs may find appropriate mentors among nursing colleagues within their agencies, specialty, professional nursing organization, or academic faculty. Colleagues from other disciplines may also become research mentors for APNs.

Regardless of the methods chosen to advance one's research skills, self-study is essential to the development of advanced research competencies. This self-study is carefully focused on the individual's specialty area and practice. For instance, in the example previously described of research efforts to determine appropriate treatment of chemotherapy extravasation (Harwood, personal communication, 1995), extensive self-study supplemented graduate education and mentorship support. Graduate work in pharmacology, chemistry, and physiology was supplemented with focused readings in areas such as doxorubicin pharmacology, free radicals and free radical scavenging techniques, and wound healing. This knowledge was used to identify potential antidotes for evaluation in a subsequent research project (Harwood et al., 1994). Determining appropriate animal models for antidote testing required focused self-study in comparative anatomy and physiology (VanSloten et al., 1982). In conclusion, the multifaceted and increasingly interdisciplinary nature of clinical practice and research will always require APNs to pursue in-depth knowledge and skills beyond their graduate education to meet research needs and other practice requirements.

SUMMARY AND CONCLUSION

Three major research competencies are required for APNs to meet the various research-related demands placed on them in today's health-care delivery system: (1) interpretation and utilization of research, (2) evaluation of practice, and (3) conduct of research. These competencies are operationalized at two levels—basic activities learned through graduate education and advanced activities acquired through postgraduate research development. As discussed earlier in this chapter, these competencies are essential to APNs as they define, implement, refine, validate, and evaluate their practice, and as they move forward to take visible leadership positions in the health-care system of the future.

REFERENCES

American Association of Nurse Executives. (1990). *Current issues and perspectives of differentiated practice*. Chicago: American Hospital Association.

American Nurses Association. (1981). *Guidelines for the investigative function of nurses*. Kansas City, MO: American Nurses Association.

Brockopp, D. Y., & Hastings-Tolsma, M. T. (1995). *Fundamentals of nursing research* (2nd ed.). Boston: Jones & Bartlett.

Brooten, D., Kumar, S., Brown, L. P., Butts, P., Finkler, S. A., Bakewell-Sachs, S., Gibbons, A., & Delivoria-Papadopoulos, M. (1986). A randomized clinical trial of early hospital discharge and home follow-up of very-low-birth-weight infants. *The New England Journal of Medicine, 315*(15), 934-939.

Brooten, D., & Naylor, M. D. (1995). Nurses' effect on changing patient outcomes. *IMAGE: Journal of Nursing Scholarship, 27*(2), 95-99.

Bruera, E., Schoeller, T., & MacEachern, T. (1992). Symptomatic benefit of supplemental oxygen in hypoxemic patients with terminal cancer: The use of the N of 1 randomized controlled trial. *Journal of Pain and Symptom Management, 7*(6), 365-368.

Burns, N., & Grove, S. K. (1993). *The practice of nursing research: Conduct, critique, & utilization* (2nd ed.). Philadelphia: W. B. Saunders.

Carter, J. H., Moorhead, S. A., McCloskey, J. C., & Bulechek, G. M. (1995). Using the Nursing Interventions Classification to implement Agency for Health Care Policy and Research Guidelines. *Journal of Nursing Care Quality, 9*(2), 76-86.

Cronenwett, L. R. (1995). Molding the future of advanced practice nursing. *Nursing Outlook, 43*(3), 112-118.

Doyle, R. L., & Feren, A. T. (1992). *Healthcare management guidelines*. Albany, NY: Milliman & Robertson.

Fallowfield, L. J., Hall, A., Maguire, G. P., & Baum, M. (1990). Psychological outcomes of different treatment policies in women with early breast cancer outside clinical trials. *British Medical Journal, 301*, 575-580.

Fawzy, F. I., Fawzy, N. W., Hyun, C. S., Elashoff, R., Guthrie, D. Fahey, J. L., & Morton, D. L. (1993). Malignant melanoma. Effects of an early structured psychiatric intervention, coping, and affective state on recurrence and survival six years later. *Archives of General Psychiatry, 50*(9), 681.

Firlit, S. L., Walsh, M., & Kemp, M. G. (1987). Nursing research in practice: A survey of research utilization content in master's degree programs. *Western Journal of Nursing Research, 9*(4), 612-616.

Fowler, F. J., Jr. (1993). *Survey research methods* (2nd ed.). Thousand Oaks, CA: Sage.

Funk, S. G., Tornquist, E. M., & Champagne, M. T. (1989a). A model for improving the dissemination of nursing research. *Western Journal of Nursing Research, 11*(3), 361-367.

Funk, S. G., Tornquist, E. M., & Champagne, M. T. (1989b). Application and evaluation of the Dissemination Model. *Western Journal of Nursing Research, 11*(4), 486-491.

Gelhar, D. K., Kobler-Miserendino, C. A., O'Sullivan, P. L., & Vessey, J. A. (1994). Research from the Research Utilization Project: Environmental temperatures. *Journal of Obstetric, Gynecologic, and Neonatal Nursing, 23*(4), 341-344.

Haller, K. B. (1990). The clinical nurse researcher role in a practice setting. In N. L. Chaska (Ed.), *The nursing profession: Turning points*. St. Louis: C. V. Mosby.

Hanson, J. L., & Ashley B. (1994). Advanced practice nurses' application of the Stetler Model for Research Utilization: Improving bereavement care. *Oncology Nursing Forum, 21*(4), 720-724.

Harwood, K., & Bachur, N. (1987). Evaluation of dimethyl sulfide and local cooling as antidotes for doxorubicin extravasation in a pig model. *Oncology Nursing Forum, 13*(1), 39-44.

Harwood, K., Strauman, J., & Gonin, R. (1994). Short-term vs. long-term local cooling after doxorubicin (DOX) extravasation: An Eastern Cooperative Oncology Group (ECOG) study. *Proceedings of the American Society of Clinical Oncology, 13*, 447. (abstract)

Hendrich, A., Nyhuis, A., Kippenbrock, T., & Soja, M. E. (1995). Hospital falls: Development of a predictive model for clinical practice. *Applied Nursing Research, 8*(3), 129-139.

Hodgman, E. C. (1983). The CNS as researcher. In A. B. Hamric & J. A. Spross (Eds.), *The clinical nurse specialist in theory and practice*. Philadelphia: W. B. Saunders.

Horsley, J., Crane, J., Crabtree, M., & Wood, D. (1983). *Using research to improve nursing practice: A guide*. New York: Grune & Stratton.

Kachoyeanos, M. K. (1995, March/April). Research or else. *MCN, 20*, 111.

Kilpack, V., Boehm, J., Smith, N., & Mudge, B. (1991). Using research-based interventions to decrease patient falls. *Applied Nursing Research, 4*(2), 50-56.

King, D., Barnard, K., & Hoehn, R. (1981). Disseminating the results of nursing research. *Nursing Outlook, 29*, 164-169.

Kinsey, D. C. (1990). Mentorship and influence in nursing. *Nursing Management, May*, 45-46.

Kirchhoff, K. T. (1993). The role of nurse researchers employed in clinical settings. *Annual Review of Nursing Research, 11*, 169-181.

Krueger, R. A. (1994). *Focus group: A practical guide for applied research* (2nd ed.). Thousand Oaks, CA: Sage.

Krueger, J., Nelson, A., & Wolanin, M. (1978). *Nursing research: Development, collaboration, and utilization*. Germantown, MD: Aspen.

Lang, N. M., & Marek, K. D. (1992). Outcomes that reflect clinical practice. In National Center for Nursing Research, *Patient outcomes research: Examining the effectiveness of nursing practice*. Bethesda, MD: Department of Health and Human Services, Public Health Service, National Institutes of Health, NIH Publication No. 93-3411.

Larsen, J. (1980). Knowledge utilization: What is it? *Knowledge Creation, Diffusion, and Utilization, 1*, 421-442.

Lombness, P. M. (1994). Difference in length of stay with care managed by clinical nurse specialists or physician assistants. *Clinical Nurse Specialist, 8*(5), 253-260.

Lydon-Rochelle, M. T., Albers, L., & Teaf, D. (1995). Perineal outcomes and nurse-midwifery management. *Journal of Nurse-Midwifery, 40*(1), 13-18.

Martin, P. A. (1995). Finding time for research. *Applied Nursing Research, 8*(3), 151-153.

Mateo, M. A., & Kirchhoff, K. T. (Eds.). (1991). *Conducting and using nursing research in the clinical setting*. Baltimore: Williams & Wilkins.

McGuire, D. B. (1992, January). *The process of implementing research into clinical practice*. Proceedings of the American Cancer Society Second National Conference on Cancer Nursing Research. Atlanta: American Cancer Society, Publication No. 92-50M-No. 3320.00-PE.

McGuire, D. B., & Harwood, K. V. (1989). The CNS as researcher. In A. B. Hamric & J. A. Spross (Eds.), *The clinical nurse specialist in theory and practice* (2nd ed., pp. 169-203). Philadelphia: W. B. Saunders.

McGuire, D. B., Walczak, J. R., Krumm, S. L., Haisfield, M. E., Beezley, A., Reedy, A. M., Shivnan, J. C., Hanson, J. L., Gregory, R. E., & Ashley, B. (1994). Research utilization in oncology nursing: Application of the Stetler model in a comprehensive cancer center. *Oncology Nursing Forum, 21*(4), 703-724.

Medoff-Cooper, B. (1994). Transition of the preterm infant to an open crib. *Journal of Obstetric, Gynecologic, and Neonatal Nursing, 23*(4), 329-335.

Meier, P. P. (1994). Transition of the preterm infant to an open crib: Process of the project group. *Journal of Obstetric, Gynecologic, and Neonatal Nursing, 23*(4), 321-325.

Mitchell, P. H., Armstrong, S., Simpson, T. F., & Lentz, M. (1989). American Association of Critical-Care Nurses Demonstration Project: Profile of excellence in critical care nursing. *Heart & Lung: The Journal of Critical Care, 18*(3), 219-237.

National Center for Nursing Research. (1992). *Patient outcomes research: Examining the effectiveness of nursing practice*. Bethesda, MD: Department of Health and Human Services, U. S. Public Health Service, National Institutes of Health, NIH Publication No. 93-3411.

National Institute for Nursing Research Priority Expert Panel on Symptom Management: Acute Pain (1994). *Symptom management: Acute pain*. Bethesda, MD: National Institute of Nursing Research, U. S. Department of Health and Human Services, U. S. Public Health Service, National Institutes of Health, NIH Publication No. 94-2421.

National League for Nursing. (1987). *Nursing theory: A circle of knowledge, Parts I and II* [videotape]. Available from NLN, 10 Columbus Circle, New York, NY, 10019.

Neidlinger, S. H., Scroggins K., & Kennedy, L. M. (1987). Cost evaluation of discharge planning for hospitalized elderly. *Nursing Economics, 5*(5), 225-230.

Nolan, M. T., Larson, E., McGuire, D., Hill, M. N., & Haller, K. (1994). A review of approaches to integrating research and practice. *Applied Nursing Research, 7*(4), 199-207.

Polit, D. F., & Hungler, B. P. (1991). *Nursing research: Principles and methods* (4th ed.). Philadelphia: J. B. Lippincott.

Ramsey, J., McKenzie, J., & Fish, D. (1982). Physicians and nurse practitioners: Do they provide equivalent health care? *American Journal of Public Health, 72*(1), 55-56.

Rossi, P. H., & Freeman, H. E. (1993). *Evaluation, fifth edition: A systematic approach*. Thousand Oaks, CA: Sage.

Rutledge, D. N., & Donaldson, N. E. (1995). Building organizational capacity to engage in research utilization. *Journal of Nursing Administration, 25*(10), 12-16.

Sandrick, K. (1993). Out in front: Managed care helps push clinical guidelines forward. *Hospitals, 67*(9), 30-31.

Shivnan, J. C., McGuire, D., Freedman, S., Sharkazy, E., Bosserman, G., Larson, E., & Grouleff, P. (1991). A comparison of transparent adherent and dry sterile gauze dressings for long-term central catheters in patients undergoing bone marrow transplant. *Oncology Nursing Forum, 18*(8), 1349-1356.

Sirkin, R. M. (1994). *Statistics for the social sciences*. Thousand Oaks, CA: Sage.

Spiegel, D., Bloom, J. R., Kraemer, H. C., & Gottheil, E. (1989). Effect of psychosocial treatment on survival of patients with metastatic breast cancer. *Lancet, 2*(8668), 888.

Stake, R. E. (1995). *The art of case study research*. Thousand Oaks, CA: Sage.

Stetler, C. B. (1985). Research utilization: Defining the concept. *IMAGE: The Journal of Nursing Scholarship, 17*(2), 40-44.

Stetler, C. B. (1994). Refinement of the Stetler/ Marram model for application of research findings to practice. *Nursing Outlook, 42*(1), 15-25.

Stetler, C. B., & DiMaggio, G. (1991). Research

utilization among clinical nurse specialists. *Clinical Nurse Specialist, 5*(3), 151-155.

Stetler, C. B., & Grady, E. (in press). Research utilization competencies: From beginner to proficient.

Stetler, C. B., Bautista, C., Vernale-Hannon, C., & Foster, J. (1995). Enhancing research utilization by clinical nurse specialists. *Nursing Clinics of North America, 30,* 457–453.

Stetler, C. B., & Marram, G. (1976). Evaluating research findings for applicability in practice. *Nursing Outlook, 24*(9), 559-563.

Stetz, K. M., Haberman, M. R., Holcombe, J., & Jones, L. S. (1995). 1994 Oncology Nursing Society research priorities survey. *Oncology Nursing Forum, 22*(5), 785-789.

Stouthamer-Loeber, M., & Van Kammen, W. B. (1995). *Data collection and management.* Thousand Oaks, CA: Sage.

Straubert, H. J., & Carpenter, D. R. (1995). *Qualitative research in nursing: Advancing the humanistic imperative.* Philadelphia: J. B. Lippincott.

Thurston, N. E., Watson, L. A., & Reimer, M. A. (1993). Research or quality improvement? Making the decision. *Journal of Nursing Administration, 23*(7/8), 46-49.

Titler, M. G., Kleiber, C., Steelman, V., Goode, C., Rakel, B., Barry-Walker, J., Small, S., & Buckwalter, K. (1994). Infusing research into practice to promote quality care. *Nursing Research, 43*(5), 307-313.

Vance, C. N., & Olson, R. K. (1991). Mentorship. *Annual Review of Nursing Research, 9,* 175-200.

VanSloten, K., Gee, M., Bachur, N., & Wiernik, P. (1982). Treatment of doxorubicin extravasation in a rat model [Abstract]. *Proceedings of the Oncology Nursing Society Annual Congress.* Pittsburgh: Oncology Nursing Society.

Whedon, M. B., & Shedd, P. (1989). Prediction and prevention of patient falls. *IMAGE: Journal of Nursing Scholarship, 21*(2), 108-114.

Wu, Y. W. B., Crosby, F., Ventura, M., & Finnick, M. (1994). In a changing world: Database to keep the pace. *Clinical Nurse Specialist, 8*(2), 104-108.

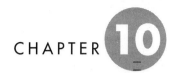

CHAPTER 10

Clinical and Professional Leadership

Beverly L. Malone

INTRODUCTION

Leadership is a core competency of the advanced practice nurse (APN). According to the ninth edition of *Merriam Webster's Collegiate Dictionary*, the word *advanced* means "being beyond others in progress or development." When nurses have moved forward educationally (obtaining a master's degree in nursing), profession-ally (obtaining certification), and clinically (in patient-focused practice), they have acquired the primary foundation for advanced nursing practice (ANP). Along with the acquisition of an ANP role comes the obligation to lead. However, although leadership is fundamental to advanced practice, the ability to lead is not distributed with the master's degree diploma, with certification, or with securing an APN position. Leadership is nurtured and developed through experiential, reflective learning, also known as risk taking. In this chapter, the concept of leadership is explored. The essential elements of leadership are defined, and how these elements are transferred into the philosophy and behavior of the APN in both clinical and professional arenas is described. Obstacles to APN leadership are examined, along with strategies to manage the obstacles and thereby move vision into the reality of outcome.

THE CONCEPT OF LEADERSHIP

In 1978, James MacGregor Burns defined leadership as being "exercised when persons with certain motives and purposes mobilize in competition or conflict with others, institutional, political, psychological, and other resources so as to arouse, engage, and satisfy the motives of followers" (p. 18). Burns indicated that leaders bring their whole being to the process. They incite, stimulate, share with, pacify, and satisfy their indispensable partners, their followers. One notes immediately the interdependent, interactional nature of leadership. Yet Jago (1982) pointed out that

> *Leadership is both a process and a property. The process of leadership is the use of noncoercive influence to direct and coordinate the activities of the members of an organized group toward the accomplishment of group objectives. As a property, leadership is a set of qualities attributed to those who are perceived to successfully employ such characteristics.* (p. 315)

By including the descriptor "noncoercive," Jago placed leadership above manage-ment, which requires the coercive employment contract for implementation. It is a fact that leadership exists without contractual arrangements or boundaries. Rather, it requires what some have described as a spiritual and transcendental relationship between the leader and followers (Keoerner & Bunkers, 1994). Kellerman (1984), referring to the feminist perspective of leadership, implied that it is authority on behalf of, not power or authority over, one's followers.

Barker (1994) defined leadership as a process whereby change occurs in which "the purposes of the leader and follower become fused, creating unity, wholeness and a collective purpose" (p. 83). Emphasizing wholeness, Koerner and Bunkers (1994) reaffirmed the spiritual, almost passionate process of "inner and outer realities being brought together in ways that assist individuals to integrate their unique inner world (values and beliefs) and outer world (life experience) into a unified whole" (p. 71). This unification does not occur without leadership.

Senge (1990) identified learning organizations as the only entities that not only survive, but grow. He described leaders as designers, stewards, and teachers responsible for building organizations in which people continually expand their capabilities to understand complexity, clarify vision, and improve shared mental models. In other words, leadership is responsible for learning.

Leadership may be simply viewed as a process of moving the self and others toward a shared vision that becomes a shared reality. In answer to the question, What is leadership?, DePree (1989) responded, "The first responsibility of a leader is to define reality" (p. 11). DePree's idea of defining reality is closely related to Senge's (1990) idea of understanding complexity and involves clarifying the shared vision and improving shared mental models. It is also an empowerment of followers. DePree (1989) described leadership as an art form that liberates (empowers) people "to do what is required of them in the most effective and humane way possible" (p. 1).

As may be noticed, throughout all of these definitions are the themes of movement, wholeness, and goals. Yet one can also trace from 1978 to more recent definitions the inclusion of integrity, empowerment, and caring, which are more directly related to leadership by APNs. Nursing is not a solo endeavor. To deliver care in an effective and humane way requires a host of learning organizations with multidisciplinary providers.

In discussing leadership for the clinical nurse specialist (CNS) role, Gournic (1989) proposed a continuum of leadership and management skills, knowledge, and processes. On opposite ends of the continuum are leadership and management. In this scenario, the CNS may be torn between the two opposing poles. This model had strong implications for CNSs in a management position, who may find that the paperwork, scheduling, and evaluation responsibilities of management tend to curtail their ability to function as a clinical leader, providing consultation, advocacy, and support to patients and staff nurses.

A different approach is to view leadership as the umbrella concept, with management as a subconcept. This model implies that leadership is at a higher developmental level than management and that to be a leader, one inherently manages others. In contrast to Gournic's (1989) model, management is not defined in terms of discrete tasks, but rather as the ability to work through others to accomplish a goal. In a higher developmental step, leadership is the ability to encourage, empower, and motivate others to desire the accomplishment of the goal, the vision.

This understanding of clinical leadership is illustrated in the case of Jill, a certified nurse-midwife (CNM) who had a vision of providing expert obstetrical care to indigent adolescents as well as professional women. Over the years, the nursing and medical staff at the hospital where Jill worked had tended to treat the two groups differently, deferring to professional women and discounting indigent adolescents. As Jill assumed the primary provider role for both groups, she began to build collegial relationships with both nursing and medical partners, clearly demonstrating her clinical expertise and continually sharing her vision of care. As the unit's primary provider, she was clinically responsible for the level of care delivered. However, clinical care cannot be delivered without administrative management, and so she found herself problem-solving with the nursing and medical staff around day-to-day management issues.

During a particular staff meeting, one of the multigravida adolescents was being discussed in unflattering terms. As Jill started to assume the advocate role, she heard the nurse manager speak passionately, yet with precision, about the unprofessional behavior of staff and its effect on the delivery of services to the young adolescent. In response to the nurse manager, a second speaker revealed his anger about children having children and admitted that his anger left him feeling ambivalent toward young mothers. Jill marveled as she witnessed her vision becoming a shared goal of the staff. She had taken the first step toward defining reality. The empowerment of the staff was a natural sequela.

In this example, both leadership and management activities are evident, but it is the affirmation by others of the vision and leader that puts leadership on a higher conceptual level than management. In this example, the CNM allowed others to share the role of advocate, facilitated an environment that permitted weaknesses and feelings to be shown and owned by members of the team, and relinquished total ownership of the vision as it became affirmed by others.

THE ESSENTIAL ELEMENTS OF LEADERSHIP

Leadership requires vision, risk taking, boundary management, use and empowerment of followers, and mentoring (Bennis & Nanus, 1985; Grohar-Murray & DiCroce, 1992; Malone, 1984).

VISION

A vision is a relative of the dream; it is not constrained by logic or time and place. However, it is the sharable vision, as opposed to the unsharable dream, that is meaningful and achievable. The vision has been the primary methodology that has allowed advanced nursing practice to exist by expanding nursing practice to effectively address clients' needs. The vision may be originally experienced as fragments of thoughts and ideas waiting to be arranged to solve a puzzle. In a study by Dunham and Fisher (1990), a nurse executive described the visioning process as follows: "I always use the analogy of the artist who sketches a scene on a piece of canvas. It doesn't have to have all the colors. A tree doesn't have to have all the leaves" (p. 3).

APNs may envision, for example, the merging of separate medical and surgical cancer units under the umbrella of a cancer center. They may clearly visualize the increased efficiency and collaborative work of the nursing and medical staff in delivering a smoother flow of care. Yet, the vision must be shared with and accepted by others if it is to move from its solitary existence, its dreamlike status, to reality (Gournic, 1989). The sharing of the vision is accomplished through communication. In fact, Spross and Baggerly (1989) described leadership as the use of communication processes to influence the activities of others toward the attainment of goals. The communication of the vision is more thoroughly discussed later in this chapter.

RISK TAKING

The second major element of leadership is risk taking. Howell and Higgins (1990) identified risk taking as one of the characteristics of successful change agents. In advanced nursing practice there is no blueprint for action, because the arena is changing so rapidly. Without a blueprint, room for mistakes must be provided (Grohar-Murray & DiCroce, 1992). With risk taking there must be a safety net and permission to fall, not necessarily fail. What others may perceive as failures are simply delays for a visionary APN.

BOUNDARY MANAGEMENT

Boundary management is the third element of leadership. Leadership is cutting-edge behavior. An edge is a boundary. It separates entities and immediately alerts a leader for the need to design transactions across this dividing line. DePree (1989) distinguished between living and dying edges. "To ignore the dignity of work and the elegance of simplicity, and the essential responsibility of serving each other is to be at the dying edge" (p. 21). The living edge is just the opposite, full of possibilities and potential relationships in service to the vision. The APN not only guards the boundary, but also extends it as a bridge in partnering with other groups and expands it as other client health-care needs are identified. The APN must know where the current boundaries of nursing practice are in order to go beyond them, and going beyond the boundaries is another way to define risk taking.

In addition to being a boundary breaker, the APN is a boundary manager, one who teaches others how to temporarily overlap boundaries with another entity while maintaining the integrity of their own boundaries. Another term for this process is *collaboration*. A CNM may delicately negotiate the boundary of collaboration between the neonatologist and the nursing staff. Perhaps it is a nurse practitioner (NP) and a CNS in two oppositional professional organizations who provide the boundary management to ensure continuous communication and collaboration across and between the two groups. Both clinical leadership and professional leadership require the negotiation of boundaries, whether those borders are drawn around patient populations or organizations.

USE AND EMPOWERMENT OF FOLLOWERS

The fourth element of leadership is the use and empowerment of followers. Using followers implies to some a traditional hierarchical system of leadership that is based more on the male model than on a woman's way of knowing (Belenky, Clinchy, & Tarule, 1986). However, Grohar-Murray and DiCroce (1992) discussed the situational approach to leadership, which includes the element of follower. This approach, defined by Stogdill in 1948 and expanded by Fiedler, Chermers, and Mahar in 1976, suggests that leadership is situationally dependent, with identified leaders and followers in interchangeable roles contingent on environmental demands. DePree (1989) used the term *roving leadership* to describe a participatory process that legitimizes the situational leadership of empowered followers through the support and approval of the hierarchical leader. This theory has great relevance for the APN, who will continually work in collaborative health-care teams that will require that the roles of leader and follower be interchangeable to meet the complex needs of the patient. However, with full appreciation of the situational approach to leadership, the role of leader extends beyond the immediate situation when the element of vision is addressed. The APN as a leader who has a vision of collaboration among health-care team members may facilitate an atmosphere that supports individuals (followers) in assuming the leadership role in various situations. The APN does not cease being the leader by empowering colleagues to appropriately assume a leadership role. In fact, this approach may be an effective way of sharing a vision.

MENTORING

The fifth element of leadership is mentoring. Mentoring is an intense, career-building, mutually beneficial relationship between two individuals of unequal power in an organization (Levinson, 1978; Yoder, 1994). The mentor, usually a senior member of the organization, is the guide, coach, advocate, and sponsor in formal and informal settings and is committed to maximizing the success of the protégé. Although the mentor and protégé are frequently uneven in terms of power, reciprocity is a primary characteristic of mentoring relationships. The protégé has the ability to give support, affirmation, and information to the mentor. One result of this give-and-take relationship is intimacy.

In today's health-care institutions, including community-based operations, a critical mass of APNs may be nonexistent or small, with a limited number of available mentors. As a result, the APN may not have access to an on-site nurse mentor, particularly if the APN is seeking a mentor with the same area of nursing concentration and credentials. For example, a certified registered nurse anesthetist (CRNA) looking for a CRNA mentor on site in a small community hospital may experience some difficulty. It is frequently the perceived isolation of the APN in health-care settings that becomes a major barrier to the survival and growth of the APN role.

One potential solution to the isolation dilemma is for the various types of APNs to begin the arduous task of tearing down the walls and boundaries that separate them. Mentoring is a powerful methodology for creating new linkages and re-aligning as well as redefining old boundaries. For example, an organization could encourage the establishment of a mentoring relationship between a CNS and a NP on the basis of the CNS's senior membership in the organization and ability to provide organizational nurturance to a new NP. Mentoring would thus be from a senior APN to a junior APN.

Where does such a proposition leave the development of specific role characteristics for the NP? Fortunately, Roche (1979) has shown the advantages of having more than one mentor. The APN should approach the acquisition of mentors as a multiopportunity process. There should be an emphasis on selecting mentors who nurture various aspects of the APN's life, including clinical, professional, cultural, personal, and spiritual. These mentors may be on and off site. Rarely can individuals find a single mentor who represents all they need and want to be.

At a professional organizational level, mentoring can be structurally arranged (Kanter, 1977). For example, upon joining an organization, each APN may be asked to identify a mentor or may be assigned a mentor. In addition, mentoring development workshops are held to teach assigned and chosen mentors how to coach and support their protégés more effectively. Rewards of recognition and achievement are then strategically placed to encourage the mentors' commitment and effort. Within the organization, an individual or a group is responsible for monitoring, evaluating, and adapting the mentoring program as necessary. With this type of process, the organization shows concern for both the mentor's and protégé's professional development.

TRANSFER OF THE ELEMENTS OF LEADERSHIP TO APNs

After identifying the essential elements of leadership, the next step is the process of transferring these elements into the philosophy and behavior of APNs. This process is divided into the following components: (1) education, (2) personal mastery, (3) communication, (4) patient-focused practice, and (5) systems thinking. These components are not listed in terms of sequencing or importance, for they may occur simultaneously or in an irregular order. In this discussion, the first component to be examined is education. The researchable question is, Does one begin the process of developing APN leadership with education or personal mastery?

EDUCATION

In graduate nursing educational settings, all of the elements of leadership—vision, risk taking, boundary management, empowerment of followers, and mentoring—need to be reflected in the curriculum, both in clinical practice experiences and discussion of theory and in the professional behavior of students and faculty. Courses that include content in advanced communication skills, organizational/systems theory, negotiation and conflict management, and power and authority in small and large groups would capture the essence of the elements of leadership. Clinical training that involves the APN in small group work as a member and facilitator provides the basic model for the APN to use to motivate and encourage work groups such as health-care teams.

In the educational arena, faculty members should be primary role models of leadership behavior. No one faculty member may possess all the essential elements at the maximum proficiency, but the elements of leadership should be identifiable and reflective of the critical mix of clinical and professional role components.

The educational base represents a primal source of the APN's leadership development, because it is within the graduate educational experience that the seeds of clinical expert power planted in earlier educational and patient care experiences are cultivated. Once the master's degree in nursing is completed and access to the real world environment begins, the clinical and professional development of APN leadership begins.

PERSONAL MASTERY

Bennis (1989) described management of the self as a critical component of ethical leadership. Without it, a leader can be a danger to society, rather than the healing, liberating force described by DePree (1989). Personal mastery is the continuous process of identifying and managing one's personal and professional boundaries with a clear vision of potential growth. APNs have to learn to manage themselves. A key ingredient of personal mastery is strong intra-personal fortitude. *Intra-personal fortitude* can be defined as strong positive self-regard that leads to endurance. The APN who lacks fortitude will view risk taking as overwhelmingly dangerous, and the likelihood of this APN's developing as a leader is diminished.

Seeking an advanced graduate degree in nursing indicates that several important intra-personal characteristics of leadership already exist in APNs: the willingness to take risks and rise above the majority of their nursing colleagues; self-confidence that they can master the advanced content and also function under often vague state regulatory statutes that are silent about the boundaries of nursing practice; and hardiness or persistence in the face of obstacles.

Intra-personal fortitude requires affirmation on a consistent basis. APNs may garner affirmation—assurance that they are who they say they are—personally, clinically, professionally, and spiritually. APNs' personal affirmation or validation comes from themselves and their family, friends, and significant others. Clinical affirmation refers to the validation of expert clinical skills, and APNs receive it from themselves, their patients, their families, the community, their nurse colleagues and other care providers, as well as system managers. Professional affirmation is acquired through involvement with other APNs, which is facilitated by active membership in professional organizations. One underused method of acquiring affirmation is for the APN to participate in self-exploration and validation through individual, group, or family therapy. This is a bold, high-risk, self-caring step reflective of a commitment to leadership development both professionally and personally.

Spiritual affirmation is the APN's belief that a stronger power than humankind has given him or her the right and authority to exist, grow, and develop. DePree (1989) spoke of leadership as a gift from God—with strings attached. The strings include the disappointments, the responsibility for the vision and its implementation into reality, and the lack of rewards for the effort. Much is required of the person to whom much is given. The spiritually affirmed leader has an unending source of motivational power and commitment to a vision that is by its nature contagious and compelling to others.

The formula for becoming an effective leader is a learning process over time. Senge (1990) did not define learning as simply acquiring more information, but rather as the continuous expansion of the ability to produce the results envisioned by the leader. In their intense search for additional expert clinical skills, APNs may not consider personal mastery a priority. As they assume more positions of leadership, the need to identify and manage their own strengths and weaknesses will become more and more necessary. Personal mastery is the continuous process of identifying and managing one's personal and professional boundaries with a clear vision of potential growth. Without personal mastery, APN leaders cannot adequately manage boundaries between APNs and staff nurses, APNs and physicians, APNs and health-care administrators, and APNs and APNs and therefore will not be able to promote collaboration between these groups. Mature boundary management is a key ingredient of successful collaboration. The evolving health-care system is seeking professionals who specialize in collaboration. The APN with personal mastery is in a strong position to be known as a specialist in the art of collaboration.

COMMUNICATION

As discussed earlier, communicating a vision is one of the key tasks of a leader. This is accomplished through clarification, repetition, and inviting others to adapt and design elements of the vision until it becomes a shared reality. Grohar-Murray and DiCroce (1992) offered some basic suggestions for effective communication, which in turn will lead to effective leadership.

1. *Clarify one's own ideas before communicating to others.* APNs will always be in positions of influence, whether as team leaders or team members. For example, the NP who is strongly advocating for a patient to the nursing staff may unintentionally project the idea that nurses are the only true advocates for patients and place all other team members in an oppositional position. Implying that only the APN and the nursing staff truly care about the patient can sow seeds of discord among team members. It is incumbent upon APNs to choose their messages with care, giving thought to their potential impact on others. An audiotape, a videotape, or an objective colleague can prove exceptionally helpful in providing feedback through practice.

2. *Consider the physical and psychological settings.* For example, a CRNA who has some disquieting comments for the lead surgeon may appropriately decide not to share them during a surgical procedure, but to schedule an appointment in office space most comfortable for a potentially difficult encounter with the surgeon.

3. *Consult with others when necessary to be exact and objective.* The APN who unintentionally provides misinformation should acknowledge and correct the error. With the title of APN comes the mixed blessing of being seen as an expert. In nursing language, *expert* means infallible, all knowing and perfect. Meeting this role expectation is impossible. The APN, even when occupying the leadership role for the entire health-care team, must be able to ask for assistance and clarification from others.

4. *Be mindful of the overtones as well as the content of the message.* This implies sensitivity to the context, sequence, and emotional underlay of what is being said as well as what is not being said. Attention to verbal and nonverbal cues is essential. When APNs have the luxury to travel in pairs, one APN can function in the role of meeting processor, paying specific attention to body language and the unspoken dynamics of the encounter, while the other functions as the primary communicator. Psychiatric CNSs excel in the processing role.

5. *Convey something of value or praise to the intended receiver of the message.* Praise tends to empower others through encouragement and reaffirmation. One strategy is for APNs to develop a written list of praiseworthy attributes and behaviors for those colleagues with whom they have the most difficulty. Some of the most highly volatile meetings have been disarmed by opening the encounter with praise and closing the encounter with praise. The critical message is sandwiched between praise statements that are positive, honest, and accurate. This allows for further consideration and digestion of the critical message by the receiver.

6. *Follow up all communication regarding a vision.* A leader's vision must be able to be shared through communication. This usually requires more than one contact with the receiver. The feedback loop is critical to the APN's successful functioning. Although the role of most APNs is filled with high-intensity activity, time must be made for feedback and follow-up. One way the APN can make the time for evaluation, reflection, and corrective or additional action is to actually schedule times for these activities as part of the workday.

7. *Be sure one's actions support one's communication.* In other words, practice what you preach. As leaders, APNs are watched for discrepancies between their philosophy (what they say they believe) and their performance (what

they do). For example, NPs who say one day that physicians should treat staff with more respect but the next day arrive at the agency without speaking to the staff are not practicing what they have preached. If this is part of patterned behavior, staff will begin to doubt the validity of the NP's words and eventually the NP as a leader.

PATIENT-FOCUSED PRACTICE

APN leadership must be clearly visible in the delivery of care to patients. Functioning primarily as practitioners, APNs may not automatically connect leadership activities with their daily care-giving practice. Yet, working effectively in multidisciplinary teams and with other nurses in various roles requires the leadership elements described earlier in this chapter: vision, risk taking, boundary management, empowerment of followers, and mentoring.

APNs must have a vision of how the health-care team can collaboratively work together in partnership with the community to provide optimal health care. To achieve this vision will require risk taking as boundaries between disciplines are crossed and colleagues are empowered to deliver care in new settings with an array of new providers. The mentoring element is of special value in relationship to patient-focused practice. It is through mentoring that the patient care and leadership expertise of the APN is transferred to other nurses and providers.

SYSTEMS THINKING

The APN cannot adequately function without systems thinking. Senge (1990) defined systems thinking as the discipline of seeing wholes. He described it as a framework for seeing interrelationships rather than isolated things, for seeing patterns of change rather than snapshots. Senge pointed out that the words *whole* and *health* come from the same root, the Old English *hal,* as in "hale and hearty." Seeing the whole of a situation allows one to identify the health of an organization and design healing strategies if necessary. Leadership requires the ability to see the whole. Once again, this ability may have existed in the clinical arena, but its transferability to the professional association setting may be difficult, particularly because it is leaders whom the APN is leading.

When clinical leadership is exercised, professional leadership is easier to develop, however. Professional leadership is built on the foundation of clinical leadership. For the APN, professional involvement is critical to survival as well as growth. In today's rapidly changing health-care environment, the unity of APNs is a primary success strategy. The organizational structure for a unified group of APNs is the professional association. Yet APNs are professionally organized not as a total group, but by patient-focused specialty areas, whose professional associations were developed separately and independently. Before the larger issue of an overall professional organizational structure for APNs can be addressed, the process of becoming a professional leader, or a leader among leaders, must be understood.

It is at this juncture that the need for mentoring supersedes the other elements of leadership. In professional associations, it is important to have a mentor who sees the system as a whole and can decipher the organizational code, provide an accessible role model, and clarify the parameters for risk taking. Finding a good mentor should be the first thing APNs who wish to develop their professional leadership abilities do. An APN's level of entry into the professional association is dependent on the mentor's power base. If the mentor is a board member or chairs a committee, the APN may sail over the anonymity stage and enter with a prime assignment that has significant meaning to the professional association. In the development of professional leadership, one of the most important steps is the mentee's first assignment in the organization. A mentor can be especially helpful in ensuring the mentee entry and access to the organization.

Kanter's (1977) description of the mentor (or sponsor) role provides additional support for the importance of this role. Mentors develop their protégés in such a way that they move effectively in and through the organization; they fight formally and informally for their protégés, helping them bypass the hierarchy of information, planning, and implementation, cutting the proverbial red tape; and they provide reflected power and status by indicating to others that their protégés have access to their resources and support. Mentoring relationships between senior and junior APNs are a relatively new occurrence in nursing. The politics of the present health-care environment demand a prudent, efficient system, like mentoring, for developing organizationally astute APNs.

A major part of seeing the organization as a whole is related to advanced communication skills, which must expand to include small and large group work. This means the ability to conduct meetings, present speeches, provide consultation, and publish information in written form. All of these skills are necessary for the development of the individual APN as well as the organization, whether clinical or professional.

There is appropriate overlap between the systems-thinking skills needed for the clinical and professional arenas. Skills developed in the clinical arena are usually generalizable to the professional one. At times, though, an APN may have difficulty transferring skills learned in the clinical setting to the professional association setting. As an example, consider the case of Addie, an APN who was eagerly looking forward to the annual meeting of her specialty association. Addie was going to present a report from the prescriptive authority committee, addressing the entire membership of the association for the first time. She was excited about the chance to make her mentor, vice president of the association, proud. Immediately before the time of Addie's presentation, however, a fellow committee member hurriedly approached her. Addie was informed that none of the committee members would be present for the report. Her colleague, representing the other committee members, wanted her to forthrightly address the sensitive issue of physicians' lack of competence when prescribing and monitoring drug treatment. She was warned that this should be handled delicately, because physicians would be present in the audience. Finally, she was told that if she did not feel up to the task, her colleague would be happy to relay her unreadiness to the rest of the committee. Perhaps most troubling was the fact that the message was delivered in an angry and sarcastic tone.

Addie approached the podium feeling apprehensive, betrayed by the absence of her committee colleagues, and unsettled by the underlying anger she felt from the messenger. Her presentation reflected her confusion; although she had successfully developed speaking and organizational skills in the clinical arena, they did not transfer at this point. Addie experienced the loss of her skills because of the intensity of the interaction and the fact that she had not seen the system as a whole, including her colleagues' reaction to her quick, well-sponsored rise in the association. She was not prepared to face issues of competition, authority, and power from fellow APNs, within the assumed safety net of her own professional APN association.

Professional leadership tends to demand more personal exposure of the leader than clinical leadership does. In the clinical arena, the patient, as the center of the organizational effort, may offset some of the negative small and large group dynamics. In the professional arena, personal battles over power and control cannot be fought behind the protective cover of the claim, "I'm just advocating for the patient."

As Addie found, a common reaction to stress is to become de-skilled and confused. The healing strategy for ethical and collaborative professional leadership is personal mastery and the use of communication skills. The APN must possess or develop the intra-personal fortitude to withstand perceived and real attacks, even from those with whom he or she is most closely associated. In the same manner, the exquisite use of communication skills is most visible in pressured situations. The APN must come to terms with the reality that one of the consequences of leadership is becoming a target for competition and envy. The ability to clarify one's behavioral options in a situation and the ability to communicate with respect for others in the most humane way possible, regardless of the circumstances, are critical to the leadership development of the APN.

THE DEVELOPMENT OF APN LEADERS

All the ingredients for leadership development have been discussed. There remains the unanswered question of sequencing, or stages of development. A model, seen in Figure 10–1, can be viewed as four concentric circles, with personal mastery as the core circle. In the next outer circle is education, representing not only the

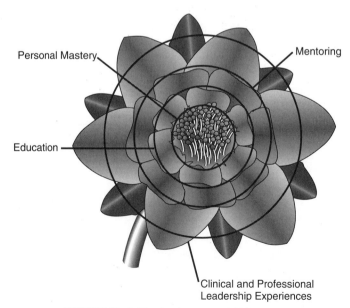

FIGURE 10–1. The development of APN leaders.

initial graduate nursing degree but also lifelong learning. The third outer circle is mentoring, and the fourth circle represents the lived experience of both clinical and professional leadership. The model unfolds like a flower from its core to its furthermost boundary of lived experience, but it has the ability to refold within itself, appearing as one circle and allowing even the fourth circle of experience to touch and reinforce the circle of personal mastery.

This global model captures the essence of leadership development. The development of leadership requires practice of the application of leadership over time. A more specific guideline for the application of leadership has been provided by Heifetz (1994), who outlined the following steps:

1. Identify the adaptive challenge. Clarify reality and begin to design the vision.
2. Regulate distress. This includes the system's distress as well as the leader's and is regulated by personal mastery and expert clinical skills.
3. Direct disciplined attention to the issue. Step 3 requires communication and expert clinical and/or systems-thinking skills.
4. Give the work back to the people. Empower followers to share the vision and implement strategies to produce outcomes.
5. Protect voices of leadership in the community. This final step represents the empowerment of followers through communication, risk taking, support, and also mentoring.

OBSTACLES AND STRATEGIES FOR OVERCOMING THEM

There are obstacles to achieving this vision of APN leadership in clinical and professional association settings. Two obstacles are the star complex and the lack of unification between and among types of APNs.

THE STAR COMPLEX

The star complex is a condition frequently associated with the experienced APN in the clinical setting. As an example, consider the case of Janice, an APN who, over the years, has become identified with superior patient-focused care. Physician colleagues and other providers consider her to be a partner in the delivery of care. In a recent conversation, a well-respected physician colleague told her how impressed he was with her practice. "In fact," he stated, "you're really not a nurse. You're different from all the other nurses I know." Janice graciously accepted this compliment, knowing that stardom, although overdue, had finally arrived. She had ascended to the heights of provider status and crashed through the nursing ceiling into a zone beyond nursing. Clearly, Janice's boundary management of herself as an APN was dormant.

APNs are particularly vulnerable to being seduced into believing they are something other (more) than a nurse. This vulnerability stems from the historical lack of recognition of nursing by physicians, other disciplines, and nurses; the need for approval and to be liked, which is a profile characteristic of most nurses and women; and a lack of personal mastery.

A primary strategy for the management of this obstacle is effective mentoring by a powerful APN with an intact nursing identity. The APN with the star complex has usually been mentored exclusively by individuals outside of nursing, such as physicians. Mentors tend to select protégés who remind them of themselves (Bowen, 1985) and then mold their protégés in their own image. The affirmation of the APN's expert clinical skills and even personal mastery are thus validated by a reference group outside of nursing. To acquire a new reference group for validation of worth requires mentoring of the APN by a member of the desired reference group.

An additional essential strategy is to use clear and concise communication skills to provide an appropriate response to a colleague who believes that it is a compliment to be identified as other than a nurse. Grohar-Murray and DiCroce's (1992) guidelines for effective communication, discussed earlier in this chapter, are applicable. An appropriate response for Janice to have made would have been, "I'm excellent at what I do; but I'm only one of many excellent nurses."

The existence of the star complex may represent a more fundamental problem for the APN than good communication skills can address. The issue is whether the APN truly desires to be identified as a *nurse*, performing at the boundaries of nursing practice and accepted by other nurses as a valued member of the nursing profession. The resolution of this issue may require counseling and/or group experiential exploration and training. Self-exploration within the context of organizations is provided by various educational organizations. For example, the A.K. Rice Institute gives individuals opportunities to focus disciplined attention on their role, particularly in terms of authority, power, and leadership, in both small and large groups (Colman & Geller, 1985). This type of experiential training may prove invaluable to APNs attempting to identify their professional reference group.

UNITY VERSUS FRAGMENTATION

With the recent emphasis on health care reform and President Clinton's support of the APN as a significant provider of care in the reformed system, the acceptance of the APN by the public has been positive. In a 1993 Gallup poll, more than 85% of the respondents reported that an NP would be acceptable as a primary care provider (American Nurses Association, 1993). In the results of the poll lie the roots of the problem of APN disunity. The report identifies the NP, rather than the APN, as acceptable to the public. The unique differences between the types of APNs can lead to fragmentation instead of a unified group known as advanced practice nurses who have distinct roles as CNMs, CNSs, CRNAs, NPs, and so on.

At different times, each subgroup of APNs has emerged as a leader for the nursing profession. Psychiatric CNSs were among the first entrepreneurial APNs to hang out their shingles, despite the litigious climate in which they could be threatened with law suits for "practicing medicine." CNMs and CRNAs have led the way in powerfully using data to justify their existence. Both groups began early to record the results of their practices, showing the quality and suitability of their care (Diers, 1992). And in the 1990s, NPs, with their flexible, community-based primary care practices, stand at the forefront of the changing health-care delivery system. The obstacle to leadership is the tendency for APNs to separate and establish the boundaries that distinguish them from one another in concrete, thereby blocking opportunities for the increased power that unity would bring.

With this tension and fragmentation, there is a leadership role for the APN. This role is not only for boundary management but also for bridging boundaries between APNs and other nursing groups and within the ranks of the APN constituency. Although the uniqueness of each type of APN must be protected, a professional structure that provides a forum for discussing issues pertinent to all types of APNs also needs to be created. This structure may be simply an annual meeting for APNs, or it may be a permanent entity residing within an existing or new professional organization. The vision to unify, practice, and collaborate is calling to every APN.

The following guidelines adapted from Heifetz (1994) may help APNs move from fragmentation to unity:

1. Because leadership, as stated at the beginning of this chapter, is a core competency for the APN, the goal of unification must be translated into a shared vision.
2. APNs and their various professional associations need a forum to explore, identify, and regulate the stress related to crossing and perhaps merging boundaries previously viewed as impenetrable. A specific example of this is the blended CNS/NP role discussed in Chapter 17. This redefinition of reality will require taking risks with and without the benefit of a safety net.
3. With a legitimate forum established, APNs will direct disciplined attention to the issue of unity.
4. Each type of APN will return to the referent professional association for continuing dialogue and support of the outcomes from the forum discussion. This involves giving the work back to the people.
5. Each APN will listen with respect and in every humane way possible to leadership voices in the APN and nursing profession communities and in the communities of care recipients, providers, payors, legislators, and citizens.
6. APNs will emerge from this systematic, inclusive exploration of unity with a clear trajectory for building a learning organization to support the continued development of APN leadership in unity.

CONCLUSION

APN leadership, both clinical and professional, is founded on clinical expertise, which is a product of education and experience. In addition, APN leadership is legitimately authorized by role and position. With APNs at the forefront of the health-care delivery system as it is currently evolving, they have the authority to lead that their clinical expertise, role, and position bring. The developmental question is the effectiveness of APN leadership. The APN's effectiveness through the filter of personal mastery is strongly linked to vision, risk taking, mentoring, and the empowerment of followers. These elements of leadership identify the effective leaders, and their absence or lack of consistent use identifies those who are less effective leaders.

As APNs contemplate the demands and opportunities for leadership the future is bringing, they need to have a clear focus on identifying, clarifying, and demystifying reality. Within today's reality lie the building blocks of tomorrow's change. APNs are change specialists operating at the boundaries of the present reality and using collaboration and affirmation as tools to place the nursing profession and health care system in a position to more effectively meet the needs of individuals, families, and global as well as local communities.

REFERENCES

American Nurses Association. (Sept 1993). Consumers willing to see a nurse for routine doctoring according to Gallup Poll. Washington, DC: ANA News Release, pp. 1–2.

Barker, A. (1994). An energy leadership paradigm: Transformational leadership. In E.I. Hein & M.J. Nicholson (Eds.), *Contemporary leadership* (4th ed., pp. 81–86). Philadelphia: J. B. Lippincott.

Belenky, M.F., Clinchy, B.M., & Tarule, J.M. (1986). *Women's ways of knowing.* New York: Basic Books.

Bennis, W. (1989). *On being a leader.* Reading, MA: Addison-Wesley.

Bennis, W., & Nanus, B. (1985). *Leaders: The strategies for taking charge.* New York: Harper & Row.

Bowen, D. (1985). Were men meant to mentor women? *Training and Development Journal, 39,* 30–34.

Burns, J.M. (1978). *Leadership.* New York: Harper & Row.

Colman, A., & Geller, M. (1985). *Group relations reader 2.* Washington, DC: A.K. Rice Institute.

DePree, M. (1989). *Leadership is an art.* New York: Doubleday/Currency.

Diers, D. (1992). Nurse-midwives and nurse anesthetists: The cutting edge in specialist practice. In L. Aiken & C. Fagin (Eds.), *Charting nursing's future* (pp. 159–180). Philadelphia: J.B. Lippincott.

Dunham, J., & Fisher, E. (1990). Nurse executive profile of excellent nursing leadership. *Nursing Administration Quarterly, 15,* 1–8.

Fiedler, F.E., Chermers, M.M., & Mahar, L.C. (1976). *Improving leadership effectiveness: The leader match concept.* New York: Wiley.

Gournic, J. (1989). Clinical leadership, management and the CNS. In A.B. Hamric & J.A. Spross (Eds.), *The clinical nurse specialist in theory and practice* (pp. 227–240). Philadelphia: W.B. Saunders Company.

Grohar-Murray, M.E., & DiCroce, H.R. (1992). *Leadership and management in nursing.* Norwalk, CT: Appleton & Lange.

Heifetz, R. (1994). *Leadership without easy answers.* Cambridge, MA: Belknap Press.

Howell, J.M., & Higgins, C.A. (1990) Champions of change: Identifying, understanding and supporting champions of technological innovations. *Organizational Dynamics, 19,* 40–55.

Jago, A. (1982). Leadership: Perspective training and research. *Management Science, 28,* 315–336.

Kanter, R. (1977). *Men and women of the corporation.* New York: Basic Books.

Kellerman, B. (1984). *Leadership: Multidisciplinary perspectives.* Englewood Cliffs, NJ: Prentice-Hall.

Keoerner, J., & Bunkers, S. (1994). Transformational leadership: The power of symbol. In E. Hein & M.J. Nicholson (Eds.), *Contemporary leadership behavior* (4th ed., pp. 71–80). Philadelphia: J.B. Lippincott.

Levinson, D.J. (1978). *Seasons of a man's life.* New York: Knopf.

Malone, B. (1984). Strategies and approaches to policymaking: A nursing perspective. *Occupational Health Nursing, 32* (1), 24–27.

Roche, G.R. (1979). Much ado about mentors. *Harvard Business Review, 57* (1), 14–28.

Senge, P. (1990). *The fifth discipline.* New York: Doubleday.

Spross, J.A., & Baggerly, J. (1989). Models of advanced practice. In A.B. Hamric & J.A. Spross (Eds.), *The clinical nurse specialist in theory and practice* (2nd ed., pp. 19–40). Philadelphia: W.B. Saunders Company.

Stogdill, R.M. (1948). Personal factors associated with leadership in a survey of the literature. *Journal of Psychology, 25,* 35–71.

Yoder, L. (1994). Mentoring: A concept analysis. In E. Hein & M.J. Nicholson (Eds.), *Contemporary leadership behavior* (4th ed., pp. 187–196). Philadelphia: J.B. Lippincott Company.

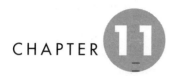

CHAPTER 11

Collaboration

Charlene M. Hanson
Judith A. Spross

INTRODUCTION

Advanced practice nurses (APNs) interact with a broad range of professionals and clients. For this reason, they must have or acquire interpersonal communication skills and behaviors that make collaboration possible. Clients assume that their health-care providers communicate and collaborate effectively. However, client dissatisfaction with care, unsatisfactory clinical outcomes, and clinician frustration can often be traced to a failure to collaborate. The ability to collaborate is a core competency of advanced nursing practice (ANP). Collaboration depends on clinical and interpersonal expertise and an understanding of factors that can promote or impede efforts to establish collegial relationships.

In this chapter, historical factors that have shaped collaboration in advanced nursing practice are outlined; a definition and characteristics of collaboration that more fully address values, interpersonal aspects, and goals are offered; factors that can affect collaborative efforts are identified; and strategies for developing and evaluating this competency are suggested. Key collaborative relationships for the APN are those with physicians, those within interdisciplinary teams, and those with other nurses. These relationships are used to illustrate aspects of this important core competency.

HISTORICAL OVERVIEW OF COLLABORATION

Over the years, there have been many reports of successful collaborative relationships involving APNs (examples include Ryan, Edwards, & Rickles, 1980; Steele, 1986; Littell, 1981; Crowley & Wollner, 1987; Hilderley, 1991; Kavesh, 1993; Dressler, 1994; Kedziera & Levy, 1994; Siegler & Whitney, 1994a). Most of them are anecdotal; few reports are found in the early research literature on APNs. In the early 1970s, the American Nurses' Association (ANA) and the American Medical Association collaborated to form the National Joint Practice Committee (NJPC, 1979). The committee was created to respond to tension and conflict between physicians and nurses that was perceived to be due to increased patient loads and cost constraints, which were placing excessive demands on both groups. The NJPC funded several demonstration projects to implement joint practice arrangements within four different hospital settings that were attempting to improve nurse-physician relationships. The NJPC identified five criteria that were considered critical to the implementation of collaborative practice arrangements in hospital settings: primary nursing, integrated patient records, encouragement of nurse decision making, a joint practice committee, and a joint record review (NJPC, 1979; Devereux, 1981). These criteria are still seen as essential components in the establishment of cooperative practice arrangements. Although the data from these NJPC projects from 20 years ago indicated improved communication and improved patient care outcomes, the work was never completed. Unfortunately, there has not been widespread implementation of the NJPC's recommendations over time (Crowley & Wollner, 1987; Fagin, 1992).

From the perspective of the physician-nurse relationship, legislative and regulatory limitations in the areas of autonomy for APNs (e.g., reimbursement and/or prescriptive authority) have been major disincentives for the implementation of collaborative roles (Fagin, 1992; Inglis & Kjervik, 1993). Although major strides have been made in some states, there continues to be a hierarchical structure to physician-nurse relationships that hampers overall collaboration between these health-care providers. APNs, especially certified registered nurse anesthetists (CRNAs), certified nurse-midwives (CNMs), and nurse practitioners (NPs), who are perceived to be practicing within medicine's domain, continue to struggle with the issue of supervision versus collaboration in their practice relationships. In addition, research by Sands, Stafford, and McClelland (1990) suggests that team members see themselves primarily as representatives of their own discipline, rather than as members of a collaborative team.

Of equal concern, some role confusion and turf issues within the nursing profession continue to exist, hampering collaboration between nurses and APNs and between the different types of APNs. An example of these tensions is the current disagreement over the convergence or divergence of the NP and clinical nurse specialist (CNS) roles. In addition, the lack of unity among various specialty professional organizations is a strong indication that team-building work needs to be done within the profession. With APNs evolving as bona fide providers of health care, collaborative practice and referral patterns between APNs that identify and strengthen nursing's contribution to innovative care modalities are critical.

A CONCEPTUALIZATION OF COLLABORATION

Collaboration can be thought of as one of several modes of interaction that occur between and among clinicians during the delivery of care. To appreciate the complexity of collaboration, it is useful to describe the variety of interactions that can occur. Over time, CNMs have been credited with creating the clearest definitions of collaboration, consultation, and referral in their practice relationships with obstetricians. These include parallel communication and functioning, information exchange, coordination, consultation, co-management, referral, and collaboration.

Parallel communication: Providers interact with a patient separately; they do not talk together before seeing a patient nor do they see the patient together. There is no expectation of joint interactions. For example, the staff RN, the medical student, and the attending physician all ask the patient about the medications the patient is taking.

Parallel functioning: Providers care for patients, addressing the same clinical problem, but do not engage in any joint or collaborative planning. For example, nurses, physical therapists, and physicians document their interventions for pain in separate parts of the patient record.

Information exchange: *Informing* may be one- or two-sided and may or may not require action or decision making. If action is needed, the decision is unilateral, not a result of joint planning.

Coordination: The establishment of structures to minimize duplication of effort and to maximize efficient use of clients' and providers' resources.

Consultation: The process whereby the clinician who is caring for a client seeks advice regarding a client concern but retains primary responsibility for care delivery.

Co-management: This refers to the process of two or more providers providing care in which each provider retains accountability and responsibility for defined aspects of care. This process usually arises from consultation in which a problem requires management that is outside the scope of practice of the referring clinician. One clinician usually retains responsibility for the majority of care (as in primary care settings) while the second provider is accountable for managing the problem that is outside the primary provider's expertise. Providers must be explicit with each other about their responsibilities. Co-management may also characterize well-functioning interdisciplinary teams.

Referral: The process by which the APN directs the client to a physician or another practitioner for management of a particular problem or aspect of the client's care when the problem is beyond his or her expertise.

With the exceptions of parallel communication and parallel functioning, these processes require some level of interaction and communication among providers. Information exchange, coordination, consultation, co-management, and referral do not require collaboration as it is described here, although collaboration is likely to enhance them.

According to the dictionary, *collaboration* means "to work together, especially in a joint intellectual effort"; it also means to cooperate with the enemy (McKechnie, 1983). The term *collaborative* is often used with other words, such as *teamwork* or *partnership*.

The description of collaboration in the ANA's (1995) Social Policy Statement informs the definition and discussion of collaboration in this chapter. ANA recognizes that the boundaries of each health profession change and that high quality care depends on the exchange of ideas and knowledge. They describe collaboration as involving the:

> *recognition of the expertise of others within and outside one's profession. . . . [it] also involves some shared functions and a common focus on the same overall mission.*
>
> (1995, p. 12)

None of these meanings adequately represent this concept as it exists, or should exist, in the provision of health and illness care. On the basis of our review of the literature and experiences, we propose the following definition of collaboration:

Collaboration: An interpersonal process in which two or more individuals make a commitment to interact constructively to solve problems and accomplish identified goals, purposes, or outcomes. The individuals recognize and articulate the shared values that make this commitment possible.

This definition implies shared values, commitment, and goals and yet allows for differences in opinions and approaches. This definition also suggests that collaboration is complex. Including the notions of shared values and commitment makes clear that collaboration is a process that evolves over time. Tjosvold (1986) and Hughes and Mackenzie (1990) emphasize the importance of goal interdependence to true collaboration. By definition, collaboration describes relationships that are positive and work well for professionals and clients. There is room for disagreement in collaborative relationships; partners develop strategies for dealing with disagreement that are mutually satisfactory and enhance collaboration. Because it is an interpersonal process, collaboration cannot be accomplished by mandate.

This broad-based definition invites exploration of the characteristics that make up a truly collaborative relationship and the personal and setting-specific attributes that are pivotal to successful professional collaborations.

CHARACTERISTICS OF EFFECTIVE COLLABORATION

Effective collaboration between and among APNs, physicians, and other nurses in an ever-changing health-care environment depends on many factors. The definition of collaboration proposed in this chapter demands a radical rethinking of how APNs are prepared and how clinicians interact to ensure positive patient outcomes. Some of the characteristics of collaboration have long been recognized and promulgated, but as the work of the NJPC indicates, clinicians and organizations have resisted adopting the philosophy and behaviors that promote collaboration. The five components of collaborative practice that the NJPC (1979) identified as critical (see earlier in this chapter) acknowledge nurse autonomy and authority for nursing practice and are still important today. Steele's (1986) analysis of collaboration among NPs and physicians revealed several characteristics: mutual trust and respect, an understanding and acceptance of each other's disciplines, positive self-image, equivalent professional maturity arising from education and experience, recognition that the partners are not substitutes for each other, and a willingness to negotiate. Hughes and Mackenzie (1990) outlined four characteristics of NP/physician collaboration: collegiality, communication, goal sharing, and task interdependence. Spross (1989), based on a review of CNS and interdisciplinary literature, described three essential elements of collaboration: a common purpose, diverse and complementary professional knowledge and skills, and effective communication processes. Although this is not an exhaustive summary of the literature on collaboration, it is clear that shared values, effective interpersonal communication, and organizational structures can promote productive alliances among clinicians and create an environment in which collaboration is valued and practiced.

The discussion of characteristics of collaboration that follows elaborates on the definition of collaboration proposed in this chapter. The ability to "make a commitment to interact constructively" suggests that there are characteristics that are prerequisites—qualities that prospective partners must bring to initial and ongoing encounters. These characteristics are a common purpose, clinical competence, interpersonal skills (or a willingness to learn them), and a sense of humor. Other characteristics such as trust, respect, and valuing each other's knowledge and skills reflect the nature of collaboration as an "interpersonal process." They are equally important but only develop fully over time. However, in order for them to develop, prospective partners must enter encounters with a commitment to respect, a willingness to trust, and an assumption that the other's knowledge and skills are valuable. In this sense, these characteristics are also prerequisites, but they are fully realized only after many constructive and productive interactions have occurred. Evans (1994) discussed collaboration as a force for achieving desired outcomes. She confirmed that clinicians who collaborate engage in a communal, intellectual effort on behalf of patients and share problem-solving, goal setting, and decision making (Evans, 1994). Thus, collaboration can occur only when prospective partners recognize that a problem can be solved only when each party's input, expertise, or participation is solicited (Stichler, 1995).

COMMON PURPOSE

The notion that a common purpose must be the basis for collaboration is well supported in the literature (Alpert, Goldman, Kilroy, & Pike 1992; Arslanian-Engoren, 1995). Even if partners have not discussed the purposes and goals of their interactions, the organizations in which they work usually have an explicit mission and goals. These can be the starting point for identifying the goals and purposes of clinical collaboration. Evans (1994) made the point that true collaboration involves a bond, a union, a degree of patient caring that goes beyond a single approach to care and represents a synergistic alliance that maximizes the contributions of each participant. Alpert et al. (1992) developed a model unit to test the concept of collaboration between doctors and nurses at Boston's Beth Israel Hospital, a 504-bed tertiary care institution. They found that collaboration is more than simply working closely next to a co-worker; rather there is a special synergy that comes from working in a true collaborative manner that allows for better overall outcomes in patient care.

Collaboration, by its very definition, implies that the participants are interdependent. Recognizing their interdependence, team members can combine their individual perceptions and skills to synthesize more complex and comprehensive care plans (Forbes & Fitzsimmons, 1993). Each member brings a particular set of skills and unique expertise to the table for a combined strength that cannot be matched by individuals working alone. Like other characteristics, the common purpose(s) that initially brought partners together may change over time. For example, the organizational goals or situation that brought two clinicians together becomes subordinate to the deep, personal commitment to work together that arises from joint efforts that result in successful patient outcomes and are interpersonally satisfying. In order to make a commitment to a common purpose and follow through on it, a broader statutory definition of professional autonomy for APNs than currently exists in many states is called for; this is necessary if the more complex autonomy of interdependent collaborators is to be exercised effectively (Forbes & Fitzsimmons, 1993; Inglis & Kjervik, 1993).

CLINICAL COMPETENCE

Clinical competence is perhaps the most important characteristic leading to a successful collaborative experience among clinical caregivers, for without it the trust and desire needed to work together are not possible. The literature clearly shows that there is not a level playing field vis à vis competence. Physicians are perceived as all-knowing, whereas nurses are portrayed as non-intellectual and second-best substitutes for excellent health care (Fagin, 1992; Petronis-Jones, 1994; Sands et al., 1990). The status of advanced nursing practice is still such that nurses must prove their competence to the profession and to society (Prescott & Bowen, 1985; Fagin, 1992).

When the clinical competence of collaborating clinicians is reliable and consistent, certain processes vital to collaboration can occur. For example, leadership is problem-based, not team- or role-based. Instead of one person always being the team leader, in a departure from the traditional "captain of the team" approach, leadership can shift among partners. Thus, the person with the most expertise, interest, or talent can respond to the particular demands of the situation or problem. The trust and respect among collaborators are such that they can count on satisfactory resolution of the problem even when they know as individuals they might have approached the issue differently. For example, it is clear that APNs are expert in educating patients about their illnesses and lifestyle choices. Thus, collaboration offers APNs very viable arenas in which to role-model innovative nursing strategies as well as to learn from the expertise of teammates. APNs need to showcase their competent and exemplary practice in order to build nursing's reputation for competence (Fagin, 1992; Lenz, 1994).

INTERPERSONAL COMPETENCE

Interpersonal competence is the ability to communicate effectively with colleagues in a variety of situations, including uncomplicated, routine interaction, disagreements, value conflicts, and stressful situations. It requires a level of self-esteem and assertiveness that nurses have begun to acquire only in the past few years. It is imperative that nurses understand and articulate what they bring to the table as members of the health-care team. The key to demonstrating interpersonal competence is the APN's ability to communicate clearly and convincingly, both verbally and in writing. This attribute was identified by Hanson, Hodnicki, and Boyle (1994) in their analysis of the attributes that physicians most valued in their NP colleagues. The ability to communicate well with physicians, other staff members, the patient, and the patient's family was highly regarded by the physicians in Hanson et al.'s study. After clinical competence, interpersonal competence may be the most important individual characteristic for APNs to focus on when moving toward collaborative roles in practice.

HUMOR

Another important aspect of the collaborative process is humor. Balzer (1993) suggested that humor in which the intent is positive can be a non-threatening, creative way to set the stage for effective communication and problem solving between disciplines. In collaborative practice, humor serves to decrease defensiveness, invite openness, relieve tension, and deflect anger. It helps individuals keep perspective and acknowledge the lack of perfection and sets the tone for trust and acceptance among colleagues so that difficult situations can be reframed (Balzer, 1993). Humor is a powerful tool that should be added to educational curricula as a support for effective communication.

TRUST

Implicit in discussions of collaboration is the presence of mutual trust, mutual respect, and personal integrity, qualities evinced in the nature of interactions between partners. In fact, distrust is often cited as a major barrier to successful collaborative relationships (Alpert et al., 1992; Evans, 1994). The development of trust and respect depends on clinical competence; it is very difficult to trust and respect a colleague whose clinical competence is questionable. Partners must recognize and appreciate their overlapping and diverse skills and knowledge

(Spross, 1989) for mutual trust and respect to develop and deepen over time. Partners observe that each other's clinical competence is consistent; that their interactions—even those that involve significant conflict over goals of care and interventions—are respectful, productive, and satisfying; and that patients benefit from their combined talents and efforts. They come to depend on each other to use good clinical judgment and to take appropriate actions.

A central theme of the development of trust is *sharing*. Partners are guided by a shared vision of the possibilities inherent in collaboration; they believe in the value of collaboration, and they are committed to achieving the relationship's potential (Krumm, 1992). Collaboration also means sharing in planning, decision making, problem solving, goal setting, and assuming responsibility (Baggs & Schmitt, 1988). Thus, even though partners' ideas, opinions, and actions might be different, their belief in each other and their shared vision permit—even value— such differences.

The issue of developing trust presents a particular challenge to APNs since it has been observed that the competence of physicians is assumed and medical incompetence must be proven while nurses must prove themselves and their competence in each new encounter (Prescott & Bowen, 1985; Fagin, 1992). APNs encounter numerous physicians in the course of practice; a lack of positive expectations and the potential assumption of incompetence of APNs until they demonstrate otherwise are major barriers to collaboration (Fagin, 1992). This means APNs require courage and fortitude to challenge such assumptions assertively when they become apparent in disconfirming or aggressive encounters with colleagues (Coeling & Wilcox, 1994).

VALUING AND RESPECTING OF DIVERSE, COMPLEMENTARY KNOWLEDGE

Respect for others' practice and knowledge is key to successful collaboration, because it enhances shared decision making. A great deal of successful collaborative work is self-driven. There must be a desire, at a very personal level, to collaborate and to value and respect others' ideas and actions, as well as a personal belief that complementary knowledge will enhance one's own personal plan for patient care. Initially, there is limited knowledge of each other; collaboration is a "conscious, learned behavior" that improves as team members learn to value and respect one another's practice and expertise (Alpert et al., 1992). Medicine and nursing, though overlapping disciplines, are culturally distinct and have diverse goals for patient care. In many cases, they complement each other in their quest to restore patients to health. Collaboration is built on the respect and valuing of the contributions of each profession to the common goal of optimal health-care delivery (Stichler, 1995).

PROCESSES ASSOCIATED WITH EFFECTIVE COLLABORATION

Recurring Interactions

In addition to the attributes discussed above, there are several processes that drive effective collaboration.

A theme implicit in the reports of those who have written about their experiences with collaboration is that establishing a trusting and collaborative relationship is a developmental process (Alpert et al., 1992; Krumm, 1992). While this notion of development over time is relevant to all aspects of collaboration, it is particularly important to establishing trust. The fact that effective collaboration is developmental and time-dependent explains why collaborative relationships are difficult to develop in organizations where there is a high staff turnover or frequent rotation of clinicians, such as house physicians. A physician wrote that the process seemed to be related to how well the nurse and physician know each other (Alpert et al., 1992).

It seems likely that a series of less complicated interactions, such as information exchange and coordination, that have been satisfactory clinically or personally contribute to the development of collaborative relationships. Team members need recurring interactions to acquire an understanding of their role requirements and functions and to develop patterns of interaction that are constructive, productive, and supportive. Several reports illustrate the developmental aspects of interactions that lead to collaborative relationships (Hilderley, 1991; Alpert et al., 1992; Dickinson, Mateo, Jackson, & Swartz, 1995). Recurring interactions help clinicians learn the similarities and differences in each discipline's practice. Understanding each other's scope of practice and responsibility enables APNs, physicians, and other colleagues to use their knowledge and skills to benefit patients.

Bridging

Krumm (1992) noted that bridging is a component of collaboration. She did not define bridging but implied that it is the ability to develop connections that support positive outcomes for individuals and populations of patients. She described one bridging skill as the "ability to recognize and rearrange boundaries within the practice setting" (Krumm, p. 24).

Two examples illustrate the concept of bridging. NPs in a gynecological practice noted the length of time it took for patients to get an appointment for colposcopy and the disadvantages to the practice of having only one physician who could do the procedure. They proposed that two of the NPs become trained to do the procedure. They outlined the precedents for such a change in practice and the benefits in terms of clinical outcomes, patient satisfaction, productivity, and cost-effectiveness. The proposal was adopted, two NPs acquired the training, and many of the advantages they anticipated have been realized. The second author, while a clinical specialist at a tertiary hospital, noted that patients who were admitted directly from the oncology clinic for a short admission were receiving their chemotherapy late at night because members of the house staff were not doing the patients' histories and physicals until last. Lengths of stay were longer, treatments that could have been prepared and given during the better-staffed day shift were burdening the evening and night staff, and patients were dissatisfied. House staff left these admissions until last because the patients tended to be clinically stable, to the interns an appropriate way of triaging their workload. The CNS and nurse manager met with the physician director of hematology/oncology to propose that short-stay chemotherapy admissions be handled differently from other admissions—an idea for which there was no precedent. All admissions were done by the interns and residents. Under the new arrangement, patients would come to the unit directly from the clinic with their admission orders written by the attending physician. Intravenous lines could be initiated immediately, prescriptions could be filled by pharmacy as the orders came down, and nurses could initiate teaching and other interventions in a timely fashion. In both cases boundaries were rearranged in ways that improved patient care and staff job satisfaction.

An important aspect of these examples is that the APNs understood both medical and nursing aspects of care. Brown (1989) called this "shuttle diplomacy." She described the CNS as the person capable of speaking the languages of both medical and nursing subcultures, understanding the problems of each, and assisting in clinical and organizational problem solving. As these examples suggest, bridging can create conditions that are conducive to collaboration. Bridging occurs when collaborators move tasks that they consider exclusively within their domain to other team members.

Consultation

Consultation (see Chapter 8) is another process that drives collaboration between clinicians. CNSs have developed this form of communication to an art form and use it very successfully to interact with nurse colleagues within the hospital setting. As APNs mature in their roles, their use of the consultation process with nurses and between APNs and colleagues in other disciplines will further augment the process of collaboration.

FORCES DRIVING AND RESTRAINING COLLABORATION

Although it is easy to discuss professional liaisons and to draw up collaborative arrangements on paper, there are many obstacles to actually implementing serious collaborative professional relationships in the workplace.

SOCIAL/SOCIETAL ISSUES

Tradition is a major obstacle to collaboration. Safriet (1992) suggested that the field of medicine staked out broad turf early on and considered any movement into this turf by nurses at any level to be unacceptable. Indeed, physicians have often viewed the expanded roles of APNs as encroaching on their domain. Thus turf issues have been a major stumbling block to successful interactions between nurses and physicians.

Although nurses are highly valued for the physical care, nurturing, and psychosocial support they provide for patients, it is clear that the physician is perceived and valued as the decision maker about treatment. Many people think of nurses as second best or as caregivers for the unfortunate or indigent. This contributes to the perpetuation of the power structure in which the physician is the supervisor and the nurse is the subordinate. Unfortunately, because of barriers to practice that are difficult to break, APNs may tend to buy into this view, which further prevents them from having a truly collaborative, collegial role in care. Lenz (1994) noted that

> *Nurses, in sync with their socialized humility, rarely act to bring their contributions to the forefront and to correct the inaccurate images held by the public. Nurses continue to suffer from false and misconstrued*

*public images of dependency, lack of intellectual challenge in the
profession, and moral questionability.*

(p. 590)

Sexism affects collaboration (Siegler & Whitney, 1994; Coeling & Wilcox, 1994). Stereotypes dominate images of nurses in the media. APNs are rarely portrayed on television and, with few exceptions, their contributions are not profiled in health-care reports in the lay press. Media bias and the nursing profession's inability to market itself adequately make nursing and ANP invisible (Fagin, 1992). Despite an influx of women into medicine, medicine is still seen as being predominantly male and nursing remains a predominantly female profession. The "doctor-nurse game," first recognized in the 1970s, continues to operate in many institutions; it is apparent, however, that the rules are changing and nurses do not want to play anymore (Stein, Watts, & Howell, 1990). Stereotypical images and the invisibility of APNs influence how nursing is viewed by both health professionals and consumers—at best nurses are viewed as kind and nice; at worst, as unintelligent and incompetent. Stereotypical mindsets are anathema to collaboration. Thus, APNs often find that they must actively counter low expectations with interactions and practices that convey their intelligence, competence, confidence, and trustworthiness.

Although not discussed in the literature, the authors have observed that successful collaboration can lead to an intimacy that arises from working closely together over time. In her sixth year in a collaborative practice, one NP compared the relationship to a marriage in terms of the interpersonal ups and downs that occurred and the challenge of dealing with the same person daily over matters of great or negligible, albeit clinical import. Thus, mature collaboration can be both rewarding and challenging.

Ethical issues are also an important consideration in collaborative arrangements. The process of ethical decision making in health care is enhanced by a collaborative approach with team input. APNs can be much more effective if they join the team as collaborators rather than as ancillary members in a hierarchical system.

Patients, as the consumers of health care, are important players in the quest for successful collaboration. Patients are sensitive to the relationships between caregivers and are quick to pick up on the lack of respect or trust between their providers. Successful collaborative practices are those in which patients easily move back and forth between providers as their care and situation dictate.

SYSTEM ISSUES

Health-care reform has helped to lead health professionals toward a more collaborative, interdisciplinary approach to practice. Consortia and group practices are becoming the norm and often are requirements in funding schemes at both the national and state levels. Managed care, toward which health-care delivery in the United States is moving, is predicated on teams of providers seeing panels of patients within a supportive network, allowing cost-effective use of the system. In the authors' view, greater strides in collaboration have been made at the grassroots level, where multidisciplinary providers care for special populations, than at the policy and formal organization levels. Community-based initiatives across many kinds of practice settings require collaborative agreements between public and private organizations. For example, CNS-driven teaching nursing home models that are run by state-operated nursing schools are carried out in privately owned nursing homes. New projects from Pew Charitable Trust, the Robert Wood Johnson Foundation, and the Kellogg Foundation are requesting proposals and implementing demonstration projects of interdisciplinary models. Health-care delivery must be collaborative in nature if resources are to be used effectively and health-care costs decreased. The move toward a more community-based, health promotion, disease prevention model of care further enhances the appropriateness of APNs as primary caregivers across several practice settings. New alliances both among ANP groups and between ANP and physician groups need to be developed and nurtured.

Technology transfer is an integral part of this shift in the approach to health care. Multidisciplinary teams will collaborate to carry out skills that were assigned to a specific discipline in times past. An excellent example of this concept is the role of the neonatal NP in the neonatal unit.

Supervision of APNs by physicians is often mentioned explicitly or implicitly in some of the literature on NPs' and CRNAs' practice and in certain nurse practice acts. The view advanced here is that supervision precludes the development of a collaborative relationship and that physicians cannot truly supervise advanced nursing practice. A study of physicians' supervision of pediatric nurse practitioners (PNPs) suggests that what is called "supervision" is actually consultation or referral as it is defined in this text (Cruikshank & Chow, 1984). The approach taken by the American College of Nurse-Midwives and further developed here is appropriate for most, if not all, ANP specialties. That approach is to define the scope of autonomous nursing management and identify high-risk populations within a particular population or practice that would require consultation, collaboration/co-management, or referral.

In the past 10 years there has been a slow but steady movement away from language requiring physician supervision and reference to protocols in state nurse practice acts. Rather, revisions of practice acts have tried to emphasize consultation, collaboration, peer review, and use of referral. However, the American Medical Association (AMA, 1995) reaffirmed a policy that supports *supervision* of APNs by physicians and claims that physicians have the responsibility for managing health-care needs of patients. Despite rhetoric to the contrary, such a policy does not promote a philosophy of collaboration and reinforces stereotypes of nurse–physician relationships.

The issues surrounding certification and practice standards are relevant to the discussion of collaboration and collegial practice arrangements of any type. State barriers to practice are fraught with concerns about a gold standard for care across disciplines and who should define that standard. There is an urgent need for nursing to standardize ANP educational programs, national certification, and state credentialing. Chapter 22 explores these issues in greater depth.

THE EFFECTS OF FAILURE TO COLLABORATE

The failure to collaborate affects all care providers as well as patients. Alpert et al. (1992) found that job satisfaction and attitude were negatively affected when collaboration failed and that territoriality and competitiveness increased.

In 1983, the National Commission on Nursing found that the lack of recognition and understanding of the nurse's role in health-care delivery by the public, by other health professionals, and by nurses themselves was considered by many to be a key contributor to the nursing profession's problems (Spross, 1989). The stance preferred by physicians is not to collaborate with anyone (Fagin, 1992); failed collaboration efforts support this stance, with the concomitant result of loss of status and esteem by other members of the team.

Knaus and Draper (1986) found improved outcomes for intensive care unit patients who were cared for by collaborative teams of physicians and nurses. The absence of collaborative relationships was associated with a higher incidence of morbidity and mortality (Knaus & Draper, 1986). The most important result of failure to collaborate is its negative effect on patient care.

SOCIALIZATION TO COLLABORATION DURING GRADUATE EDUCATION

As part of the socialization process toward building collaboration, it is important that APNs add to the communication skills they learned in their undergraduate nursing programs. ANP curricula need to offer a foundational framework for collaborative interactions throughout the entire graduate program. Course objectives and specific content should be based on the characteristics of effective intra- and interdisciplinary collaboration and the development of skills to achieve this goal. Professional roles and issues courses need to include content that profiles not only the role sought by the student, but also the roles of the health-care providers with whom the student will interact, such as physicians, other nurses, and social workers. Content that leads the novice through team interaction, networking, and conflict negotiation, and other concepts that build personal self-esteem and confidence are crucial. The theme of collaboration can be woven throughout the major coursework as well as the graduate core curriculum by including objectives that build collaborative skills within other class requirements. For example, an objective for a role development core course that requires the student to build a collage depicting collaborative relationships within nursing would help the student grasp the concept of collaboration.

The curriculum should include content on group dynamics, role theory, organizational theory, change theory, and negotiation strategies to prepare learners for collaborative roles. Students should discuss examples of collaboration and non-collaboration from their own clinical experiences and should be able to identify what factors accounted for success or failure. Furthermore, students need to be aware of the forces, both positive and negative, that influence collaborative efforts. It is important that APNs be able to articulate the roles of nurse, NP, CNS, CNM, and CRNA and to explain the nursing profession to consumers and non-nurse health care providers.

Innovative classroom strategies that allow for interactions, such as role-playing; storytelling; and, most important, interdisciplinary seminars in which students can learn to walk a mile in each other's shoes, are extremely worthwhile. Students need opportunities to debrief with peers and faculty positive and negative experiences of collaboration. This is vital if students are to be able to analyze the personal, social, and organizational variables that affect collaboration. Furthermore, it is very important for students to observe faculty in collaborative relationships with their interdisciplinary peers. New funding initiatives that allow for interdisciplinary education in both the classroom and the clinical setting offer great promise for improved collaborative relationships between health provider disciplines.

Clinical placements for APN students have the potential to set the stage for long-term successful collaboration between APNs and physicians. The key is careful assessment of sites during the pre-placement phase in order to match APN students and students from other disciplines with preceptors who support collaboration. Good interdisciplinary clinical educational experiences should not be characterized by parallel processes but by true team approaches to the diagnosis, management, and education of clients and families. Faculty who practice collaboratively with colleagues play a key role in setting up these experiences and can serve as important role models and mentors. Supportive debriefing via journals, patient rounds, and postclinical seminars is an excellent way to instill the concepts of collaboration into long-term student learning, especially when efforts to collaborate are unsuccessful or unsatisfactory.

Final preceptorships and practica offer additional opportunities for APN students to try out collaborative relationships with physicians and to practice newfound collaborative skills. Collaboration between nurses and doctors requires recognition of complementary skills; as nursing and medical educational endeavors move toward interdisciplinary models, there is a need to restructure curricula in order to better understand training and education strategies in non-nursing education models (Evans, 1994; Fagin, 1992). The resurgence of interdisciplinary training for physicians and nurses for primary care practices should have a positive effect on collaboration.

IMPLEMENTING COLLABORATION

In *The Fifth Discipline: The Art and Practice of the Learning Organization*, Senge (1990) uses the metaphors of a superlative basketball team and a fantastic jazz ensemble to illustrate the power of people working in collaboration. It is clear that it takes more than professionals with expert skills, who may have different strengths, working side by side. Senge discusses the energy and power that are produced when teams become aligned to purpose, when they are able to combine energies and harmonize to produce a synergistic effect. Although individuals may come with great skills and expertise, it is the shared vision and the commonality of purpose that lead to success and improved outcome (Senge, 1990). These ideas, based on team efforts, can be easily transferred to collaborative teams that are striving to achieve high-level patient outcomes and goals for successful clinical practice relationships.

ASSESSMENT OF PERSONAL FACTORS

Professionals bring many personal attributes to a professional partnership. Personal characteristics such as clinical and interpersonal competence and well-developed communication skills are vital to the collaborative relationship. Good clinical judgment and a well-developed sense of ethics promote trust. In addition, the valuing of diverse opinions and respect for others' points of view are basic to the association. A good sense of humor is a plus! Most important for a good collaborative experience is a truly shared vision of the desired outcome. There needs to be a mutual willingness to strive for results that meet the expectations of both parties.

Successful professional collaboration requires work and practice in the same way that personal relationships require time and effort. Self-assessment is one important component to think about when embarking on a new professional relationship or evaluating the success or failure of current or potential collaborative relationships. The self-directed questions in Table 11–1 may help team members identify their personal strengths and weaknesses vis à vis collegiality.

According to Senge (1990), practice is the hallmark of teamwork. Successful professional relationships, be they basketball team, a team of primary care physicians and nurses, a birthing center group, or a team of anesthesiologists and CRNAs, need continued work and practice to grow and succeed.

In *The Seven Habits of Highly Effective People*, Covey (1989) offered another perspective on moving toward a higher level of interdependence with colleagues. He portrayed interdependence as a higher level of performance than independence. Only individuals who have gained competence and confidence in their own expertise are able to move beyond autonomy and independence toward the higher synergistic level of collaboration. Collaboration appears to have the same meaning as interdependence in Covey's work. This view is provocative as a means to move beyond the barriers of the hierarchical domain toward a truly interdisciplinary team practice in which the client is the real winner.

ASSESSMENT OF ORGANIZATIONAL FACTORS

Administrative leadership plays a key role in the development of collaborative relationships between organizational members. Facilities that place physicians as authority figures over all other health-care personnel set up hierarchies that are difficult to overcome. Administrators who support team and interdisciplinary administrative models and who are good communicators themselves can do a great deal to forward the momentum of new collaborations. Increased acuity of illness in both in-patient and out-patient settings is an obstacle to collaboration. As professionals move from one crisis to another, there is little time to sit down, communicate, analyze data, and make joint decisions (Spross, 1989). The lack of time to communicate is still seen as a barrier to collaboration (Coeling & Wilcox, 1994).

Power inequities between medicine and nursing are most often discussed. However, power issues also exist among nurses. Elitist stances by APNs set up hazardous roadblocks to collaboration with staff nurses. Balancing power differences between groups equalizes the hierarchical differences between members and makes collaboration possible if there is sufficient expertise among players (Stichler, 1995).

Differing philosophies and standards of care within organizational settings can cause conflict between team members and need to be resolved early (Spross, 1989). As roles become more interdisciplinary, these discrepancies will become less distinct. The common vision of desired patient outcomes makes collaboration between the APN and the nursing administrator a natural occurrence (Krumm, 1992).

TABLE 11–1. PERSONAL STRENGTHS AND WEAKNESSES QUESTIONNAIRE

Am I clear about what my role is in the partnership?
What do I expect to gain or lose by collaborating?
What do others expect of me?
Do I feel good about my contribution to the team?
Do I feel self-confident and competent in the collaborative relationship?
Are there anxieties causing repeated friction that have not been addressed?
Has serious thought been given to the boundaries of the collaborative relationship?

STRATEGIES FOR SUCCESSFUL COLLABORATION

Many of the barriers to successful collaboration occur because of values, beliefs, and behaviors that have, until recently, gone unchallenged in society and in the organizations in which nurses practice. There is a need for radical change if the conditions conducive to collaboration are to become the norm. APNs may feel like they are the only ones with an active commitment to collaboration (Spross, 1989). Of all the competencies required for advanced practice, collaboration may be the most difficult to accomplish because it is mediated by social processes (Siegler & Whitney, 1994b) that are ingrained in the larger culture. Efforts to change the environment to one that is more collaborative involve proving oneself over and over and challenging colleagues' behaviors that restrain attempts to work together. These intrapersonal demands, along with the clinical demands of one's job, can be exhausting. Therefore APNs need to evaluate the potential for collaboration when seeking employment opportunities. Questions about how clinicians work together—the interpersonal climate as well as organizational structures that support collaboration—should be a high priority. A realistic appraisal of the existence of or potential for collaboration is needed to determine whether APNs can provide the standard and quality of care that are characteristic of advanced nursing practice and whether they can expect a reasonable level of job satisfaction.

INDIVIDUAL STRATEGIES

The strategies Norton and Grady (see Chapter 12) offer for developing and implementing the change agent competency are equally important for collaboration. APNs should actively seek opportunities to promote a collaborative climate.

One strategy is for APNs to showcase their exemplary nursing practices to help both other health professionals and consumers better understand their strengths as health-care providers (Fagin, 1992). In today's health-care environment, participating in critical pathway development is one way to do this. Within advanced nursing practice, it is useful for nurses to role-model their practice strategies for other nurses to facilitate intra-nursing collaboration and consultation. One way to share excellence in practice is to include in grand rounds or team conferences the opportunity for each care team member to describe his or her own decision making about patients and suggest new strategies for care to the team. Furthermore, Garcia, Bruce, Niemeyer, and Robbins (1993) suggested that integrated patients' records provide a means to communicate formally about patient care. Joint review and audit of patient care is an important component of collaboration in practice.

Working together on joint projects is another way to facilitate good collaboration. Collaborative research and scholarly writing projects as well as community service projects that tap the strengths of various members open people's eyes to the benefits of collaboration. Federal and private agencies are currently supporting interdisciplinary collaborative studies. Reporting the results in the literature will illustrate the considerable advantages of collaborative interactions. In addition, social opportunities at conferences and receptions allow camaraderie to grow and help reinforce the bond between members of the partnership (Fitzpatrick et al., 1990; Hanson, 1993). These strategies move across lines from personal life to organizational settings and from education to practice arenas. New models that foster joint medical and nursing care are needed in primary care as well as within specialty practice in all settings.

ORGANIZATIONAL STRATEGIES

Fagin (1992) and Hanson (1993) identified several strategies that lead toward successful collaboration at all levels. First, there needs to be a move toward interdisciplinary educational programs that allow for face-to-face interaction between medical and nursing students. This will require definitive changes in the structure of clinical hours as well as sequencing of content. Given the entrenched bureaucracies involved, this will be a difficult task requiring stronger interactions between schools of medicine and schools of nursing. Health-care providers need to be learning about health policy issues from a perspective that offers broad-stroke solutions to health-care issues. Faculty in both nursing and medicine need to be evaluating and treating patients and supervising students together. It is important to introduce joint appointments of nursing faculty to medical school clinics to give faculty opportunities to role-model ANP care and build rapport (Fitzpatrick, Wykle, & Morris, 1990).

National and state medical and nursing organizations must endorse the shift toward a more interactive model (Fagin, 1992; Hanson, 1993). Strategies that facilitate this shift, such as retreats, social interactions, communication workshops, joint practice committees, and sensitivity training sessions, are imperative. Again, sharing exemplary nursing innovations is a major factor. Until strategies for this type of change are instituted, barriers to successful interprofessional collaboration will remain.

EXEMPLARS OF SUCCESSFUL COLLABORATIVE PRACTICE

Several examples of the positive effects of collaboration have been identified throughout this chapter. As team practice becomes the norm, more positive effects will emerge. The following are just two examples of successful collaborative practice.

THE NP IN PRIMARY CARE

For several years, Syntex Corporation has sponsored a Nurse Practitioner of the Year Award to honor NPs who have achieved high levels of success in their practice. The letters of the physicians and nurses who nominate successful NPs for the award all seem to say the same thing: The individual exhibits a high level of collaboration. The following is a composite of the nomination letters received by Syntex from physicians:

I would like to tell you about MQ, a nurse practitioner who is a member of our group primary care practice. Mary is an extremely competent nurse practitioner and an able diagnostician. I would trust her to care for my own wife and children. She is totally committed to her patients, strives to give them the best possible care, and has many of the same values and ideas about good patient care that my physician partner and I do. Although Mary carries her own panel of patients very successfully, she seems to want and need to consult with me and our other physicians if she is concerned about a complex patient. We all function as a team and we have all learned from Mary's nursing expertise, as she has from ours. All of us work together to give high-quality care. Most importantly, Mary is a team player; all the members of our group practice enjoy her quick wit and willingness to share her expertise. At first, one of the partners did not want a nurse practitioner to join the group, but Mary won him over with her professional and interpersonal competence. I guess that the most important quality that I would share is that Mary is a people person; she works hard to communicate at a high level and it pays off. We trust her as a professional colleague and a friend.

THE CRNA AS A MEMBER OF AN INTERDISCIPLINARY TEAM

LC is a nurse anesthetist assigned to the cardiopulmonary surgical team in a major medical center. The interdisciplinary anesthesia team is made up of anesthesiologists, anesthesia residents, nurse anesthetists, student nurse anesthetists, and anesthesia technicians. As a nurse anesthetist, LC has an individual role as well as a team role in meeting the goal of optimal patient care. Although the anesthesiologist is the senior consultant on the team, LC provides leadership by coordinating the direct patient care and follow-up with nursing administrators and the staff nurses in the postoperative and discharge phases of the patient's stay. Her collaborative role with the CNS in the pulmonary intensive care unit (ICU) allows for critical interface between the operative team and the pulmonary ICU staff, the patient, and the patient's family.

CONCLUSION

Collaborative relationships are not only professionally satisfying (e.g., Alpert et al., 1992; Fagin, 1992), they improve access to care (e.g., Waugaman & Foster, 1995; Siegler & Whitney, 1994a) and patient outcomes (e.g., Rubinstein, Josephson, Wesland, et al., 1984; Knaus & Draper, 1986). While APNs collaborate with many individuals within and outside nursing and do so successfully, APNs may find that one of their most important collaborative relationships—those with physicians— may also be the most challenging. Despite the fact that there are many successful individual APN–physician collaborative practices, many with data to demonstrate their beneficial effects on health care, tradition and stereotypes are often powerful influences on policy-making and in health care and professional organizations, such as hospitals or the AMA.

In the current health-care environment, collaboration may flourish, regardless of the barriers identified. To meet the demands for cost effectiveness and quality, clinicians from all disciplines are meeting together to discuss the care they provide and to define ways to deliver it so as to maximize quality and minimize duplication of effort. It is these interactions that foster the trust and respect required for mature collaboration. They enable collaborators to recognize their interdependence and value the input of others, thus creating a synergy that improves the quality of clinical decision-making (Stichler, 1995). APNs will find that their success as clinicians and leaders often depends on their proficiency as collaborators.

REFERENCES

Alpert, H., Goldman, L., Kilroy, C., & Pike, A. (1992). 7 Gryzmish: Toward an understanding of collaboration. *Nursing Clinics of North America, 27,* 47–59.

American Medical Association. (1995). *Board of Trustees Report 6-A-95.* Chicago: Author.

American Nurses' Association. (1995). *Nursing's social policy statement.* Washington, DC: Author.

Arslanian-Engoren, C. M. (1995). Lived experiences of CNSs who collaborate with physicians: A phenomenological study. *Clinical Nurse Specialist, 9* (2), 68–73.

Baggs, J. G., & Schmitt, M. C. (1988). Collaboration between nurses and physicians. *Image 20,* 145–149.

Balzer, J., (1993). Humor—a missing ingredient in collaborative practice. *Holistic Nursing Practice, 7* (4), 28–35.

Brown, S. J. (1989). Supportive supervision of the CNS. In A. B. Hamric & J. A. Spross (Eds.), *The clinical nurse specialist in theory and practice* (2nd ed., pp. 285–286). Philadelphia: W. B. Saunders Company.

Coeling, H., & Wilcox, J. (1994). Steps to collaboration. *Nursing Administration Quarterly, 18* (4), 44–55.

Covey, S. R. (1989). *The seven habits of highly effective people.* New York: Simon & Schuster.

Crowley, S. A., & Wollner, I. S. (1987). Collaborative practice: A tool for change. *Oncology Nursing Forum, 14* (4), 59–63.

Cruikshank, B., & Chow, T. (1984). Physician supervision/collaboration as reported by PNPs in practice settings. *Pediatric Nursing, 10* (1), 13–18.

Devereux, P. (1981). Nurse/physician collaboration: Nursing practice considerations. *Journal of Nursing Administration, 9* (9), 37–39.

Dickinson, C. P., Mateo, M., Jackson, D., & Swartz, W. (1995). OB-GYN consultants and Sharp, the birthplace: An exemplar of nurse-midwife and obstetrician independence and integration. *Advanced Practice Nursing Quarterly 1* (2), 40–48.

Dressler, D. (1994). The critical care clinical nurse specialist in joint practice with physicians. In A. Gawlinski & L. Kern (Eds.), *The clinical nurse specialist in critical care* (pp. 51–61). Philadelphia: W. B. Saunders Company.

Evans, J. A. (1994). The role of the nurse manager in creating an environment for collaborative practice. *Holistic Nursing Practice, 8* (3), 23–31.

Fagin, C. (1992). Collaboration between nurses and physicians: No longer a choice. *Nursing and Health Care, 13,* 354–363.

Fitzpatrick, J., Wykle, M., & Morris, D. (1990). Collaboration in care and research. *Archives in Psychiatric Nursing, 4* (1), 53–61.

Forbes, E., & Fitzsimmons, V. (1993). Education: The key for holistic interdisciplinary collaboration. *Holistic Nursing Practice, 7* (4), 1–10.

Garcia, M.A., Bruce, D., Niemeyer, J., & Robbins, J. (1993). Collaborative practice: A shared success. *Nursing Management, 24* (5), 72–79.

Hanson, C. M. (1993). Our role in health care reform: Collegiality counts. *American Journal of Nursing, 93* (12), 16A–16E.

Hanson, C. M., Hodnicki, D. R., & Boyle, J. S. (1994). Nominations for excellence: Collegial advocacy for nurse practitioners. *Journal of the American Academy of Nurse Practitioners, 6,* 471–476.

Hilderley, L. (1991). Nurse-physician collaborative practice: The clinical nurse specialist in a radiation oncology private practice. *Oncology Nursing Forum, 18,* 585–591.

Hughes, A., & Mackenzie, C. (1990). Components necessary in a successful nurse practitioner-physician collaborative practice. *Journal of the American Academy of Nurse Practitioners, 2* (2), 54–57.

Inglis, A., & Kjervik, D. (1993). Empowerment of advanced practice nurses: Regulation reform needed to increase access to care. *Journal of Law, Medicine & Ethics, 21* (2), 193–205.

Kavesh, W. (1993). Physician and nurse practitioner relationships. In M. Mezey & D. McGivern (Eds.), *Nurses, nurse practitioners: Evolution to advanced practice* (pp. 171–184). New York: Springer Publishing.

Kedziera, P., & Levy, M. (1994). Collaborative practice in oncology. *Seminars in Oncology, 21,* 705–711.

Knaus, W., & Draper, E. (1986). An evaluation of outcomes from intensive care in major medical centers. *Annals of Internal Medicine, 104,* 410–418.

Krumm, S. (1992). Collaboration between oncology clinical nurse specialists and nursing administrators. *Oncology Nursing Forum, 19* (1, Supplement), 21–24.

Lenz, C. (1994). Multidisciplinary community-based education and practice. In J. C. McCloskey & H. K. Grace (Ed.), *Current issues in nursing* (pp. 586–602). St. Louis, MO: C. V. Mosby.

Littell, S. (1981). The clinical nurse specialist in private medical practice. *Nursing Administration Quarterly, 6* (1), 77–85.

McKechnie, J. L. (Ed.). (1983). *Webster's new universal unabridged dictionary.* New York: Simon & Schuster.

National Joint Practice Commission [NJPC]. (1979). *Brief description of a demonstration project to establish collaborative or joint practice in hospitals* (pp. 2–6.) Chicago: Author.

Petronis-Jones, R.A. (1994). Nurse-physician collaboration: A descriptive study. *Holistic Nursing Practice, 8* (3), 38–53.

Prescott, P., & Bowen, S. (1985). Physician-nurse relationships. *Annals of Internal Medicine, 103,* 127–133.

Rubenstein, L., Josephson, K., Wieland, G., English, P., Sayre, J., & Kane, R. (1984). Effectiveness of a geriatric evaluation unit. *New England Journal of Medicine, 311,* 1664–1670.

Ryan, L., Edwards, R., & Rickles, F. (1980). A joint practice approach to the care of persons with cancer. *Oncology Nursing Forum, 8* (1), 8–11.

Safriet, B. J. (1992). Health care dollars and regulatory sense: The role of advanced practice nursing. *Yale Journal on Regulation, 9* (2), 417–487.

Sands, R., Stafford, J., & McClelland, M. (1990). "I beg to differ": Conflict in the interdisciplinary team. *Social Work in Health Care, 14* (3), 55–72.

Senge, P. M. (1990). *The fifth discipline: The art and practice of the learning organization.* New York: Doubleday.

Siegler, E. L., & Whitney, F. W. (1994a). *Nurse physician collaboration: Care of adults and the elderly.* New York: Springer Publishing Company.

Siegler, E., & Whitney, F. (1994b). Social and economic barriers to collaborative practice. In E. Siegler & F. Whitney (Eds.), *Nurse-physician collaboration: Care of adults and the elderly* (pp. 21–32). New York: Springer Publishing.

Spross, J. A. (1989). The CNS as collaborator. In A. B. Hamric & J. A. Spross (Eds.), *The clinical nurse specialist in theory and practice* (2nd ed., pp. 205–226). Philadelphia: W.B. Saunders Company.

Steele J. E. (Ed.). (1986). *Issues in collaborative practice.* Orlando: Grune & Stratton.

Stein, L. I., Watts, D. T., & Howell, T. (1990). The doctor–nurse game revisited. *New England Journal of Medicine, 322,* 546–549.

Stichler, J. F. (1995). Professional interdependence: The art of collaboration. *Advanced Practice Nursing Quarterly, 1* (1), 53–61.

Tjosvold, D. (1986). The dynamics of interdependence in organizations. *Human Relations, 39,* 517–540.

Waugaman, W. R., & Foster, S. D. (1995). CRNAs: An enviable legacy of patient service. *Advanced Practice Nursing Quarterly, 1* (1), 21–28.

CHAPTER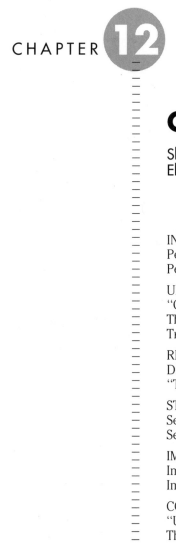

Change Agent Skills

Sheila F. Norton
Elizabeth M. Grady

The wedge of change was driven to the head rendering what was solid mass to fragments, things cemented and held together by the usages of years burst asunder . . . and what was rock became but sand and dust.

(Charles Dickens, *Martin Chuzzlewit*, p. 20)

INTRODUCTION

Change is a messy, emotional, disorganized business when it is planned. Even worse is unplanned change—the unanticipated chaos of passivity, or the result of a band-aid approach when what is needed is system problem-solving. This chapter aims to improve the advanced practice nurse's (APN's) ability to identify situations needing to be changed, facilitate planned change, understand and address unanticipated results, and enhance a working comfort level with the interaction of self, others, and organizations. It is designed to be reread as the APN gains experience in clinical practice and with organizations.

The authors are two nurses: SFN, an experienced, master's-prepared nurse-midwife currently at work on a doctorate in education; and EMG, a highly experienced academician and consultant in organizational development. We have had our share of successes and failures in our efforts to promote change and advocate for improvement in the health care system and nursing education. We do not write from the perspective of "experts" on change in the manner of "do what I have done and you too can succeed as I have." Our aim is to make change agent skills understandable and accessible, and we frequently include ourselves in the text because we continue to work on the skills described. Openness to experience and enhanced self-knowledge, a passion for one's work, and the courage of one's convictions are essential to continued development as a change agent.

The concepts of change and power are linked consistently in the literature. All definitions of power contain elements of control and freedom (Oshry, 1972), ideas essential to change. In his treatise on power, Rollo May (1972) defined power as the ability to cause or prevent change. The reader will find that Chapter 10 provides additional consideration of the relationship between change and power. Although this chapter focuses on the APN as a change agent and the knowledge, skills, personal characteristics, and disposition toward risk-taking required, the reader should consider the influences of power and powerlessness on this essential advanced practice competency.

PERSPECTIVES ON NURSES AND APNs AS CHANGE AGENTS

At one time, the profession believed that hope for change lay with the BSN-prepared nurse: once all nurses were college graduates, desired reforms in the profession and in health care would occur (Brown, 1948). Texts have been published since the 1970s exhorting the nurse to become a "change agent" (Brooten, Naylor & Hayman, 1978). What was not emphasized in these early notions of BSN-prepared nurses as change agents was the development of intrapersonal and interpersonal processes and skills needed and acquired along the continuum of beginning student, graduate nurse, and expert clinician. APNs are now expected to provide the leadership necessary, both to effect change in clinical and organizational environments and to model these processes and skills for nurses in basic practice.

For readers who doubt the professional desirability or personal likelihood of change agency for the APN, it is instructive to consider how much of nursing practice depends on the abilities of nurses to facilitate change. The notion of change is embedded in everyday nursing practice at all levels. The study of change is part of basic education for practice. Nurses study body systems and function; changes as a result of illness, surgery, or stress; what interventions change body systems toward health; and finally, perhaps most importantly, how illness changes the individual. Nurses learn the therapeutic use of self in assisting the individual toward physical and psychosocial health. Within basic nursing education, skills and techniques are used: to change patient ignorance to knowledge of health promotion and illness management; to encourage health-promoting behaviors in place of self-neglectful ones; to change the course of individual lives through disease prevention, screening, and treatment; and to reframe the course of chronic illness and dying through rehabilitative and palliative care.

Therefore, it is no surprise that APNs, while expanding the depth and breadth of practice expertise, would also focus on change. In addition to effecting change for individual patients, the APN also directs efforts at changing systems in which individuals are cared for. Clinical nurse specialists (CNSs) have always expected that they would foster change in nursing practice using such clinical *and* organizational skills as direct practice, consultation, collaboration, role-modeling, and research (Hamric & Spross, 1983, 1989). For nurse practitioners (NPs), nurse anesthetists (CRNAs), and nurse-midwives (CNMs), change in nursing practice has come about largely through the direct-care role and accompanying legislative and regulatory changes. These APNs have assumed responsibility for skills formerly performed exclusively by physicians (diagnosis and treatment, provision of anesthesia during surgery, and delivery care as well as labor support in obstetrics) and are practicing in settings outside larger organizations (private practices, clinics, health centers, birthing centers, and homes). Today, APNs of all specialties can be found in settings ranging from primary to tertiary care, as well as in the home and community.

The common focus of change along the continuum from basic to advanced practice, from single-provider private practices to medical center careers, is the question "What will improve care?" In basic practice, change in the individual is emphasized with a focus on such aspects as comfort, teaching, medication, visitors, and coordination of care. This is accomplished through the nurse-patient relationship—the therapeutic use of self. In advanced practice the nurse takes a broader view: "What will improve the care for this group of patients as well as this individual?" Change in this case could focus on research utilization, policy development, organizational systems, hospital staff bylaws, third-party reimbursement, consumer advocacy, and efforts to change entrenched attitudes. APNs practice in settings in which therapeutic use of self is also applied to the organization and those working within it.

Some formal educational programs, in particular CNS curricula, are explicit in their expectations of change agency, and course work is directed toward this goal. Other educational programs such as nurse-midwifery emphasize the elements of changed clinical practice but provide less formal theory about how to understand organizations and create change within them. Other programs seem to focus simply on expanding nursing practice: they lack both explicit expectations for fostering change and related course work. As educational programs organize curricula around APN competencies, all APNs will be prepared to be change agents. As APNs assume different positions and specialties, the position description and nature of the practice will determine the extent to which change agent skills are emphasized.

PERSPECTIVES ON CHANGE IN THE HEALTH CARE SYSTEM

Nurses in basic and advanced practice must contend not only with patients' changing conditions, new protocols and policies, and new technology but with rampant change in the health-care system itself. The only thing certain about the settings in which care is provided is that they are dynamic. There is a more explicit "business" model for health care, diversity in third-party-payer models, governmental initiatives, the increased professionalization of non-MD provider groups, and the use of unlicensed personnel.

Change, not stability, characterizes the work in nursing and in health care, a formerly predictable field. Nurses at all levels and in all settings must develop a working comfort with change in order to respond flexibly and plan effectively in ever-changing environments. The nursing profession must be prepared to meet change and to create it, not remain merely a recipient.

Much is still written, certainly good work is being done, but why does it feel incomplete? Although theories are useful as frameworks within which to understand change, the authors maintain that not enough has been made explicit about the internal processes necessary to understand ourselves as potential change agents. "Progress is a nice word," Robert F. Kennedy once noted, "but change is its motivator and change has its enemies" (quoted in Boughn, 1994). Those of us less comfortable with change do not have a choice, for it will happen despite our objections, and in bigger leaps in less time with less notice! Such an agenda requires a theoretical understanding of change, the development of a disposition toward risk-taking, and the wise use of strategies to facilitate change. Graduate programs preparing APNs need to integrate theoretical content and clinical experiences with supportive faculty consultation so that students may begin and refine the acquisition of personal understanding, development, and wisdom with regard to change.

UNDERSTANDING CHANGE

Change is "to make different in some particular: alter; to undergo transformation, transition or substitution; to pass from one phase to another" (Webster's 10th Collegiate Dictionary, 1993). Changes can be simple or complex, minute or enormous, short-term or long-term, received well or badly. Many of us work hard to limit the amount of change we must contend with in our lives, some actively seek it, some deny it. Many of us are terrific at accepting and flexing with changes imposed on us but see ourselves as unlikely to initiate change. For some, change is a cause for anger or anxiety—"How could they do this to me?"—or a sense of losing "control" of a situation over which we really had none. We can spend a lot of energy simply coping with change. Telling graduate nursing students that they will be "change agents" can create much anxiety. Students ask, "What will this mean for me? for my practice?" Some may say, "I don't want to be a change agent—I just want to see patients." Becoming an agent for change can be intimidating—especially for those of us who have become good at accepting changes made for us, good at flexibility, good at compliance.

Among advanced practice skills and abilities defined by the National Council of State Boards of Nursing's Position Paper (1993) are the identification of alternative possibilities as to the nature of a health-care problem and the selection of appropriate treatments. If one employs the common focus of change in nursing, "What will improve care?," the APN's answer has to do with organizational problems and solutions, as well as complex individual clinical problems requiring specialized knowledge and skills. APNs have the autonomy to "practice at the edges of the expanding boundaries of nursing's scope of practice . . . [their] expanded practice and knowledge base . . . is also characterized by a complexity of clinical decision making and a skill in managing organizations and environments that is greater than that required for the practice of nursing at the basic level" (American Nurses' Association, 1995, p. 16). The APN in any setting must be prepared to understand organizational structures and processes as well as complex clinical problems in order to function adequately in any advanced practice role.

"CHANGE MUST BE THE NORM, NOT CAUSE FOR ALARM" (Peters, 1988, p. 464)

Kurt Lewin (1951) has often been cited by authors writing about change in basic and advanced practice nursing. He offered an understandable, three-stage conceptualization of a complex process that has endured. Unfreezing (stage 1) involves "breaking the habit—disturbing the equilibrium." This sets the stage for change, raising discontent and highlighting discrepancies between the real and the ideal through new or disconfirming information. The disequilibrium thus created establishes the motivation for change, if defensiveness can be avoided. Moving (stage 2) means developing new responses based on new information; thus people change attitudes, feelings, values, and behaviors. Refreezing (stage 3) means reaching a new status quo, stabilizing and integrating new behaviors with the proper support available to maintain the change.

Although Lewin's conceptualization remains a useful introduction to understanding change process, it is too simple and relatively static to be useful to APNs. In the 1990s and beyond, organizational change is less likely to lead to new, "refrozen" states than were changes of preceding decades. Organizations must be prepared to make changes rapidly and thoughtfully or risk falling behind and becoming noncompetitive. APNs need an eclectic theoretical background and clinical experiences that enable them to analyze the change process. This analysis includes the interaction of structural changes, the effects on people within the system, and the resulting "down-time" or nonproductive time during which the changes are integrated. Readers may find it useful to review some of the change literature commonly cited in nursing (Caffrey, 1994; Clare, 1993; Goren & Ottaway, 1985; Manion, 1995; Strunk, 1995; Watson & Phillips, 1992).

Given our experiences and the corporate context in which much of health care is delivered, the authors take a different approach—one we believe particularly addresses the needs of APNs and their educators. Kanter et al.'s (1992) model captures the nature and complexity of change in the contemporary corporate environment. Bridges' (1991) work addresses affective responses to any change— intrapersonal, interpersonal, or organizational. These perspectives are useful in the analysis of a need for change, organizational change one experiences, and anticipation of potential effects of change. APNs may "try on" the various theories to find one or a combination that "fits" with their world views and the organizational variables they face as they work toward change in their settings.

THE "BIG THREE" MODEL

Kanter, Stein, and Jick (1992) developed a model of change that accounts for the enormous complexity of contemporary organizational life. This model considers separately the contingencies and variables that change agents must contend with in facing today's and tomorrow's challenges. It is referred to as the "Big Three" Model because it describes three types of *orientation* to change, three *forms of change*, and three *roles in the change process*.

Orientation

Orientation refers to the level of the organizational structure at which change is occurring and the accompanying direction an organization's response to change ("motion" or "movement") will take. The three types of movement identified in the model are *macroevolutionary, microevolutionary,* and *revolutionary*. The first is oriented toward the external environment. *Macroevolutionary* movement is a response to forces outside the organization. For example, a historically successful health maintenance organization (HMO) finds itself dropped as an option from a number of employer insurance plan offerings because of lower premiums charged by increasingly successful competitors. Managed care corporate executives immediately begin making changes in the organization's approach to providing health care services. This could take the form of special premium discounts or different marketing strategies. It may also take the form of internal cost-cutting measures, redistribution of resources, or the closing of less profitable programs.

Microevolutionary, the second type of orientation, is movement that occurs as internal organizational parts come in contact with each other in the process of implementing changes that have been made at the top. For example, once corporate executives determine what internal response will occur as a result of external change, departmental and area managers of the HMO set up meetings, committees, and task forces to determine how the different areas will interact given the new executive mandates. Included in this organizational review is a plan for communication of changes to individuals and working groups. Coordination among these separate parts is essential if the changes are to be successful.

The third type of orientation, *revolutionary,* is movement at the individual level. It is defined as change of a political nature and involves the redistribution of power and resources as a result of change. This occurs as people struggle for influence over decisions that affect their interests and jockey for positions of power in a newly configured organization. Both the loss of a formerly reliable corporate policy and the need to cut costs in the face of diminished income are likely to threaten the financial and personal security of employees. In anticipation of layoffs and promotions, employees may change their behavior, becoming competitive, antagonistic, angry, or depressed. At the HMO, for example, support staff watch warily as departments "re-engineer" and supervisory staff change. Each individual must form a new relationship with those in immediate authority. Distrust and decreased morale follow the awarding of contested positions and pink slips. "Teamwork" becomes a forgotten concept.

Forms of Change

Forms of change refer to the actions taken, and the factors or characteristics that "look different," as a result of change. Three forms of change or action focus are *identity, coordination,* and *control. Identity* changes in an organization occur in response to environmental opportunities or pressures. Often the organization becomes a different entity entirely, both legally and publicly. The HMO leadership in the aforementioned example may decide to specialize in care for a particular population or concentrate its services in a particular region. Thus the HMO may change its name, CEO, or other high-level staff. The second action focus, *coordination* changes, refers to the internal rearrangements in size, shape, habits, and culture resulting from deliberate attempts to reshape or revitalize the organization. For example, three formerly different departments in the HMO—obstetrics, pediatrics, and nutrition—are consolidated into one large unit. Coordination changes involve how the individuals and departments now function together within the organization. *Control* changes refer to changes in ownership or governance: new persons in key leadership roles. This change results in a new dominant group with shifts and replacement of formal supervisory staff and informal leaders within the newly consolidated unit.

Roles in the Change Process

The three action roles devised by Kanter et al. follow the same three levels of implementation described earlier for orientation and form. *Change strategists* deal with macro forces. They operate at the top level of organizations and are responsible for developing vision, initiating change, and establishing and maintaining the corporate view and links to the market and stakeholders. APNs who are responsible for a clinical program, those in private practice, or those in nurse-managed centers are likely to be visible change strategists.

Persons who are chiefly concerned with the internal development of the organization, translating the corporate vision for change recipients, are filling the role of *change implementors.* They make change happen and are in the middle of the change and of the organizational hierarchy. Many APNs in larger organizations can be found in this position—for example, a unit-based CNS who acts as a bridge between staff nurses and a medical specialty's or nursing director's innovations in practice or policy. Another example would be a nurse-midwifery service director who reports to both the Chief of Obstetrics and the VP for Nursing. Implementors represent the corporate vision to those responsible for operationalizing it; they also represent the recipients' needs and responses to those in charge. This is similar to Brown's (1989) early description of CNSs as "shuttle diplomats."

Members of the organization who are most strongly affected by the change fill the role of *change recipients.* The effectiveness of the corporate vision of change and its implementation are illustrated by recipients' reactions to a change effort. Change recipients reflect the effectiveness of strategists and implementors in the way the change is operationalized. Internal politics of the organization, including who exercises control and who resists it, are highlighted at this action role level.

Table 12–1 provides a summary of this model.

TRANSITIONS

The "Big Three" model for change is primarily a structural one, dealing with factors outside the individual. It does not deal in depth with the affective experience of

TABLE 12–1. KEY CHANGE MAKERS

	Role and Mindset	Orientation to Change (Kind of Motion)	Action Focus	Typical Organizational Level	Dominant Stage of Involvement
Change strategist	Visionary Instigator Corporate view	External environment	Ends Corporate values and business results	Top	Unfreezing
Change implementor	"Project image" Translator Division or department	Internal coordination	Means Overcoming resistance "Project image"	Middle	Changing
Change recipient	User and adapter Institutionalizer Personal view Operational	Distribution of power and proceeds	Means-end congruence Personal benefits	Bottom	Refreezing

Reprinted with the permission of The Free Press, an imprint of Simon & Schuster from THE CHALLENGE OF ORGANIZATIONAL CHANGE: How companies experience it and how leaders guide it by Rosabeth Moss Kanter, Barry Stein, Todd D. Jick. Copyright © 1992 by Rosabeth Moss Kanter, Barry Stein, Todd D. Jick.

change, yet this may be critical in enabling changes to be implemented and adopted. Bridges' (1991) work distinguishes transitions from changes and provides insights on this dimension of change for APNs. Change is an external, situational phenomenon, whereas transition is an internal, psychological phenomenon. He maintains that "change" works only if "transition" occurs. This theory acknowledges the affective responses to change (individuals and groups) and proposes strategies for coping.

The transition process consists of three overlapping phases: an ending, the "neutral zone," and a beginning. Transitions start with an ending in which old relationships and routines are broken as a result of the external forces of change. This ending is a "letting go." Any important (or not so important) life change involves letting go. This is a tough phase because people do not like endings, yet beginnings depend on them. One reason people are uncomfortable with endings is that they require attending to losses and the grief that accompanies loss. Who has to let go? What is over for everyone? Individual losses must be acknowledged and dealt with sympathetically. A change agent must expect and accept various signs of grief within a group experiencing loss such as anger, anxiety, or sadness. While people struggle with their losses, change agents can provide clear information, mark the ending symbolically when possible, and treat the past with honor and respect.

Further progress in transition depends on moving through a second phase, "the neutral zone," where everything is perceived to be "up in the air." Transition ends with a new beginning, as new relationships and routines become established. Bridges' "neutral zone" represents a time of redefinition. Feeling neither here nor there, individuals experience a wide variety of affective responses. People may feel anxious, lonely, out of control, and without motivation as they move through the neutral zone. It is a time of polarization and confusion, as the ground shifts beneath their feet. The work of the neutral zone focuses on gaining or restoring balance and enhancing feelings of personal control. Organizationally, it is important that policies and short-term goals be consistent with the organization's new direction. Individuals can be reassured that a wide range of difficult emotional responses are normal in these circumstances. Attention to providing opportunities for continued growth or progress, such as specialized training in a new area or access to college or graduate courses, can also assist in this effort. Most importantly, it is a time to do things differently and better. New patterns of thought emerge; they can be encouraged and supported by vehicles such as retreats, brainstorming sessions, policy reviews, and other activities that encourage creativity and experimentation. Above all, people must be kept informed. At such a time it is virtually impossible to overcommunicate.

Bridges' last phase, a new beginning, differs from a "start" because starts engage the mind only and beginnings engage the mind and heart. One can design a start but must nurture and support a beginning. Beginnings take people out of the static and difficult but less risky neutral zone. They ratify endings and present new directions and challenges. Change agents can help people in the beginning phase by explaining the purpose or expected outcome of the change, painting a picture of how it might look and feel, phasing in the outcome, working from a plan, and giving everyone a part to play in the plan and the outcome. Such approaches build an individual investment in both the process and the goal.

As pointed out earlier in this chapter, the APN works within a changing environment and will be a recipient of change as well as its agent. For example, the new APN bids goodbye to student colleagues, faculty, and former mentors at graduation. This ending is a requirement for career progress. Whether one has a position or is still seeking one, the time between graduation and becoming integrated in a work setting is a "neutral zone," neither here nor there. Obtaining and beginning a job provides a gradual progression from the second phase into a "new beginning" as one learns the ropes and gains confidence in one's ability to perform well. Perception of one's knowledge and skills can follow a parallel track: feeling confident as a new graduate, then despair at realizing all one doesn't yet know, and finally the "new beginning" of confident clinical practice as successes add up. One does well to keep Bridges' (1991) stages of transition in mind as applied to the self as well as to others. An APN who has a solid foundation in change theory fulfills an important prerequisite to becoming a change agent. A further requirement is possession of the disposition toward risk-taking.

RISKING CHANGE

APNs with sound knowledge of change and transition theories who possess good interpersonal skills do not automatically become effective change agents. It is essential to have a disposition toward risk-taking. The nursing profession appears to value risk-taking but does not cultivate it. Few if any learning opportunities are designed explicitly for demonstrating the inclination to take a risk in nursing education at the basic or advanced level. The authors have considered personal opportunities and challenges involving risk-taking and have observed others acting in the role of change agent. It is our conclusion that the disposition is born of a constellation of factors that cause or allow a person to take a risk. Risk-taking is a behavior that results when one possesses heightened interpersonal competence, critical commitment,* and courage.

DISPOSITIONS TOWARD CHANGE

Heightened interpersonal competence comes from working at relationships. The individual who continually reflects on and refines behavior in relationships with others deepens capacities for authenticity and mutuality. These capacities foster the ability and willingness to be vulnerable. Expert caring is provided by the individual with heightened interpersonal competence because she† can turn her consciousness toward another and experience joy in relatedness (Noddings, 1984).

Authenticity is reliable, believable self-knowledge, including recognition of biases, limitations, and sensitivities as well as of strengths. The authentic person is conscious that her perceptions are exclusively her own—viewed through a unique lens. She is cognizant of her own way of being in the world and maintains or regains this centeredness within relationships.

Mutuality is a full appreciation of the "other." The other's views are sought, respected, and valued. Expressions of difference are encouraged and celebrated. Persons in mutual relationships are aware of and acknowledge each other's way of being in the world, soliciting and offering feedback. In mutual relationships we acknowledge our connections, recognizing that we are all part of each other's stories.

Vulnerability is allowing oneself to be susceptible to feeling hurt or inadequate. It involves knowing when one is in need and asking for support without feeling diminished. It is part of the challenge of day-to-day caring that lies at the heart of nursing practice.

With heightened interpersonal competence, an individual gains self-awareness, acceptance, and the confidence that others believe in her and will support her. This in turn enhances a sense of her own credibility and the potential that she will take a risk.

Critical commitment comes from devotion to a cause or a sense of duty. It involves acting with sustained initiative on one's beliefs, both personal and professional. The individual who acts with critical commitment analyzes and acknowledges fully the potential consequences of taking a particular stand, including error and failure. Critical commitment demands that one "walk the talk" that gives meaning to the work of advanced practice in nursing. This factor encourages both self-discipline and self-respect. With critical commitment comes a moral imperative that propels an individual towards risk-taking behavior.

When the psychological factors of heightened interpersonal competence—the existential foundation of caring and critical commitment—are present, an individual needs only courage to take a risk. **Courage** is the quality of mind that equips the individual to face danger or hardship without flinching. Courage manifests itself in the resolute and frequently optimistic manner in which individuals deal with ambiguity and uncertainty. Persons with courage engage readily in taking risks with confidence and hope in the outcome.

---

*The concept of critical commitment is adapted from Madelon V. Baranoski (1994) with permission.
†The feminine form is used deliberately here because of power imbalances in health care systems that make it particularly difficult for women to develop these capacities.

Risk-taking has many forms and levels: to know oneself better, to connect emotionally with patients or colleagues, to remain with an unpopular but just cause, or to violate the rules that no longer serve a patient or family's needs. Developing this disposition is not a linear process but a kaleidoscopic experience involving reflection, opportunity, and practice. Whether a risk is taken to change one's interactions, improve an aspect of patient care, or improve large organizational systems, the constellation of factors here described must be present in some measure.

"TAKE A RISK, MAKE A DECISION, PAY THE PRICE" (Helen Mannock, personal communication, 1959)

Risk-taking behaviors differentiate those APNs who will be recognized as change agents from other knowledgeable professionals. By learning to take risks, the individual enlarges her behavioral repertoire, making possible more spontaneity and flexibility in responding to anger, conflict, resistance, and other human reactions to change. APNs can build and refine their competencies through nursing education, advance practice education, clinical experience, and reflection on what works and what does not. In taking risks that are not always successful, the APN gains confidence in the ability to survive setbacks and return to risk another day. The acknowledgment of the potential costs as well as benefits of risk-taking is an important component of change agency. The APN who aspires to be an agent for change can actively contribute to this process via a number of strategies, which follow.

STRATEGIES

SELF AND OTHERS

Competencies such as assertiveness, including attention to anxiety, anger, and irrational thinking, and conflict negotiation are generally useful in all aspects of life but are a necessity to the APN who wishes to facilitate change. This section addresses the characteristics and skills developed within the self that are reflected in one's interactions with others.

Actively listening to our patients in the process of care is a respected and valued competency of nurses in both basic and advanced practice. Nurses are experienced listeners when dealing with patients' concerns and issues. We are sometimes less effective listeners when dealing with the concerns of professional colleagues or when receiving feedback on our own behaviors. Listening demands self-discipline and focus, as well as openness and trust. Enhanced self-knowledge arises from acting, eliciting the responses of trusted others, reflecting, and modifying behavior as warranted. Active listening is an important component of effectiveness in practice, especially advanced practice.

Assertiveness

Competence in assertiveness is essential to advanced practice. The ability of APNs to consider their own needs, feelings, and rights in interactions with others is critical to positive interpersonal outcomes. People cannot be interpersonally competent if they are not appropriately assertive. Nurses are usually seen as being, and believe themselves to be, interpersonally competent, yet nurses are often, as a result of sex and occupational role socialization, not generally assertive. Frequently, nurses are out of touch with their own rights, needs, and feelings because orientation toward "the other" is so deeply ingrained from social learning and reinforced by nursing education (Ashley, 1976; Herman, 1976). Nurses' behaviors often demonstrate great respect for patients and professional colleagues while simultaneously showing a diminished or absolute lack of self-respect. To regain or heighten self-respect one may need to (re)assess personal limits and boundaries, one's ability to ask for what is wanted or needed, and how much one is willing to risk.

Ideally, such interpersonal work is undertaken in a group dedicated to assertiveness training and led by an expert. It is possible, however, to gain insight into one's responses and behavior that are either nonassertive or aggressive without group work. It may be more difficult because external support for internal change is enormously helpful. In any event, individual consciousness can be raised in a number of ways, including solitary reading and reflection. One might consider a contract with a trusted colleague for reading, discussion, and debriefing of behavior changes and their results. If behavior is to change toward being more assertive, one must allow the time and permit oneself to unlearn old behaviors while acquiring new ones. The metamorphosis will take months, not minutes, for it is not a matter of deciding "I will be assertive today" and being so. Learning assertiveness demands reflection, practice, and risk-taking.

One way to begin is by exploring an assertive philosophy, an example of which is found in Table 12–2 (Jakubowski-Specter, 1976). It is essential to differentiate assertive behavior from nonassertive, aggressive, or indirect aggressive behavior.*

---

* In psychiatric terms, this is sometimes called passive-aggression. Assertiveness training avoids psychiatric diagnoses, focusing instead on behaviors, in this case indirect as opposed to directly aggressive behavior.

TABLE 12–2. TENETS OF AN ASSERTIVE PHILOSOPHY

1. By standing up for our rights, we show we respect ourselves and achieve respect from other people.
2. By trying to govern our lives so as to never hurt anyone, we end up hurting ourselves and other people.
3. Sacrificing our rights usually results in destroying relationships or preventing ones from forming.
4. Not letting others know how we feel and what we think is a form of selfishness.
5. Sacrificing our rights usually results in training other people to mistreat us.
6. If we don't tell other people how their behaviors negatively affect us, we are denying them an opportunity to change their behavior.
7. We can decide what's important to us; we do not have to suffer from the "tyranny of the should and should not."
8. When we do what we think is right for us, we feel better about ourselves and have more authentic and satisfying relationships with others.
9. We all have a natural right to courtesy and respect.
10. We all have a right to express ourselves as long as we don't violate the rights of others.
11. There is more to be gained from life by being free and able to stand up for ourselves and from honoring the same rights of other people.
12. When we are assertive, everyone involved usually benefits.

From Jakubowski-Specter, P. (1976). Self-assertive training procedures for women. In D. Carter & E. Rawlings (Eds.), *Psychotherapy with women: Treatments towards equality.* Courtesy of Charles C Thomas, Publisher, Springfield, Illinois.

A simple criterion to apply to behavior is the concept of rights. Assertive people identify and protect their own rights and those of the other in a situation. Nonassertive people violate their own rights and consequently invite others to do so. Aggressive people are concerned exclusively with their own rights and violate others' rights. Indirect aggression is the violation of another's rights, sometimes while seeming to be protective or helpful, or it can occur without direct interaction. Because women are always supposed to be "nice," this can be the form aggression takes in women-dominated settings. Indirect aggression, such as gossip, is difficult to identify and can be troublesome to handle assertively. Under these circumstances, it is important to trust your own responses in a particular situation and analyze it for violations of rights by yourself or another. If you have a vague "bad" feeling about something (e.g., upset stomach, sadness, crying, bad mood), try to get at its origins. If you have difficulty with another's behavior, it is important to inquire about its meaning to that person ("When you said 'this is a bad idea,' what did you mean in terms of the strategies we've been developing in prior meetings?") and state your own boundaries ("I would prefer in the future that if you object to the ideas we're generating, please tell me in a timely fashion rather than surprising me at the next meeting.")

Assertiveness is situation-specific. Although most people behave in ways that are primarily assertive, nonassertive, or aggressive, we are all capable of behaviors of each type. Situations shape the different behavioral responses. In improving one's assertiveness, it is helpful to identify the specific situations of most concern and what it is about them that prevents assertive behavior. Most people find their potential assertions blocked in some way by anxiety, anger, or irrational thinking. Through role-playing in groups or through real-life practice and reflection, these obstacles can be reduced and assertive behaviors developed.

Anxiety can be assessed via a device known as the Subjective Unit of Disturbance Scale (SUDS) (Wolpe & Lazarus, 1966). Use of the scale can help to track relative anxiety about one's actions in particular situations. The scale ranges from 0, complete comfort, to 10, intolerable anxiety.* In assertiveness training, students are asked to recall three or four specific situations with which they are involved and concerned and award each situation a SUDS number from 1 to 10. An example follows:

Janet is an experienced adult nurse practitioner who is comfortable in her own practice with an established caseload of patients with hypertension, diabetes, and asthma. She occasionally makes presentations at continuing education offerings that require public speaking to colleagues and peers. Although she considers herself fairly quiet and somewhat shy, she is committed to bringing her experience to newer practitioners. She has just been invited to speak to her largest audience yet and is trying to decide whether to accept.

Also on Janet's mind are Mr. and Mrs. Potter. When either name appears on her appointment schedule, Janet can feel herself tense up. Mr. Potter takes copious notes at all their visits, and at subsequent appointments he pages back in his notebook to point out: "But on April 5th you said this—now what are you saying? Don't you know what you're doing?" Janet has found herself beginning to second-guess her own decisions and knows this can't go on.

When Janet attends an assertiveness training course at the adult education program in her town, she is asked to describe and rate one or two instances in which

---

*The original scale of 0–100 was adapted by E. M. Grady (1980).

she finds herself anxious or distressed in anticipation of an interaction. She rates her public speaking decision as a 6, and the Potters as a 4.

Taking the lowest SUDS rating first, the trainer works with Janet to develop potential strategies and responses to the Potters. The next step is role-playing the responses, with the Potters' possible reactions played by someone else. The expectation is that once Janet has explored the range of her responses and the Potters' reactions and has decided how to handle them, she will be better able to decide on a strategy to use in the office and to use it with confidence. A further benefit is that once one anxiety-producing interaction is dealt with, others may be reduced on the SUDS scale because of increased confidence in one's ability to handle the issues.

Anger presents a challenge to all of us, but it is especially difficult for women because of cultural expectations and socialization (Lerner, 1985; Miller, 1986). It is important to recognize that we are moved in relationships by emotions—they are powerful initiators of behavior. Anger is a genuine and legitimate emotion. Anger usually stems from an inability to express an experience—a feeling of not being heard or an inability to hear another. It usually coexists with other recognizable emotions such as hurt, disappointment, or humiliation. More than anything else, anger is a feeling of vulnerability. Although anger is generally viewed negatively, it can actually open up opportunities for better working relationships with others. The expression and engagement of real feelings enables individuals to search for mutual understanding and recognition. If your self-assessment suggests that anger is a barrier to heightened interpersonal competence, Lerner (1985) is an excellent self-help resource.

The connections that women and nurses value so much are damaged and lost when anger cannot be expressed or resolved. APNs can establish productive and positive relationships with colleagues by expressing their own feelings of anger in appropriately assertive ways and encouraging others to do likewise. Such behaviors are healthy and liberating.

Irrational thinking (Ellis & Harper, 1975) is negative self-talk that leads to self-defeating, unassertive behaviors. When we think irrationally, something everyone does at times, we display excessive concern about an interaction or relationship and exaggerate its effects. This can happen in one's professional or personal life. For example, one's first response might be: "Why should I bother to make the effort of explaining this man's social situation to his primary physician; doctors never listen anyway." or "Those attending this collaborative practice meeting don't understand the first thing about how an APN functions or even how we're educated. *I'm* not going to call attention to myself, get embarrassed, and be labeled a trouble-maker in trying to explain. Let someone else do it!"

Disciplined thinking is the examination of our own feelings and their appropriateness. This type of thinking can lead to a reasoned consideration and choice to feel differently, which can enhance assertive behavior. In following the above example one might say, "That's pretty negative thinking; besides, I won't be happy with myself unless I try to explain. Here goes!" or "OK, maybe I won't speak up this time. I wonder who's in charge of the agenda? I bet that other uncomfortable-looking APN would like to see better information provided here. I'll call her later."

Negotiating Conflict

Essential to interpersonal effectiveness is tolerance for the inevitable conflicts that we all experience in organizational life. Conflict is relational, situational, and moral (related to values). It may have special meaning for women whose socialization regarding conflict is similar to that regarding anger: that it is to be dreaded or denied and responded to by accommodating, soothing, or mediating behaviors. Instead, women and nurses must, in Miller's words, "reclaim conflict" (Miller, 1986, p. 125) and undertake "respectful engagement" with each other, with colleagues in other disciplines, and within organizations. Thus, learning how to negotiate in conflict situations also helps in dealing with anger.

Conflict always has consequences, many of which are positive (win-win situations, expanded flexibility). It can be analyzed and managed, whether it is a simple interpersonal disagreement or a departmental turf battle. Change agents have many opportunities to engage in conflict negotiation, both as players in conflicts and as neutral third parties. Although interpersonal conflicts have many origins, most can be tied to failure to define common goals, unclear definitions of responsibility, the inability or unwillingness to see and admit interdependence, or the inability to appreciate how one's role contributes to the "big picture" of the organization as a whole.

When people differ with regard to structural issues such as roles, policies, and practices, they can usually employ cognitive problem-solving processes successfully. If, on the other hand, the conflict involves personal antagonisms in which people become angry, defensive, distrustful, or resentful, cognitive processes are useless. These situations demand that one come to terms with feelings. This means accepting and owning one's negative responses, allowing those of the other, and attempting to understand their origins as they interfere with managing the conflict. This permits the restructuring of one's perceptions of what is at stake and thus moving forward. Such processes are primarily affective.

Conflicts are likely to involve structural and relational issues, and both cognitive and affective processes must be applied to manage them. Personality clashes, misunderstandings, and power struggles are endemic to organizational life. In health care, clinical work among different groups of providers creates situations in which appropriate patient care may depend on resolving conflict. Nurses, particularly leaders such as APNs, must develop the skills to deal with conflict.

Since 1985, the Harvard Negotiation Project* has provided the public with much insightful information about conflict negotiation. Fisher & Ury (1981) offer a model of great strength and simplicity, that of principled negotiation. Principled negotiation is a method in which participants decide issues on their merits rather than as a trade-off between getting what you want and getting along with people. Thus negotiators are "hard" on the merits of a conflict and simultaneously "soft" on each other as persons. The method includes four "principles." The parties involved should be able to separate the *people* from the problem, focus on *interests* not positions, invent *options* for mutual gain, and insist on using objective *criteria*—that is, the use of agreed-on independent standards.

When separating people from the problem, negotiators must talk about themselves, not accuse each other. It is essential that "I" rather than "you" statements be made. Listening is necessary to appreciate another's perspective; it becomes a fine art in which individuals seek clarification and verify that the message heard was the one that was sent. Listening is both auditory and visual. When nonverbal

* Located at Harvard Law School but open to negotiation and mediation professionals and students from outside Harvard University.

behavior is not consistent with the speaker's words, the listener attempts to understand the discrepancy.

Nurses' skill in their use of self provides a solid foundation on which to build conflict negotiation skills. We usually see negotiation as a consideration of two opposing positions. We need to reframe any negotiation as a consideration of mutual interests and expanding available options. Fisher & Ury (1981) encourage us to explore shared interests and to recognize that people who hold incompatible positions can and often do have compatible interests (e.g., keeping a practice or a program alive, safe patient care). In this spirit, people can consider the problem thoroughly before rushing to a solution or insisting on a single answer. A full consideration of alternatives becomes possible.

In addition, negotiators can invent options through brainstorming without making any decisions. This is called "expanding the pie" and creates even more possibilities for alternative agreements. Such processing helps the parties look forward, not backward.

Lastly, objective criteria are a must in principled negotiation. When criteria such as cost, efficiency, moral (ethical) standards, or patient welfare are employed, conflicting parties are yielding to principle—not pressure. Every negotiation should be framed as a joint search for objective criteria. For example: "If the patient is not better in two days with a normal temperature and white count, then we will do this. Agreed?"

SELF, OTHERS, AND ORGANIZATIONS

Strategies discussed in this section are those actions that can be taken specifically to facilitate organizational change. They include utilizing more than one perspective in analyzing organizations, or reframing (Bolman & Deal, 1991), coalition-building (Kanter, 1983), and managing change (Jick, 1993).

Reframing

Bolman and Deal (1991) offer leaders and change agents a tool for looking at organizational situations from more than one vantage point. They present four analytic frames from four major schools of organizational thought: the structural, human resource, political, and symbolic. Frames are windows on the world, lenses that bring the world into a particular focus. Bolman and Deal's thesis is that we tend to look at the organizational world predominantly, but not exclusively, through one of these frames. Such frames influence what we see, understand, and do, and how effective we are.

The *structural frame* evolved from efficiency studies and sociology; it emphasizes designing solutions to reflect specific goals, strategies, environment, technology, and people. Coordination and control are essential to effectiveness, and problems can be solved through restructuring or developing new systems.

The *human resource frame* is based in social psychology. Organizations exist to serve human needs; the need is mutual—organizations need ideas, energy, and talent and people need work opportunities and salaries. A good fit between the individual and the organization benefits both; a poor fit benefits neither. In this frame, people are the most important resource in the organization.

Political science research is the source for the *political frame*. The frame can be summarized by five propositions: organizations are coalitions; there are enduring differences among individuals and groups; decisions involve allocation of scarce resources; conflict is central and power the most important resource; and organizational goals and decisions emerge from bargaining, negotiation, and jockeying for position among various interest groups. In the political frame, various groups and individuals are in constant conflict and negotiation for resources and are exercising what power and influence they have to affect organizational direction.

The *symbolic frame* evolved from social and cultural anthropology and dispenses with the traditional assumptions of rationality, certainty, and linearity of decision-making found in the other frames. In this frame, organizations are viewed as cultures with rituals, ceremonies, stories, heroes, and myths. Central assumptions in this frame are that the meaning of an event is more important than what happened; the same event can have different meanings for different people; many significant organizational events and processes are ambiguous and uncertain; faced with ambiguity and uncertainty, human beings create symbols and rituals to reduce confusion, increase predictability, and provide direction; and many events and processes are more important for what they express than for what they produce. Symbolic culture includes the invisible and unexpressed rules that a newcomer encounters on entering an organization.

These frames are not diagnostic tools. Rather, knowledge of them enables us to take several perspectives on the same organizational event or problem. To the extent that we are able to be aware of and integrate visions of reality other than our predominant one, we will better appreciate the complexity of organizational life. These four frames should be used to develop a comprehensive view of organizations and as sources of useful information when dealing with others whose predominant frames are different from our own. Once all four frames are within our conceptual grasp, the APN can select one or more that best applies to fit or analyze a particular situation.

As an example, we will consider the increasing flow of CNSs back to school to obtain NP skills and certification. The structural frame perspective raises many questions. What goal or strategy is served by this change? What new system or program requires this group of APNs to retool their skills? Is it based on an analysis of outcomes? Who or what is coordinating the change organizationally? What systems are affected by the loss of the CNS role? Attempting to answer the questions raised by the structural frame reveals that there are significant gaps in understanding what is driving the move.

If we turn to the human resource frame, we take a different view. Have the organizations within which CNSs work become so different that the CNS now needs NP skills and knowledge? Is the decision based on a sound analysis of patient, organizational, staff, and CNS needs? Are these organizations now hiring NPs in place of CNSs because their skills and knowledge base are more appropriate? How will the organization and the CNS benefit from the new certification? It does not seem as though human resource needs are driving this move either.

With the political frame we may be closer to our desired understanding. Power is the most important resource, and in large health-care institutions, it is a scarce commodity among nursing staff. The prospect of obtaining NP certification and therefore legislative recognition, third-party reimbursement, and prescriptive authority has to be an extremely attractive option to CNSs as a means of gaining more power in an institution. Even if the CNS does not recognize this, nursing administration may instruct CNSs under their supervision to return to school and obtain this certification, thereby gaining power for the nursing department itself. Is anyone examining potential losses in power?

Finally, the symbolic frame provides us with a perspective that allows us to analyze the meaning of NP certification to the CNS. Is it possible that in the media coverage of health care reform and the oft-repeated need for primary care providers, the CNS role seemed invisible to those fulfilling it? In obtaining NP certification, are CNSs now NPs, or are they CNSs with NP skills? What happens to their specialty knowledge? —to their acute care or rehabilitation skills? Where will they belong, and where do they want to be? What does this change mean to CNSs?

Use of all the frames to examine this particular shift in advanced practice preparation suggests that the trend has not been fully analyzed. A more detailed application of the frames would probably yield further cost-benefit assessments.

Bolman and Deal claim that choosing a frame involves a combination of analysis, intuition, and artistry. They offer a table to facilitate the analysis of conditions under which each frame can contribute to organizational effectiveness (Table 12–3).

Coalition-Building

An essential skill in any change agent's repertoire is coalition-building. We all need interpersonal support to do successful work, and we build coalitions (a political act) by cultivating allies within our work settings. Furthermore, coalition-building is a key strategy in shepherding APN-friendly laws and regulations through state and federal legislatures.

Rosabeth Kanter (1983) offers a model for securing support and "spreading the risk" when undertaking a change effort. She suggests that the would-be changemaster engage in four key activities: clearing the investment, making cheerleaders, horse-trading, and securing blessings. Clearing the investment means eliciting preliminary agreement and support from one's immediate boss for an initiative. This is a first step, for without such an agreement further investment might be wasted. With such an agreement in hand the change agent is in a position to promote the idea with as many stakeholders of the issue as possible, contacting each individually. This is the process of making cheerleaders. Once cheerleaders are on board, horse-trading, or promising a reward or favor later for support now, can be undertaken. This is analogous to "doing your homework." Blessings are

TABLE 12–3. CHOOSING A FRAME

Question	Structural Frame	Human Resource Frame	Political Frame	Symbolic Frame
How important are commitment and motivation?	Unimportant	Important	?	Important
How important is the technical quality of the decision?	Important	?	Unimportant	Unimportant
How much ambiguity and uncertainty are present?	Low to moderate	Moderate	Moderate to high	High
How scarce are resources?	Moderately scarce	Moderately abundant to abundant	Scarce (or getting scarcer)	Scarce to abundant
How much conflict and diversity are present?	Low to moderate	Moderate	Moderate to high	Moderate to high
Are we working top down or bottom up?	Top down	Top down	Bottom up	Top down or bottom up

267

more likely to be secured from higher-level executives or legislators when a proposed initiative is packaged with administrative agreement and other cheerleaders.

Although this strategy is usually successful, it is not fail-safe. It is subject to the vicissitudes of organizational and political life, including changes in leadership, power shifts or imbalances, and other factors. One may not wish to be so explicit about one's change strategy. Informal wisdom among experienced change activists suggests that sometimes it is better to go ahead and do something and apologize afterward for not going through channels, rather than ask permission up front.

Managing Change

Change can constitute improvement of what is, moving from one state to another in a controlled and timely fashion, as slow evolution, or in chaos. Change agents can be involved in managing change in several ways, according to Jick (1994). He labels such involvement as envisioning, enabling, and implementing change.

Envisioning change is the development of a vision of the future should particular changes occur. Change must be "seen" and its direction charted in the mind before anything happens. Individuals or groups are charged with the vision task, to shape an organization or a structural unit within it. Vision is tied inextricably to a philosophy that lays out guiding values and principles for the work. Vision relates to a desired future for an organization, a preferred "big picture." Change influencers can develop their own visions and opportunistically find occasions to discuss and gain support for them. An example of this is the invention and use of the term "advanced practice" and the efforts being made to include the many different practices and professional groups under this term. It was necessary to "see" that the different groups had shared interests and goals that went beyond the immediate specialty or certification. It was important to invent language to use to refer to this idea. Once these were accomplished, then collective consciousness could develop and become part of APNs' identities.

The activities of *enabling* are those which represent strategic choices on rolling out or unfolding the change: pace, scope, depth, publicity, supporting structures, and who drives the change. These choices are made by change strategists but will affect all persons within the change agent's sphere of influence. An APN who wants to institute a practice change would consider several factors: how quickly all relevant clinicians could learn the practice; how complex the new practice is and how different it is from current practice; whether there should be a pilot or test case; how this new practice relates to past practice changes or those to follow; how the usual management processes and routine channels get used or bypassed in the effort; and lastly, what key individuals will be involved in driving the change, such that ownership occurs at the appropriate organizational levels.

A relevant example of enabling is the development of a strategy to include local office-based APNs under the hospital bylaws that currently allow only CNMs to obtain hospital privileges. The strategy must include input from CNMs who currently have privileges. It must address concerns that might be raised by nurse managers and hospital staff not familiar with an office-based NP or CNS role. Communication with the bylaws committee, nursing administration, and physician and nursing staff must occur continuously as negotiations proceed.

Implementation is the how of the change process. How do we get the change through? How do we get these people to change? How are we doing? Implementing is "simply" making it happen. Acknowledging that there is no foolproof process for managing change, Jick offers an inventory of ingredients for consideration in his "Ten Commandments of Implementing Change" (Jick, 1993, p. 195)*:

1. *Analyze the organization and its need for change.* Such an analysis involves consideration of the organization's work, its external environment, and its perceived strengths and weaknesses. The history of the organization must also receive consideration.
2. *Create a shared vision and common direction.* This should reflect the organization's philosophy and help articulate what it hopes to become. Implementors have the task of translating the vision to the grassroots so they can appreciate its potential implications for their work or positions.
3. *Separate from the past.* It is important to isolate the structure and the practices that no longer work and determine to move beyond them.
4. *Create a sense of urgency.* People will not go along with change that they see no need for. Currently, the health care system/nonsystem appears to be providing lots of urgency for caregivers as well as other major players. APNs can capitalize on this urgency to focus their practice.
5. *Support a strong leader role.* Desired change does not happen without strong leadership. In these chaotic times, many organizations do not depend on one leader but utilize leadership teams.
6. *Line up political sponsorship.* Once leadership is identified, support must be generated. This is similar to coalition-building, mentioned earlier.
7. *Craft an implementation plan.* A map of the change effort with specific timelines is necessary. It will need to detail clear responsibilities for the various organizational roles.†
8. *Develop enabling structures.* Structures that will facilitate and highlight change are necessary. Consider pilot programs, retreats, training workshops, and new reward systems.
9. *Communicate, involve people, and be honest.* A change announcement must be timely, brief, specific, and concise. The necessary follow-up communication must involve listening, repeating, explaining across communication styles, and responding to concerns and resistance.
10. *Reinforce and institutionalize the change.* The commitment to change must be obvious. The new culture must begin to show itself through the reinforcement of new behaviors.

This list is not the magic formula for success. If you are an implementor for a change agenda, however, you do have a guide to the issues in these recommendations. If you are a strategist in a small part of a large organization, or for a small organization in its entirety, the guide still holds.

IMPLICATIONS

IMPLICATIONS FOR EDUCATION

If change agency is a valued competency in nursing, then nursing educational programs need to be explicit about its value and develop educational strategies for

---

*Adapted and reprinted by permission. From Todd D. Jick, Implementing Change, case no. 491–114. Boston: Harvard Business School, 1991. In *Managing Change: Cases and Concepts* by Todd D. Jick. Burr Ridge, IL: Richard D. Irwin, Inc., 1993. Copyright © 1991 by the President and Fellows of Harvard College.

†The reader may find it useful to pursue "responsibility charting" as described by Beckhard and Harris (1992), which clarifies the behavior that is required to implement each change task, action, or decision and the persons accountable for the behavior (in Beckhard & Pritchard, 1992).

preparing nurses as change agents. This would mean beginning in basic nursing with fundamentals such as the psychology and sociology of organizations, assertiveness, and beginning conflict negotiation skills. Traditional nursing values of service and silence would be replaced by active questioning and action to improve patient care. Students should expect to see faculty modeling risk-taking behaviors in clinical practice and academic organizations. Experiences of disapproval, resistance, or aggression should be debriefed thoroughly in a manner that provides safe expression of the difficult feelings these responses can raise.

Advanced practice education would build on this basic foundation with organizational theory, change theory, and enhanced conflict negotiation skills. Clinical opportunities for risk-taking and subsequent reflection on outcomes would be integrated into the further development of practice skills. In the absence of safe settings and mentors for debriefing difficult experiences at the basic level, APN programs must provide this vital preparation for the real world of health care. Faculty would need expertise in these areas as well as specialty clinical knowledge and skill. Academic administrators and faculty would likely benefit from ongoing educational opportunities in organization and change theory, assertiveness training, conflict negotiation, and safe settings in which to debrief difficult emotional experiences.

These implications for education are broad strokes. The sky is the limit if nursing truly values educating its novice practitioners so that both RNs and APNs are prepared to participate actively in the changing health-care environment. In today's environment, success will depend on the revision of all of nursing's more traditional expectations. Education is where it happens first.

IMPLICATIONS FOR PRACTICE

Upon graduation and certification, the new APN is expected to have a set of knowledge and skills that can be applied to providing patient care in a chosen specialty and setting. With the educational background suggested earlier, the novice APN is truly in a position to change practice, and the clinical practice area is perhaps the easiest and most logical one in which to contemplate initiating change. Initiating change requires self-empowerment and the exercise of leadership. In the exercise of one's own leadership, one begins to discriminate among effective and inadequate leadership styles. This in turn may lead to the APN's initiation of changes in the leadership or directorship of a committee, practice, or other organization. Once changes made to benefit groups of patients occur, change initiators do not remain invisible. Contributing to productive change creates opportunities for initiating more change through invitations to participate on committees and developing a reputation for "getting things done."

CONCLUSION

First things learned are the hardest to forget. Traditions pass from one generation to the next. We need to change.

(From Matty Rich, *Straight Out of Brooklyn,* "Epilogue," MGM Films, 1991)

Everything begins somewhere, no less the skills and internal fortitude to facilitate change. It is important to see the strategies and actions described here as part of a continuum of nursing/APN practice and not as fully developed capabilities that the new graduate automatically possesses.

"UPPER-CASE" AND "LOWER-CASE" CHANGE AGENTS

Some characteristics, dispositions, and skills are brought to basic nursing education from previous life or work experience and are further refined in practice. Sometimes it is not until advanced practice education or a position after graduate school that one is disposed to risk-making change. Gaining heightened interpersonal competence, consolidating critical commitment, and developing courage are highly individualized processes that are never linear. This reality has implications for education, practice, and the future of the profession.

Just as there are different paths for developing change agent characteristics and skills, there is also a continuum of locations where the APN facilitates change. Not all APNs choose to be *Change Agents* who exercise leadership publicly. Many find significant satisfaction as *change agents* through improving patient care on a smaller scale. The ideas, exercises, and strategies found in this chapter will serve to strengthen one's efforts no matter where they are made. In time, a comfortable niche is found, or a heretofore unknown drive is discovered and pursued perhaps locally or nationally.

FOR THE FUTURE

Change agency is a complex kaleidoscope of theoretical, practical, psychological, personal, organizational, and intuitive knowledge and skill. This means that the aspiring agent for change can begin anywhere and follow her own path. The range of opportunities to create change is infinite and depends only on the desires, disposition, and skills of the APN. Nursing and advanced practice need all change-makers at whatever point they are working to assist in the huge endeavor of making nursing as viable and visible a profession in the future as it has been a vocation in the past.

One need only begin.

REFERENCES

American Nurses Association. (1995). *Nursing's social policy statement.* Washington, D.C.: ANA.

Ashley, J. A. (1976). *Hospitals, paternalism, and the role of the nurse.* New York: Teachers College Press.

Baranoski, M. V. (1994). The voice of nursing: The power of care. Speech given at New England Medical Center, Boston, May 4, 1994.

Beckhard, R., & Pritchard, W. (1992). *Changing the essence: The art of creating and leading fundamental change in organizations.* San Francisco: Jossey-Bass.

Bolman, L., & Deal, T. E. (1991). *Reframing organizations: Artistry, choice, and leadership.* San Francisco: Jossey-Bass.

Boughn, S. (1994). Why do men choose nursing? *Nursing and Health Care, 15*(8).

Bridges, W. (1991). *Managing transitions: Making the most of change.* Reading, MA: Addison-Wesley.

Brooten, D. A., Naylor, M. D., & Hayman, L. L. (1978). *Leadership for change: A guide for the frustrated nurse.* Philadelphia: J. B. Lippincott.

Brown, E. L. (1948). *Nursing for the future.* New York: Russell Sage Foundation.

Brown, S. J. (1989). Supportive supervision of the CNS. In A. B. Hamric & J. A. Spross (Eds.), *The clinical nurse specialist in theory and practice.* Philadelphia: W. B. Saunders.

Caffrey, R. A., & Caffrey, P. A. (1994). Nursing: Caring or codependent? *Nursing Forum, 29*(1), 12-17.

Clare, J. (1993). A challenge to the rhetoric of emancipation: Recreating a professional culture. *Journal of Advanced Nursing, 18,* 1033-1038.

Dickens, C. (1953). *Martin Chuzzlewit.* London: Collins.

Ellis, A., & Harper, R. A. (1975). *A new guide to rational living.* Englewood Cliffs, NJ: Prentice-Hall.

Fisher, R., & Ury, W. (1981). *Getting to yes: Negotiating agreement without giving in*. New York: Penguin Books.

Goren, S., & Ottaway, R. (1985). Why health-care teams don't change: Chronicity and collusion. *Journal of Nursing Administration, 15*(7, 8), 9-16.

Grady, E. M. (1980). Resocializing professional nurses: The case for assertiveness training. Unpublished Doctoral Dissertation, Case Western Reserve University.

Hamric, A. B., & Spross, J. (1983). *The clinical nurse specialist in theory and practice*. Philadelphia: W. B. Saunders.

Hamric, A. B., & Spross, J. A. (1989). *The clinical nurse specialist in theory and practice* (2nd ed.). Philadelphia: W. B. Saunders.

Herman, S. J. (1976). *Becoming assertive: A guide for nurses*. New York: D. Van Nostrand.

Jakubowski-Spector, P. (1976). Self-assertive training procedures for women. In D. Carter & E. Rawlings, (Eds.), *Psychotherapy with women: Treatments toward equality*. Springfield, IL: Charles C Thomas.

Jick, T. D. (1993). *Managing change: Cases and concepts*. Burr Ridge, IL: Irwin.

Kanter, R. M. (1983). *The changemasters: Innovation and entrepreneurship in the American corporation*. New York: Simon & Schuster.

Kanter, R. M., Stein, B. A., & Jick, T. D. (1992). *The challenge of organizational change: How companies experience it and leaders guide it*. New York: Free Press.

Lancaster, J., & Lancaster, W. (1982). *Concepts for advanced nursing practice: The nurse as change agent*. St. Louis: C. V. Mosby.

Lerner, H. G. (1985). *The dance of anger*. New York: Harper & Row.

Lewin, K. (1951). *Field theory in social science*. New York: Harper & Row.

Manion, J. (1995). Understanding the seven stages of change. *American Journal of Nursing, 95*(4), 41-43.

May, R. (1972). *Power and innocence*. New York: W. W. Norton.

Miller, J. B. (1986). *Toward a new psychology of women* (2nd ed.). Boston: Beacon Press.

National Council of State Boards of Nursing. (1993). *Position Paper on the Regulation of Advanced Nursing Practice*.

Noddings, N. (1984). *Caring: A feminine approach to ethics and moral education*. Berkeley: University of California Press.

Oshry, B. (1972). Power and the power lab. In W. W. Burke (Ed.), *New technologies in OD development*. Bethel, ME: NTL Institute.

Peters, T. (1988). *Thriving on chaos*. New York: Alfred A. Knopf.

Strunk, B. L. (1995). The clinical nurse specialist as change agent. *Clinical Nurse Specialist, 9*(3), 128-132.

Watson, J. & Phillips, S. (1992). A call for educational reform: Colorado nursing doctorate model as exemplar. *Nursing Outlook, 40*(1), 20-26.

Webster's 10th collegiate dictionary. (1993). Springfield, MA: Merriam-Webster.

Wolpe, J., & Lazarus, A. A. (1966). *Behavior therapy techniques*. New York: Pergamon.

Additional Readings

Alberti, R. E., & Emmons, M. L. (1974). *Your perfect right: A guide to assertive behavior*. San Luis Obispo, CA: Impact Publishers.

Belenky, M. F., Clinchy, B. M., Goldberger, N. R., & Tarule, J. M. (1988). *Women's ways of knowing: The development of self, voice, and mind*. Basic Books.

Bowditch, J. L., & Buono, A. F. (1994). *A primer on organizational behavior* (3rd ed.). New York: Wiley.

Bridges, W. (1980). *Transitions: Making sense of life's changes*. New York: Addison-Wesley.

Fisher, R., & Brown, S. (1988). *Getting together: Building relationships as we negotiate*. New York: Penguin Books.

Fisher, R., Kopelman, E., & Schneider, A. K. (1994). *Beyond Machiavelli: Tools for coping with conflict*. Cambridge, MA: Harvard University Press.

Haddon, R. M. (1989). The final frontier: Nursing in the emerging health-care environment. *Nursing Economics, 7*(3), 155-161.

Hamer, M., & Champy, J. (1993). *Reengineering the corporation: A manifesto for business revolution*. New York: Harper Business.

Heifitz, R. A. (1994). *Leadership without easy answers*. Cambridge, MA: Harvard University Press.

Lange, A. J., & Jakubowski, P. (1976). *Responsible assertive behavior*. Champaign, IL: Research Press.

Muff, J. (1982). Altruism, socialism, and Nightingalism: The compassion traps. In J. Muff (Ed.), *Socialization, sexism, and stereotyping: Women's issues in nursing*. St. Louis: C. V. Mosby.

Reverby, S. M. (1987). *Ordered to care: The dilemma of American nursing, 1850–1945*. Cambridge, UK: Cambridge University Press.

Senge, P. (1990). *The fifth discipline: The art and practice of the learning organization*. New York: Doubleday/Currency.

Tishman, C. (1994). What makes a good thinker: A look at thinking dispositions. *Education: The Harvard Graduate School of Education Alumni Bulletin, 39*(1).

Weisbord, M. R. (1987). *Productive workplaces: Organizing and managing for dignity, meaning and community*. San Francisco: Jossey-Bass.

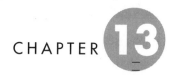

CHAPTER 13

Ethical Decision-Making Skills

Juanita Reigle

INTRODUCTION

Various factors, including changes in inter-professional roles, advances in medical technology, and heightened economic constraints, have increased the complexity of ethical issues in the health-care setting. Nurses in all areas of health care routinely encounter disturbing moral issues, yet the success with which these dilemmas are resolved varies significantly. Because nurses have a unique relationship to the patient and family, the moral position of nursing in the health-care arena is distinct. As the complexity of issues intensifies, the role of the advanced practice nurse (APN) becomes particularly important in the deliberation and resolution of complicated and difficult value choices. It is a basic tenet of the central definition of advanced nursing practice (ANP; see Chapter 3) that ethical decision-making skills are part of the core competencies of all APNs.

CHARACTERISTICS OF ETHICAL DILEMMAS IN NURSING

In this chapter, the terms "ethics" and "morality" or "morals" are used interchangeably. An ethical or moral dilemma occurs when two (or more) morally acceptable courses of action are present and to choose one prevents selecting another. The agent experiences tension because the moral obligations resulting from the dilemma create differing and opposing demands (Beauchamp & Childress, 1994; Purtilo, 1993). In some moral dilemmas, the agent must choose between equally unacceptable alternatives—that is, both may have elements that are morally wrong. The various perspectives, values, and beliefs of patients, families, and members of the health-care team often lead to differing but morally defensible positions (Rushton, 1988).

Although the scope and nature of moral dilemmas experienced by nurses reflect the varied clinical settings in which they practice, some general themes emerge when examining ethical issues in nursing practice. A recent survey conducted by the American Nurses Association Center for Ethics and Human Rights identified 10 priority issues confronting nurses in practice. The issues most frequently mentioned by the respondents were issues of cost-containment that jeopardized patient welfare; end-of-life decisions; breaches of patient confidentiality; incompetent, illegal, or unethical practices of colleagues; pain management; use of advance directives; informed consent for procedures; access to health care; issues in the care of persons with human immunodeficiency virus (HIV) infection or acquired immunodeficiency syndrome (AIDS); and providing "futile" care (Scanlon, 1994). Other issues encountered by nurses include ethical conflicts associated with the patient-physician-nurse relationship; patient autonomy; truth-telling; quality of life (including symptom management); refusal of treatment; and organ transplantation (Aroskar, 1989; Calkins, 1993; Omery, Henneman, Billet, et al., 1995; Solomon, O'Donnell, Jennings, et al., 1993; Viens, 1994; Winters, Glass, Sakurai, et al., 1993).

Issues that traverse acute and non-acute health care settings include quality of life and symptom management (Calkins, 1993; Omery et al., 1995; Solomon et al., 1993; Winters et al., 1993). It is not surprising that these issues are central moral concerns for nurses. Typically the nurse monitors the patient, interprets symptoms, and administers medication to provide optimal relief of undesirable and intolerable symptoms. Pain relief and symptom management become problematic for nurses when physicians appear to be reluctant to prescribe adequate amounts of medication to alleviate the patient's pain and suffering (Omery et al., 1995; Solomon et al., 1993). Balancing chronic illness, symptom management, and quality of life challenges nurses to confront the subsequent themes surrounding the patient-physician-nurse relationship such as informed consent, truth-telling, and decision-making at the end of life (Winters et al., 1993).

Dilemmas of justice, such as the fair distribution of health-care resources and access to care, are prevalent in community health nursing (Aroskar, 1989). Situations in which the community lacks adequate resources or funds to meet the needs of families are issues for both the individual practitioner and society. Although these issues require the attention of the entire society, community health nurses manage individual dilemmas by relying on nursing colleagues for support and by focusing on the contextual needs of the patient rather than societal needs (Aroskar, 1989).

In contrast, a study of primary care nurse practitioners (NPs) indicated that they interpreted their moral responsibilities as balancing obligations to the patient, family, colleagues, employer, and society (Viens, 1994). However, the NPs thought that attending to societal needs, such as responsibilities for research protocols and cost-containment, conflicted with ethical obligations to the individual patient. These conflicting loyalties generated moral distress in the primary care NPs and resulted in inconsistent decision-making (Viens, 1994). In addition to external factors, the qualities present in the NP-patient relationship also influenced the response of the NPs to the dilemma. For example, when caring for a patient with AIDS, the NP may struggle with entering the patient in a research protocol that provides no benefit to the patient but may advance medical knowledge. In this case, the nature of the NP-patient interaction, such as development of the relationship over time, may influence the nurse's moral response (Viens, 1994). Therefore, the manner in which the NP balances the conflicting responsibilities to the patient and society reflects both the central values inherent in the nurse-patient relationship and the NP's accountability to society.

EXPECTATIONS OF NURSES

PROFESSIONAL PRACTICE

Nurses just entering the profession and nurses with many years' experience rely on the *Code for Nurses* for guidance and direction in professional issues (American Nurses Association, 1985). The *Code* serves a worthy function by describing the profession's philosophy and the general ethical obligations of the professional nurse. However, the *Code* describes broad guidelines that more reflect the profession's conscience than provide clear directions for specific clinical situations. In this sense, the *Code* delineates the nurse's overriding moral obligations to the patient but offers little specific help in balancing competing demands from the institution and other health care professionals. One of the main moral dimensions of the *Code for Nurses* is the concept of advocacy.

Generally, professional nurses understand their moral obligations through the concept of patient advocacy. In this model, the patient is the central focus, and members of the health care team act to support and achieve the patient's informed choices (Millette, 1993). Patient advocacy implies a duty to equalize the power imbalance between the patient and others in the health care setting. Although the intentions of the advocate role are to promote patient autonomy, self-actualization, and uniqueness, nurses often feel powerless to effect these outcomes (Gadow, 1980; Veatch & Fry, 1987).

Erlen and Frost (1991) examined nurses' perceptions and experiences in influencing ethical decisions related to the care of patients. When confronted with an ethical dilemma, nurses reported feelings of powerlessness, helplessness, and vulnerability. The attempt to exert any influence on an outcome or resolution was silenced by a perception of physician dominance and control. In other words, the nurses perceived themselves as lacking authority and power over the resolution of moral dilemmas. Several factors contributed to perceptions of powerlessness. When information was withheld or an awareness of available choices was lacking, individuals were unable to make reasoned and comprehensive decisions. Erlen and Frost (1991) reported that nurses in the study were unaware of alternatives or opportunities to change the outcome of the dilemma.

When the lack of knowledge regarding suitable options is coupled with the inability to clearly communicate an understanding of the moral dilemma, effective resolution of the issue is seriously hindered. Open communication is a fundamental element of collaboration, and successful resolution of moral issues is best achieved in an environment that fosters shared decision-making. In a collaborative practice environment, the contributions of all participants are encouraged and valued. Such an environment stimulates moral reasoning and supports the identification of alternatives and acceptable solutions (Pike, 1991). Ineffective, ambiguous, and elusive patterns of communication erode the mutual trust and respect essential to the collaborative milieu.

Too frequently nurses remain silent or simply talk with nursing colleagues when experiencing moral dilemmas. In many health care settings the overriding presumption is that the physician controls the direction and resolution of moral issues. Moral distress occurs when institutional constraints prevent the nurse from following the morally correct course of action (Jameton, 1984). However, as nurses gain clinical knowledge and learn new ways to relate to physicians, the communication of moral concerns increases and nurses choose to take action (Erlen and Frost, 1991).

APN PRACTICE

Although many experienced nurses can successfully negotiate moral dilemmas and achieve satisfactory outcomes, the ethical decision-making skills exhibited by the APN reflect a broader range of development. The purpose of this chapter is to define and clarify these skills. As stated earlier, most nurses view their role as moral agents from the position of individual patient advocacy. However, the sense of moral agency may not be reflected in the nurse's actions. In one study of pediatric nurses, most nurses limited participation in raising and addressing ethical issues to within the immediate health-care team. On the other hand, nurses with graduate education were more likely to take an active role in communicating ethical issues and addressing broader organizational concerns (Martin, 1989). This sense of responsibility and accountability for confronting ethical issues tends to increase with formal education (Crisham, 1981; Duckett, Rowan-Boyer, & Ryden, et al., 1992; Martin, 1989; Rest, 1986).

Beyond the role of patient advocate, the APN advocates for a process of ongoing, rather than episodic, ethical inquiry. This process of moral reflection sanctions open discussions of values and divergent views and is realized through the reciprocal exchanges of information between members of the health-care team and the patient. Throughout this process, the APN incorporates the skills necessary to facilitate dialogue, mediate disputes, analyze options, and design optimal solutions. Therefore, the ethical decision-making skills of the APN move the resolution of moral dilemmas beyond individual cases toward the cultivation of an environment in which the moral integrity of individuals is respected. Development and preservation of this ethical environment is the key contribution of the APN. The following case illustrates the varying perspectives and roles of the patient, family, APN, and members of the health-care team.

Mrs. Howard, an elderly, diabetic, African-American woman presented to the emergency room with necrotizing fasciitis of her left lower leg secondary to a minor traumatic injury she had received several days earlier. She was admitted to an acute care unit, and antimicrobial therapy was initiated. She agreed to undergo surgical exploration, debridement, and drainage. Despite aggressive treatment, the infection continued to rapidly progress and became gangrenous. The physicians recommended that Mrs. Howard undergo an amputation of her lower left leg. They stated that her underlying chronic illnesses, diabetes and hypertension, as well as the severe anaerobic infection placed her at significant risk of developing sepsis. Mrs. Howard refused to undergo the amputation, stating that she "would rather die than have her leg cut off." She said she would pray that God would "do the right thing" and heal her or take her to her "Savior." Although Mrs. Howard was widowed, she had two adult children. Her daughter supported her mother's refusal, but Mrs. Howard's son disagreed. He told the physicians that his mother didn't understand that she would be able to function capably with only one leg, and that he would sign the consent form for the surgery.

The nurse caring for Mrs. Howard was uncomfortable with the patient's refusal, but supported Mrs. Howard's right to refuse even beneficial surgery. Although Mrs. Howard demonstrated all the elements of decisional capacity, the surgeons expressed concerns regarding their legal liability in following a "medically unreasonable" decision. The physicians were influenced by the son's explanation that Mrs. Howard simply did not understand the level of functional capacity she could achieve after surgery. Attempts to convince Mrs. Howard to undergo the surgery deteriorated into threatening remarks by her son, who stated, "If you don't sign the form then I will!" and distant and impartial comments by the physicians such as "We'll do whatever you want us to do." Mrs. Howard became more agitated and defiant, and the nurses caring for her began to question her decisional capacity. At this point, the nurses on the unit consulted the clinical nurse specialist (CNS) to help define the issues and develop an acceptable plan for the nurses to follow.

This case illuminates the multiple dilemmas that can originate from one situation. The staff nurse must balance respecting the patient's informed refusal with the professional and personal value of providing optimal care. The surgeon is concerned for Mrs. Howard's welfare and is uneasy about the legal implications of not performing the needed surgery. Mrs. Howard's son is distressed with his mother's refusal and dismisses her decision as illogical and impaired. Finally, Mrs. Howard is angry and exasperated with the health-care team and her son for questioning her capacity and decision.

The case could easily be limited to a question of capacity. Once Mrs. Howard is determined to have decisional capacity (which she does possess), the caregivers could render care accordingly and her son would have to adjust to his mother's decision. However, the disturbing remnants of the dilemma would linger, creating an atmosphere of unaddressed discomfort. In this case, the moral integrity of many individuals in the dilemma was challenged. Thus, to create an environment that preserves and protects the moral qualities and values of its members, all layers of a dilemma must be addressed. The APN facilitates the process of addressing the remaining issues. For example, the staff nurse must now find acceptable ways to provide care in less than optimal circumstances. Because Mrs. Howard's beliefs are not congruent with the nurse's value system, the APN should facilitate a discussion between Mrs. Howard and the staff nurse. Together with Mrs. Howard, the nurse must retrieve the elements of her professional values that maintain her moral integrity without jeopardizing Mrs. Howard's choice. For example, one value the nurse can still act on is to provide comfort and care. The nurse can discuss with Mrs. Howard acceptable means for palliation and pain relief that would not conflict with the patient's religious beliefs. This action empowers the nurse to discover more imaginative and humanized ways to provide care without violating core values. The APN helps the nurse to accept Mrs. Howard's decision and accept the options. Once the issue is addressed the nurse can leave it behind and accept that the issue received the deserved attention. Attention to the remaining doubts and questions encourages agents to act again when faced with a moral dilemma (van Hooft, 1990).

As just illustrated, clinical cases in which ethical dilemmas arise often emerge from clinicians' differing realities and incompatible interpretations of the situation. Differences also exist in the outcomes pursued by the individuals involved in the conflict. The APN must guide a process in which all parties can hear the other's perspectives and negotiate acceptable solutions. It is not essential that the parties interpret previous decisions similarly. Instead, the APN facilitates dialogue so that each person's concept of reality is acknowledged and the meanings of particular occurrences are shared.

ETHICAL THEORIES

Although ethical decision-making in health care is extensively discussed in the bioethics literature, two dominant models are most often applied in the clinical setting. The analytical model of decision-making is a principle-based model. In this model, ethical decision-making is guided by theories, principles, and rules (Beauchamp & Childress, 1994; Fowler, 1989). In cases of conflict, the principles or rules in contention are balanced and interpreted with the contextual elements of the circumstance. However, the final decision and moral justification for actions are based on an appeal to principles. In this way, the principles are both binding and tolerant of the particularities of specific cases (Beauchamp & Childress, 1994).

The principles of respect for persons, autonomy, beneficence, nonmaleficence, and justice are commonly applied in the analysis of ethical issues in nursing. The *Code for Nurses* embraces the principled approach and underscores the first moral obligation of nursing as respect for persons (Fowler, 1989). The emphasis on respect for persons throughout the *Code* implies that it is not only a philosophical value of nursing but a binding principle within the profession.

Although ethical principles and rules are the cornerstone of most ethical decisions, the principle-based approach has been criticized as too formalistic and rigorous for many clinicians (Ahronheim, Moreno, & Zuckerman, 1994). Critics argue that this approach to moral problems reduces the resolution of a clinical case to simply balancing principles. Consequently, when conflicts among principles occur, the description of the principle is inadequate to provide guidance for resolving the dilemma (Ahronheim et al., 1994; Beauchamp & Childress, 1994).

The second approach to ethical decision-making is the casuistic model, in which current cases are compared with paradigm cases (Ahronheim et al., 1994; Beauchamp & Childress, 1994; Fowler, 1989; Jonsen & Toulmin, 1988). The strength of this approach is that dilemmas are examined in a context-specific manner and then compared with an analogous earlier case. The fundamental philosophical assumption of this model is that ethics emerges from human moral experiences (Ahronheim et al., 1994; Jonsen & Toulmin, 1988). The casuists approach dilemmas from an inductive position and work from the specific case to generalizations, rather than from generalizations to specific cases (Ahronheim et al., 1994; Beauchamp & Childress, 1994).

Some concerns arise when evaluating a casuistic model for ethical decision-making. As a moral dilemma arises, the selection of the paradigm case may differ among the decision-makers, and thus the interpretation of the appropriate course of action will vary. Furthermore, casuists have no mechanisms, other than the reliance on previous cases, to justify their actions. The possibility that previous cases were reasoned in a faulty or inaccurate manner is not considered or evaluated (Beauchamp & Childress, 1994).

Other theories, such as utilitarianism, Kantianism, virtue-based theory, and care-based theory, provide alternative processes for moral reflection and argument (Beauchamp & Childress, 1994). In particular, the ethics of care has emerged as relevant to nursing (Cooper, 1989). The care perspective constructs moral problems as issues surrounding the intrinsic needs and corresponding responsibilities that occur within relationships (Cooper, 1989; Gilligan, 1982). Moral reasoning involves empathy and emphasizes responsibility rather than rights. The response of the individual to a moral dilemma emerges from the affiliative relationship and the norms of friendship, care, and love (Beauchamp & Childress, 1994; Cooper, 1991).

Although every ethical theory has some limitations and problems, an understanding of contemporary approaches to ethics and bioethics is valuable in achieving a moral resolution. Moral reasoning more often reflects a blend of the various theories rather than the application of a single theory. The APN can gain an understanding of the prevailing ethical theories through formal and informal education.

FOUNDATIONS FOR ETHICAL DECISION-MAKING

THE NURSE-PATIENT RELATIONSHIP

The changing health care environment has placed extraordinary demands on nurses in independent practice settings as well as in acute care settings. The limitations of time, reimbursement, and resources conflict with nursing's moral imperatives of involvement, connection, and commitment. The relationship of caring practices to the patient's recovery process is reflected in the definition of nursing. According to the American Nurses Association (ANA), nursing integrates objective scientific knowledge of diagnosis and treatment with the philosophy and science of caring to facilitate health and healing (American Nurses Association, 1995). To understand and deal with human responses, the nurse must focus on the patient as a unique human being rather than a disease. Therefore, the essence of nursing's professional accountability is embedded in the relationship between the nurse and the patient and family.

The first encounter between the nurse and patient is often polite, constructed, and somewhat ritualistic. The nurse adheres to rules or standards that serve to establish a trusting foundation for subsequent encounters. Unfamiliar environments, pain, suffering, and sudden or chronic illnesses increase vulnerability and suppress opportunities for the patient and family to regain control. Behaviors common in most health-care settings, such as removal of personal clothing or restrictions on family visitation, further dehumanize and disempower the patient and family. The APN initiates a trusting environment by establishing feelings of certainty and security for the patient. Describing the environment, others' roles, the plan of care, or general routines will give the patient a sense of predictability about his or her surroundings. Confidence and comfort in the health-care setting increases as the patient perceives the APN and other caregivers as competent and qualified professionals.

It is important for patients to understand their reciprocal responsibilities within the health-care team. A comprehensive and accurate evaluation of the patient is impossible if information is withheld or intentionally concealed. The APN should explicitly identify the shared expectations of truthfulness and honesty. The patient's commitment to truthfulness and openness must be balanced with the health-care team's obligation to be truthful (also known as veracity) and respect for patient confidentiality. Because the nurse provides intimate physical care and is entrusted with sensitive and personal information, the importance of preserving privacy and confidentiality is heightened in the nurse-patient relationship. The explicit dialogue between the APN and patient or family defines the expectations of each party and thus enables all parties to communicate values and openly address both clinical and ethical issues. In this way, the APN positions the patient and family in an empowered capacity, which is an essential step for collaborative decision-making.

THE NURSE-PHYSICIAN RELATIONSHIP

Nurses and physicians define, perceive, analyze, and reason through ethical problems from distinct and often opposing perspectives. These differing approaches may create conflict between the nurse and physician, further separating and isolating the perspectives. The physician either may be unaware of the nurse's differing opinion or does not recognize this difference as a conflict (Grammelspracher, Howell, & Young, 1986). Conflicts are intensified when the physician does not agree with the nurse that certain details and specifics of the situation are important or simply does not feel accountable to resolve the conflict with the nurse (Grammelspracher et al., 1986; Haddad, 1991). The APN must first deal with the inter-professional communication problems between the nurse and physician before seeking resolution of ethical problems.

Although open communication is a necessary component of the collaborative environment, it is not sufficient. Physicians and other members of the health-care team must understand the nurse's role and responsibilities. In the traditional hospital setting, many physicians view the nurse as subordinate and functioning primarily to carry out the physician's orders (Grammelspracher et al., 1986). In some cases, physicians perceive their authority as threatened when nurses expand their education and assume more autonomous roles as NPs and APNs (Haddad, 1991). On the other hand, respect may increase as the physician perceives the APN as more competent and accountable than other nurses. Successful collaboration between nurses and physicians is grounded in communication, cooperation, competence, accountability, and trust (Baggs & Schmitt, 1988). A clearer understanding of the values and perspectives that each profession brings to the decision-making arena will enhance the formation of a collaborative environment.

VALUES CLARIFICATION

Personal and Professional Values

Individuals' interpretations and positions on issues are a reflection of their underlying value system. Value systems are enduring beliefs that guide life choices and decisions in conflict resolution (Uustal, 1987). Because values influence behaviors, actions, and choices, an awareness of personal values generates more consistent choices and behaviors.

Professional and personal communication is based on individual interpretations of the facts, meanings, and significance of the information. The therapeutic options that are offered and the practices in which the APN participates are based on personal and professional values. Self-examination of personal values enables the APN to consciously examine, analyze, and understand internalized moral convictions that guide decisions. Values clarification is an approach to examining the influence that values have on decision-making and behavior (Uustal, 1987). This process enables the APN to appreciate and articulate the personal and professional values that influence behavior as well as to recognize and respect the values of other health-care team members. Values clarification and values education are practical and effective strategies to expand the health-care team's awareness of each other's professional beliefs. The mutual understanding of professional value systems will generate a greater understanding of how each profession views the ethical problems it faces. This is an important first step to developing a collaborative approach to moral reasoning.

Patient Values

Values also underlie the decisions of patients and families. Through the process of values clarification, the APN can guide the patient and family toward the recognition and appreciation of previously unconscious value choices. Careful examination of the patient's values enhances treatment decision-making and clarifies the motivation underlying the individual's expressed wishes and treatment preferences for the APN and other health-care professionals (Doukas & McCullough, 1991). As health-care professionals gain an understanding of factors that guide a person's decisions, treatment plans that reflect the patient's value preferences are more easily developed.

An example of the importance of values clarification centers around the use of advance directives. Advance directives were developed to document, prior to a person's loss of decision-making capacity, that person's stated wishes regarding end-of-life treatment. However, it is not unusual for the caregiver to find an advance directive of little benefit when decisions to withhold or withdraw treatment arise. Without a clear understanding of the values underlying the patient's choices, the formation of a suitable treatment plan is complex and speculative. In addition, the surrogate decision-maker often is unsure of the interpretation intended by the patient. If, however, discussions regarding the patient's value preferences are held with the health-care professional in addition to completion of the advance directive form, a plan that reflects the patient's choices is more likely to emerge.

The APN is in an ideal position to initiate discussions with patients regarding treatment choices. This is particularly true when the APN practices in an out-patient setting and follows the same individual over long periods of time. Because such discussions often are lengthy, intense, and involved, the out-patient setting lends itself to a more favorable and relaxed milieu. Discussions that reveal underlying values encourage a prospective examination of issues such as terminal care, chronic illness, quality of life, aggressive treatment, and the interests of family members (Pawlik-Plank, 1994).

A clinical tool that complements an advance directive is the values history. Several models of the values history have been proposed, and all concentrate on uncovering the individual's core values and beliefs regarding health-care decisions (Doukas and McCullough, 1991; Kielstein & Sass, 1993). Regardless of the form chosen, the values history enhances the patient's autonomy beyond the boundaries of current advance directives. Table 13–1 provides an example of a values history form.

TABLE 13–1. VALUES HISTORY FORM*

Section 1
    A. Written legal documents
        Living will
        Durable power of attorney
        Durable power of attorney for health-care decisions
        Organ donations
    B. Wishes concerning specific medical procedures
        Organ donation
        Kidney dialysis
        Cardiopulmonary resuscitation (CPR)
        Respirators
        Artificial nutrition
        Artificial hydration
    C. General comments

Section 2
    A. Your overall attitude toward your health
    B. Your perception of the role of your doctor and other health caregivers
    C. Your thoughts about independence and control
    D. Your personal relationships
    E. Your overall attitude toward life
    F. Your attitude toward illness, dying, and death
    G. Your religious background and beliefs
    H. Your living environment
    I. Your attitude concerning finances
    J. Your wishes concerning your funeral
    K. Optional questions

*Questions excerpted from the Values History Form, The Center for Health Law and Ethics, The University of New Mexico, Albuquerque, NM.

ETHICAL DECISION-MAKING PROCESS

One procedural framework nurses can use in ethical decision-making is to adapt the nursing process as a framework to organize and guide the gathering of morally relevant information (Table 13–2). This framework enables the APN to systematically organize the facts and contextual particularities of a dilemma. Although a framework provides structure and suggests a method of examining and studying the ethical issues, the essential component to resolution of ethical dilemmas is moral action. Simply knowing the right course of action does not guarantee that a person has the motivation or courage to act (Rest, 1986). Successful resolution of moral issues requires a blend of knowledge, conviction, emotions, beliefs, and individual character (van Hooft, 1990).

PROBLEM IDENTIFICATION

Ethical dilemmas often are first recognized by the intense emotional reactions they elicit. Emotions are present in all clinical settings, but when personal or professional values are questioned or trespassed, the instinctive response is to react with anger or frustration. Although this is a helpful gauge to awaken an awareness that something may be amiss ethically, too often the individual becomes entangled in the emotions and is unable to move toward an awareness of the consequences for others. It is frequently this point at which the differing parties become polarized and embedded in a particular viewpoint. A difficult but important step in problem identification is to allow and encourage the individuals in conflict to openly express their emotions. This action demonstrates that the perspectives and the emotional responses to the issue are legitimate and meaningful (Fisher & Ury, 1981). As a facilitator, the APN should recognize, understand, and acknowledge the emotions of all parties.

TABLE 13–2. USE OF THE NURSING PROCESS IN ETHICAL DECISION-MAKING

Step	Description
1: Assessment	Problem identification
	Information gathering
	Medical facts
	Nursing facts
	Values, rights, and obligations of parties
	Other relevant factors
	Culture
	Religion
	Relationships
	Other contextual features
2: Plan	Strategies for resolution
	Collaboration
	Compromise
	Accommodation
	Coercion
	Avoidance
3: Implementation	Initiate a moral action
4: Evaluation	Process
	Outcome

Many conflicts that arise in the clinical setting generate powerful emotional responses yet may not be ethical issues. Ethical issues involve some form of controversy concerning moral values (Ahronheim et al., 1994). It is essential that the APN distinguish and separate moral dilemmas from other issues such as administrative concerns, communication problems, or lack of clinical knowledge. Identifying the cause of the problem and determining why, where, and when it occurred, as well as who or what was affected, will help clarify the nature of the problem (Beare, 1989). For example, an APN may be called by less-experienced staff to resolve a dilemma in pain management. The less-experienced nurse's interpretation is that the physician ordered an inadequate dose of an analgesic to manage the patient's symptoms. The nurse requested an increased dosage for the patient, but the physician refused. The APN may determine that the severity of the disease process requires the addition of another analgesic to enhance the effects of the original medication ordered. The issue encountered was not a moral issue but instead reflected problems with nurse-physician communication and the lack of knowledge regarding appropriate pharmacological management.

INFORMATION GATHERING

Once the ethical problem is identified, the APN implements a process to gather and examine the morally relevant facts. The various ways in which illness or injury constrict one's everyday life influences the interpretation of what encompasses a morally relevant fact. Generally, information such as the medical and nursing facts; the values, rights, and obligations of the patient and others; legal factors; and cultural and religious factors should be gathered when initiating the decision-making process. However, these facts are insufficient if not tempered with the contextual features of each case. Only after the unique conditions of the case are considered can an ethically acceptable solution be identified.

Take, for example, the case of Mrs. Howard. Although her son did not have legal authority to consent to the surgery, he had a substantial interest in his mother's well-being. Their relationship was in jeopardy because both parties were locked in their positions and did not see each other's interests. Without deserved attention to the implications of Mrs. Howard's decision for her relationship with her son, a mutually acceptable solution could not be found.

STRATEGIES FOR RESOLUTION

Moral discussions and deliberation can take the form of a debate that degenerates into an assault. One party presents an argument, the other party disputes it, the original party defends, and the second party attacks (Zaner, 1988). Breaking this cycle of destructive interactions is central to arriving at solutions that are resourceful and constructive. Resolutions are most effective when the parties in dispute create the solution.

When the APN is directly involved in the conflict situation, the skills of negotiation are most useful in moving toward a satisfactory settlement. In many cases, the APN must serve as a facilitator for the parties in dispute and apply the strategies involved in mediation. The key difference between these roles is the level of active involvement in deciding the goals and strategies. As a negotiating party, the APN suggests solutions and identifies acceptable plans (Beare, 1989). In the role of a mediator, the APN guides the process but does not offer opinions or solutions (Ostermeyer, 1991). The process and steps used in negotiation and mediation overlap in many ways, and in both approaches the parties in conflict discover and determine the acceptable solutions (Beare, 1989; Ostermeyer, 1991).

The skills of negotiation and mediation are integral to exploring others' perceptions of any situation. The following strategies for negotiation are useful when the APN is facilitating resolution between two parties or when the professional or personal values of the APN collide with the values of others. The key role of the APN in the resolution of moral dilemmas is to guide and stimulate communication between the differing parties.

The objective of successful negotiation and mediation is to achieve a mutually satisfactory solution. In reality, however, that is not always possible. The issues of time, cost, resources, the level of moral certainty, and the perceived value of the relationship play important roles in the strategy used and likelihood of reaching a desired outcome (Spielman, 1993). These issues are addressed later under "Barriers to Resolution."

Collaboration

Collaboration is the preferred strategy for achieving a moral resolution. Because it is a fundamental competency of the APN, the steps involved in collaboration will be discussed in some detail. This section focuses on identifying and cultivating the elements necessary for collaboration around ethical problems. Additional methods to foster a collaborative environment are discussed in Chapter 11.

The first step in the process of collaboration is to help the disputing parties agree on the issue in conflict and to understand both the cognitive and the emotional perspectives of each party. Because emotions maintain a significant position in moral dilemmas, it is important to provide an environment in which the parties can release unexpressed emotions. An effective method to help others resolve anger or frustration is to listen in a nonjudgmental manner and avoid reacting to the criticisms (Fisher & Ury, 1981). Discussions that occur after the release of emotions are more rational and productive because the emotions have been expressed in an explicit and unambiguous manner (Fisher & Ury, 1981). The APN encourages the parties to discuss their perception of the problem, recognize their emotions, and identify their expectations for resolution (Krouse & Roberts, 1989).

This first step toward moral resolution is particularly difficult, because persons in power are often less interested in and less likely to acknowledge the perspectives of those with lesser power (Welton, 1991). This situation is not uncommon in health-care environments that traditionally have sanctioned physicians with greater authority and power than nurses. When nurses' ethical reasoning and moral actions are constrained, they react with anger, frustration, and moral outrage (Pike, 1991). The outrage intensifies as nurses sense a violation of their moral integrity. To eliminate this power imbalance, the responsibility and accountability of all parties in the negotiation process must be openly acknowledged and agreed on. In this way the APN establishes the ground rule of mutual respect and frames the process in a collaborative and shared model of decision-making.

The second step toward successful collaborative moral resolution is to engage all involved parties in active interactions and consensus building (Krouse & Roberts, 1989). Information presented should be questioned, analyzed, and examined. It is important to focus on the interests of each party rather than the positions. Interests can be identified by asking the questions Why? and Why not? (Fisher and Ury, 1981). As differing interests emerge, the varying perspectives should be acknowledged with confidence and hopefulness (Ury, 1993). The parties must listen to each other but not necessarily agree on the other's view or on what is being said. From this stage of active communication and interaction, the process of consensus-building begins.

The third step in negotiating or mediating a moral resolution involves formulating a decision and developing a plan of action. The objective of both negotiation and mediation is to generate options and solutions that are consistent with all parties' principles and achieve an outcome that is mutually satisfying (Ostermeyer, 1991; Ury, 1993). During this phase, the parties explore options and together decide on a plan of action. Initially this joint negotiation may seem unlikely, particularly when both parties are attached to their own positions. However, it is possible for the APN to facilitate progression through complex situations by using communication skills such as reframing, identifying shared interests and needs, and examining the differences (Fisher & Ury, 1981; Smeltzer, 1991).

Successful negotiations of ethical issues often result in improved interpersonal relationships. As relationships improve and decisions are negotiated, the power inequity so prevalent in the health-care setting declines, and patients perceive more control over their care (Krouse & Roberts, 1989). The goal is to keep focused on the ability and responsibility of all parties to make informed decisions (Ostermeyer, 1991). An environment in which information is shared openly and decision-making is considered a process rather than an isolated event will empower all parties to construct creative and morally satisfactory action plans.

In the case of Mrs. Howard, the APN successfully facilitated discussions between the nurse and patient that centered on acceptable means to alleviate the pain associated with a gangrenous leg. The APN enabled the patient and nurses to focus on the current issues without agreeing on the prior event (Mrs. Howard's refusal). It was important for Mrs. Howard to feel respected and valued as a decision-maker, and the collaborative process emphasized her role as a full partner in reaching a resolution. Because independence and control were important elements to Mrs. Howard, a plan for patient-controlled analgesia was instituted.

Although implementation of a collaborative process for the resolution of moral dilemmas is most desired, other approaches to manage conflict may be employed. The choice to employ another strategy for resolution may be deliberate or inadvertent. In any case, there are distinct advantages and disadvantages with other methods, and the APN should recognize these factors.

Compromise

When both parties possess a high level of moral certainty in their positions and are committed to preserving the relationship, they may choose to bargain and to have each party relinquish some control over the decision. Compromising and bargaining are time-consuming because each party must determine what are acceptable trade-offs. Because time in the clinical setting is limited, both parties must value the relationship and share in the decision-making process (Spielman, 1993).

Problems are resolved through compromise when both parties are willing to waive some components of their moral position and embrace a position of cooperation (Spielman, 1993). For example, a chronically ill patient with dilated cardiomyopathy may refuse in-hospital management of the heart failure but agree to a short-term solution, such as a trial of intravenous therapy at home.

The clinical context in which NPs and nurse-midwives (CNMs) practice most often requires collaboration or compromise as approaches to moral resolution. In these conditions the patient and clinician maintain high degrees of commitment to the relationship. In addition, most encounters are non-emergent, and thus time is available for engaging in compromise and collaboration.

Accommodation

In some cases, one party will accommodate and simply agree to support the other's position. This approach may indicate that, to one party, the issue in question was too insignificant for him or her to strive for a mutually acceptable solution (Spielman, 1993). Accommodation frequently occurs when the issue is trivial, time is limited, or one party holds a high level of commitment to preserving the relationship with the other participant (Spielman, 1993).

Accommodation is sometimes employed as a tactic in negotiation. The concession is made to dissipate friction and additionally to imply that a reciprocal action is expected in future negotiations with the other party. However, accommodation is an inappropriate strategy when used routinely to gain acceptance or merely to avoid conflict.

In the case of Mrs. Howard, the nurse adapted her moral posture to accommodate the patient's position. This approach may have reflected the nurse's uncertainty about her own moral position, the limited time to arrive at a decision, or the underlying desire to maintain a relationship with the patient.

Coercion

A coercive and controlling approach may be used when time is short, such as in an emergency, or when the party has little commitment to the relationship. This approach is often aggressive and competitive and reflects a high degree of commitment to a particular moral position (Spielman, 1993). Because control of the decision is assumed by one party and the differing perspectives are discounted, this approach damages the self-esteem of the other party and results in a sense of powerlessness and moral outrage (Pike, 1991).

An environment in which a coercive and controlling approach is prevalent generates a power imbalance that accentuates vulnerability. Vulnerability damages self-esteem, constrains independence, and restricts choices (Copp, 1986). In this environment relationships have little importance, and it is unlikely that the group with authority will actively pursue empowering the vulnerable group. Change can occur in this climate, but it often emanates from the constrained party. Redefining one's position (i.e., from victim to involved decision-maker) and acknowledging accountability and responsibility for reaching collaborative resolutions are strategies to alter a coercive environment (Pike, 1991).

Although a coercive approach is aggressive and often undesirable, it sometimes is necessary. For example, when a child of Jehovah's Witness parents must emergently receive a blood transfusion and the parents refuse to give consent for the treatment, legal approval is sought. Time, in this case, is limited, and the caregivers are convinced of the moral rightness of their views, just as the parents are convinced of their moral position. Because the child's well-being depends on prompt action, the caregivers are limited to a coercive approach for resolution. In this case, the law coerces or compels the parents to permit treatment of the minor child.

Avoidance

Participants may avoid, ignore, or deny the dilemma when the moral issue is perceived as trivial or conversely is deeply felt by one party and highly charged emotionally. Avoidance is also seen when time is short (Spielman, 1993). If a decision is unnecessary, it may be appropriate for a participant to withdraw from the process of decision-making. However, this strategy often is employed when the participant abdicates moral accountability. The APN should consciously monitor avoidance behaviors and pursue the rationale for this technique. It is likely that the individual who practices this technique regularly avoids conflict and would benefit from additional knowledge, support, and role-modeling of approaches to conflict management.

EVALUATION

The evaluation of ethical decision-making should focus on two areas: the process and the outcome. Process evaluation is important because it provides an overview of the moral disagreement, the interpersonal skills employed, the interactions between both parties in conflict, and the problems encountered during the phases of resolution. Whether the APN was the facilitator or a party in conflict, a deliberate and reflective evaluation of the process of resolution should occur (Olczak, Grosch, & Duffy, 1991). It is useful for the APN to assess the type of issue, the inter-relational and situational variables, the conceptual shifts that occurred during the process, and the strategies used by both parties during the negotiation phase (Olczak et al., 1991). As the APN reflects on the process, attention should be given to how similar situations could be anticipated and resolved in the future. Deliberate and consistent review of the process will help the APN assess various approaches to the resolution of ethical dilemmas and identify the onset of moral conflict earlier.

Evaluation of the outcome is also critical because it acknowledges creative solutions and celebrates moral action. Other components of the outcome evaluation include the short-term and long-term consequences of the action taken and the satisfaction of both parties with the chosen solution (Olczak et al., 1991). Unfortunately, a successful process does not always result in a satisfactory outcome. Occasionally the outcome reveals the need for changes within the institution or health-care system. The APN may choose to become involved in advancing these identified changes or identify appropriate resources to pursue the desired objectives. The goal of the outcome evaluation is to minimize the risks of a similar event by identifying predictable patterns and thereby averting recurrent and future dilemmas.

BARRIERS TO RESOLUTION

A number of variables influence how moral issues are addressed and resolved in the clinical setting. The APN must respond to the barriers that inhibit the development of a morally responsive environment.

The APN often relies on other nurses and caregivers to recognize ethical issues and initiate dialogue with professional colleagues. In some situations, nurses are uncertain, fearful, insecure, or simply unable to articulate their moral concern (Pike, 1991). The issues of continuity of care and knowing the patient and family are significant problems in acute care settings. The APN must address these barriers and educate other caregivers in ways to articulate ethical concerns. Through role-modeling the APN can illustrate ways to identify and clarify moral problems as well as guide others through the process of moral action. An environment that supports ethical reasoning and judgment will foster action.

Although other strategies can yield successful resolutions, the approaches of collaboration and compromise are usually more satisfactory to all parties. Unfortunately these methods require more time from the patient and health-care team. Because time is usually short, the benefits of collaboration or compromise are seldom realized. To overcome this barrier, the APN may need to resolve the dilemma in stages, with the most central issue addressed first. In the case of Mrs. Howard, a decision about her capacity and the surgery were most essential. The issues surrounding continued care and her son's concerns could be addressed less immediately. It would also be wise for the APN to identify resources both within and outside the institution to assist with the process of resolution. The recognition of a moral dilemma does not commit the APN to conducting and managing the process of resolution. Instead, the APN should engage the appropriate resources to address the identified needs.

In many situations, such as in rural clinics, resources within the organization are not available. Without another professional colleague to help decipher the problem, the APN is sometimes left with little more than intuition. The guidelines from professional organizations regarding the APN's moral obligations are helpful in providing some direction for action. APNs practicing in isolation should network with colleagues and establish resources for providing direction in ethical reasoning.

Moral resolution and open reflection cannot occur in an environment that devalues the perspectives of some professionals. When one group of individuals is empowered to act and other parties are constrained, a distrustful and hostile environment results. Because vulnerability presents opportunities for empowerment, the APN can advocate for change by working to empower the oppressed group.

DEVELOPING ETHICAL DECISION-MAKING SKILLS

The skills needed to identify, articulate, and address ethical dilemmas are complex and diverse. Particular strategies, such as those used in values clarification, negotiation, and mediation, provide a foundation for the practice aspects of ethical decision-making. The APN must understand the theoretical elements of biomedical ethics and be aware of relevant cases and law to interpret moral issues in the health-care setting. Both the practice and knowledge aspects must be combined with compassionate and assertive communication skills. The APN can acquire and develop these skills in a variety of ways.

EDUCATION

Although professional nurses develop beginning ethical decision-making skills in their initial education and student experiences, the formation of ethical reasoning and a sense of moral agency develops in practice and is formalized during academic preparation. As nurses gain clinical experience, their abilities to recognize and be comfortable with addressing ethical issues increase. Ethical reasoning and clinical judgment share a common process, and both serve to teach and inform the other (Solomon et al., 1991). The importance therefore, of clinical practice cannot be overemphasized.

In some format, either continuing education or graduate education, the APN should be introduced to and undergo a process of values clarification. Values clarification will enable students to define and analyze their personal and professional beliefs, attitudes, and value systems. In addition to personal and professional growth, students can apply the strategies of values clarification to facilitate the decision-making of patients and surrogates in the clinical setting. This approach also is useful during the process of negotiation, in which the APN guides both parties in conflict to identify interests.

Graduate education also should expose students to general ethical theories, principles, rules, and decision-making frameworks. Because the APN will apply the theoretical principles in actual encounters with patients, it is imperative that consideration of the contextual factors in specific situations be strengthened. A portion of graduate ethics education should involve discussion of clinical cases involving moral issues. These cases should reflect typical clinical issues encountered by the APN rather than issues that receive extensive media attention yet occur infrequently.

Successful resolution of ethical dilemmas is directly related to the success of the negotiation process. The strategies used in mediation and facilitation often are utilized in managing moral conflicts and should be included in graduate education (Beare, 1989). However, the art of mediation and negotiation lies in the process of successfully navigating a conflict, arriving at consensual agreement, and strengthening each party's respect for the other (Ostermeyer, 1991). Ideally, graduate students should be provided precepted opportunities to guide patients, families, and other health-care professionals through a collaborative pattern of moral resolution.

Public policies and legal guidelines may infringe on the process of ethical decision-making. It is not unusual to find profound importance attached to the interpretation of current law surrounding the issue in conflict. Misinterpretation of the legal reaction in precedent-setting cases may diminish the chances of successful negotiation. APNs should be familiar with relevant case law in their particular area of practice as well as pertinent state and federal policies and guidelines. Information on legal and policy guidelines may be offered during graduate practicum experiences in the area of clinical concentration.

Although the foundation for ethical decision-making skills should be provided during graduate education, continuing education programs also are effective and necessary forums to provide current information in a rapidly changing health-care environment. Ethical issues are dynamic and reemerge in altered forms. The APN must keep abreast of changing trends, and continuing education programs meet this need.

Probably the most important component of continued learning and the development of ethical reasoning is the application of the various models in clinical practice. As with most skills, experience and practice reinforces knowledge and provides opportunities to construct an approach and manner of moral action that is comfortable and acceptable to the APN's interpretation of moral agency.

Professional organizations delineate standards of performance that reflect the responsibilities, obligations, duties, and rights of the members. These standards serve as guidelines for professional behavior and define the desired conduct. Although the general principles are relatively stable, professional organizations often reflect on contemporary issues and assume a proactive posture on pivotal concerns. One example is the ANA's position statements on active euthanasia (American Nurses Association, 1994). This position statement holds that active euthanasia violates the *Code for Nurses,* and the ANA opposes the participation of the nursing profession in such an act (American Nurses Association, 1994). Both the novice and the experienced APN must be familiar with the profession's position on topics relevant to the area of practice. Some degree of involvement with professional organizations is necessary to strengthen the APN's voice in guiding the profession's moral accountability to the public.

DEVELOPMENT OF SKILLS

Acquiring the skills and competence to facilitate the resolution of moral dilemmas is an evolutionary process. Because ethical decision-making is not exclusively based on theoretical knowledge, moral reasoning must be tempered with clinical reality. As APNs gain the necessary knowledge and skills in ethical decision-making, their involvement should intensify and become more extensive. Once an advanced nursing role is assumed, the APN accepts the function of a full participant in resolution of moral dilemmas rather than simply an interested observer or one of many parties in conflict.

Initially, the APN serves several functions when moral dilemmas arise in the clinical setting. The responsibilities of the novice APN are to recognize the problem as an ethical infringement and to seek clarification and illumination of the concern. The novice APN earns credibility and gains self-confidence by bringing the issue to the awareness and attention of others. If the issue remains a moral concern after clarification, the APN may seek additional help to pursue resolution. For example, an elderly woman admitted to an in-patient psychiatric unit for depression may be labeled as incompetent and therefore unable to refuse electroconvulsive therapy. The psychiatric CNS may identify this as an ethical dilemma and seek additional information, such as the woman's *functional* capacity and the process involved in the determination of incompetence. If concern remains after the additional information is acquired, the CNS may seek additional resources to address the dilemma with the psychiatrist and the patient.

The dedication and courage to pursue ethical issues until resolution is achieved or options are exhausted is an essential behavior of both the novice and the more experienced APN. Often the inequities or infringements to other persons are enough to motivate moral action. However, moral action is sometimes risky, and it requires courage and motivation to pursue troubling cases. Motivation is an internal factor exemplified through behaviors and actions of the person seeking resolution to ethical issues. Moral action may be required to change the course in present as well as future situations. Therefore, the importance of moral action should not be underestimated, and it should be recognized, fostered, and valued by others.

Often, the more experienced APN has developed professional working relationships with colleagues that are based on trust and mutual respect. Because the preservation of relationships is a significant goal in working toward collaborative decision-making, the experienced APN can select strategies that build on this commitment. Clearly, resolutions that originate from collaborative processes are more satisfactory, generate more creative solutions, and strengthen relationships (Spielman, 1993). This feeling of solidarity empowers others to explore and participate in the ethical decision-making process.

The experienced APN may initiate informal learning opportunities for nurses and other professional colleagues. Ethics rounds and case review are two ways to attract others in the discussion of moral issues. During this educational process, the APN empowers others by providing knowledge, role-modeling, and both a closer look and the larger picture (Copp, 1989).

The experienced APN anticipates situations in which moral conflicts occur and recognizes the more subtle presentations of moral dilemmas. For example, the health-care team may avoid informing a family or patient of an error in administration of a thrombolytic agent that resulted in a retroperitoneal bleed following cardiac catheterization. Although this complication was discussed as a risk of the catheterization procedure, the bleeding was exacerbated secondary to the medication error. During morning rounds, the APN addressed the importance of disclosure of the error, and the physicians reluctantly agreed to disclose the error. In this case, the APN practiced preventive ethics and fostered a practice environment that confronts rather than avoids simmering issues.

PREVENTIVE ETHICS

As noted, ethical decision-making skills enable the APN to focus on identifying the values in conflict and developing a course of action suitable to the parties in dispute. This approach, however, concentrates on the resolution of current and ongoing issues rather than preventing the recurrence of moral dilemmas (Forrow, Arnold, & Parker, 1993). An additional important role of the APN is to extend the concept of ethical decision-making beyond the traditional and immediate model and move toward a paradigm of preventive ethics.

Preventive ethics is derived from the model of preventive medicine (Forrow et al., 1993). When value conflicts arise, resolution is more difficult because one value must be chosen over another. Preventive ethics emphasizes that all important values should be reviewed and examined prior to the conflict so that situations in which values may differ can be anticipated (Forrow et al., 1993). In other words, the goals of the health-care team should be articulated as clearly as possible to avoid potential misinterpretations. For example, a CNM should have an understanding of the patient's values regarding aggressive treatment of the premature neonate. On the other hand, the CNM's moral and legal obligations should be openly discussed so that the patient and professional appreciate and recognize each other's values and moral positions.

In addition to the early examination and ongoing dialogue of values, a conscientious inspection of other factors that influence the evolution of moral dilemmas is required. The roles and responsibilities of all parties must be clearly defined to expose any existing power imbalance. During this process the issues of powerlessness and collaborative practice surface as areas in which the APN can influence change.

Perceptions of powerlessness influence how active the staff nurse will become in the resolution of ethical dilemmas. The APN's role clearly necessitates empowering the staff and patients to overcome and avoid the destructive feelings of vulnerability (Copp, 1986). One of the most effective strategies for empowering others is that of role-modeling and teaching (Copp, 1986). The APN should not only apply the skills of critical thinking but should demonstrate those skills to other nurses and members of the health-care team. Asking and helping nurses and patients to identify, explore, and analyze values and assumptions will cultivate skills in critical reflection and invite the consideration of alternative interpretations of the issue. In this way, the APN helps clarify the interests and obligations of others in ethical decision-making.

By providing knowledge, promoting a positive self-image, and preparing others for participation in decision-making, the APN empowers individuals. The skill of the APN is not used to resolve moral dilemmas single-handedly but to mentor others to assume a position of moral accountability and engage in shared decision-making. This process of enhancing others' autonomy and providing opportunities for involvement in reaching resolution is a key concept in preventive ethics (Forrow et al., 1993). Although many ethical issues will develop with little warning, the practice of preventive ethics will improve the delivery of morally responsible, innovative, and humanistic patient care.

CREATING AN ETHICALLY SENSITIVE ENVIRONMENT

An environment that encourages patients and caregivers to raise their own questions and value the critical exchange of ideas will nourish the resolution of important moral questions. Thoughtful ethical decision-making arises from an environment that supports and promotes collaboration among members of the health-care team, patients, and families. A collaborative practice environment in turn supports shared decision-making, shared accountability, and group participation, and it fosters relationships based on equality and mutuality (Pike, 1991). The APN is integral in the development and preservation of a collaborative climate that inspires and empowers individuals to respond to moral dilemmas.

When the APN assumes a posture of empowerment, an atmosphere of moral accountability develops. An ethical environment fosters early identification of issues and anticipation of possible dilemmas. The ability to predict areas of conflict and develop plans in a proactive, rather than reactive, manner will avert some potentially difficult dilemmas (Benner, 1991; Forrow et al., 1993).

CONCLUSIONS

Ethical decision-making skills are an art and a science. The APN is in a key position to assume a more decisive role in managing the resolution of moral issues. The skills of problem identification, values clarification, negotiation, collaboration, and evaluation empower the APN to critically analyze and direct the decision-making process. The identification of patterns in the presentation of moral issues will enable the APN to engage in preventive strategies to improve the ethical qualities of patient care.

REFERENCES

Ahronheim, J. C., Moreno, J., & Zuckerman, C. (1994). *Ethics in clinical practice*. Boston: Little, Brown and Company.

American Nurses Association. (1985). *Code for nurses with interpretive statements*. Kansas City, MO: Author.

American Nurses Association. (1994). *Position statement on active euthanasia*. Washington, D. C.: Author.

American Nurses Association (1995). *Nursing's social policy statement*. Washington, D. C.: Author.

Aroskar, M. A. (1989). Community health nurses: Their most significant ethical decision-making problems. *Nursing Clinics of North America, 24*(4), 976.

Baggs, J. G., & Schmitt, M. H. (1988). Collaboration between nurses and physicians. *Image: Journal of Nursing Scholarship 20*(3), 145.

Beare, P. G. (1989). The essentials of win-win negotiation for the clinical nurse specialist. *Clinical Nurse Specialist, 13*(3), 138.

Beauchamp, T. L., & Childress, J. F. (1994). *Principles of biomedical ethics* (4th ed.). New York: Oxford University Press.

Benner, P. (1991). The role of experience, narrative and community in skilled ethical comportment. *Advances in Nursing Science, 14*(2), 1.

Calkins, M. E. (1993). Ethical issues in the elderly ESRD patient. *ANNA Journal, 20*(5), 569.

Cooper, M. C. (1989). Gilligan's different voice: A perspective for nursing. *Journal of Professional Nursing, 5*(1), 10.

Cooper, M. C. (1991). Principle-oriented ethics and the ethic of care: A creative tension. *Advances in Nursing Science, 14*(2), 22.

Copp, L. A. (1986). The nurse as advocate for vulnerable persons. *Journal of Advanced Nursing, 11*(3): 255-263.

Crisham, P. (1981). Measuring moral judgment in nursing dilemmas. *Nursing Research, 30*(2), 104.

Doukas, D. J., & McCullough, L. B. (1991). The values history. *Journal of Family Practice, 32*(2), 145-150.

Duckett, L., Rowan-Boyer, M., & Ryden, M. B., et al. (1992). Challenging misperceptions about nurses' moral reasoning. *Nursing Research, 41*(6), 324.

Erlen, J. A., & Frost, B. (1991). Nurses' perceptions of powerlessness in influencing ethical decisions. *Western Journal of Nursing Research, 13*(2), 397.

Fisher, R., & Ury, W. (1981). *Getting to yes*. New York: Viking Penguin.

Forrow, L., Arnold, R. M., & Parker, L. S. (1993). Preventive ethics: Expanding the horizons of clinical ethics. *Journal of Clinical Ethics, 4*(4), 287.

Fowler, M. D. M. (1989). Ethical decision-making in clinical practice. *Nursing Clinics of North America, 24*(4), 955.

Gadow, S. (1980). Existential advocacy: Philosophical foundation of nursing. In S. F. Spickler, S. Gadow (Eds.), *Nursing: Images and ideals* (pp. 79-101). New York: Springer.

Gilligan, C. (1982). *In a different voice*. Cambridge, MA: Harvard University Press.

Grammelspracher, G. P., Howell, J. D., & Young, M. J. (1986). Perceptions of ethical problems by nurses and physicians. *Archives of Internal Medicine, 146*, 577.

Haddad, A. M. (1991). The nurse/physician relationship and ethical decision making. *AORN Journal, 53*(1), 151.

Jameton, A. (1984). *Nursing practice, the ethical issues*. Englewood Cliffs, NJ: Prentice-Hall.

Jonsen, A. R., & Toulmin, S. (1988). *The abuse of casuistry: A history of moral reasoning*. Berkeley: University of California Press.

Kielstein, R., & Sass, H. M. (1993). Using stories to assess values and establish medical directives. *Kennedy Institute of Ethics Journal, 3*(3), 303.

Krouse, H. J., & Roberts, S. J. (1989). Nurse-patient interactive styles: Power, control, and satisfaction. *Western Journal of Nursing Research, 11*(6), 717.

Martin, D. A. (1989). Nurses' involvement in ethical decision-making with severely ill newborns. *Issues in Comprehensive Pediatric Nursing, 12*, 463.

Millette, B. E. (1993). Client advocacy and the moral orientation of nurses. *Western Journal of Nursing Research, 15*(5), 607.

Olczak, P. V., Grosch, J. W., & Duffy, K. G. (1991). Toward a synthesis: The art with the science of community mediation. In K. G. Duffy, J. W. Grosch, & P. V. Olczak (Eds.), *Community mediation* (pp. 329-343). New York: The Guilford Press.

Omery, A., Henneman, E., Billet, B., et al. (1995). Ethical issues in hospital-based nursing practice. *Journal of Cardiovascular Nursing, 9*(3), 43.

Ostermeyer, M. (1991). Conducting the mediation. In K. G. Duffy, J. W. Grosch, & P. V. Olczak (Eds.), *Community mediation* (pp. 91-104). New York: The Guilford Press.

Pawlik-Plank, D. M. (1994). Framing treatment options: A method to enhance informed consent. *Clinical Nurse Specialist, 8*(4), 174.

Pike, A. W. (1991). Moral outrage and moral discourse in nurse-physician collaboration. *Journal of Professional Nursing, 7*(6), 351.

Purtilo, R. (1993). *Ethical dimensions in the health professions* (2nd ed.). Philadelphia: W. B. Saunders.

Rest, J. R. (1986). *Moral development: Advances in research and theory*. New York: Praeger.

Rushton, C. H. (1988). Ethical decision making in critical care, Part 1: The role of the pediatric nurse. *Pediatric Nursing, 14*(5), 411.

Scanlon, C. (1994). Survey yields significant results. *American Nurses Association Center for Ethics and Human Rights Communiqué, 3*(4), 1.

Smeltzer, C. H. (1991). The art of negotiation. *Journal of Nursing Administration, 21*(7/8), 26.

Solomon, M. Z., Jennings, B., & Guilfoy, V., et al. (1991). Toward an expanded vision of clinical ethics education: From individual to the institution. *Kennedy Institute of Ethics Journal, 1*(3), 225.

Solomon, M. Z., O'Donnell, L., & Jennings, B., et al. (1993). Decisions near the end of life: Professional views on life-sustaining treatments. *American Journal of Public Health, 83*(1), 14.

Spielman, B. J. (1993). Conflict in medical ethics cases: Seeking patterns of resolution. *Journal of Clinical Ethics, 4*(3), 212.

Ury, W. (1993). *Getting past no.* New York: Bantam Books.

Uustal, D. (1987). Values: The cornerstone of nursing's moral art. In M. D. M. Fowler & J. Levine-Ariff (Eds.), *Ethics at the bedside* (pp. 136-153). Philadelphia: J. B. Lippincott.

van Hooft, S. (1990). Moral education for nursing decisions. *Journal of Advanced Nursing, 15,* 210.

Veatch, R. M., and Fry, S. T. (1987). *Case studies in nursing ethics.* Philadelphia: J. B. Lippincott.

Viens, D. C. (1994). Moral dilemmas experienced by nurse practitioners. *Nurse Practitioner Forum 5*(4), 290.

Welton, G. L. (1991). Parties in conflict: Their characteristics and perceptions. In K. G. Duffy, J. W. Grosch, & P. V. Olczak (Eds.), *Community mediation* (pp. 105-118). New York: The Guilford Press.

Winters, G., Glass, E., & Sakurai, C. (1993). Ethical issues in oncology nursing practice: An overview of topics and strategies. *Oncology Nursing Forum, 20*(Suppl. 10), 21.

Zaner, R. M. (1988). *Ethics and the clinical encounter.* Englewood Cliffs, NJ: Prentice-Hall.

PART III

ADVANCED PRACTICE ROLES: THE OPERATIONAL DEFINITIONS OF ADVANCED NURSING PRACTICE

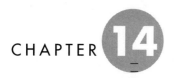

CHAPTER 14

The Clinical Nurse Specialist

Deborah McCaffrey Boyle

INTRODUCTION

The clinical nurse specialist (CNS) role is probably the most debated of the advanced nursing practice (ANP) roles and has generated considerable discussion and controversy (Williams & Valdivieso, 1994). The American Nurses' Association's (ANA, 1976) early definition of the CNS serves as the authoritative historical template for discussion of this ANP role. This definition stated,

> *The clinical nurse specialist (CNS) is a practitioner holding a master's degree with a concentration in specific areas of clinical nursing. The role of the CNS is defined by the needs of a select client population, the expectation of the larger society and the clinical expertise of the nurse. By exercising judgment and demonstrating leadership ability, the CNS functions within a field of practice that focuses on the needs of the client system and encompasses interaction with others in the nursing and health care systems serving the client. The function of the CNS is unique with respect to the particular use of clinical judgment and skills regarding client care, service as an advocate when the client is unable to cope with a particular situation, and influence for change as necessary in the nursing care and in the health care delivery system. The CNS is obligated to operate within and affect nursing care delivery systems and the total health care delivery system. While roles may change by circumstances for a certain period of time, this practitioner ceases to be recognized as a CNS when the patient-client-family ceases to be the basis of practice.*

(ANA, 1976, p. 5)

ACKNOWLEDGMENT: The author would like to acknowledge the contributions of clinical nurse specialist colleagues Elizabeth Abrahams, Deirdre Carolan, and Linda Schakenback to the preparation of this chapter.

The inclination of some advanced practice nurses (APNs) whose practice is not based on ongoing interactions with patients and families to refer to themselves as CNSs furthers the confusion and controversy over this role.

A thorough review of the evolution of the CNS role is provided in Chapter 1. However, for the purposes of the in-depth look at the CNS role provided in this chapter, it is important to establish that this author and this book's editors strongly believe that the CNS role can be clearly differentiated from other ANP roles and that, despite these tumultuous times, it remains an important and viable advanced practice role. Although the classic hospital-based CNS is referred to most often in this chapter, this is not intended to exclude CNSs in other settings.

DEFINITION OF THE CNS

In its 1980 Social Policy Statement, the ANA included an abbreviated version of its earlier conceptualization of the CNS role, describing the CNS as "a registered nurse who, through study and supervised clinical practice at the graduate level (master's or doctorate), has become an expert in a defined area of knowledge and practice in a selected clinical area of nursing" (p. 23). This statement was significant, because it was the first time a definition of an ANP role mandated graduate preparation. However, like the initial 1976 definition, it leaves unanswered questions about the operationalization of the CNS role.

The multifaceted nature of the CNS role requires a multifaceted description. Hamric (1989) described this diverse role as including three primary components:

1. *Attainment of primary criteria for job performance,* including graduate specialty study in nursing, certification, and a practice focus on the patient and family;
2. *Enactment* of subroles, including expert clinical practitioner, educator, consultant, and researcher; and
3. *Proficiency in selected skills and competencies that influence subrole success,* such as facilitation of change, collaboration, clinical leadership, role modeling, and patient advocacy (Fig. 14–1).

It is this emphasis on managing and mastering multiple subroles and their concomitant proficiencies that most clearly differentiates the CNS from other APNs. This blending of skills should also be apparent to the numerous consumers who receive a CNS's services.

PARAMETERS INFLUENCING CNS ROLE PERFORMANCE

Before considering the specifics of CNS practice, it is important to understand the parameters that have influenced, and continue to influence, role implementation. Four role performance issues have affected the state of CNS practice and help to differentiate the CNS role from other ANP roles. These key distinguishing issues include the evolution of the role, the nature of the consultee relationship, functional clarity, and justification.

Evolution of the Role

The CNS role was conceived as a way of keeping nurses with advanced education in direct patient care. Creation of the role can be likened to the creation of a

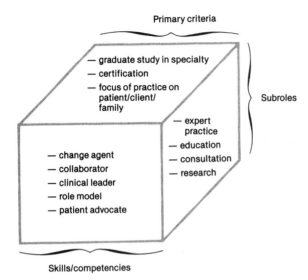

FIGURE 14–1. Defining characteristics of the clinical nurse specialist role. (From Hamric, A. B. (1989). History and overview of the CNS role. In A. B. Hamric & J. A. Spross (Eds.), *The clinical nurse specialist in theory and practice* (2nd ed., pp. 3–18). Philadelphia, PA: W. B. Saunders Company.)

clinical ladder to be climbed by exemplary and committed bedside nurses who sought both graduate education and a role that allowed them to stay in the clinical nursing arena. Empowerment of nurses, improvement of nurse-physician relationships, organizational enhancement of nursing practice, and strengthening of nursing service lines were other goals envisioned for this role decades ago.

Before the late 1960s, nurses with graduate education had only education or administration positions available to them. The position of CNS, clinical expert and resource for staff, was unlike other career path opportunities for graduate level nurses at that time. CNSs' graduate education focused on an advanced and expanded theoretical and experiential knowledge base in a clinical specialty and enabled them to remain in clinical practice and expand their nursing proficiency in their chosen area. The CNS role created practice possibilities at a higher level in the nurse's respective specialty and with more autonomy than that of the staff nurse role.

One of the unique features of the development of the CNS role was its primary evolution in acute care hospitals where nursing is a 24-hour operation. Since CNSs could not be in the clinical setting for 24 hours, their effectiveness depended on establishing partnerships with nurses in staff and supervisory positions across three shifts and the seven days of the week. To ignore this aspect of nursing care delivery would risk having two different standards of patient care—one that was met when the CNS was available and one in which patients and families did not benefit from the CNS's expertise. In addition to collaborating with nursing staff across shifts, CNSs perhaps needed to invest more time than other APNs in developing policies, procedures, and guidelines so that patients would receive appropriate care regardless of the CNS's physical presence in the setting. CNSs experienced with these aspects of advanced nursing practice are likely to continue to be useful as APNs deal with issues of accountability across settings of care.

Distinguishing the functions of the CNS, especially those related to direct practice, has been and remains an issue. Hamric and Taylor (1989) asserted,

> *The CNS is a nontraditional nurse with expanded boundaries. The role does not fit the usual conception of staff nurse, head nurse or supervisor and as a consequence, the CNS does not "belong" in the same way that staff nurses belong to a nursing unit. (p. 43)*

This "not belonging," the inability of others in the work setting to categorize the CNS as a staff nurse, supervisor, or even medical staff member, means CNSs face a special challenge. They have to constantly explain who they are and what they do (Fenton, 1984). Since, even within an institution, two CNSs might function differently (a desirable characteristic) because of program needs or level of staff expertise, staff could not develop a standard set of role expectations that would define CNS work, regardless of the specialty or who was in the CNS role. Such expectations existed for staff nurses, supervisors, and physicians. CNSs who are well prepared in their educational programs for the role know about this challenge and are equipped to address it.

With the exception of psychiatric CNSs, this evolution of the CNS role has been different from that of the roles of nurse practitioner (NP), certified nurse-midwife (CNM), and certified registered nurse anesthetist (CRNA) whose direct practice contributions have been visible and valued. The direct practice of these other APN roles often led to diversification of settings in which APNs practiced, expanded job responsibilities, credentialing for advanced nursing practice, changes in statutes, and reimbursement for services by third party payers. While credentialing in advanced nursing practice is often one of the criteria for APN licensure and reimbursement, and certification in selected CNS specialties has been available from the ANA for many years, benefits such as statutory changes and reimbursement for CNSs have been slow to develop and marginalized CNSs. Unfortunately, in many states, legal, regulatory, and reimbursement criteria continue to be factors that separate CNSs from other ANP roles. This lack of recognition of CNSs in regulations and health policy has rendered CNSs as a group relatively invisible to consumers and legislators, when compared with nurses in other APN roles. This may be partly explained by the consultation subrole. It should be remembered, however, that physicians and insurers had vested interests in evaluating the contributions of NP and CNM care, which led policy makers to fund studies evaluating their effectiveness (Spross, 1995; see also Chapter 26). As a role that evolved almost entirely within the nursing profession, historically CNSs were not perceived to be a threat to physicians or payers, and this at least partially explains why there are fewer data on CNS and patient outcomes than is true of other APN roles (Spross, 1995).

All of the above factors need to be considered in any discussion of the CNS as an advanced practice role and should encourage caution in a rush to merge CNS and NP roles.

The Prominence of the Consultation Subrole in CNS Practice

An expectation of the CNS's advanced clinical preparation was the availability of an expert to mentor staff nurses and enhance their clinical skills and judgment. This expectation along with the need to affect care across shifts through partnership with other nurses, meant that consultation activities often dominated CNSs' practices. Through consultation CNSs would influence the care of more patients and families than they could interact with directly. The primary means of doing this would be consultation, role modeling, and the establishment of structures (i.e., care plans, policies, and specialty orientation) that could shape nursing practice and the care of patients.

CNSs have encountered obstacles to exercising this influence, however. Some do not have the theoretical background to understand the dynamics of and engage in, formal consultation. In other cases, structures are not in place to assist staff in knowing how and when to use their consultative services. In addition, many staff nurses have not been schooled in using the consultative services of an APN. Barron (1989) noted that most staff nurses view their peers and physicians as appropriate consultants. Complicating this phenomenon is many nurses' belief that they must "know it all" and that consulting another expert nurse in a formal manner implies failure, inadequacy, or incompetency.

Born of a need to integrate a higher level of nursing and specialty knowledge into the clinical practice activities of staff, CNSs have found that their interacting with staff nurses is critical since staff are often unclear on how and when to use their services.

This emphasis on CNS consultation probably fit better with functional or team leader models of staff nursing practice where accountability for patient care rested in the team leader or head nurse. It may have been easier, in these circumstances, to allow the CNS to take over and be accountable for a patient's care, thus retaining the direct care component vital to any APN role. In fact, assuming responsibility for the care of patients for a shift was seen as a strategy for demonstrating the CNS's clinical practice competence and role-modeling desired clinical behaviors for staff (Felder, 1983; Koetters, 1989). As primary nursing took hold, with its emphasis on the primary nurse's accountability for patient care across shifts and hospitalizations, it became more difficult for many CNSs to retain the direct practice subrole. The emergence of consultation, not direct care, as the prominent contribution of CNSs meant that CNSs were not directly linked to patient outcomes. This failure to link CNSs with accountability for patient outcomes or costs meant that, in some organizations, CNS positions disappeared when organizations restructured to cut costs (Hamric, 1992). Some administrators were successful in linking CNS consultation activities with clinical or fiscal productivity (Malone, 1989).

Functional Clarity

Although there is philosophical agreement on which role components are necessary to enact the CNS role effectively, there is little agreement on the operationalization of the CNS role in the clinical setting (e.g., how CNSs perform, where they should target their interventions, and optimum reporting responsibilities). Comparing the commonalities and distinctions between CNSs and NPs, Fenton and Brykczynski (1993) found significantly more role ambiguity in CNSs as a primary distinguishing characteristic. When there is no clear consensus among the CNS, administration, and staff nurses on the CNS's functions, role implementation is thwarted (Sparacino, 1986).

A critical issue is who the primary customer of the CNS is or should be—patients and their families or staff nurses (Hamric, 1989; Page & Arena, 1994; Wolf, 1990). According to the ANA (1976), position statement, the patient and family are the primary foci of CNS practice. CNSs have two means of effecting change in patient/family care, however. They may serve as direct instruments of change, providing direct care interventions to high-risk, multiproblem patients and their families, or they may serve as indirect instruments of change, influencing the direction and quality of the staff nurse's problem solving as work unfolds with the patient and family (Fig. 14–2). Another example of an *indirect* mode of effectiveness is the CNS's mediation of change through systems intervention such as policy implementation or modification and creation of interdisciplinary teams or special programs to meet the needs of a defined patient problem. Elder and Bullough (1990) documented that most CNSs spend half of their time in indirect care activities.

The importance of good relationships with staff nurses and other caregivers has been consistently emphasized as a way of improving patient care (Koetters, 1989; Barron, 1989). CNSs who act with little or no interface with staff nurses undermine the contributions of this ANP role to patient care. The mentoring of other staff is an expected attribute that distinguishes the CNS from the NP, CNM, and CRNA. This is not to say that other APNs do not assume mentorship responsibilities. CNSs, however, have an inherent and ongoing responsibility to mentor staff in solving various clinical problems so that they are not needed (either directly or indirectly through consultation) for these problems in the future. Assisting staff with mastery of clinical problem solving is imperative for the CNS to succeed. In theory, such mentoring could eliminate the need for CNS positions. However, as staff become more proficient, the kinds of problems that arise are more complex or new clinical and programmatic needs arise that require CNS intervention.

Justification

The unexpected dominance of the consultation subrole in CNS practices meant that much of their impact on care was invisible unless CNSs systematically documented consultations and their outcomes. Despite the interface with numerous customers

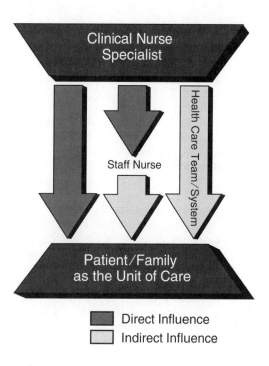

FIGURE 14–2. How CNSs influence patient care.

arising from consultation, CNSs often lament that they are "spread very thin." This reality has given rise to a certain degree of questioning about CNS role performance, as characterized by the query, "So, just what is it you do?" The absence of ongoing and summated performance documentation by CNSs has perpetuated this questioning.

Despite early calls for role documentation and evaluation (Hamric, 1983), many CNSs have assumed that their worth is known and appreciated by those who make decisions about job necessity in their organization. This avoidance of quantifying and qualifying months of work not only reinforces role ambiguity but also ignores an excellent opportunity to systematically market what CNSs do by disseminating performance results (Boyle, 1995). Inadequate documentation promotes the "invisibility of advanced practice" in the health-care arena (Hamric, 1992). In the health-care climate that has evolved, every position is scrutinized for its contribution to clinical and fiscal goals. CNSs' documentation of activities and outcomes to justify the role has been an issue and is more important than ever. In addition, the ability to target, and demonstrate achievement of, outcomes is a critical competency for the CNSs in the evolving health-care system. Further thoughts on approaches to improving documentation and evaluation are offered later in this chapter (see also Chapter 26).

PROFILE OF CURRENT PRACTITIONERS

CNSs are the largest group of APNs (see Chapter 1) but they have the fewest number of certified individuals in their ranks (ANA, 1993). Unlike CRNAs and CNMs, CNSs do not have a single national organization that oversees credentialing, standards of practice, certification, and education. To a limited extent ANA and the respective specialty organizations have addressed these ANP issues for CNSs. The lack of a national organization for CNSs (until 1995) and the fact that CNSs come from a wide variety of specialties have made it difficult to gather aggregate data on CNSs and their practices. Since CNSs usually belong to their specialty organizations, the author conducted an informal survey of national specialty nursing organizations. This survey revealed that APNs in CNS positions represent a small percentage of the total memberships of most specialty organizations (Table 14–1). Readers are encouraged to learn about the *newly created* National Association of Clinical Nurse Specialists and its goals (Beecroft, 1996).

A recent survey of all 50 state boards of nursing to clarify educational preparation for APNs yielded some interesting findings (Ray & Hardin, 1995). In only 11 states did 100% of individuals using the title of CNS have a master's degree or higher education (Table 14–2). Twenty-eight state boards of nursing have no mechanism in place to track APNs. Regulation of APNs by state varies according to four levels of verification, including designation/recognition, registration, certification, and licensure (Ray & Hardin, 1995).

Lack of reimbursement for services has created utilization barriers to optimum integration of the CNS into the U.S. health-care delivery system (see Chapter 22). Attainment of reimbursement is an important step toward increased recognition of CNSs' contribution to patient care. Pearson (1994) reviewed the statewide variability in the legal authority, prescriptive authority, and reimbursement of all APNs. Because these statutes, rules, and regulations are being challenged on an ongoing basis, the information here becomes dated quickly.

Federal reimbursement for CNSs' service varies by state discretion and federal

TABLE 14–1. NUMBER OF CLINICAL NURSE SPECIALISTS (CNSs) BY PROFESSIONAL SPECIALTY ORGANIZATION*

Organization	Total Membership	% of Membership with Master's Degree or Higher	No. of CNSs	% of Membership Who Are CNSs
Academy of Medical-Surgical Nurses	2,700	—	1,871	69
American Association of Critical Care Nurses	77,835	10	2,800	4
American Nephrology Nurses Association	9,309	10	370	4
Association of Operating Room Nurses	47,800	6	1,096	2
Association of Rehabilitation Nurses	9,455	18	435	5
Association of Women's Health, Obstetric and Neonatal Nurses	24,000	19	1,200	5
Emergency Nurses Association	24,500	13	140	1
National Association of Orthopaedic Nurses	9,000	9	1,710	19
Oncology Nursing Society	24,651	16	1,616	7

*Data retrieved from phone survey, November 1995; national offices of specialty organizations queried about members identifying themselves as CNSs in role identification listing in membership rosters; data unavailable in some organizations; numbers represent approximations in % categories.

program. Medicare Part B reimburses CNSs who practice in rural areas, Medicaid reimbursement is dictated by state mandate, the Civilian Health and Medical Program of the Uniformed Services reimburses certified psychiatric CNSs only, and the Federal Employee Health Benefit Program reimburses for interventions, performed by a CNS (Mittelstadt, 1993). The transition to capitated care across the United States will reduce the necessity for traditional reimbursement of CNSs' services. If CNSs can justify their importance in collaborating in care delivery and creating patient care delivery models that are both high in quality and cost-effective, their value in the economically driven health-care market will increase.

DESCRIPTION OF PRACTICE: THE SUBROLES OF THE CNS

The aspect of the CNS role that most differentiates it from other APN roles is subrole enactment. This emphasis on multidimensional expertise, including expertise in clinical practice (with both direct and indirect care responsibilities), education, research, and consultation, substantially increases the CNS's potential sphere of influence, but it also fosters role ambiguity and time management dilemmas. This is particularly true in today's evolving health-care market, in which, because they are viewed as in-house experts on change facilitation, many CNSs are being consulted to help with fostering a climate of receptiveness to change in their organization, in addition to meeting their many other obligations.

Harrell and McCullough (1986) explained that, paradoxically, the same knowledge base and role freedom that empower the CNS to solve problems creatively are the major source of their role stress and role confusion. Particularly for the neophyte CNS, expectations of simultaneous enactment of subroles may be overwhelming (M. M. Brown & Wilson, 1987; Robichaud & Hamric, 1986). Priority setting is crucial, because it affects the CNS's overall productivity, reduces stress, and provides positive role-modeling behavior to the nursing staff.

TABLE 14–2. STATE BOARD OF NURSING SURVEY OF MASTER'S DEGREE
REQUIREMENT FOR CLINICAL NURSE SPECIALIST (CNS) TITLING

States with 100% of CNSs with a master's degree	
Kansas	North Dakota
Louisiana	Oregon
Maryland	South Carolina
Nebraska	Virginia
Nevada	Wyoming
New Mexico	
States with <100% of CNSs with a master's degree	
Kentucky	(76.6%)
Alabama	(44.6%)
North Carolina	(34.0%)

Note: States not listed had no data available. Data from Ray, G. L., and Hardin, S. (1995). Advanced practice nursing: Playing a vital role. *Nursing Management, 26,* 45–47.

Acknowledging the dynamic nature of health care and the practice setting's reactions to this ongoing change, the CNS must be flexible. This flexibility should be demonstrated in the CNS's use of the appropriate subrole(s) to respond to identified needs in a timely manner. Before discussing the four classic subroles of the CNS, it is important to emphasize that although they are described as distinct entities, in reality their boundaries are overlapping. It rarely happens that practice is not enhanced by education, consultation not offered without the knowledge of practice, research not implemented without prior consultation, and education not delivered without drawing on knowledge and skills from four areas: expert practice, consultation, education, and research. Hence while considering the following discussions of the critical elements of each CNS subrole, the reader should be aware of each subrole's synergy with the others.

EXPERT PRACTITIONER

The expert practitioner subrole significantly influences proficiency in the other three subroles (educator, researcher, and consultant) and greatly determines the acceptance of the CNS by colleagues and other consumers. Several authors have described this phenomenon (Baird, 1985; Menard, 1987; Hamric, 1989; Koetters, 1989; Sparacino & Cooper, 1990).

> *Expert practice is the prime mechanism by which the CNS gains entry into patient situations and sustains that activity.*
>
> (Sparacino & Cooper, 1990, p. 15)

> *The expert practitioner subrole is really the sine qua non of the CNS role.*
>
> (Hamric, 1989, p. 10)

> *The CNS must be clinically competent and be the expert in practice. The mandate is absolute. Clinical competency is essential to survival and to fulfilling implementation of the role. The CNS will never gain*

the true acceptance of senior level clinicians, nursing and medical,
without clinical competency based on practice.

(Baird, 1985, p. 54)

Sparacino (1986) described the expert practitioner subrole of the CNS as being characterized by a high level of discriminative, clinical judgment; advanced knowledge and skill, including expertise in the humanistic and technical aspects of care; and innovation and creativity. Koetters (1989) further characterized the direct care role of the CNS as having two components: care that is regularly and systematically provided (e.g., the neuroscience/rehabilitation CNS sees all head injury patients daily to provide selected aspects of care) and care that is episodic. Both Koetters (1989) and Malone (1989) noted that when CNSs provide direct care they are often accomplishing other purposes in addition to accomplishing specific patient outcomes and refinement of the CNSs' own expertise. Such purposes might include teaching staff or assessing a system problem at the level of care delivery.

The CNS performs the expert practitioner subrole by (1) *integrating specialty knowledge*, (2) *demonstrating his or her specialty skill*, (3) *taking a holistic orientation* to clinical practice, and (4) *documenting* practice (Fig. 14–3). The reader will note the similarity between these four core elements of practice and Brown's description of APN practice in Chapter 6.

Integrating Specialty Knowledge

Specialty knowledge in nursing emanates from a base of specialization and advanced nursing therapeutics. The CNS's clinical expertise depends on mastery of both the principles of medical treatment of the specialty population and the nursing care of the population. Hence the CNS is expected to understand the biology and science of the physical and psychosocial concerns as well as nursing care issues such as comfort, patients' adjustment and adherence to therapies, and family coping. This is the essence of nursing practice. If CNSs articulated only the medical aspects of the patient's condition and did not interpret and integrate them into

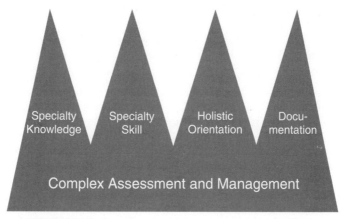

FIGURE 14–3. Core elements of the expert practitioner subrole.

nursing care, there would be little difference between them and medical staff or physician assistants.

Demonstrating Specialty Skill

To demonstrate *specialty skill* is to put knowledge into practice. Integration of national standards of care into the practice setting is a primary responsibility of the CNS. This includes identifying policies that affect nursing practice; defining, maintaining, and interpreting standards of practice; and evaluating policies essential to the delivery of nursing care services (Nuccio et al., 1993). This the CNS does, while also assimilating the many variables that influence the patient's individualized plan of care.

Demonstrating the practical relevance of specialty knowledge is a critical determinant of CNS influence. As explained, if CNSs possess theoretical knowledge but do not have the experience and skill to translate that knowledge into practices staff nurses can use, the CNSs' suggestions will be ignored or devalued until such skills are demonstrated (Sparacino and Cooper, 1990).

Taking a Holistic Orientation to Practice

Taking a *holistic orientation* to care means viewing the patient from the biopsychosocial perspective. In addition to clinical expertise, this requires skill in communication, counseling, conflict resolution, and triage. Within a health-care system characterized by problems with continuity, a multiplicity of professional caregivers, and the foreign language of medical care, CNSs serve as translators and negotiators for both the staff (e.g., to articulate gaps in service implementation) and patients and families.

The CNS also performs a vital liaison role, bringing the many diverse groups of providers together to optimize care. Through their team orientation to care, CNSs often provide group leadership and a collaborative approach to care planning (Spross, 1989). Although staff nurses routinely act as coordinators of patient care, CNSs assist in mobilizing forgotten team members whose expertise may benefit patient recovery (e.g., a physical therapist or speech pathologist), transition to other health-care settings, family adjustment, or the dying process. Critical care CNSs have formally adapted these liaison responsibilities into their conceptual model of care (Boggs & Smith, 1994).

Documenting Practice

Documentation of CNS practice is critical and occurs at three levels. The first level is that which affects individual patients. CNSs document their interventions on the patients' records. CNSs' documentation of interventions with patients is a communication tool that reflects their holistic and interdisciplinary orientation to patient care. Through their documentation they demonstrate their synthesis of clinical, scientific, and experiential knowledge and its application to specific patient problems. This is one way to tie CNS interventions to patient outcomes and make CNS practice visible. Documentation also reflects the CNS's respect for and use of other clinicians' knowledge of the patient. Through their documentation, CNSs model strategies for making many aspects of nursing practice and all nurses' contributions to patient care more visible. Finally, CNSs are in a unique position to influence the selection and use of appropriate patient assessment tools, particularly when used to collect outcome data (Harris & Warren, 1995), which is important to the next level at which documentation occurs.

The second level is related to systemwide aspects of care. Through case studies, chart audits, or other mechanisms, CNSs may translate their clinical experiences with individual patients or specialty populations, and those of staff nurses, into data that can be used by administrators to justify changes in staffing patterns, program initiation, or continuing education needs (Prouty, 1983). Selection of valid and reliable tools for documenting patient care (e.g., pain assessment) that are clinically and practically useful can facilitate the routine retrieval of data that can be used for clinical and programmatic improvements (Harris & Warren, 1995). The ability to identify, select, and introduce standardized tools for capturing clinical data should be a hallmark of the CNS's approach to assessing and documenting data needed for unit or systemwide practice (see Chapter 9).

The first two levels are related to the third level of documentation, evaluation of the CNS role, which is discussed in some detail later. Case Study 1 illustrates the many aspects of the CNS's direct practice subrole.

CASE STUDY 1

Mr. S was an 84-year-old retired engineer who had been diagnosed with multiple myeloma over 10 years ago and was now being admitted to the oncology unit after falling at home and experiencing increasing confusion. During his first night, he was disoriented and agitated, and the nursing staff spoke to the oncology CNS the following morning, concerned about his safety and mental status. The CNS and the staff nurse spoke with Mr. S's family about the events leading up to this admission. They reported a worsening of confusion over the past week that had required his wife to be at his side constantly.

The CNS performed a Mini–Mental Status Exam and reoriented the patient to his hospital environment, reassuring him that she would try to get him home as soon as possible. With his family, the CNS discussed the need to seek more information about the cause of his confusion in an attempt to try to reverse it, but in the meantime, the CNS and staff were concerned about his safety. The family orchestrated a schedule to sit with the patient over a 24-hour period, because the nursing staff and family did not want to use restraints on the patient. Outside the patient's room, the CNS discussed with the staff nurse the possible etiologies for his confusion. Review of laboratory results indicated that the confusion was probably the result of hypercalcemia due to advancing myeloma. Removing the patient from his usual environment and the institution of sleeping medications could exacerbate this disorientation. A protocol for Haldol administration and the need for frequent checks to assess the degree of agitation the patient was exhibiting was discussed with the staff nurse. The CNS placed a note documenting her assessment of Mr. S's altered mental state (including the results of the Mini–Mental Status Exam) in the chart. The staff nurse then spoke with the attending oncologist about this plan of care to reduce the patient's confusion. The CNS called the Gerontology CNS to determine which sedatives had the fewest untoward effects in the elderly, so that in addition to Haldol, a safe sleeping medication could be prescribed by the physician for the patient. Treatment of hypercalcemia was begun.

The following morning, the patient's confusion had decreased and the degree of agitation was minimal. The CNS met with the family, sought their feedback on the patient's care thus far, and reviewed the patient's treatment plan. Resolving signs and symptoms that characterize improvement in hypercalcemia were identified for the staff nurse and placed on the Kardex. Later that day, the CNS spoke privately with the patient's wife and daughter about how difficult it must have been for them to see this successful, articulate man acutely confused and not recognizing his family. The CNS monitored the patient's progress with the staff during the remainder of his hospitalization, documented her interventions, and worked closely with the social work staff on discharge planning. The staff nurses' documentation reflected their grasp of the patient's complex clinical condition.

EDUCATOR

Clayton (1984) noted that CNSs' practice of remaining vigilant for new, relevant information and then sharing this information in an effective and timely manner with their colleagues is one of their most effective teaching interventions. There are many consumers of CNSs' educational expertise. This fact is in part responsible for the high value placed on the CNS educator subrole by administrators and staff nurses (Nuccio et al., 1993; Scherer, Jezewski, Janelli, Ackerman, & Ludwig, 1994). Because of the range of real and potential users of their educational expertise, some CNSs focus on this subrole to the exclusion of the other three. When this occurs, the CNS role is not being operationalized. When professional education becomes the sole focus of the CNS, ambiguity heightens. How is the CNS different from a staff development nurse? The CNS's classroom must remain the bedside.

CNSs' Integration of Staff Education into Their Practice

CNSs' proficient integration of the staff educator subrole into the multifaceted realm of their practice is readily apparent. First, patient-focused instruction is the mainstay and most differentiating characteristic of the CNS education role from those of staff development educators and academicians. Collaborative discussion of patient problems, individualized assessment, and joint decision making are the hallmarks of conjoint patient-specific care planning and staff learning. Teaching may be structured or impromptu; it often occurs on site, but may also occur on the phone.

Second, the educator subrole is actualized concurrently with the other subroles. As mentioned earlier, the subroles of the CNS do not have rigid boundaries. Hence, in responding to a request for clarification about why a clinical event has transpired, expert practitioners integrate patient-specific data and their knowledge of research findings to support what is occurring clinically and give attention to the consultee's need for clarification and reinforcement of teaching. The most important operational event occurring in these situations is role-modeling or apprenticeship. Rather than solving the problem in isolation, the CNS creates a situation that enables staff to intervene on their own in similar situations in the future. Nurse educators who are not in CNS positions usually lack both this patient-specific framework from which to teach and concurrent implementation of several subroles (Priest, 1989).

Third, consumers of CNSs' educational expertise are numerous and wide-ranging (Fig. 14–4). The most frequent recipients of CNS teaching are the *internal*

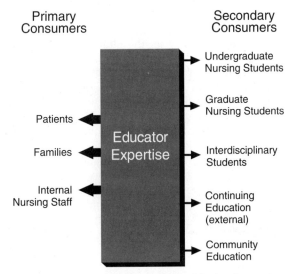

FIGURE 14–4. Consumers of CNSs' educational expertise.

nursing staff with whom the CNS practices. In a survey of 313 nursing directors of hospitals in New York State, Scherer et al. (1994) elicited perceptions of critical care CNSs. Of the 10 survey items regarding CNS educator role functions, the four expectations ranked the highest by the nursing administrators included that the CNS

- *Remains current in the critical care nursing field;*
- *Functions as a role model to professional and nonprofessional nursing staff;*
- *Assists staff members in gaining and retaining clinical knowledge and skills; and*
- *Disseminates new information and/or research through scholarly publications or presentations. (Scherer et al., 1994)*

All of the above-mentioned education actions serve as stimuli to improve the overall quality of patient care (Sparacino, 1986). Internal nurse colleagues within the CNS's work setting receive informal and formal education in the form of bedside teaching, rounds, in-services, specialty orientation, courses, and workshops (Priest, 1989).

In addition, the CNS may be asked to assist with *other disciplines'* continuing education needs such as house staff, physical therapist, and others. *Undergraduate and graduate nursing students* may be taught in the classroom or be precepted by CNSs in their clinical settings. *Continuing education to serve the community* or region may also be offered by CNSs as an outreach effort or as a revenue-producing effort. Participation in these external programs helps CNSs market their institutions in general and their specialty programs and nursing in particular.

Patients, families, and the lay community are the remaining focus of CNSs' educational interventions. In the practice setting, the CNS may intervene directly or indirectly with patients or families who have specific learning needs or require novel approaches to educational planning. For specific patients and families, the CNS may intervene directly by performing a more in-depth assessment of barriers impeding teaching than do the staff. Is the staff's frustration about the patient's inability to learn related to physiological, psychological, social, readiness, or cultural variables? Another responsibility of the CNS in patient/family education is follow-up. It doesn't make sense to create and orchestrate and then forget to evaluate! Was the intervention effective? Did the wife demonstrate necessary skill in performing the dressing change and recite indices of worsening infection at home? The CNS may also influence patient education by creating or collating supportive materials to offer or reinforce instructions given by staff nurses. The CNS's complex assessment, planning, and evaluation in collaboration with staff nurses offers an invaluable opportunity for role modeling at the bedside, which in turn enhances staff nurses' competency for future episodes of care.

Development of new patient/family educational tools and programs is another example of the CNS's education involvement. The CNS's clinical experience yields data on patients' and their families' concerns, confusion, and needs for clarification. Although many colleagues often collaborate on the creation of these written, audiovisual, and computer-based materials, the CNS's clinical base provides needed structure for these projects. This is similar in scope to community-based education programs. In their review of health maintenance programs (i.e., support groups, outpatient consultation clinics, and community education programs), Mullin, Opperwall, and White (1995) identified CNSs' instrumental role in identifying, planning, and evaluating the programs, as well as in driving system changes to make the programs flourish.

As the reader may gather, the CNS's educator subrole is itself multifaceted and requires proficiency in learning theory and practice for both professional and nonprofessional consumers.

CASE STUDY 2

The orthopedic/neuroscience CNS was consulted for assistance by a staff nurse unfamiliar with how to perform an ingress/egress irrigation for a hand infection. First, the CNS and staff nurse visited the patient and together assessed her hand and dressing. Then, at the nurses' station, the CNS and staff nurse discussed the patient's care, not only addressing the specifics of the dressing change but also reviewing key concepts of wound infection, impaired wound healing, and the patient's disease process. After this brief review of infection, the CNS explained the rationale behind wound irrigation and drew a picture of the system so that the staff nurse could visualize the irrigation process. The CNS also shared some trouble-shooting tips and patient parameters the nurse should assess in the coming days. The CNS and staff nurse then returned to the patient's room, where the CNS coached the staff nurse through the irrigation startup. After this collaborative effort, the staff nurse stated better understanding of the irrigation process and increased confidence in her ability to teach the patient this process. The following day, the CNS and staff nurse outlined major points to reinforce with the patient as the patient attempted to master this procedure in preparation for discharge.

As a result of this request for help, the CNS determined that the other members of the nursing staff needed to learn from this situation and would benefit from some on-site education. She developed an educational poster that illustrated ingress/egress irrigation, listed its principles, and displayed it in the nurses' station. The poster included a reference sheet that identified key points as well as practical tips for trouble-shooting. The goal of both these informal and formal venues for teaching was to help staff master this component of patient care so that in the future they would be able to undertake this procedure without assistance from the CNS, with the exception of cases having unusual characteristics.

CONSULTANT

Consultation is the provision of assistance to enhance the consultee's ability to master a given situation (see Chapter 8). Consultation requires availability, willingness, insight, clinical expertise, communication skills, and a nonjudgmental attitude on the part of the CNS. There is considerable agreement that the consultative component of the CNS role is a highly valued role function and that nursing administrators, in particular, view skill in the consultant subrole as vitally important to CNSs' effectiveness (Naylor & Brooten, 1993; Scherer et al., 1994). Like the educator subrole, the consultant subrole includes numerous intervention options, ranging from a patient-specific request for help to a systems analysis (Fig. 14–5).

Consultation for a Patient Problem

Effective consultation on a *complex patient problem* requires sensitivity to boundary and territory issues. Ownership of the identified problem is important to assess, because it affects sensitivity and receptiveness to suggested interventions made by the CNS. This is particularly true if the CNS identifies the patient problem via active

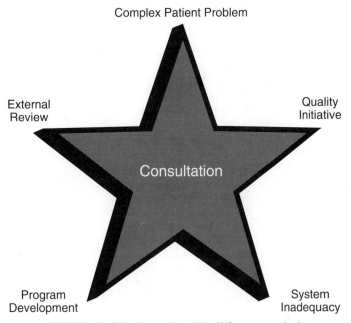

FIGURE 14–5. Problems for which CNSs are consulted.

case finding (as in the case of patient rounds) and the staff has not identified the need for the CNS's assistance. Prevention and amelioration of complications are important aspects of consultation to quantify (Gurka, 1991). Hence negotiation is a crucial component of consultation and emanates from leadership ability and expertise. Particularly in conflict situations, the CNS can role-model team-building skills and demonstrate positive ways to disagree and negotiate (Boyd et al., 1991).

Consultation for Quality Improvement

Never before has the *quality imperative* been so emphasized for CNSs as in these times of health care reengineering. Partnerships among quality improvement department managers and other experts are vital to CNS performance. Just as they do in their educator and researcher subroles, CNSs bring a practice-based frame of reference to the quality problem at hand. They are instrumental in the initial identification of the quality indices in question. According to Siehl (1982), "The role of the CNS is to assist nurses and other health professionals find the balance between what is and what ought to be" (p. 754). This establishes the CNS as an ongoing assessor of the culture of quality in the practice setting.

From identification to intervention, CNSs are instrumental in unraveling the quality puzzle, particularly as solutions are posed. Using their knowledge of the setting, the staff, the patient population, and the desired outcomes, CNSs help choreograph a quality initiative to improve care. The American Association of Critical-Care Nurses (1990), for example, has identified outcome indicators for critically ill patients. They include the absence or control of nausea, pain, and dyspnea and effective communication and patient and family coping. Attainment of these nationally based standards is the outcome goal for critical care CNSs and their work with staff. It is the fact that they offer a micro view in addition to a macro view of care delivery that differentiates CNSs from other quality consultants.

Elaborating on Benner's (1984) work on expert nurses, Fenton (1985) identified a new area of skilled performance for CNSs with a quality focus. The recognition of a generic recurring event or problem that requires a policy change is not infrequent for CNSs. Because of their specialty knowledge and experience that crosses many boundaries in the health care setting, they are invaluable for solving *quality deficits throughout the system*. The emergence of CNSs as case managers speaks to their ability to intervene effectively in systems of care (see Chapter 20). CNSs who specialize in wound and skin care, gerontology, and psychiatry, for example, can help evaluate system needs as they relate to documented problems with utilization and costs incurred with specialty beds, managing confused patients while minimizing restraint use, decreasing hospital costs for sitters, and the behavioral and pharmacological management of suicidal in-patients as these factors affect length of stay.

Unit-specific CNSs have comparable opportunities to enhance hospital- or systemwide quality initiatives. These might include implementation of weaning protocols to decrease critical care length of stay by the acute care CNS, consulting on hospitalwide chronic pain management pathways by the oncology CNS, implementation of a fall prevention program by the gerontologic CNS in collaboration with the orthopedic/neurological CNS, and increasing servicewide compliance with isolation precautions related to TB exposure by the medical CNS. These examples show that CNSs are skilled at blending both cost and quality of care in the overall quality process. This component of the consultant subrole is so vital that CNSs who cannot cite considerable productivity in this area are most certainly vulnerable to job elimination.

Program Development

Formal *program development* is often a response to quality initiatives and system inadequacies. Programs may result from changing trends in the patient population base, length-of-stay mandates, or technologically driven self-care requirements. Options include creating a formal program to solve a problem within the organization or devising a supportive project to enhance continuity of care and continuation of a quality initiative. Examples might include the creation of a case management program for symptomatic HIV-positive patients or the establishment of an outpatient nurse-directed clinic to reinforce new ostomy teaching or central line dressing care for elderly clients. All of these are responses to quality shortfalls.

CASE STUDY 3

Over lunch, the critical care and gerontology CNSs were discussing the increased incidence of skin impairment in their respective patient populations. They also discussed staff nurses' lack of appreciation for the importance of early intervention in high-risk patients. In a monthly meeting of the CNS group, they determined that several other CNSs were seeing the same phenomenon. The group decided to undertake a systemwide quality initiative on skin care. First, the group made plans to conduct a hospitalwide prevalence study. On two predetermined days, skin assessments were performed on every adult medical-surgical patient to evaluate the pervasiveness of skin alterations in the in-patient population. With the help and training of staff nurses who collaborated with the CNSs on this undertaking, the CNS group revealed a lower than average overall prevalence rate of all stages of pressure ulcers but a higher than national average of nosocomial skin alterations that required intervention. In addition, there were no consistent, stage-related interventions for skin alteration—a random approach seemed the norm for treating pressure ulcers that ranged from hyperemia to Stage 4 lesions. Hospital charges also revealed that the institution was paying over $500,000 a year on nonreimbursable specialty bed products.

These data were communicated to respective units to heighten their sensitivity to the nature of this problem. The CNS group created skin care standards and guidelines with an algorithm for intervention selection. Discussions with product evaluation and purchasing personnel resulted in the elimination of egg crate mattresses and chair rings from hospital supplies. A mandate was also approved that if a specialty bed was desired, an order from one of the CNSs must accompany the request. In one year's time, costs for specialty beds were reduced to $25,000, and the overall nosocomial skin ulcer rate was lowered. Recent and ongoing endeavors to support this quality initiative included a "Bed Fair" for staff nurses, where local bed vendors as well as other skin care product vendors were invited to demonstrate their products. Nurses attended this offering throughout the day and had the opportunity to learn about a variety of product options related to compromised skin. Skin care nursing staff liaisons were also established on each unit so that the CNS group had a unit-based collaborator to consult with as intervention approaches were discussed and deliberated. Ongoing evaluation was planned in the form of repeat prevalence surveys as well as review of cost savings data. A multidisciplinary team was formed to oversee the continued monitoring of skin care housewide. The team was composed of representatives from the CNS group, unit managers, rehabilitation personnel, and physicians.

RESEARCHER

Although uniformly perceived as the subrole the CNS has the least time for implementation of, the researcher subrole facilitates the improvement of the quality of nursing care by scholarly inquiry and application of science to clinical practice (see Chapter 9). Felder (1983) noted that, at the very least, CNSs should be able to interpret, evaluate, and communicate to nursing staff the nursing research findings pertinent to their fields of specialization. Hence, CNSs' assimilation of research into the context of their proficiency is a vital element of quality enhancement and professional growth.

A perceptual problem that precludes CNSs' active participation in research activities is the assumption that it's only worth participating in research if one is a principal investigator. To counter this perception, McGuire and Harwood (1989) described three levels of research involvement by CNSs. This distinction, based on level of involvement and expertise, is critical to inspiring CNSs to view themselves as critical thinkers, planners, and investigators to meet their responsibilities for ensuring appropriate clinical care. Utz and Gleit (1995) believed levels of involvement in research are useful since factors such as years of advanced nursing practice, research preparation and experience, and the priorities of the employing institution influence how much time and resources the CNS can invest in research and scholarly activities.

Establishing a practice climate of *clinical inquiry* is a realistic first step for implementing the CNS's research subrole. Getting staff in the habit of asking "I wonder why?" or "What is the basis for why we do this?" is an important prerequisite to research awareness and synthesis.

Research *utilization* involves integration of completed research into daily clinical practice, a skill valued by administrators (Scherer et al. 1994) and further described in Chapter 9. Formation of a research journal club is one way of stimulating clinical inquiry and use of research results (Tibbles & Sanford, 1994).

Research *facilitation* implies support of others' research, either directly or indirectly, by consulting on research methodology or evaluating the appropriateness of setting utilization. By knowing the practice environment, the CNS can facilitate research implementation and address operational constraints that may influence research outcomes. This is particularly true of the evaluation of medical research and its impact on nursing resources (Engelking, 1992).

In *investigating* a patient care issue, CNSs may undertake a formal research endeavor. However, this more advanced level of the researcher subrole is often performed by those who are experienced in the CNS role, are doctorally prepared, or have mentors and collaborators available to guide the research effort. The time commitment required of an original research project can affect execution of other subroles. Thus, staff must know when and how to call for the CNS's assistance if the CNS expects to allocate more time to a research project. Often, staff can be an important part of the research team, supporting the project, communicating the research agenda to peers, and fostering enthusiasm for the unit's participation in the nursing research trial.

CASE STUDY 4

In doing her rounds in four intensive care units, the critical care CNS noted that each unit drew laboratory blood samples from arterial lines differently. She discussed this observation with the Critical Care Practice Committee, and a consensus was reached that a consistent standard of practice was needed. With the CNS's guidance, the committee generated some questions: What procedures are being currently used? How much blood needs to be drawn off an arterial line before a quality laboratory sample can be obtained? Can all laboratory blood samples be obtained from an arterial line? What does the literature say? The committee undertook a literature search and found two studies that cited two different methodologies and varied conclusions. Hence, it was decided that research utilization could not be implemented when sound, valid conclusions were not available. A clinical investigation was designed, approved, and implemented as a joint effort between the practice committee, composed of staff nurses and the CNS. The CNS's facilitation of the research process extended well beyond mentoring the research proposal development process. She conducted negotiations with both nursing and laboratory personnel regarding human resource needs for the study and obtained physician support. Thinking through data collection as well as procedural issues was critical to the success of the study. Funding for the research, data analysis, and clerical support was secured. The members of the Critical Care Practice Committee communicated the study's purpose and methodology to their peers and found them to be enthusiastic and supportive. The CNS monitored compliance with the research protocol during data collection and took on the responsibility for data analysis. With the CNS's stewardship, the committee drew conclusions and developed a global standard of practice for acute care. Poster presentations and article submission evolved as a joint effort to market this effective collaborative research endeavor.

SCOPE OF PRACTICE/ROLE BOUNDARIES

The borders of CNS practice can best be described as fluid, because of the overlap of practice and interests in patient care among CNSs and staff nurses, physicians, social workers, pharmacists, physical therapists, counselors, and nurse managers, to name a few of the colleagues with whom the CNS interacts. Each of the CNS's primary subroles, expert practitioner, educator, consultant, and researcher, brings him or her together with co-workers and other interested parties who have a comparable investment in some aspect of clinical practice, scholarship, deliberation, and investigation. Naturally, this gives rise to some degree of territoriality and resistance.

RELATIONSHIPS WITH PHYSICIANS

CNSs share common ground with physicians in relation to the physiological recovery of the patient. This includes management of symptom distress, skin and wound care programs, extubation and weaning parameters. In addition, they share concern about comprehension, informed consent, coping, and end-of-life decision making.

Interpersonal conflict between nurses and physicians characterizes nursing's history. There are numerous factors that influence physicians' attitudes toward nursing staff and thus the degree of conflict between them and nursing personnel: the culture of medical decision making in which physicians were trained, whether they were exposed in their formative years to mentors who valued and relied on nursing expertise in the clinical setting, the gender role expectations of their family and culture, their expertise about the patient problem in question, and the degree of physician empowerment within the health care setting. These dynamics were recently implicated as barriers to the integration of novel nursing roles (Katzman & Roberts, 1988). Societal expectations and gender role attributions (e.g., doctors are men, women are nurses) are thought to contribute to the medical profession's ongoing influence over nursing roles and functions.

The CNS-physician relationship does not transcend the general nurse-physician issues, it seems. Katzman and Roberts (1988) identified one of these general issues as nurses' subordination of their professional judgment about patient care to the decision-making power of the physician. Without prescriptive privileges, CNSs must rely on physician collaboration to direct some components of patients' care plans. If there is disagreement about the plan of care, negotiation is often arduous and stressful for both the CNS and any staff nurses involved. Subtle undermining of CNS authority by verbal inequities (such as nurses being addressed using first names and physicians being addressed as Dr. [surname]) promotes a subordinate posture.

To counter this overall negative portrayal of the CNS-physician relationship, it is important to cite instances where inter-professional synergy creates an ideal patient care environment. This collaboration is being driven in part by health care institutions and practitioners reexamining nurse-physician relationships as they influence outcomes of care (Fagin, 1992). Indeed, there are many instances where CNS-physician interdependence is effective and serves as a model for others to emulate. As mentioned at the beginning of this chapter, Hamric (1989) identified five skills CNSs use to enact their four classic subroles. Their skill in **collaboration** is appropriate to discuss at this juncture.

The term *collaboration* is often used in the nursing literature as though it needed no distinct definition because it has a shared meaning in our culture (Baggs & Schmitt, 1988). Spross (1989) noted, however, that three elements are essential for collaboration to be operational: a common purpose or mission, the existence and recognition of divergent and complementary skills and contributions, and effective communication. Unfortunately, collaboration that incorporates all three of these elements is rare, yet effective collaboration requires them (Spross, 1989). Also, the absence of conflict does not necessarily imply collaboration. With physicians, CNSs must start by analyzing their collaborative potential. Do physicians share a common purpose? Is there mutual respect for complementary expertise? Is communication ongoing, two-way, and proactive?

Collaboration that minimizes nurse-physician conflict requires skill that is enhanced by the CNS's identification of gaps in one of the three aforementioned elements essential to collaboration. This may include clarification of the purpose of the care intervention, demonstration of complementary knowledge, and effort to improve communication. For example, the CNS might propose,

"Tom, can we find time today to talk about Mrs. White's rigors from the platelets and amphotericin infusions? I'm concerned that none of the premedications we're giving her are helping; in fact, the rigors are worsening. Is our goal here to at least decrease their intensity if not stop them altogether? I'd like to talk with you about two other things we can do to make her more comfortable: the efficacy of extremity wraps reported in the research literature in reducing shivering associated with amphotericin B and another possibility for premedication. She is so debilitated that I'm concerned this worsening symptom distress is compromising her limited physical and emotional reserves. When can we sit down?"

This interchange demonstrates a CNS's attempt to collaborate with a physician to accomplish medical and nursing goals. The mission of care was addressed, a complementary level of expertise was presented, and two-way communication was solicited. It is important to view collaborative role development with physicians as an evolutionary process (Arslanian-Engoren, 1995). When perceptions, education, culture, and work setting constraints are addressed, collaboration can be achieved.

RELATIONSHIPS WITH SOCIAL WORKERS

The major patient care areas of concern to both CNSs and social workers involve psychological and social support. Each discipline brings its own theory base and skill to the patient's bedside, and these can indeed complement each other. Over two decades ago, Mullaney, Fox, and Liston (1974) listed responsibilities that CNSs and social workers share, and these remain the same in the 1990s. The CNS and social worker are jointly responsible for helping the patient adjust to the hospitalization, assisting the patient and family in accepting the physical and emotional aspects of illness and disability, and providing a detailed analysis of the impact and consequences of the illness on the patient and family.

Territorial reactions ensue when either party claims an intervention made by the other as its exclusive purview. For example, a social worker may have received her graduate education in a program that emphasized psychosocial counseling, with little attention to discharge planning. One CNS who intervened to provide psychosocial support to a patient and his wife after an emergency amputation and then asked the social worker to answer the wife's question about insurance coverage was berated for having the audacity to counsel a patient and then triage an inappropriate request to the social worker. In this case, the social worker's turf was seriously invaded, and she perceived her expertise to be devalued. These are perceptual issues that surface when role negotiation is not facilitated at the outset of new role relationships.

A certain amount of duplication and overlap will exist. The goal of role negotiation is to establish what unique aspect of psychological and social support each discipline brings to the problem-solving or preventive endeavor. CNSs may find themselves frequently asked, "When do I call you to help with a support issue, and when do I call the social worker?" It is advisable that they discuss this question with a social worker colleague and then, together with the colleague, articulate to the staff their unique and complementary roles. First, it should be clarified to staff that calling either the CNS or the social worker for help does not preclude the need for the other's assistance. Then the CNS can explain,

"If your nursing judgment tells you that the patient's or family's emotional distress or anxiety stems from a problem with understanding, comprehension, a knowledge gap, or confusion, then it would be appropriate to call me. I might be able to address the educational issue that is prompting the emotional distress. If, however, you feel what you are seeing emanates from overall adjustment problems or coping difficulties, or the patient has a premorbid psychological history, or there are numerous relatives enmeshed in a family crisis, it would be best to call the social worker."

The skill in **role-modeling** that Hamric (1989) observed in CNSs is demonstrated in this scenario, as staff observe the CNS resolve a potentially conflictual situation. Also, staff see the CNS consult a colleague within the team, which portrays the message "You don't have to know it all." Boundary issues need to be addressed up front. If CNSs can't work out the gray areas in question, how can they expect staff to know whom and when to call for help (Welch-McCaffrey, 1988)?

A particularly beneficial skill to role-model, when appropriate, is assertive communication in conflict situations. An ideal and effective form of such communication is a timely, nonemotional request for clarification. For example, the CNS might ask the social worker, "Mrs. Jones tells me that you told her the home care nurse would do all of her dressing changes and that she doesn't need to learn this. We've been working on this teaching for two days now, getting her ready to go home. Can you clarify why you told her this, as that's not my understanding of how this process works?" Because of the myriad of patient needs and colleagues who have parallel interests and investments in patient care, no CNS can escape the necessity of becoming proficient at negotiating conflict. However, when the CNS is skilled in this area, an astute and confident demeanor is presented to team members and modeled for others to emulate. Furthermore, the effective use of conflict negotiation skills establishes the CNS as an above-board player and reduces the likelihood of undermining behavior by others in the future (see Chapter 12).

RELATIONSHIPS WITH PHARMACISTS

Drug therapy is the shared context between CNSs and pharmacists. This being the primary domain of pharmacists, the CNS's expertise and suggestions in this area could be perceived as threatening. Yet, the pharmacist's in-depth knowledge of pharmacodynamics and pharmacokinetics and the CNS's knowledge of patients' clinical responses to medications, self-care capabilities, requirements, and constraints are the basis for a natural alliance of their complementary talents.

The third skill of CNSs that Hamric (1989) identified, **patient advocacy,** can be demonstrated here. McMillan, Heusinkveld, and Spray (1995) surveyed 637 master's-prepared nurses in oncology clinical practice and found that the respondents ranked "Serve as a client and family advocate" as the highest item on the direct caregiver subscale. Although the medical diagnosis leading to the patient's admission remains the focus of concern, the CNS's knowledge of the patient's comorbidities, demands in the home setting, and past problems with adherence to therapies helps to create a pharmacological plan of care that minimizes toxicities, unrealistic expectations regarding pill taking, and out-of-pocket expenses associated with polypharmacy. CNSs' orientation toward "knowing the patient" often enhances their intervention planning (Jenny & Logan, 1992).

RELATIONSHIPS WITH OTHER APNs

Partnerships among APNs strengthen nursing's overall clinical authority base in an institution. When the trauma, critical care, and orthopedic/neurological CNSs jointly monitor barriers to patient transfer within the hospital, including medication requirements, infection rates, and rehabilitative outcomes and their costs, their concerted effort creates a powerful lobby for the creation of a novel CNS-driven critical pathway. When the geriatric and psychiatry CNSs do nursing rounds on all elderly patients on medical units accompanied by the respective nurse managers and key staff, this team empowers unit-based resources to master problematic situations before the onset of a crisis. These examples illustrate that clinical leadership is a shared phenomenon in which credibility and collaboration positively influence the behavior of others (Gournic, 1989).

Just as the CNS professes to the nursing staff that they don't have to know it all, neither does the CNS. Girouard (1983) noted that new CNSs must learn early on that they will never have all the knowledge they need for any given situation and that they must be willing to admit ignorance. Appropriate consultation with other CNSs and APNs sets the stage for staff nurse adoption of similar behavior. The inability to know one's knowledge limits and admit "I don't know" is closely related to low self-esteem, perfectionism, and fears of losing leadership status to another. There is room for more than one clinical leader, and this should be the reality when there is more than one CNS in an institution.

Even though CNSs and other APNs in an institution develop strong alliances, boundary issues may arise. These must be addressed if consumers are expected to know why, when, and how they should use their services. The **clinical leadership** skill Hamric (1989) observed in CNSs is a key factor here.

The designation "clinical leader" is a powerful one, implying a significant amount of formal and informal influence with team members. Classic CNSs in staff positions are ideal leaders. They are pacesetters who are visionary and yet practical, effective communicators and yet competent listeners, and morale builders as well as "corrections officers." Many CNSs and APNs vie for this esteemed label and find it difficult to share it.

When a patient's condition requires transfer to another specialty unit, the CNS's body of specialty knowledge is less pertinent, and insecurity can arise. This is particularly true when patients are transferred to the critical care unit. Not knowing the intricacies of critical care nursing, the medical-surgical CNS must rely on the critical care CNS for clarification, and the family now depends on the intensive care unit nursing staff for debriefing. An unconscious "impostor phenomenon," or fear of inadequacy, may arise in the CNS (Arena & Page, 1992). Thus, lack of knowledge, fear of inadequacy, and renegotiating relationships with patients and their new caregivers are two factors in this scenario that must be addressed.

RELATIONSHIPS WITH STAFF NURSES AND NURSE MANAGERS

Expertise is what many nurses strive for in their specialty. Knowing when and how to respond when a patient is "going bad," choosing how to approach an occluded central line and then achieving success, implementing a new restraint method for use with an agitated child, comforting a husband who remained uncommunicative throughout his wife's illness and then, when she is dying, asks them to take care of her—these are all examples of a proficiency that mark the staff nurse an "expert." The presence of another expert with a more formal title and a master's degree in hand may threaten the expertise and confidence the staff nurse has worked hard to achieve.

Ideally, CNSs identify staff nurses who are informal leaders and create alliances with them early on in their employment. Even with good intentions and efforts, competition and conflict can arise in CNSs' relationships with expert staff nurses.

Turning an adversarial relationship with a staff nurse into a collegial one is an excellent example of role success, particularly if the staff nurse is an informal leader on the unit (Welch-McCaffrey, 1990a, 1990b). CNSs can mobilize staff nurses who feel threatened or are resistant by engaging them as partners on clinical projects or revisions of standards of care, soliciting their advice, and designating them as clinical resources for select unit problems. A special relationship evolves between the mentor and protégé whereby the alliance creates an atmosphere for professional growth. The staff nurse attempts to emulate, rather than reject, characteristics of the professionally powerful CNS.

Working out boundary and territory issues with other nurses draws on the fifth skill Hamric (1989) observed in CNSs: **facilitation of change.** Strunk (1995) identified that facilitating change is an integral part of each CNS subrole. The CNS's very clinical presence predicts a change effort. The change may be a better way to manage dyspnea, a creative protocol to dress a fungating breast lesion, the creation of an agitation critical pathway in the critical care units, or any number of things. Such changes require staff nurses to practice in a different way. Some staff welcome advice and suggestions to modify practice, whereas others cling to existing norms as a safety net. Much of the staff's reaction to change is influenced by the nurse manager's own receptiveness.

In essence, the CNS's job is to rock the boat. The nurse manager is the CNS's most important ally in this effort (Barron, 1989; Spross, 1989; Baird & Prouty, 1989). If the CNS and the nurse manager do not share a vision of the importance of cultivating a climate of change, role strain for both will ensue. The CNS may applaud change, while the manager may desire maintenance of the status quo and thus sabotage efforts to foster transition. A power struggle may be a hidden agenda in this process. Role competition may foster the nurse manager's rivalry with the CNS, leading the nurse manager to second-guess the CNS's decisions (Galassi & Wheeler, 1994).

In today's health care environments, two leaders are often required to manage the health care product. Indeed, Prouty (1983) and Baird and Prouty (1989) spoke to the importance of clinical and administrative leadership. One leader is required to monitor and manage the business of the unit, the division, the program, the office, or the agency, while another is required to improve the quality of the health care product. If they have respect for each other's expertise, the nurse manager and CNS can cultivate a richness in care delivery that is best served by two distinct experts who have complementary responsibilities.

FALLACIES ABOUT CNS PRACTICE

A review of what CNSs are *not* helps to clarify what they are. There are five common fallacies about CNS practice that undercut the clarity of the CNS role and subsequent role negotiation. CNSs must recognize these misperceptions themselves before they can be clarified with consumers and critics.

THE CNS WILL BE WELCOMED WITH OPEN ARMS

Many CNSs believe that the health care system will welcome them with open arms. CNSs who fail to acknowledge the realities of resistance, territoriality, and boundary issues, be they novices or experts in their respective areas, will unknowingly alienate colleagues for a variety of reasons.

First, the title "specialist" itself implies a certain elitism, connoting a higher level of expertise than that possessed by the core of existing workers. This is an issue for many specialized and experienced clinicians who perceive themselves to be experts and feel threatened by a nurse with the formal title. Other indices of professional status that cause jealousy include "getting to do the fun things" (Baird, 1985), having a flexible schedule, wearing street clothes, having a different pattern of interaction with physicians, and having more autonomy.

Second, the presence of the CNS implies change. The CNS who has arrived to rock the boat may not be the new employee of choice, particularly for long-standing personnel. Also, in these times of turbulence and dramatic change in health care, staff nurses may resent the arrival of another leader when another worker bee is what seems most needed.

CNSs must expect to encounter resistance. Before starting their positions, CNSs must meet with team members and begin to assess their expectations and discuss areas of potential overlap. Such information can help CNSs determine if there is a good fit. After taking a position these issues should be revisited early on and negotiations regarding relationships and parameters of practice begun. Meetings with representative groups of nursing staff (by shift, by unit, by committee, etc.) will help reveal needs, misconceptions, and feelings about the role's implementation. Once these perceptions are communicated, explanation and clarification can occur. Reassuring team members that they will be included in the change effort will reduce their anxiety. By conceptualizing change as a team endeavor, CNSs further promote an image of themselves as a collaborator, rather than an independent practitioner.

THE CNS IS ALWAYS AVAILABLE

Consumers of the CNS's services tend to think their project is the only thing the CNS has on his or her plate. This belief is perpetuated by the multirole nature of the CNS position: because the CNS's work is diffused across many boundaries, colleagues and other users of the CNS's expertise are not aware of the other projects and responsibilities making claims on the CNS's time and tend to think the CNS is available on an unlimited basis for their needs. This expectation is also perpetuated by many CNS's hesitancy to say no to requests for help. They may see a request for help as an opportunity to improve the working relationship with a colleague, or they may see repeated calls for help for the same problem as proof of their indispensability (when really they imply only the consultee's unwillingness to assume responsibility for change and integration of new knowledge). When CNSs try to be all things to all people, they exacerbate the demands their roles place on them. Project goals and deadlines get delayed, and when this happens, it is not long before people begin asking, "Just what is it you do?"

CNSs can make sure they don't get themselves into this position by clearly delineating to their consumers the constraints placed on their time by practice requirements, project deadlines, and service needs. They must limit their acceptance of additional responsibilities in the face of these real constraints, for an inability to follow through is a complaint frequently made about individual CNS performance. Negotiation of quarterly goals with the CNS administrator may help

CNSs learn to set realistic goals and understand their professional limitations. When asked to participate in yet another endeavor, the CNS can decline on the basis of current responsibilities or can possibly negotiate a later date for taking on the new project.

THE CNS IS INTERCHANGEABLE WITH OTHER ROLES

Another misperception is that the CNS is interchangeable with the clinical manager, data collector, project coordinator, staff nurse, or other expanded roles, such as case manager, as required by system need. When the need for one of these roles arises, it is frequently assumed that the CNS can fill in as an organizational pinch-hitter. This expectation does not seem to be placed on the NP, CRNA, or CNM.

There are a variety of reasons why this unreasonable expectation occurs for the CNS. One is the perception that the CNS's usual work is not of utmost importance and thus can be forgone for a more critical administrative need. The CNS may be perceived to have ample time to assume additional responsibilities. In addition, ongoing experience practicing in numerous subroles lends credence to the CNS's capability in assuming other health care roles. However, this perception of "use fluidity" only perpetuates role ambiguity and minimizes the critical nature of the clinical availability and consultation that are hallmarks of traditional CNS role enactment. Ways to dispel the myth of the CNS's interchangeability are similar to ways to redress the lack of recognition of CNSs' work and are mentioned in the next section.

HARD WORK WILL BE RECOGNIZED

CNSs often assume that their co-workers know what they do and appreciate the effort they put into the role. This is far from the truth, however.

First, many CNSs deny the need to validate, evaluate, and disseminate their role achievement. Rather than view evaluation as extra work, CNSs must perceive it as necessary to the marketing of the effectiveness of their role (Boyle, 1995; Brooten & Naylor, 1995; Hamric, 1989). The current emphasis on cost containment in health care is causing many CNSs to become more focused on patient outcomes, documenting the effectiveness of interventions quantifying the cost savings and revenue they generate (McFadden & Miller, 1994).

Second, the CNS must view education of his or her colleagues to apprise them of his or her work responsibilities as an ongoing necessity, because the reality of being spread thin is a consistent one. Continued education of consumers and co-workers about the obligations of the CNS role underscores the heterogeneity of the role. This is of particular importance when intensive involvement by the CNS is not an option on all units or for all consumers who use the CNS's expertise.

The strategies CNSs can use to correct the misperception that their role is interchangeable with other roles and to obtain recognition for their work are closely intertwined. Summarizations of projects and yearly reports must be distributed to colleagues who are power brokers and have an investment in knowing the results of the CNS's endeavors. This helps clarify just what the CNS does and gives specific value to work that may have a nebulous quality when only spoken of in general terms. Work quantification also paints a portrait of what wouldn't be done in the organization if the CNS were not present. This is important particularly for those most interested in continuous quality improvement, customer satisfaction, and benchmarking.

"ONCE A CNS, ALWAYS A CNS"

"Once a CNS, always a CNS," it is claimed. It is critical that CNSs see their title as a functional job description, rather than an indefinite professional role attribute indelibly marking them with the title for life. Hamric (1989) wrote, "Unfortunately, the title has been seen by some nurses as a professional attribute, a mark of their achievement of a graduate clinical education or clinical expertise, rather than as a discrete work role with describable functions" (p. 7). The use of the CNS title by master's-prepared nurses not functioning in the CNS role only heightens the ambiguity of the CNS role and further confuses the public and other health care providers.

Measures to address this fallacy should begin at the individual level. CNSs who leave their positions or whose positions are restructured to preclude a direct care role must be willing and able to give up the title. CNS position descriptions should link CNS activities to patient outcomes, some of which are accomplished through direct intervention with patients. At the policy level, CNSs need to be recognized as ANP providers in legislation, regulation, and insurance contracts.

Each CNS should articulate and confront the specifics of CNS job performance at his or her own institution, particularly if an inappropriate use of the title is ongoing or proposed. On a broader level, these distinctions can be debated at meetings of specialty organizations, nursing education commissions, and the broad bodies representing nursing nationally. Avoiding these discussions perpetuates the ambiguity of the CNS role and thus threatens it with extinction.

COMPETENCIES OF CNSs

Think for a moment of a CNS you have emulated and respected, a CNS mentor in graduate school, perhaps, or a current colleague. What are the competencies of this person to whom you so favorably respond? CNS exemplars often exhibit significant proficiency in the following 10 skills, which actualize the eight core competencies described in Part II of this book.

ACTIVE CASE FINDING

One method of actualizing *clinical practice expertise* (Chapter 6) is ***active case finding,*** whereby the CNS articulates the appropriateness of a CNS intervention and then follows through. This may occur informally in patient care rounds, or it may take place during the change-of-shift report, as, for example, the CNS proposes to the team, "I'll stop by and talk with the patient about his concerns in taking this new drug. It sounds like he's worried about unusual side effects, and how he would manage them living alone in a rural area." Active case finding often is required when potential consumers of CNS consultation are not sure when to call for help or when CNSs know certain patients are at risk for something staff are unfamiliar with. An important part of active case finding is reporting back to key team members what was identified and offered as a proposed plan. This educates colleagues about the positive effects of using CNS services.

EXPERTISE IN CHRONIC ILLNESS CARE

As CNSs are discovering, there is a growing need for them to be skilled as ***chronicity experts.*** Clinical decision making across settings and over the disease trajectory will be a central component of the CNS's practice in the future. Even critical care CNSs acknowledge the need to follow through and report long-term effects of immobilization, resuscitation, and intubation. It is this current emphasis on the long-term continuum of nursing care delivery that mandates expanding knowledge about recovery and survivorship. Also, in the future, fewer nurses will be acute care, hospital-based nurses (Boyle, 1994). CNSs will be much more community focused and proficient in chronic care as they assist staff and interdisciplinary teams to optimize care in the home, office, and extended care settings. Creating opportunities now to enhance communication and collaboration among the staff in hospitals, clinics, and home settings will serve as a template for the future, when chronic illness care will occur more often in communities than in hospitals.

INTERPERSONAL COMPETENCE

Interpersonal competence supports the CNS core skills of direct care (Chapter 6), expert guidance and coaching (Chapter 7), collaboration (Chapter 11), and change agency (Chapter 12). A fine-tuned, intuitive, and responsive communication style is vital to professional success. Like starting an IV, being an effective communicator is a skill that must be developed. CNSs who are interpersonally competent are active listeners. Through eye contact and body language they portray an attitude of interest and concern, and they ask questions and voice acknowledgment of the message being relayed. They also are skilled in summarizing and paraphrasing elements of an interaction, resolving conflict, providing supportive counseling, and using touch.

SKILLED CLINICAL INQUIRY

Skill in ***clinical inquiry*** is mandatory, because it transcends both quality and research initiatives. It is instrumental in operationalizing consultation research and competencies (Chapters 8 and 9). CNSs model this questioning attitude to staff and support the staff's emulation of this behavior. Again, this skill is apparent in both formal and informal milieus as individual cases are being discussed or when a group process is facilitated. Asking "I wonder why?" or "Is there a better way?" stimulates critical thinking on behalf of the group charged with problem solving. Consultation outcomes benefit by the provision of an open forum for problem solving that invites discussion by all invested in the patient care dilemma at hand. Other opportunities for clinical inquiry include using research and experiential knowledge to create standards of practice, develop clinical pathways, and create novel clinical programs for patients and their families.

SKILLED DOCUMENTATION

Skill in ***documentation*** assists the CNS in many arenas, but it is particularly critical as the foundation of *research* identification, interpretation, synthesis, and utilization—core competencies of APN practice (Chapter 9). Documentation is the instrument for translating assessment and intervention data to colleagues, which in turn enhances their education about CNS roles. In addition, the written word is a powerful tool for identifying the dimensions of a researchable topic, providing feedback, posing a new idea, or presenting the end results of an exhaustive quality initiative or the collated summary of a year's worth of work. Both qualitative and quantitative data sources are invaluable to describe the CNS's and nursing staff's work. For example, use of Likert scales to report the degree of symptom distress before and after CNS intervention illustrates the impact the CNS makes on a clinical episode of care and lays the foundation for a wider scale research project. The marketing of what the CNS does goes nowhere if the documentation remains isolated, however. Various reports need to be disseminated to key people so that the CNS's achievements are made visible.

SKILL IN ANTICIPATING THE FUTURE

Skill in ***anticipating the future*** positions the CNS for indispensability. Communicating trends within their specialties and citing influences that will change clinical practice in the coming decades place CNSs in a position of authority as the organizations in which they work ponder their future needs. Being seen as a *clinical and professional leader* is a critical competency for the CNS as the evolution of health care continues (Chapter 10). Political savvy and the use of active strategies to influence policy position CNSs to be effective advocates for patients and nurses in the health-care market. Tracking technological advances and anticipating human resource requirements enable CNSs to contribute to timely and efficient transfer of knowledge to practice. Keeping an astute eye on the future empowers CNSs by giving them knowledge of "what can be" in creating a preferred future for consumers, CNSs, and the organizations in which they work.

ROLE ASSERTION

Collaboration (Chapter 11) is a mandatory proficiency in any APN role. However, in CNS practice, it requires astute sensitivity and, at times, a willingness to take a stand to introduce how the CNS may enhance outcome planning. ***Role assertion*** often occurs in a more formal group context as CNSs advocate for the appropriate use of their expertise specifically or nursing expertise in general. In negotiating projects, programs, and new prototypes for care delivery, CNSs relate nursing's contribution to care and innovation, thereby enlightening colleagues. This supports Fenton's (1985) citing of skill in interpreting the role of nursing in specific clinical patient care situations to nursing and other professional staff as a competency of CNSs within the consulting role domain. CNSs may also counter colleagues' misperceptions about their role or nursing's role.

AWARENESS OF LIMITS

In trying to facilitate role acceptance, however, CNSs must be careful not to overextend themselves. Skill as a ***limits accountant*** is needed. This means that CNSs must undertake active and ongoing review of their own role expectations to ensure there is no undue role strain and role overload associated with ongoing consultative responsibilities. This skill is an evolving one, requiring vigilance and proficiency. For the novice CNS, their supervisors (Brown, 1989) or APN colleagues can help.

Staff nurses may need help in evaluating their overextension from meeting the needs of patients and families and reacting to the demands of system redesign. Being asked to do more with less, in a shorter amount of time and with a different blend of resources, decreases staff nurses' resilience and hence requires a long, close look at limits. When staff don't tally their limitations and stress escalates, the CNS's capability to promote necessary quality endeavors is affected. Helping staff set limits benefits the CNS's consultative practice as well.

FACILITATION OF CHANGE

Change facilitation has been mentioned numerous times in this chapter, being the key to successful CNS role actualization (Chapter 12), as it is to the actualization of any APN role. Acknowledgment of factors such as barriers, driving forces, and rewards or limitations perceived to be associated with change is part of the CNS's planning process when the work group is asked to make modifications in their activities. Because change occurs across a continuum, rather than at a time-limited end point, CNSs are continually involved in it. Effective change also evolves from a group effort, and thus CNSs must develop the ability to be a resource broker to mobilize colleagues in the redesign effort.

ETHICAL DECISION MAKING

Engelking (1995) cited nursing's role in bridging the gap between high-tech and humanistic nursing care in the future, particularly as the genetics revolution takes hold in health care. Warnick, Sullivan, and Smith (1988) described what hospital-based nursing will be like in 2020. One of the critical roles for all nurses they identified was that of ***ethics consultant.*** Ethical decision making at the bedside and in more formal venues was projected to be increasingly important for all nurses. Skill in ethical decision making is one of the core APN competencies (see Chapter 13). CNSs' liaison role places them in the middle of debates on the myriad of ethical issues arising from practice. Having firsthand knowledge of the patients and families involved in the ethical decision-making process, CNSs can articulate dilemmas and opportunities within a situation.

ISSUES IN DEVELOPING THE CNS ROLE

There are three issues critical to the continued success of the CNS role in the future: increased attention to evaluation, enhancement of opportunities for professional development to retain seasoned CNSs in their role, and awareness of trends to be ready for the future.

THE NEED FOR MORE OUTCOME DATA ON THE CNS ROLE

Although *evaluation* may be perceived as something to be avoided at all cost, CNSs must welcome it. They need to view evaluation as necessary and helpful in marketing their effectiveness (Boyle, 1995; Hamric, 1989). In addition, evaluation is a critical strategy for increasing functional role clarity, enhancing CNS visibility and consequently ensuring survival of the CNS role.

All of these efforts are aimed at justification for, and validation of, the CNS's presence in the health care system. In a recent Oncology Nursing Society survey of oncology APNs, subscale items describing the administrative and coordinating activities of advanced practice oncology nurses "justifying continuation of the clinical nurse specialist/nurse practitioner position through ongoing documentation and reporting" were ranked within the top 10 role priorities (McMillan et al., 1995). There is a consensus in the literature that the multiple contributions the CNS makes to his or her organization cannot be captured by the use of only one evaluation mechanism (Menard & Wabschall, 1987). However, various models have been reported to assist with evaluation methods (see Chapter 26). What is most important in the evaluation effort is that CNSs "just do it" (Hamric, 1992). Rather than wait for the ideal method to be published, CNSs need to begin chronicling their practice now so others can begin to appreciate the magnitude of their contributions to the system.

Consensus exists in the literature that not one unilateral reporting mechanism is available to capture the multiple contributions CNSs make to their given organization (Menard & Wabschal, 1987). However, various models have been reported to assist with evaluation methodologies (see Chapter 26). Some of these noteworthy studies will be mentioned here. Boyd et al. (1991) communicated their project in CNS role substantiation by describing their instrument review, including submission of paradigm cases, revenue production, publications, grant proposals, weekend coverage, serious occurrence reviews, and clinical logs. One of the outcomes of this group's evaluative efforts was their ability to support the investment in hiring CNSs who could economically combine four important roles into one position. Ferraro-McDuffie, Chan, and Jerome (1993) implemented a quarterly fiscal report to clarify the financial worth of CNS practice by citing cost savings and revenue generation data. Aiken, Taggart, and Tripoli (1993) described a time documentation tool designed to record quantitative and qualitative facets of the CNS role. Peglow et al. (1992) shared an evaluation instrument that utilized a process-outcome evaluation methodology.

CNS ROLE MATURITY AND PROFESSIONAL DEVELOPMENT

CNSs have focused on the novices among their ranks, to the neglect of the needs of the seasoned CNS, including developmental needs for retention, career advancement, and role satisfaction (Oda, Sparacino, & Boyd, 1988). **Role maturity** should be a concern not only for CNSs themselves but also for administrators who risk the loss of a veteran APN who is mentor, motivator, change agent, and evaluator. Hamric and Taylor's (1989) work on CNS role development suggested that peer support and administrative support are variables that facilitate role development. Variables that promote longevity in the CNS role should be a priority on today's nursing research agenda (Fitzpatrick et al, 1991).

Leaders of CNSs need to be able to support CNSs' autonomy while at the same time offering supervision (see Chapter 24). Characteristics of optimum supervisors include a noncontrolling style, inclusion of CNSs in change forums, encouragement of broadening the CNS's sphere of influence, and facilitation of mentor relationships. S. J. Brown (1983; 1989) created a conceptual model for CNS supervision that delineated an ideal synergy among supervision, CNS achievement, and enhanced patient care (Figure 14–6).

Several authors have reported interventions that retain experienced and com-

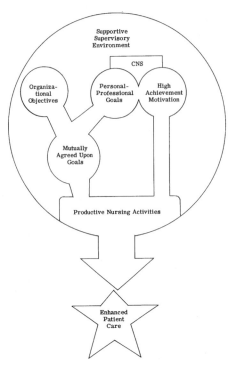

FIGURE 14–6. Conceptual model of clinical nurse specialist (CNS) supervision. (From Brown, S. J. (1983). Administrative support. In A. B. Hamric & J. A. Spross (Eds.), *The clinical nurse specialist in theory and practice* (pp. 149–170). New York: Grune & Stratton.)

petent CNSs. Hamric and Taylor (1989) suggested the creation of clinical ladders to facilitate continued role maturity and to reward exemplary practice. Oda et al. (1988) recommended the options of sabbaticals and monetary recognition for exemplary performance and entrepreneurship. Hazelton, Boyum, and Frost (1993) suggested offering modules on marketing strategies, financial management, business law, and organizational structure to enhance CNSs' existing clinical knowledge.

THE NEED TO BE ORIENTED TO THE FUTURE

Developing an eye for current trends that will intensify in the ***future*** is an invaluable skill to ready CNSs for an evolving health care market. Table 14–3 lists projected considerations and related opportunities for CNS practice in the coming decades. In particular, their expanded health orientation (versus an illness orientation) to care delivery readies CNSs for the wellness focus to health care that will be paramount in the near future (Fenton & Brykczynski, 1993). This focus on wellness will include those with chronic illnesses. Wellness, for them, might mean optimal functioning and avoiding hospitalization.

Their competency in enacting numerous subroles enables CNSs to explore entrepreneurial career options (Hazelton et al., 1993). Transformational CNS leaders use skills and proficiencies similar to those they use to promote subrole enactment

TABLE 14–3. FUTURE DEVELOPMENTS AND OPPORTUNITIES IN THE EVOLUTION OF THE CLINICAL NURSE SPECIALIST (CNS) ROLE

Hamric (1992)	Galassi and Wheeler (1994)
• Increasing patient complexity • Increasing delivery of care in alternative settings • Changing professional practice models • Combining of advanced practice roles • Certification and reimbursement for advanced practice • Articulation of advanced practice behaviors in new practice models • Increasing collaborative practice with physicians	• CNS skill prioritization to match organizational need • Differentiation of advanced practice skill level • Outline of patient selection criteria (e.g., complexity, risk) requiring CNS intervention • Delineation of consultative expertise within one's specialty (e.g., pain control, new product evaluation) • Health promotion and wellness • Patient/family education

in readying colleagues for an evolving future. The transformational leader embraces innovation and a commitment to both personal and professional growth. Critical attributes in this process include visioning, empowerment, charisma, vulnerability, knowledge, concern, and courage (Gurka, 1995; also see Chapter 10).

On a more concrete level, preparing themselves for an environment of increasing managed care is probably one of the most proactive stances CNSs could take. A critical review of the CNS role to support rigorous cost containment along with quality enhancement in an expanding capitated environment positions the CNS now for the reality of the future. This requires quantification of both individual efforts and success at mobilizing multidisciplinary teams (Madden & Ponte, 1994). A certain degree of occupational restructuring is called for to cultivate critical alliances and effective partnerships to move into the coming decades (Styles, 1990). Once again, flexibility, demonstrated in relation to the core elements of the CNS role, is the descriptor of choice.

Finally, CNSs have and will continue to become increasingly aware of the importance of political savvy to advance role acceptance. Tribett (1994) outlined important variables to assess as the CNS works within a political context of health care. One important element of political savvy is realizing the critical need to market the CNS role and its impact on patient outcomes.

CONCLUSION

CNS practice has been marked by evolution, exploration, and evaluation. However, the clinical imperative of this role is nonnegotiable. As Sparacino and Cooper (1990) observed,

> *Clinical nurse specialists, skilled as clinicians, will continue to struggle to frame their practice. Although CNSs cannot succeed merely as a result of clinical expertise, these skills and the discrimination one brings to the bedside form the bedrock that gives meaning or brings merit to all else that the clinical nurse specialist does. (p. 22)*

A complex, critical role in both the health care system of today and that of the future, the CNS role is best served by ongoing evolution and continued refinement. As the future unfolds, the history of the CNS role as one that is flexible and responsive to shifting patient and organization needs will continue to make it a desirable position for organizations to maintain and for APNs to seek. Its survival depends on linking the CNS's expertise to patient and system outcomes. Therefore, CNSs must reclaim their direct practice subrole and systematically document and evaluate their work.

REFERENCES

Aiken, J., Taggert, J., & Tripoli, C. (1993). Evaluation and time documentation for the CNS. *CNS, 7,* 33–38.

American Association of Critical Care Nurses. (1990). *Outcome standards for nursing care of the critically ill.* Laguna Niguel, CA: Author.

American Nurses' Association. (1980). *Nursing: A social policy statement.* Kansas City, MO: Author.

American Nurses' Association. (1993). Advanced practice nursing: A new age in health care. In *Nursing facts.* Washington, D.C., Author.

American Nurses' Association, Congress on Nursing Practice (1976). *Description of practice: Clinical nurse specialist.* Kansas City, MO: Author.

Arena, D. M., & Page, N. E. (1992). The impostor phenomenon in the clinical nurse specialist role. *Image: Journal of Nursing Scholarship, 24,* 121–125.

Arslanian-Engoren, C. M. (1995). Lived experience of CNSs who collaborate with physicians: A phenomenological study. *Clinical Nurse Specialist, 9,* 68–74.

Baggs, J. G., & Schmitt, M. H. (1988). Collaboration between nurses and physicians. *Image: Journal of Nursing Scholarship, 20,* 145–149.

Baird, S. B. (1985). Administrative support issues and the oncology CNS. *Oncology Nursing Forum, 12*(2), 51–54.

Baird, S., & Prouty, M. (1989). Administratively enhancing CNS contributions. In A. B. Hamric & J. A. Spross (Eds.), *The clinical nurse specialist in theory and practice* (2nd ed., pp. 261–284). Philadelphia: W. B. Saunders Company.

Barron, A. M. (1989). The CNS as consultant. In A. B. Hamric & J. A. Spross (Eds.), *The clinical nurse specialist in theory and practice* (2nd ed., pp. 125–146). Philadelphia: W. B. Saunders Company.

Beecroft, P. C. (1996). Combining the energy of CNSs. *Clinical Nurse Specialist, 10,* 1.

Benner, P. (1984). *From novice to expert.* Menlo Park, CA: Addison-Wesley.

Boggs, R. L., & Smith, S. L. (1994). Defining the critical care clinical nurse specialist: A collaborative practice model. In A. Gawlinski & L. S. Kern (Eds.), *The clinical nurse specialist in critical care* (pp. 3–10). Philadelphia: W. B. Saunders Company.

Boyd, N. J., Stasiowski, S. A., Catoe, P. T., Wells, P. R., Stahl, B. M., Judson, E., Hartman, A. L., & Lander, J. H. (1991). The merit and significance of clinical nurse specialists. *Journal of Nursing Administration, 21*(9), 35–43.

Boyle, D. M. (1994). New identities: The changing profile of patients with cancer, their families and their professional caregivers. *Oncology Nursing Forum, 21,* 55–61.

Boyle, D. M. (1995). Documentation and outcomes of advanced nursing practice. *Oncology Nursing Forum, 22,* 11–17.

Brooten, D., & Naylor, M. D. (1995). Nurses' effect on changing patient outcomes. *Image: Journal of Nursing Scholarship, 27,* 95–99.

Brown, M. M., & Wilson, C. (1987). Time management and the CNS. *Clinical Nurse Specialist, 1,* 32–38.

Brown, S. (1989). Supportive supervision of the CNS. In A. B. Hamric & J. A. Spross (Eds.), *The clinical nurse specialist in theory and practice* (2nd ed., pp. 285–298). Philadelphia: W. B. Saunders Company.

Brown, S. J. (1983). Administrative support. In A. B. Hamric & J. A. Spross (Eds.), *The clinical nurse specialist in theory and practice* (pp. 149–170). New York: Grune & Stratton.

Clayton, G. M. (1984). The clinical nurse specialist as leader. *Topics in Clinical Nursing, 6,* 17–26.

Elder, R. G., & Bullough, B. (1990). Nurse practitioners and clinical nurse specialists: Are the roles merging? *Clinical Nurse Specialist, 4,* 78–84.

Engelking, C. (1992). Clinical trials: Impact, evaluation and implementation considerations. *Seminars in Oncology Nursing, 8,* 148–155.

Engelking, C. (1995). The human genome exposed: A glimpse of promise, predicament and impact on practice. *Oncology Nursing Forum, 22*(2) (suppl), 3–9.

Fagin, C. (1992). Collaboration between nurses and physicians: No longer a choice. *Nursing and Health Care, 13,* 354–363.

Felder, L. A. (1983). Direct patient care and independent practice. In A. B. Hamric & J. A. Spross (Eds.), *The clinical nurse specialist in theory and practice* (pp. 59–72). New York: Grune & Stratton.

Fenton, M. V. (1985). Identifying competencies of clinical nurse specialists. *Journal of Nursing Administration, 15*(12), 31–37.

Fenton, M. V., & Brykczynski, K. A. (1993). Qualitative distinctions and similarities in the practice of clinical nurse specialists and nurse practitioners. *Journal of Professional Nursing, 9,* 313–326.

Ferraro-McDuffie, A., Chan, J., & Jerome, A. (1993). Communicating the financial worth of the CNS through the use of fiscal reports. *CNS, 7,* 91–97.

Fitzpatrick, E., Sullivan, J., Smith, A., Mucowski, D., Hoffman, E., Dunn, P., Trice, M., & Grosso, L. (1991). Clinical nursing research priorities: A Delphi study. *Clinical Nurse Specialist, 5,* 94–98.

Galassi, A., & Wheeler, V. (1994). Advanced practice nursing: History and future trends. In S. M. Hubbard, P. E. Greene, & M. K. Knobf (Eds.), *Oncology nursing: Patient treatment and support* (Vol. 1, pp. 1–10). Philadelphia: J. B. Lippincott.

Girouard, S. (1983). Theory-based practice: Functions, obstacles and solutions. In A. B. Hamric & J. A. Spross (Eds.), *The clinical nurse specialist in theory and practice* (pp. 21–37). New York: Grune & Stratton.

Gournic, J. L. (1989). Clinical leadership, management, and the clinical nurse specialist. In A. B. Hamric & J. A. Spross (Eds.), *The clinical nurse specialist in theory and practice* (2nd ed., pp. 227–248). Philadelphia: W. B. Saunders Company.

Gurka, A. M. (1991). Process and outcome components of clinical nurse specialist consultation. *Dimensions of Critical Care Nursing, 10,* 169–175.

Gurka, A. M. (1995). Transformational leadership: Qualities and strategies for the clinical nurse specialist. *Clinical Nurse Specialist, 9,* 169–174.

Hamric, A. B. (1983). Role development and functions. In A. B. Hamric & J. A. Spross (Eds.), *The clinical nurse specialist in theory and practice* (pp. 39–56). New York: Grune & Stratton.

Hamric, A. B. (1989). History and overview of the CNS role. In A. B. Hamric & J. A. Spross (Eds.), *The clinical nurse specialist in theory and practice* (2nd ed., pp. 3–18). Philadelphia, PA: W. B. Saunders Company.

Hamric, A. B. (1992). Creating our future: Challenges and opportunities for the CNS. *Oncology Nursing Forum, 19,* 11–15.

Hamric, A. B., & Taylor, J. W. (1989). Role development of the clinical nurse specialist. In A. B. Hamric & J. A. Spross (Eds.), *The clinical nurse specialist in theory and practice* (2nd ed., pp. 41–82). Philadelphia, PA: W. B. Saunders Company.

Harrell, J. S., & McCullough, S. D. (1984). The role of the clinical nurse specialist: Problems and solutions. *Journal of Nursing Administration, 16*(10), 44–48.

Harris, M. R., & Warren, J. J. (1995). Patient outcomes: Assessment issues for the CNS. *Clinical Nurse Specialist, 9,* 82–86.

Hazelton, J. H., Boyum, C. M., & Frost, M. H. (1993). Clinical nurse specialist subroles: Foundations for entrepreneurship. *Clinical Nurse Specialist, 7,* 40–45.

Jenny, J., & Logan, J. (1992). Knowing the patient: One aspect of clinical knowledge. *Image: Journal of Nursing Scholarship, 24,* 254–258.

Katzman, E. M., & Roberts, J. I. (1988). Nurse-physician conflicts as barriers to the enactment of nursing roles. *Western Journal of Nursing Research, 10,* 576–590.

Koetters, T. (1989). Clinical practice and direct patient care. In A. B. Hamric & J. A. Spross (Eds.), *The clinical nurse specialist in theory and practice* (2nd ed., pp. 107–124). Philadelphia: W. B. Saunders Company.

Madden, M. J., & Ponte, P. R. (1994). Advanced practice roles in the managed care environment. *Journal of Nursing Administration, 24*(1), 56–62.

Malone, B. (1989). The CNS in a consultation department. In A. B. Hamric & J. A. Spross (Eds.), *The clinical nurse specialist in theory and practice* (2nd ed., pp. 397–412). Philadelphia: W. B. Saunders Company.

McFadden, E. A., & Miller, M. A. (1994). Clinical nurse practice: Facilitators and barriers. *Clinical Nurse Specialist, 8,* 27–33.

McGuire, D. B., & Harwood, K. V. (1989). The clinical nurse specialist as researcher. In A. B. Hamric & J. A. Spross (Eds.), *The clinical nurse specialist in theory and practice* (2nd ed., pp. 169–203). Philadelphia, PA: W. B. Saunders Company.

McMillan, S. C., Heusinkveld, K. B., & Spray, J. (1995). Advanced practice in oncology nursing: A role delineation study. *Oncology Nursing Forum, 22,* 41–50.

Menard, S. W. (1987). The CNS as practitioner. In S. W. Menard (Ed.), *The clinical nurse specialist: Perspectives on practice* (pp. 81–100). New York: John Wiley & Sons.

Menard, S. W., & Wabschall, J. M. (1987). Evaluation of the CNS. In S. W. Menard (Ed.), *The clinical nurse specialist: Perspectives on practice* (pp. 189–212). New York: John Wiley & Sons.

Mittelstadt, P. C. (1993). Federal reimbursement for advanced practice nurse services empowers the profession. *Nurse Practitioner, 18,* 43–49.

Mullaney, J. W., Fox, R. A., & Liston, M. F. (1974). Clinical nurse specialists and social workers: Clarifying the roles. *Nursing Outlook, 22,* 712–718.

Mullin, M. H., Opperwall, B. C., & White, S. L. (1995). Clinical nurse specialist development of health maintenance programs: Quality improvement and cost reduction. *Clinical Nurse Specialist, 9,* 45–49.

Naylor, M. D., & Brooten, D. (1993). The roles and functions of clinical nurse specialists. *Image: Journal of Nursing Scholarship, 25,* 73–78.

Nuccio, S. A., Costa-Lieberthal, K. M., Gunta, K. E., Mackus, M. L., Riesch, S. K., Schmanski, K. M., &

Westen, B. A. (1993). A survey of 636 staff nurses: Perceptions and factors influencing the clinical nurse specialist role. *Clinical Nurse Specialist, 7,* 122–128.

Oda, D. E., Sparacino, P. S., & Boyd, P. (1988). Role advancement of the experienced clinical nurse specialist. *Clinical Nurse Specialist, 2,* 167–171.

Page, N. E., & Arena, D. M. (1994). Rethinking the merger of the clinical nurse specialist and the nurse practitioner roles. *Image: Journal of Nursing Scholarship, 26,* 315–318.

Pearson, L. J. (1994). Annual update of how each state stands on legislative issues affecting advanced nursing practice. *Nurse Practitioner, 19,* 11–53.

Peglow, D., Klatt-Ellis, T., Stetler, S., Cutillo-Schmitter, T., Howard, J., & Wolff, P. (1992). Evaluation of the clinical nurse specialist practice. *CNS, 6,* 28–35.

Priest, A. R. (1989). The CNS as educator. In A. B. Hamric & J. A. Spross (Eds.), *The clinical nurse specialist in theory and practice* (2nd ed., pp. 147–167). Philadelphia: W. B. Saunders Company.

Prouty, M. P. (1983). Contributions and organizational role of the CNS: An administrator's viewpoint. In A. B. Hamric & J. A. Spross (Eds.), *The clinical nurse specialist in theory and practice* (pp. 171–186). New York: Grune & Stratton.

Ray, G. L., & Hardin, S. (1995). Advanced practice nursing: Playing a vital role. *Nursing Management, 26,* 45–47.

Robichaud, A., & Hamric, A. B. (1986). Time documentation of CNS activities. *Journal of Nursing Administration, 16*(1), 31–36.

Scherer, Y. K., Jezewski, M. A., Janelli, L. M., Ackerman, M. A., & Ludwig, M. A. (1994). Nursing administrators' perceptions of critical care clinical nurse specialists. *Clinical Nurse Specialist, 8,* 138–144.

Siehl, S. (1982). The clinical nurse specialist in oncology. *Nursing Clinics of North America, 17,* 753–761.

Sparacino, P. A. (1986). The clinical nurse specialist. *Nursing Practice, 1,* 215–228.

Sparacino, P. S., & Cooper, D. M. (1990). The role components. In P. S. Sparacino, D. M. Cooper, & P. A. Minarik (Eds.), *The clinical nurse specialist: Implementation and impact* (pp. 11–40). Norwalk, CT: Appleton & Lange.

Spross, J. A. (1989). The CNS as collaborator. In A. B. Hamric & J. A. Spross (Eds.), *The clinical nurse specialist in theory and practice* (2nd ed., pp. 205–226). Philadelphia: W. B. Saunders Company.

Spross, J. (1995). Advanced nursing practice in transition: Core competencies and diverse roles. In speech given at the 25th anniversary of the Alpha Chi Chapter of Sigma Theta Tau, Boston College, Chestnut Hill, MA.

Strunk, B. L. (1995). The clinical nurse specialist as change agent. *Clinical Nurse Specialist, 9,* 128–132.

Styles, M. M. (1990). Clinical nurse specialists and the future of nursing. In P. S. Sparacino, D. M. Cooper, & P. A. Minarik (Eds.), *The clinical nurse specialist: Implementation and impact* (pp. 279–284). Norwalk, CT: Appleton & Lange.

Tibbles, L., & Sanford, R. (1994). The research journal club: A mechanism for research utilization. *Clinical Nurse Specialist, 8,* 23–26.

Tribett, D. (1994). The CNS as change agent in today's political health care environment. In D. Gawlinski & L. S. Kern (Eds.), *The clinical nurse specialist in critical care* (pp. 228–238). Philadelphia: W. B. Saunders Company.

Utz, S. W., & Gleit, C. J. (1995). Current developments in research-based interventions: Enhancing and advancing the clinical nurse specialist role. *Clinical Nurse Specialist, 9,* 8–11.

Warnick, M., Sullivan, T., & Smith, D. (1988). *Nursing 2020: A study of the future of hospital based nursing* (Publication No. 14-2217). New York: National League for Nursing.

Welch-McCaffrey, D. (1988). Role performance issues for the oncology clinical nurse specialist. *Cancer Nursing, 9,* 287–294.

Welch-McCaffrey, D. (1990a). Indices of success [editorial]. *Clinical Nurse Specialist, 4,* 200.

Welch-McCaffrey, D. (1990b). The oncology clinical nurse specialist in a tertiary care referral center. In P. S. Sparacino, D. M. Cooper, & P. A. Minarik (Eds.), *The clinical nurse specialist: Implementation and impact* (pp. 87–107). Norwalk, CT: Appleton & Lange.

Williams, G. A., & Valdivieso, G. C. (1994). Advanced practice models: A comparison of CNS and NP activities. *Clinical Nurse Specialist, 8,* 311–318.

Wolf, G. A. (1990). Clinical nurse specialists: The second generation. *Journal of Nursing Administration, 20*(5), 7–8.

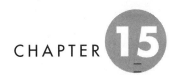

CHAPTER **15**

Primary Care Nurse Practitioner

Diane L. Hanna

INTRODUCTION

This chapter provides an overview of the primary care nurse practitioner (NP) role. With a renewed emphasis on primary health care, this advanced practice nursing (APN) role is gaining widespread attention in today's health-care system. This chapter explores the evolution of primary care NP roles and settings. Primary care NP practice as it relates to the Institute of Medicine (IOM) definition of primary care is discussed. Skills and competencies in primary care NP practice are described. Exemplars of a pediatric and family NP practicing in an urban and rural setting are provided to demonstrate the integration of NP skills and competencies in diverse primary care settings. To conclude the discussion of this APN role, comments about functional role preparation and key issues for primary care NPs are offered.

PROFILE OF THE PRIMARY CARE NURSE PRACTITIONER ROLE

Primary care NPs have been recognized as pioneers in advanced nursing practice. The first primary care NP role, that of pediatric NP, focused on the care of children and was conceived to increase access to pediatric primary care (Ford and Silver, 1967). Since then, a variety of primary care NP roles have evolved, emphasizing care to specific populations such as families, adults, the elderly, and women.

In general, these roles evolved over time as the ability of nurses in advanced practice to address the needs of varied populations was recognized. Frequently, the primary care NP role has been one acknowledged for increasing access to care for underserved populations (Clawson and Osterweis, 1993). With growing concerns over rising health costs, NPs have come to be recognized as cost-effective providers of quality primary care (Brown and Grimes, 1993; U.S. Congress, Office of Technology Assessment, 1986).

Overlapping of specialty areas, multi-specialization, and varied titling state by state make it difficult to determine the number of primary care NPs in the nation. Policymakers at both the state and federal levels have cited the difficulty in obtaining accurate information on NPs in the workforce (Virginia Joint Commission on Health Care, 1994; Washington Consulting Group, 1994). To address this need, the National Center for Nursing Research [now the National Institute of Nursing Research (NINR)] of the National Institutes of Health (NIH) and the Division of Nursing of the Health Resources and Services Administration (HRSA) initiated and funded a study of certified NPs and clinical nurse specialists (CNSs) (Washington Consulting Group, 1994). Survey data were collected from February to June 1993. NPs in this study included all nationally certified or state-recognized NPs in the United States. Data from three national certifying bodies was utilized, including the American Nurses Credentialing Center, the National Certification Board of Pediatric NPs and Nurses, and the National Certification Corporation for the Obstetric, Gynecological, and Neonatal Nursing Specialties. Those states that *did not* require national certification for licensure were also sampled.

The survey revealed that some NPs were certified by more than one organization, held certification in more than one specialty, or were licensed in more than one state. Some of the APNs surveyed held dual certifications as both NP and CNS. Adjusting for these factors, the NINR/HRSA study estimated a total of 29,965 certified NPs in the United States (Washington Consulting Group, 1994, p. 10). In this national survey, the following NP specialties were defined: family, adult, pediatric, obstetric/gynecological, gerontological, neonatal, and school NPs. The following accounted for the largest groups of primary care NPs: family (22.2%), pediatric (18.4%), obstetric/gynecological (16.9%), and adult (16.8%). The reader is referred to the NINR/HRSA survey report for an in-depth discussion of additional data such as employment status, geographic distribution by location of practice, sociodemographic characteristics of populations served, and scope of practice (Washington Consulting Group, 1994).

PRIMARY CARE NURSE PRACTITIONER PRACTICE

What do family, adult, pediatric, obstetric/gynecological, gerontological, and other primary care NPs have in common? The answer to this question lies in a more in-depth analysis of the terms "primary care" and "nurse practitioner." Definitions of primary care have evolved over time. As a part of a 2-year study on the future of primary care, the IOM has developed a definition of primary care. The definition is intended to help health professionals, policymakers, educators, and the public confront the rapid changes underway in health care as the future of primary care is reemphasized in the United States. The IOM Committee on the Future of Primary Care (1994) offers this updated definition:

> *Primary care is the provision of integrated, accessible health care services by clinicians who are accountable for addressing a large majority of personal health care needs, developing a sustained partnership with patients, and practicing in the context of family and community. (p. 1)*

Within this definition, definitions of the italicized words clarify the nature of services, those involved in the delivery of care, and the nature of the relationship between clinician and patient. Each of the italicized terms in the IOM definition is summarized and explained in the IOM document *Defining Primary Care* (Institute of Medicine, 1994).

Of note is the broad base of input into this definition of primary care. The IOM Committee on the Future of Primary Care is composed of 19 members representing medicine, nursing, dentistry, health professions educators, health insurers, public health professionals, health-care administrators, health economists, and health-care consumers. Both nurse practitioners and physician assistants are represented on the committee. The definition reflects a broad perspective of health care. It is based on a 1978 IOM definition but emphasizes the importance of the patient-clinician relationship in the context of family and community. It also recognizes the facilitation of primary care delivery by teams and integrated delivery systems.

An overview of the italicized terms in the IOM definition of primary care (1994) assists in describing the role of NPs in primary care:

> ***Integrated*** care refers to "the provision of comprehensive, coordinated, and continuous services" that addresses any health problem at any stage in the

life cycle, combines health services and information to meet a patient's needs, and provides care over time by an individual or team of professionals ("clinician continuity") with effective and timely communication of health information ("record continuity").

Accessibility describes the ease with which the care can be attained. Here, there is a specific emphasis on the elimination of barriers to care. Patient barriers include geographic location, administrative hurdles, reimbursement, culture, and language.

Health-care services encompasses all of those services aimed at promoting, maintaining, or restoring health in all care settings (e.g., hospitals, offices, schools, and homes).

Clinician is defined as "an individual who uses a recognized scientific knowledge base and has the authority to direct the delivery of personal health services to patients."

Accountable applies to both individual clinicians and the systems in which they operate. They are accountable for the care provided, including quality of care, patient satisfaction, efficient use of resources, and ethical behavior.

Majority of personal health-care needs is interpreted as a competency to manage the large majority of patient health problems without restriction by problem or organ system. Consultation or referral to other health professionals is made if further evaluation or management is needed.

Sustained partnership refers to a relationship between patient and clinician continued over time. It is based on mutual trust, respect, and responsibility.

Patient is an individual seeking care for illness, health promotion, and disease prevention.

Context of family and community references an understanding of the circumstances and facts surrounding a patient. Living conditions, resources, family dynamics, work situation, and cultural background are considered when patients are evaluated. In a broader sense, community refers to the population potentially served whether or not its members are patients. A group residing in a defined geopolitical boundary, enrollees in a health plan, and a neighborhood with a common heritage are all examples of community. Here the emphasis is on an awareness of public health trends within a community (e.g., leading causes of morbidity and mortality, immunization rates) and their implications for health promotion and disease prevention strategies. (Institute of Medicine, 1994, pp. 16–17)

This updated IOM definition of primary care encompasses much of the essence of advanced nursing practice with its emphasis on accountability, a holistic approach to patient care, inclusion of health promotion and disease prevention activities, and description of a patient-clinician relationship "predicated on the development of mutual trust, respect, and responsibility" (Institute of Medicine, 1994, p. 17). A primary care NP certainly brings these attributes and activities to the primary care setting. Indeed, Brown identifies the use of a holistic framework and forming partnerships with patients as two of the major characteristics of the APN style of care. Brown provides an in-depth discussion of these characteristics in Chapter 6.

By engaging in the *nursing* process in the primary care setting (i.e., data collection, assessment, planning, implementation, evaluation) with defined advanced practice skills and competencies, an NP can effectively provide primary care. The population of patients for which the NP is prepared to provide care (e.g., families, adults, children, women, the elderly) serves to differentiate the types of primary care NPs in practice (e.g., family NPs, adult NPs, pediatric NPs including school NPs, obstetric-gynecological NPs, women's health-care NPs, and gerontological NPs). The American Nurses Association (ANA) documents concerning the scope and standards of primary care NP practice also reflect the integration of primary care delivery and the nursing process in this APN role (American Nurses Association, 1985, 1987).

The concept of *integrated, accessible health-care services* described by the IOM also underscores the importance of a team approach in primary care delivery with collaboration between the professionals providing health services. Traditional medical models of care delivery have emphasized the diagnosis and treatment of disease, i.e., curing. Nursing models of care have emphasized developmental and systems theories in considering human responses to illness, i.e., caring over time. Using a holistic approach to assessment and treatment, the primary care NP addresses illness, promotes health, and prevents disease. Interpersonal skills, patient and family education, and counseling are critical elements of practice. The provision of care from nursing and medical models through a collaborative approach to clinical practice can enhance the comprehensiveness and quality of care rendered. Many of the skills and competencies in primary care NP practice are based on knowledge of common acute and chronic health problems encountered in primary care settings. By employing expert clinical reasoning and utilizing diverse management approaches (see Chapter 6), the NP renders appropriate cost-effective primary care.

At times, the complexity of health-care problems may exceed the NP's scope of practice. In these instances, consultation with physicians or other appropriate team members is indicated. Here, the diagnosis and treatment of disease is still integrated with nursing expertise related to the patient's experience of illness. Again, the importance of a team approach to care is emphasized. By the same token, medical practitioners and other professionals on the primary care team may and should consult NPs when issues concerning adherence to therapy, patient and family responses to illness, and health promotion strategies arise. Thus, the collaborative efforts of both medical and nursing professionals on primary care teams can assure the provision of high-quality, comprehensive, and holistic patient care (Baldwin, 1994; Clawson and Osterweis, 1993; Fagin, 1992).

SKILLS AND COMPETENCIES IN PRIMARY CARE NURSE PRACTITIONER PRACTICE

Given this overview of the scope of primary care NP practice, its differentiation from medicine and general nursing practice, and the differentiation of various NP roles in primary care, a closer examination of practice skills and competencies deepens understanding of the role. APNs in primary care NP roles bring a variety of skills and competencies to their practice that build on a foundation of basic nursing education. These skills and competencies, initially introduced in basic and graduate education programs, are continually developed through clinical experience and ongoing professional education. Hamric cites the synergistic impact of graduate education and clinical practice experience on APN development in Chapter 3. She also identifies a set of core competencies enacted in each APN role, which include:

- Clinical practice expertise
- Expert guidance and coaching of patients, families, and other care providers
- Consultation
- Research interpretation and utilization
- Clinical and professional leadership
- Collaboration
- Change agent skills
- Ethical decision-making skills

NP educators have referred to three areas of NP competencies in primary care: management of health and illness status, teaching and counseling, and organizational and role competencies (National Organization of Nurse Practitioner Faculties, 1995). These broad categories encompass the set of skills and competencies identified by Hamric in defining ANP. Of note is the more recent integration of organizational and role competencies into NP curricula. This APN competency is critical for the NP in today's rapidly changing health-care environment. An overview of each of the competency areas follows.

MANAGEMENT OF HEALTH AND ILLNESS STATUS

Primary care services encompass the entire life span and primary care NPs may be broadly prepared to care for patients at any stage of life (e.g., FNPs) or may have a particular population focus in their practice (e.g., PNPs). No matter what the focus, primary care NPs are involved in the management of health and illness status using the nursing process.

Advanced patient history-taking and physical assessment skills are critical tools for primary care NPs during the data collection stage of the nursing process. Effective interpersonal relationship and communications skills enhance the NP's ability to obtain a comprehensive history. A working knowledge of cultural diversity provides an important foundation for this process. Particular attention is paid to personal health habits, stressors, genetics, and an assessment of health risk factors to identify appropriate health promotion and disease prevention strategies.

Evaluating the subjective and objective data collected requires critical thinking and diagnostic reasoning skills on the part of the primary care NP. These aspects of clinical decision making are required not only in the identification of problems but in the further evaluation and management of health needs of primary care clients. Specific health promotion needs based on stages of physical and psychosocial development may be assessed. Much of primary care NP practice involves the diagnosis and management of acute self-limiting, minor illnesses and stable chronic diseases. However, primary care practice requires an ability to recognize signs and symptoms of complex and unstable health problems requiring medical or other consultation. It also calls for the recognition of emergency situations with subsequent initiation of effective emergency care.

Following the assessment phase of the nursing process, primary care NPs may plan for care in the form of additional diagnostic studies, specific therapeutic measures, and patient education and counseling strategies. Guidelines for practice can help to guide the clinician in planning for appropriate intervention. The efficacy and safety of therapy over time as well as the client's health goals, risk factors, and illness experience are also considered as plans are developed.

Further diagnostic tests (e.g., laboratory studies or radiography) may be required to more accurately assess the patient's health status. Age-specific screening examinations may be recommended as a part of clinical preventive service guidelines. Specific therapeutic measures may encompass both pharmacological and non-pharmacological therapies. If pharmacologic therapy is initiated, the NP determines the appropriate treatment and counsels the patient about drug regimens and side effects (National Organization of Nurse Practitioner Faculties, 1995).

Many of the primary care NP's therapeutic recommendations may be non-pharmacological (e.g., specific dietary or activity recommendations, stress management strategies). In fact, primary care NP practice has been recognized for its utilization of more non-pharmacological therapies than traditional medical practice (U.S. Congress, Office of Technology Assessment, 1986). Patient education and counseling strategies in the management of health and illness status include anticipatory guidance related to normal growth and development for patients and families as well as potential changes they may experience in terms of specific health problems. Additional teaching and counseling competencies enacted in NP practice are discussed in the following section.

Once plans of care are developed and implemented, the primary care NP uses expected outcome criteria to evaluate the effectiveness of interventions. Scheduling phone or office follow-up visits to appropriately monitor clients is an important aspect of ongoing evaluation. When outcome criteria are not achieved, the plan of care is revised accordingly, and further consultation may be indicated (National Organization of Nurse Practitioner Faculties, 1995).

TEACHING AND COUNSELING

As mentioned in the discussion of health and illness management, teaching and counseling competencies are critical elements of NP practice. The U.S. Congress Office of Technology Assessment (OTA) study (1986) recognized that an emphasis on these activities helped to differentiate NP practice from that of other primary care providers.

Teaching and counseling in NP practice is based on a variety of psychosocial theories such as learning theory, communication theory, and family dynamics. Competency in this aspect of practice may be reflected in a variety of ways. For example, the NP demonstrates competency in patient education by capturing a patient's readiness to learn and providing an environment that promotes learning. Interactions with patients in ways that are non-judgmental and culturally sensitive facilitates a sense of partnership in the primary care setting.

The explanation of a client's condition, treatment choices, and rationale for procedures is another important competency in this aspect of practice. The NP helps patients to understand their own body and symptoms and responds to their questions. Relevant lifestyle adjustments and other measures for health promotion are also discussed. When combined, these strategies can help to maximize the patients' participation in their own care. As a patient counselor, the primary care NP may assess and support patients experiencing crisis, loss, or grief situations and determines whether referral to mental health professionals may be indicated (National Organization of Nurse Practitioner Faculties, 1995).

Teaching and counseling activities become the backbone of health promotion and disease prevention activities. Once lifestyle patterns are assessed and risk factors for illness and injury are determined, the NP is positioned to work with the patient to identify and individualize appropriate health promotion strategies. Exercise, nutrition, stress management, injury prevention, safe sexual practices, and elimination of smoking and other substance abuse habits are areas frequently addressed. Again, creating a partnership with the client lays the groundwork for prioritizing risk reduction strategies and planning realistic interventions that contribute to success. Expert guidance and coaching in APN practice is also discussed in Chapter 7.

ORGANIZATIONAL AND ROLE COMPETENCIES

A more general set of skills related to the NP role and the individual, groups, and organizations that it relates to, make up this third area of practice competencies. Here, an understanding of the NP role, health policy, change and conflict theory, business and marketing, and professional leadership is a critical foundation (National Organization of Nurse Practitioner Faculties, 1995). Of the three areas of competencies described, organizational and role competencies may require the most experience and professional maturity to develop. Organizational and role competencies require an ability to see the big picture. In an era of rapid change through marketplace reform and dynamic health policy debates, the ability to market the NP role to managed care systems and policy makers is an example of a broad organizational and role competency critical to the profession's future.

At the patient care level, an NP demonstrates organizational and role competency through the coordination of care to meet multiple client health needs and requests. The importance of the interdisciplinary team and collaboration in primary care has been cited. The primary care NP assists in the development of such a team to provide optimal therapy. Establishing priorities for care and ensuring continuity of care is yet another example of organizational and role competency in patient care. Finally, serving as a role model, mentor, and preceptor for novice practitioners is a critical way to ensure a viable future for the NP role (National Organization of Nurse Practitioner Faculties, 1995).

From a broader health policy perspective, participation in professional organizations as well as health legislation and policy-making activities can result in important strategies to improve the health of populations. NPs have an important perspective to share through analysis of contemporary health policy and its impact on consumers, providers, and the nation. Historically, NPs have advocated for the needs of underserved populations in the health policy arena. In an era of rapidly evolving health-care systems, this continues to be of major importance.

EXEMPLARS

Having considered the scope of primary care NP practice along with some of its skills and competencies, specific examples are provided to demonstrate how an NP can assist in meeting the primary care needs of a particular community. The following two exemplars demonstrate two very different practice settings. However, in both situations, the same basic skills and competencies are required for effective primary care delivery.

URBAN PEDIATRIC NURSE PRACTITIONER PRACTICE

Jane is a pediatric NP caring for children in a low-income urban community. This community once thrived as part of a major industrial center but had been devastated by factory closings and a declining local economy. Recent health status indicators for this urban area reveal increasing rates of teen pregnancy. There is growing concern in the community about substance abuse, school dropouts, and community violence.

This setting is a challenging one, but Jane feels that by working with children and families through the community Child Health Clinic she might be able to help them deal with the risks that poverty introduces to their health. The clinic is a public-private venture jointly funded by the local health department, the community hospital, and various charitable organizations in the greater metropolitan area. It serves as a source of primary care to many Medicaid children from the community now enrolled in a statewide managed care program. The clinic also provides services to non-Medicaid recipients using a sliding-scale fee.

Jane sees a variety of infants, children, and adolescents who come to the clinic for both well-child visits and acute/episodic health problems. Her care entails thorough health assessments by history-taking, physical assessment, and appropriate diagnostic studies or screening examinations. She then recommends appropriate interventions (both pharmacological and non-pharmacological) for the child. These are in keeping with established clinical guidelines used in the clinic. Much of Jane's time is spent discussing normal childhood growth and development with parents as well as effective parenting skills, nutritional needs, and age-specific injury prevention guidelines. If the child is ill, she describes ways to monitor the child's health status.

At times, Jane may consult with the clinic pediatrician about acute health problems or abnormal health screening findings. For children and families with complex health problems, she may also consult with other members of the clinic team for further evaluation and management. Public health nurses are available for home assessment and case management services, and the clinic social worker provides additional outreach services. A nutritionist and eligibility worker from the Women, Infant, and Children's nutrition program are on site to address nutritional needs in depth.

Jane also engages with this community outside the walls of the clinic. This enhances her credibility and acceptance among this low-income population. On occasion she is asked to assist with health-screening examinations for the local Head Start program. Recently there has been growing concern about unmet needs for child health services in the greater urban area. As a respected primary care provider for an underserved community, Jane has been asked to serve on a local Child Health Task Force. She will work with other health-care providers and community leaders to identify ways to more effectively use public and private resources in addressing children's health needs. Together, they hope to promote a healthier future for the community at large.

RURAL FAMILY NURSE PRACTITIONER PRACTICE

With 3 years of experience as a family NP at the Mountain Breeze Rural Health Center, Mary realized how much she had developed as a primary care provider.

She had worked as a public health nurse for 10 years in this coal mining and industrial community of Appalachia and was familiar with its poverty and limited access to health care. In fact, the mountains themselves, with narrow winding roads, posed one of the major barriers to care in this area—transportation.

Before the local family physician of 40 years retired, Mary had been able to pursue her NP education through a master's degree program offered by the state university satellite program on the community college campus 40 miles away. The hour commute to school grew long, but that trip was short when compared with the additional 300 miles traversed by teleconferencing to provide for interaction with faculty on the main campus. Mary was fortunate to have been the recipient of a state scholarship for her graduate education. For this educational funding she had agreed to practice in a medically underserved area of the state. This was easy for Mary because Appalachia had been home to her for all of her life.

Anticipating the loss of their longstanding physician, the community had worked hard to support the establishment of a rural health center in the area. Mary was well known to the local citizens as a public health nurse, and they readily accepted her in her new role as an NP. The nearest hospital, 30 miles away, had recently been engaged in the development of rural health networks and provided physician coverage in the center 3 days per week. The retiring family physician had been a real asset for Mary to work with in her first year following graduation as she made the transition to her new role. Now, on the 3 days per week that physicians were on site, she could be sure that patients requiring more complex medical management were scheduled. These days also provided an opportunity to review and discuss other patient management issues and to develop skills and knowledge related to the medical aspects of her practice.

Mary's days at the center were always full but never predictable. She cared for many adults with chronic health problems such as diabetes and hypertension. She devoted much of her effort to working with patients and their families on improved nutritional status and other health promotion strategies. One of her diabetic patients had recently started insulin therapy. After teaching him how to monitor his glucose at home, she was able to adjust his initial insulin therapy over the phone. The phone proved to be a valuable tool for her practice because many families had no regular source of transportation to the clinic. As the only female primary care provider in the area, Mary found much of her time devoted to women's health care. Women found it easy to share their concerns with her, and Mary frequently discussed family health problems with them during these visits.

One afternoon a week, Mary left the clinic and made rounds on patients in the local nursing home. She worked closely with the staff there to identify ways to assist this geriatric population in maintaining as much independence as possible. She also enjoyed occasional trips to the local high school to assist with sports physicals. From time to time she was invited to be a speaker at the employee health seminars held at the nearby packaging plant.

Her work was rewarding and there were many challenges ahead. She had recently discussed the area's low childhood immunization rates with local leaders. They were now developing a proposal for a mobile health unit to increase access to immunizations and other primary preventive services to remote sections of the tri-county area. Mary was asked to portray some of this Appalachian community's health needs to a contingency of state and federal legislators visiting the area. She hoped to make a compelling case for a mobile health unit so that funding for the project could be secured.

FUNCTIONAL ROLE PREPARATION

From the exemplars, it is clear that the scope of primary care NP practice is broad and requires a high level of clinical competency and professional accountability. Students in graduate NP education programs must develop a solid foundation of knowledge in primary care and management skills in order to facilitate more autonomous clinical practice than was required in their previous generalist nursing roles. They must understand the professional accountability that is assumed when undertaking this advanced practice role and demonstrate a commitment to continuous professional growth and development. Skills as a team member are also essential to the primary care NP because the role calls for collaboration with a variety of health professionals (Hanson, 1993) (see also Chapter 11).

To prepare students for collaborative practice, interdisciplinary approaches to education should be undertaken (Baldwin, 1994). In the classroom, clinical content can be effectively presented by NPs, physicians, and other members of the primary care team as one way to facilitate understanding of the perspective and expertise that each brings to patient care. Clinical experiences for students are also enhanced by an interdisciplinary approach. By seeing first-hand how collaborative approaches to patient care can facilitate cost-effective, comprehensive care, students will be better prepared for interdependent primary care practice.

In addition to basic role and clinical competencies developed in primary care NP programs, an understanding of other professional practice issues related to advanced nursing practice is critical. NPs must be familiar with statutes and regulations governing practice in their state as well as appropriate licensing and professional credentialing procedures. Résumé development and interview and contract negotiating skills are important tools for securing a rewarding clinical practice position. Familiarity with risk management procedures and appropriate professional liability coverage will help to provide protection from costly malpractice litigation. If clinical practice involves caring for patients in institutional settings (e.g., hospitals or nursing homes), NPs may have to obtain clinical privileges before being permitted to practice at these sites. Finally, an understanding of the practice setting's billing and reimbursement policies and procedures is essential for the development of economically sound primary care practice (see Chapters 22 and 24).

The emphasis on cost-effectiveness of care will continue to grow as managed care markets expand. NPs must have an understanding of cost-efficient practices and clinical decision-making skills to be able to establish appropriate priorities in clinical care. In busy practice settings, the use of telephone triage and management skills is another tool in addressing both acute and chronic health problems. The NP may require additional guidance and experience to develop telephone interview and follow-up skills. An ongoing emphasis on clinical preventive services for health promotion and disease prevention promotes cost-effective care (Ryan, 1993). The NP must learn ways to incorporate these services into routine patient visits and seize teachable moments with clients for effective health education.

Marketplace forces and health policy debates continue to create rapid change in primary care delivery systems. The primary care NP must understand the forces that are driving change and the ways they may shape practice in the future. Furthermore, APN students should begin to develop an understanding of how they can influence health policy to assure that quality health-care services are made accessible, affordable, and available to all.

ISSUES FOR THE FUTURE OF PRIMARY CARE NURSE PRACTITIONERS

Since the inception of the role in the mid-1960s, primary care NPs have received growing attention from health policymakers and have gained increasing familiarity with health-care consumers. The needs of underserved populations that spurred the development of the movement over 25 years ago are equally pressing today. Studies repeatedly affirm that NPs can substantially increase access to these populations (Osterweis and Garfinkel, 1993). More recent efforts to contain costs in health-care delivery systems emphasize the need for cost-effective providers of primary care. Numerous studies have documented that NPs can meet the challenges of increasing access to high-quality, cost-effective care (Brown and Grimes, 1993; Nichols, 1992; U.S. Congress, Office of Technology Assessment, 1986). However, continued attention to several practice issues will be required for promoting the utilization of NPs in primary health-care delivery systems.

NPs have been limited by restrictions on their scope of practice, prescriptive authority, and eligibility for reimbursement (Safriet, 1992). The literature makes numerous references to these "barriers to practice" and efforts to address them. The committed efforts of NP leaders at state and national levels, combined with support from nursing organizations to educate policymakers and effect change in these areas, have been commendable. However, much remains to be done to remove remaining legal and regulatory restrictions to practice (see Chapter 22). Furthermore, ongoing professional vigilance to protect the gains of the past is required. Professional unity with APNs, coalition building, and strong organizational leadership at the state and national levels are critical to achieve these goals. NPs in primary care practice must be willing to invest in these organizations and activities to protect their professional futures.

Along with attention to the removal of practice barriers, NPs must maintain a high level of awareness of the forces that are driving change in the health-care delivery system today. Failure of the federal government to achieve significant reform in our health-care system has focused attention on the growing role that states will assume in this regard. NP involvement in the development of state and federal programs and policies affecting health-care delivery is essential. Perhaps even more formidable than government-initiated reforms are the changes in health-care delivery being driven by marketplace reform. As health care moves from a cost-reimbursed delivery system to competitive managed care, NPs must be positioned to market themselves to the health-care business community as cost-effective primary care providers (Ryan, 1993; Spitzer, 1984) (see Chapter 23).

In this era of rapidly changing health-care delivery, there has been renewed interest in the concept of interdisciplinary collaboration and teamwork in primary care (Baldwin, 1994; Fagin, 1992; Hanson, 1993; Mundinger, 1994) (see Chapter 11). Mundinger (1994) suggests that a collaborative practice model of NPs and physicians working together to deliver primary care is the best because it "reduces cost while enhancing quality and comprehensiveness" (p. 213). These factors are important to today's climate of many patients with few resources. As Hanson (1993) observes, "Our earliest efforts to establish our professional identity as NPs focused on gaining independence and autonomy from physicians"; this was a critical step. Now, to move forward in cooperation with other health-care professions, "we need to shift our practice ideal from complete autonomy toward a more collegial, interdisciplinary paradigm'' (p. 16A). Ryan (1993) concurs and urges that as our health-care system becomes increasingly interdependent, ''research must be encouraged to determine the most cost-effective mix of nurses and physician providers in various practice settings, in emerging delivery systems, and with different populations'' (p. 45). This concerted move toward a collaborative practice model strengthens the NP's place in the provision of primary health care for the future.

CONCLUSION

As stated earlier, primary care NPs have been recognized as pioneers in NP practice. This APN role was conceived to enhance access to cost-effective health care for underserved populations. The climate in the provision of health-care services is favorable to all APNs but most assuredly NPs as the nation moves toward prepaid, managed systems of care. With a renewed emphasis on primary care in today's health-care delivery system, the demand for primary care NPs is increasing. The IOM's updated definition of primary care (Institute of Medicine, 1994) encompasses much of the essence of advanced practice nursing and highlights the major role of NPs in primary care delivery.

The skills and competencies of primary care NP practice have been described to provide a more comprehensive overview of this advanced practice role. They can be categorized in three areas: management of health and illness status, teaching and counseling, and organizational and role competencies. As with other APN roles, the continued professional development of NPs will lead to greater proficiency in each of the competencies over time. Given the dynamic nature of the NP role, this description of competency should not be considered to address the entirety of NP practice.

Our health-care system, no doubt, will continue to evolve with marketplace and policy reforms shaping its future. NPs will assume a critical role in the primary care workforce of the future if they take an active role in developing health policy and care delivery systems today. Both professional unity and interdisciplinary collegiality must undergird these efforts.

REFERENCES

American Nurses Association. (1987). *Standards of practice for the primary health care nurse practitioner.* Washington, D. C.: American Nurses Association.

American Nurses Association. (1985). *The scope of practice of the primary health care nurse practitioner.* Washington, D.C.: American Nurses Association.

Baldwin, D. C., Jr. (1994). *The role of interdisciplinary education and teamwork in primary care and health care reform.* Rockville, MD: Department of Health and Human Services, Bureau of Health Professions.

Brown, S. A., & Grimes, D. E. (1993). *Nurse practitioners and certified nurse midwives: A meta-analysis of process of care, clinical outcomes,* and cost-effectiveness of nurses in primary care roles (#NP-85). Washington, D. C.: American Nurses Association.

Clawson, D. K., & Osterweis, M. (Eds.). (1993). *The roles of physician assistants and nurse practitioners in primary care.* Washington, D. C.: Association of Academic Health Centers.

Fagin, C. M. (1992). Collaboration between nurses and physicians: No longer a choice. *Academic Medicine, 67*(5), 295-303.

Ford, L. C., & Silver, H. K. (1967). The expanded role of the nurse in child care. *Nursing Outlook, 15,* 43-45.

Hanson, C. M. (1993). Collegiality counts: Our role in health care reform.'' *American Journal of Nursing, 93*(12), 16A-E.

Institute of Medicine, Committee on the Future of Primary Care (1994). *Defining primary care: An interim report.* Washington, D. C.: National Academy Press.

Mundinger, M. O. (1994). Advanced practice nursing—Good medicine for physicians? *New England Journal of Medicine, 330*(3), 211-214.

National Organization of Nurse Practitioner Faculties (1995). *Advanced practice nursing: Nurse practitioner curriculum guidelines and program standards.* Washington, D. C.: National Organization of Nurse Practitioner Faculties.

Nichols, L. M. (1992). Estimating costs of underusing advanced practice nurses. *Nursing Economics, 10*(5), 342-351.

Osterweis, M., & Garfinkel, S. (1993). The roles of physicians assistants and nurse practitioners in primary care: An overview of the issues. In M. Osterweis & S. Garfinkel (Eds.), *The roles of physician assistants and nurse practitioners in primary care* (pp. 1-9). Washington, D. C.: Association of Academic Health Centers.

Ryan, S. A. (1993). Nurse practitioners: Educational issues, practice styles, and service barri-

ers. In M. Osterweis & S. Garfinkel (Eds.), *The roles of physician assistants and nurse practitioners in primary care* (pp. 41-49). Washington, D. C.: Association of Academic Health Centers.

Safriet, B. (1992). Health care dollars and regulatory sense: The role of advanced practice nursing. *Yale Journal on Regulation, 9*(2), 149-220.

Spitzer, W. O. (1984). The nurse practitioner revisited: Slow death of a good idea. *New England Journal of Medicine, 310*(16), 1049-1051.

U.S. Congress, Office of Technology Assessment (1986). *Nurse practitioners, physician assistants, and certified nurse midwives: A policy analysis* (Health Technology Case Study 37). Washington, D. C.: U.S. Government Printing Office.

Virginia Joint Commission on Health Care (1994). *Optimum use of nurse practitioners* (SJR 164). (Available from Joint Commission on Health Care, Old City Hall, 1001 East Broad Street, Suite 115, Richmond, VA 23219).

Washington Consulting Group (1994). *Survey of certified nurse practitioners and clinical nurse specialists: December 1992, final report.* Washington, D. C.: Health Resources and Services Administration, Division of Nursing.

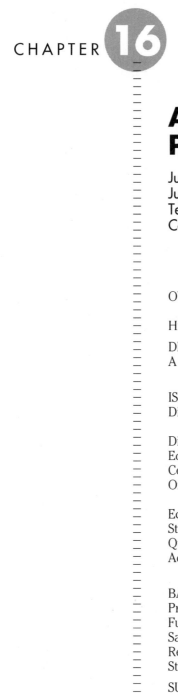

CHAPTER 16

Acute Care Nurse Practitioner

Judy Wright Lott
Judith D. Polak
Terry Boyle Kenyon
Carole A. Kenner

OVERVIEW OF THE ACUTE CARE NURSE PRACTITIONER ROLE

The acute care setting is a relatively new arena for the nurse practitioner (NP) in terms of formal standards and education. The acute care NP (ACNP) provides the same services as any other NP, but the scope of practice includes acute and critically ill patients. The purpose of the ACNP is to provide advanced nursing care to patients who are acutely or critically ill in a variety of settings. This care is continuous and comprehensive and is provided in a collaborative model involving patients, significant others, nurses, and other health-care providers. The ACNP serves as a patient case manager in acute care settings and may also provide education, consultation, leadership, and research. The ACNP's specialty body of knowledge is derived from specific acute and critical care phenomena experienced by the patient population of the specialty area. The ACNP assesses complex, acutely ill patients through health history-taking, physical and mental status examination, and risk appraisal for complications. Diagnostic reasoning and advanced therapeutic interventions, consultation, and referral to other nurses, physicians, and providers are intrinsic components of this role. ACNPs incorporate and apply appropriate theories to guide their practice. The short-term goal is stabilization of the patient, minimizing complications and providing physical and psychological care measures. The long-term goal is the restoration to maximum health potential and evaluation of risk factors for achieving this outcome. Acute care advanced nursing practice can take place in all types of settings that require the use of complex technologies, including hospitals—primarily intensive care units, trauma centers, and emergency departments—thus creating the ACNP role (American Nurses Association and American Association of Critical-Care Nurses [ANA/AACN], 1995; Keane & Richmond, 1993). As this role has emerged, advanced practice nurses (APNs) have begun to network with interdisciplinary colleagues to help further develop the role and the settings in which the role can be successfully integrated (Harrigan & Perez, in press). There is an acute need for this information sharing because this role is still evolving, in contrast with the roles of most other APNs.

The role of NPs in ambulatory care has been well documented since the 1960s. Many studies have demonstrated their impact, the quality of care they provide, the cost-effectiveness of this care, and patient satisfaction with their services (Kubala & Clever, 1974; Prescott & Driscoll, 1980; Spitzer et al., 1974; see Chapter 26). The role of the ACNP has not been as extensively documented in the literature because it is a relatively new role. The neonatal NP (NNP) role, which originated in the late 1970s, is the oldest ACNP role. This chapter explores the role of the NP in the acute care setting. It discusses the history of the role and evolution of educational programs, delineates the ACNP's scope of practice, identifies current issues, and examines future direction and expansion of the role. The reader will note that the term ACNP will be used to include titles such as tertiary NP, critical care NP, and pediatric intensivist.

HISTORY OF THE ACNP ROLE

Neonatal Nurse Practitioner

As noted, the first documented role of the ACNP was the NNP, developed in the late 1970s in response to a substantial undersupply of neonatal specialist physicians

(Silver & McAtee, 1988; Watkins, Kirchoff, Hartigan, & Karp, 1992). Traditionally, medical care in the neonatal intensive care unit (NICU) in teaching hospitals was provided by pediatric residents. The residents devoted a majority of their total training time to the neonatal service. The needs of the patients and hospitals were adequately met, but such training poorly served the educational goals of the pediatric residents. In response, the Residency Review Committee of the Accrediting Council of Graduate Medical Education established new guidelines to limit the total time a resident could devote to neonatal intensive care. At the same time, there were cutbacks in the numbers of pediatric residents due to a perceived overabundance or a maldistribution of pediatricians in the United States, coupled with increasing acuity and complexity of patients. These factors resulted in shortages of bedside medical care providers in NICUs. Additionally, there was a desire for more autonomy and responsibility by bedside neonatal nurses. Highly skilled and experienced neonatal nurses were educated to perform a wide range of activities, such as providing selected medical services, transporting critically ill infants, and resuscitating infants in the delivery room (Clancy & Maguire, 1995; Watkins et al., 1992).

The education, titles, certification, and scope of practice of these early NNPs varied widely, depending on local custom, hospital policy, or the state nurse practice act. Education of these nurses was institutionally based, with primary responsibility assumed by neonatologists and previously "trained" NNPs. As the demand for NNPs increased in the early 1980s, there was a need for more educational programs to prepare them. Unfortunately, this need was not met within existing nursing graduate education programs. The majority of NNP education programs were hospital-based or operated under the auspices of medical departments. Because these programs were not university-based and were not affiliated with nursing programs, they awarded a continuing education units "certificate" rather than graduate credit upon completion. Requirements for entry and type and amount of preparation received varied widely.

The National Association of Neonatal Nurses (NANN) has responded to its members' concerns regarding inadequate numbers of NNPs for the rapidly growing advanced practice market, the lack of NNP programs in its specialty across the country, the inconsistency in educational preparation of students, and the variable competence of program graduates. The NANN issued a position statement supporting graduate education as the entry level for the NNP and developed "Program Guidelines for Neonatal Nurse Practitioner Educational Preparation" (National Association of Neonatal Nurses, 1994). Two areas specifically addressed and delineated in the guidelines were general curriculum content recommendations and entry-level competency statements. The primary goal of this document was to facilitate the development and evaluation of graduate NNP programs. Additionally, it provides a guide for academic programs as they evolve, and it can also be used by accrediting, regulatory, and certifying bodies in the evaluation of NNP programs.

The NNP role has, to some extent, survived the test of time. There is now greater national demand for NNPs to serve the needs of institutions providing care to preterm and critically ill newborns. It is hoped by the authors that other ACNP roles continue to develop, using the experiences learned through the evolution of the NNP role.

Other ACNP Roles

The history of other ACNP roles is less clear because they have only recently emerged in response to the perceived health-care needs of specific populations. In the early 1980s, also in response to cutbacks in pediatric residency programs, the role of the "hospital NP" in pediatrics was developed (Murphy, Gitterman, & Silver, 1985). In collaboration with pediatricians, these nurses managed the care of a group of assigned children on the pediatric floor. Their education was also institutionally based, although modeled after standard pediatric NP certificate programs.

Silver and McAtee (1988) proposed to correct the undersupply of physicians, residents, and fellows in specialty practice with the use of NPs in the hospital setting. These NPs would receive augmented training in order to assume many of the functions and activities of physician residents and fellows. The goal of this proposal was to provide high-quality acute care in the face of physician reductions, particularly in teaching hospitals. To meet this goal, acute care nurses were educated in areas such as managing and prescribing care that had up to this time been the purview of the physician. Silver and McAtee (1988) envisioned nurses utilizing increased skills and greater decision-making responsibilities to admit patients to the hospital, complete the history and physical examination, and assess initial clinical status and subsequent changes in the patient's condition. These nurses would also write relevant medical orders, perform a variety of diagnostic and therapeutic tests, order and interpret laboratory studies, and counsel patients and their families in collaboration with physicians.

Swan (1993) described a new role for the ACNP. In 1989, the Hospital of the University of Pennsylvania opened an Admissions Evaluation Center staffed by NPs in collaboration with the Department of Anesthesiology. The shared goals of the center were to optimize the health of the patient before a surgery or procedure; plan the most appropriate care management; assess patient's preoperative and postoperative health-care needs, including discharge planning and follow-up care; and reduce patient and family anxiety through teaching and planning. Major clinical functions of these NPs include history-taking and physical examinations; performing pre-anesthesia evaluations; providing patient and family education; obtaining laboratory, electrocardiographic, and radiological data; identifying at-risk individuals in need of pre-admission discharge planning; initiating contacts with social services; and discharge planning. Because it is possible to foresee the growth of this type of ACNP, one can imagine the further cost- and time-effectiveness achieved with collaboration among the other in-patient APNs such as certified registered nurse anesthetists (CRNAs).

The ACNP role did indeed proliferate in the early 1990s because of cutbacks in medical education, hospital cost-containment measures, expanded graduate nursing education programs, and cutbacks in general medical education programs (American Association of Critical-Care Nurses [AACN], 1995; Clochesy, Daly, Idemoto, Steel, & Fitzpatrick, 1994; Ingersoll, 1995; Keane & Richmond, 1993). Since the 1970s there has been a move by the American Academy of Pediatrics (AAP) to educate pediatric residents more in primary care than in acute, critical care of pediatric patients; this was one impetus for the creation of the NNP role. In addition, many hospitals have expanded their specialty services even though they have cut back on the amount of house staff they train. Non-academic institutions are also expanding services and have needed to find a way to provide sufficient coverage. Hospital administrators are looking for the best way to provide that coverage; one solution is to prepare NPs to practice in acute care settings. All of these factors within the recent economic and political health-care environment have been instrumental in the movement of the NP into the acute care setting to fill perceived gaps in the health-care system (Keane & Richmond, 1993).

Now there are ACNPs working not only in NICUs but also in pediatric ICUs, emergency rooms, and various adult medical-surgical specialties. Thus far, little documentation about the planning, development, implementation, or evaluation of these roles is available. ACNPs working in various specialties must provide needed documentation and standardization of their roles. The American Association of Critical-Care Nurses (AACN) and the American Nursing Association (ANA) have published *Standards of Clinical Practice and Scope of Practice for the Acute Care Nurse Practitioner* (ANA/AACN, 1995). This document identifies standards of care and professional performance for the ACNP, based on the nursing process. It includes standards for assessment, diagnosis, outcome identification, planning, implementation, and evaluation. The standards are listed in Table 16–1 and should be used as a guide for further development of the ACNP role.

DESCRIPTION OF THE ACNP ROLE

In general, the ACNP role has not been clearly established or defined. The scope of practice is primarily determined by patient population, setting, state legislation, nurse practice acts, and professional standards of practice set forth by specific specialty organizations. The purpose of the ACNP is to provide advanced nursing care across the continuum of acute care services to patients who are acutely and critically ill (ANA/AACN, 1995).

The role of the ACNP varies from specialty to specialty and from institution to institution. As this role continues to expand, it must be standardized as much as possible. Although the wide variation in patient populations will continue to dictate some differences, essential components of the role need to be identified and clearly described. In general, the ACNP has clear responsibilities within the organization; competency in the skills of assessment, management, and advanced diagnostic and therapeutic interventions; specialized knowledge consistent with the needs of patients in the acute care setting; strong linkages with medicine; and primary

TABLE 16–1. STANDARDS FOR ACUTE CARE PRACTITIONERS

Standard I. Assessment
The acute care nurse practitioner collects the patient data.

Standard II. Diagnosis
The acute care nurse practitioner analyzes the assessment data in determining diagnoses.

Standard III. Outcome Identification
The acute care nurse practitioner identifies expected outcomes individualized to the patient.

Standard IV. Planning
The acute care nurse practitioner develops a plan of care that prescribes interventions to attain expected outcomes.

Standard V. Implementation
The acute care nurse practitioner implements the interventions identified in the multidisciplinary plan of care.

Standard VI. Evaluation
The acute care nurse practitioner evaluates the patient's progress toward attainment of expected outcomes.

Adapted with permission from ANA/AACN (1995). *Standards of clinical practice and scope of practice for the acute care nurse practitioner* (pp. 19–23). Washington, D. C.: American Nurses Publishing.

responsibility and authority for a full range of patient care activities (Keane & Richmond, 1993).

The ACNP role generally can be divided into two major forms. In one form the focus is on episodic care of patients on a particular unit during hospitalization for acute care problems. The second form involves case management of patients throughout their hospitalization. As an example of the episodic focus, an ACNP working in the cardiac ICU would manage, in collaboration with a physician, the health care of a patient admitted to the cardiac ICU with an acute myocardial infarction but would transfer the care of that patient to another provider when the patient's condition no longer warranted intensive care. On the other hand, an NNP commonly manages the patient's care from the time of admission to the NICU until discharge of the patient from the hospital. Although different, these models each have advantages and disadvantages. The episodic care model provides the ACNP with an excellent opportunity to become highly skilled and knowledgeable about a specific condition in a delimited setting. However, this model does not provide long-term continuity for the nurse and patient. The case management model provides the ACNP with a broader patient focus that requires knowledge and expertise beyond the initial condition, and it does provide opportunities for long-term continuity of care. This model works well in specialties with a more homogeneous population in which patients remain on one unit for a longer time. The type of practice model should be thoroughly researched before the ACNP role is introduced, and the differences should be considered in light of the needs of the patient, the needs and availability of ACNPs, and the institution's mission and services. The case management model is the preferred focus, although the episodic model is more common. The case management model fits with the current trends in health care delivery, which focus on a continuum of care (Harrigan & Perez, in press).

Case management involves individualized and ongoing care with continuity provided to the patient and family during hospitalization, throughout discharge to home, and at follow-up (Liljeblad, 1993). ACNPs based on general medical, surgical, and pediatric units with homogeneous populations can still utilize this systematic approach to patient care through their organized, consistent, collaborative approach to caregiving. When ACNPs are unit-based, their goal is to facilitate and coordinate a patient's hospital stay to provide quality care efficiently and cost-effectively. ACNPs work in settings that are generally considered high-intensity, such as the emergency rooms; neonatal, pediatric, and adult ICUs; and some other various acute care in-patient settings (Clochesy et al., 1994; Dale, 1991; Murphy, Gitterman, & Silver, 1985; Richmond & Keane, 1992; Spisso, O'Callahan, McKennan, & Holcroft, 1990).

Specific responsibilities may include admission of patients to the hospital in collaboration with a physician, completion of history and physical examination, assessment of initial clinical status and subsequent changes in the patient's condition, performance of a variety of diagnostic and therapeutic tests and procedures, ordering and interpretation of laboratory or radiology studies, patient and family education, and preparation for discharge. In addition, ACNPs in specialty areas with long-term patient care responsibilities provide health promotion and maintenance and may also provide resource information and respond to telephone inquiries from ancillary personnel, families, and patients (Gleeson, McIlvain-Simpson, Boos, Sweet, Trzcinski, Solberg, & Doughty, 1992).

A TYPICAL DAY IN THE LIFE OF AN ACNP: THE NEONATAL NP

Although the specific responsibilities vary widely with the actual setting, there are many similarities in jobs held by ACNPs. Because the NNP is the oldest of the ACNP roles, it will be used as an exemplar for the ACNP. The NNP role has the best-defined scope of practice of all ACNP roles. The NNP uses an advanced neonatal knowledge base, physical examination skills, and diagnostic interventions to define the plan of care in collaboration with the neonatologist and nursing staff. The NNP then implements the plan through writing appropriate orders and continually evaluating the infant. The NNP communicates with the family through routine telephone calls and visits at the bedside, maintains collegial relationships with multidisciplinary team members, and responds to sudden changes that develop in the infant's condition (Liljeblad, 1993). NNPs generally follow a daily "routine," although their activities may differ with the level of patient acuity and need for emergency care. This routine may include receiving regular sign-out (report) from their colleagues on the status of patients, followed by assessment of patients, participation in patient-focused rounds with the health-care team, participation in radiology rounds to assess or review patient x-rays, attendance at educational offerings (such as grand rounds, morbidity and mortality conference, nursing lectures), and direct patient management with diagnosis, interpretation of clinical findings, laboratory data, and radiological data. NNPs are responsible for writing all orders on patients on their service and for writing progress notes, procedural notes, and admission, interim, transfer, or discharge summaries. NNPs work closely with nursing staff as well as with other multidisciplinary team members to provide care to their patients. In addition to managing these aspects of the job, the NNP also has to be prepared to handle emergency admissions (from labor and delivery or transfer) and may also be responsible for coordinating simple or complex hospital discharges. Often NNPs are responsible for emergency situations outside their actual unit, such as attendance at high-risk deliveries for management of at-risk neonates. NNPs may also manage healthy newborns in the newborn nursery or may be called to assist with procedures (within the realm of their practice) on a pediatric floor.

Like the primary care NP, the NNP must be adept at time management. However, unlike the primary care NP, the NNP deals with the ongoing hour-by-hour maintenance care of a particular infant or group of infants with acute health-care problems. Because of the nature of illnesses seen in the NICU, a major component of the NNP's day is frequent patient reassessment. This allows the NNP to evaluate and modify therapeutic modalities, assess patient status, and make or update plans according to significant clinical findings. This continuous availability enhances the patient's care. RNs providing bedside care consider this a positive benefit to the NNP service because their concerns are addressed as they occur and do not have to wait.

The role of the NNP also is unique in that the majority of the NNP's patients remain in the NICU until discharge. The predominant model of care used by NNPs to care for their patients is primary care. NNPs manage a patient's care from admission to discharge or transfer to another facility. In the case of a very preterm infant or an infant with a severe illness that will require extensive hospitalization, this primary care model results in a long-term relationship with the neonate and family. Preterm or critically ill neonates are a unique population, requiring acute management of their initial illness and subsequent complications. However, they also require the type of care that would be considered primary care, such as well-child care, preventative care, parental education, care of chronic conditions that develop as sequelae to prematurity or therapy, and care of minor illnesses throughout their hospitalization. This type of management makes up a large part of the NNP role. As a consequence, NNPs deliver both acute and primary care to their patients, a fact that has confused other ACNPs. Typically, NNPs maintain a caseload of patients in various stages of their illness and recovery. Thus, an NNP may have a caseload of 6 to 10 patients, some of whom are acutely ill and some of whom are less acutely ill. Preterm or critically ill infants frequently move back and forth between periods of acute illness and periods of relative stability during their hospitalization. Because the NNP has cared for the infant since admission and well knows the patient's history and baseline health status, the NNP is better able to detect subtle or early signs that the infant is becoming more acutely ill or is not progressing satisfactorily. This ongoing relationship with the neonate and family constitutes one of the most satisfying aspects of the NNP role.

It would be helpful if the definitions of primary and acute care were based on the type of care provided, rather than on the setting in which the care is provided. King and Ackerman (1995) pointed out that the term "acute care" may not adequately address the scope of practice and the clinical expertise necessary for practice in a particular area or to define the field of specialization. It is highly important that the type of practice model being used to describe the ACNP role be clearly described in discussions of this role to prevent misconceptions about its scope of practice. It is the opinion of the authors that the lack of understanding of ACNP practice has created some confusion in legislation, practice, and education of the ACNP. Having the type of care so closely identified with its setting may preclude development of other appropriate ACNP roles and prevent some of the most satisfying components of the ACNP role from being recognized or developed.

The NNP uses a holistic approach to the management of patients, making sure to evaluate the patient's physical health status as well as the psychosocial and developmental needs of the patient. Because NNPs manage acutely ill patients, they are frequently responsible for communicating with patient's family members as well. It is vitally important for NNPs to use their communication skills to keep the patient and family updated. Good communication is an important tool that helps to decrease patient and family anxiety; good communication also is useful in educating patients and families so that they understand what is expected for the patient's care and outcome.

Often the NNP also has other responsibilities, including providing education for staff, meeting the rigors and challenge of participating in clinical research, or consulting with outside consultants or other professional colleagues. Patient management is always the priority for NNPs, and it is sometimes difficult to balance these other responsibilities and maintain high-quality patient management. However, these other activities should be an essential part of the NNP's job. It is these other responsibilities, in addition to the unique nursing skills, that make NNPs so valuable and clearly distinguish this role from that of resident physicians, with whom NNPs often work. It is also important for NNPs to be involved in designing and conducting research, because they are in a unique position to facilitate useful, needed nursing research, which then strengthens the scientific basis for neonatal nursing care. Thus, it is beneficial that NNPs have "off-service" time to pursue scholarly activities. Scholarly activities are important to the long-term survival and development of the role. How these activities are carried out may vary according to individual interest, institutional resources, and patient care needs. These activities, along with the holistic, comprehensive view that NPs bring to patient care, are what set the ACNP role apart from the roles of resident physicians, who tend to focus on management of the patient's physical problems. Resident physicians rarely "care" for the family or the psychosocial issues. These latter activities of the ACNP are similar to the activities of their APN colleagues.

ISSUES IN THE DEVELOPING ACNP ROLE

ACNPs face many issues in their daily work situations and in the further evolution of the ACNP role. ACNPs, by virtue of the setting in which they function, are faced with some unique issues that may differ from those of NPs in primary care settings. These issues include differentiation of the ACNP from other APNs and resident physicians, education and certification requirements for the role, organizational placement (collaboration with physicians versus supervision by physicians), economic viability and marketability of the role, quality assurance or evaluation of the effectiveness of the role, performance of advanced diagnostic and therapeutic interventions, and staffing and scheduling. These issues are addressed in this section.

DIFFERENTIATION OF THE ACNP FROM OTHER ANP ROLES AND THE PHYSICIAN ASSISTANT ROLE

The NP role differs from the other ANP roles in the type of care given. NPs give advanced nursing care that includes medical management in collaboration with physicians and other health-care team members. The ACNP role differs from other NP roles primarily by the type and acuity of the patient as well as the setting in which care occurs. Other NPs, such as pediatric NPs, women's health NPs, and family NPs, typically work in ambulatory or out-patient care areas. The primary focus of the care provided by these NPs is health maintenance, health promotion, prevention of illnesses, and care of minor illnesses. As noted earlier, ACNPs provide advanced nursing care across the continuum of acute care services to acutely and critically ill patients of a designated patient population. The primary focus of the ACNP is diagnosis and management of acute illnesses; however, ACNPs may also provide health promotion and maintenance care. It is important to recognize that these differences may not be so distinct in actual practice, because ACNPs may also provide some "primary" care services (particularly in the case of the NNP, as noted earlier), and primary care NPs may initiate "acute" care services.

In contrast to the clinical nurse specialist (CNS), the ACNP tends to be unit-based and primarily provides direct patient care. The American Nurses Association (in press) defines the CNS as a clinical expert who advocates for a specific nursing speciality. The CNS provides direct patient care and acts as a consultant, educator, and researcher. The ACNP provides comprehensive assessment, diagnosis, and care management for a specific population of clients. This practitioner may promote wellness, prevent illness or complications, and provide acute or chronic care (American Nurses Association [ANA], in press). The ACNP will prescribe the treatment plan that may be carried out by other nurses or, in some instances, physicians. The CNS historically has functioned as the unit educator and consultant for problematic patient care issues. In some settings, CNSs have not maintained a direct patient practice, although that is a clear expectation of the CNS role (see Chapter 14). The CNS might be located on a specific unit such as a neonatal CNS, whereas other CNSs work across departments, such as maternal-child CNSs who work with obstetrics, neonatal, and pediatric staffs. Often CNSs conduct patient support groups or focus on patient education. The role differentiations between these two APNs are not always this clear-cut because of institutional variations and the skills of each APN.

APNs, including the ACNP, are different from physician assistants (PAs). There are differences in philosophy, education, experience, scope of practice, approach to the patient, and relationship with the physician. PAs are educated to assist physicians; their role allows no independent or autonomous functions. Legally, PAs must work *under the supervision of physicians.* The ACNP collaborates with a physician and provides advanced nursing care using the nursing process as a foundation for assessment and therapeutic intervention. The ACNP's practice includes the holistic approach of nursing rather than focusing on the disease or illness, as is common in the medical model.

DIFFERENTIATION OF THE ACNP AND HOUSE OFFICER ROLES

It is vitally important to understand that ACNPs are not simply replacement staff for resident house officers. Although it is true that ACNPs often work alongside house staff, providing them with a vital resource and role model, ACNPs should not be viewed or treated as a member of the house staff. They should be valued for the unique contribution they make as APNs who bring to their role both the advanced nursing skills and medical competencies needed to provide consistent and high-quality patient management.

Many physicians see ACNPs as physician extenders only. They feel that the role permits the assignment of tasks that the busy physician derives little benefit from or is inclined to put off (commonly known as "scut work"). These tasks include maintaining relationships with families' referring physicians, scheduling appointments, arranging for discharge, and other duties that are related to patient care but are not direct patient care. If physicians do not recognize the difference between the ACNP and the house officer role, they have no reason to support the role, which they see as "costing" more to provide care that could just as easily be provided by resident physicians. Physicians could also view ACNPs as competing with physicians, although the close collaboration required for the ACNP role makes this less likely than in the primary NP role.

ACNPs, by virtue of their education and in-depth clinical experience, should be viewed as experts and should be capable of functioning with physician collaboration, not supervision. Resident physicians vary in their level of experience and interest in specialty areas. They rotate through various departments as part of their continuing education. However, an appropriately prepared ACNP with ongoing experience in the specialty area continues to gain expertise in the patient care in that area. Collaboration between resident physicians and ACNPs provides both with the opportunity to learn from each other, thus enhancing patient care, collegiality, and education. Although ACNPs and residents may collaborate regarding issues of patient management, the resident and the ACNP ultimately answer to the physician in charge. At this point in the evolution of the ACNP role, the physician in charge may have "a little to say" about the ACNP's practice. This function may look like "supervision," especially with regard to what had been traditional medical responsibility. This situation is more a reflection of the lack of ACNPs who have practiced, written about, and defined the scope and nature of ACNP practice. As more ACNPs are prepared and acquire experience, this situation will change. This change must start with the educational process.

EDUCATION FOR THE ACNP ROLE

As health-care needs change, nursing roles also change. It is often after the creation of a particular new APN role that nursing education programs recognize the need to provide appropriate specialty education programs at the master's level to prepare graduates for these roles. Better communication between administrators of clinical areas and faculty of nursing programs is needed to better facilitate appropriate specialty education. Administrators, nurses in the specialty area, and faculty need to plan for a new role, including educational components, before implementation of the role. This planning has not been uniform, and it has created much of the confusion about the role of the ACNP, as well as the lack of standardization of ACNP competencies.

Because of wide variations in practice areas, the education of ACNPs has been inconsistent. As mentioned previously, many initial ACNPs received on-the-job, apprentice, hospital-based training. The primary educators were physicians with the help of previously trained practitioners. Education focused on technical skills and implementation of standing orders. There was little or no didactic education, and graduates had little or no standing to practice outside their hospital department.

Today, graduate education is the accepted preparation for ACNPs. The graduate ACNP curriculum generally consists of core master's-level courses such as nursing theory, leadership, research, and health-care policy and core clinical courses. Clinical courses focus on patient and family assessment, clinical decision-making, and case management skills (ANA/AACN, 1995; National Association of Neonatal Nurses [NANN], 1994). Students spend varying amounts of time in clinical practice, depending on their specialty and requirements for certification. King and Ackerman (1995) proposed that the curriculum for ACNPs include three major areas: concepts and issues inherent to professional socialization, common knowledge for all APNs, and specialty practice knowledge (see also Chapter 4).

Clochesy et al. (1994) described different participants and their functions in an ACNP program. Leadership for the program is provided by an academic program coordinator, an interagency liaison, and an advisory committee. The academic program director is responsible for curriculum development, course development, teaching, coordinating clinical experiences, and mentoring students in the new role. The interagency liaison facilitates communication between the school and hospital clinical sites. The advisory committee, with multidisciplinary membership, makes recommendations to the faculty about the student's clinical experiences and placement. This committee may also make recommendations to hospitals about role development and implementation. All of these participants are responsible for program evaluation.

Keane and Richmond (1993) made recommendations for the ACNP, or tertiary NP as they called this specialist. These recommendations were based on the belief that this type of practitioner must have a clinical specialty with in-depth knowledge of the specialty population of patients that would be served, and that holistic principles of advanced practice nursing must be included to differentiate this from medical practice. Their recommendations were to ensure that the following content areas were covered in an ACNP education: advanced physical and clinical assessments of the patient and family unit; advanced clinical decision-making, which would include laboratory and diagnostic test interpretation; pharmacological principles (both general and specific) principles of case management, cost-benefit analysis of technology in care settings; collaborative practice issues; mobilization of community resources; and a thorough knowledge of societal, political, and economic issues that affect the ACNP role and health-care delivery (Keane & Richmond, 1993). To cover these areas in education, experts are needed to share the knowledge. This sharing requires collaboration between faculty and practitioners in the development and implementation of educational programs.

The most important resources for ACNP programs are the ACNPs themselves. Practitioners are needed to serve as faculty, preceptors, and researchers. Given the relatively small pool of these newly emerging practitioners, accommodation between education and service must be negotiated to provide enough ACNPs to serve as preceptors, educators, and developers of curricula and research for practice. As new programs develop, educators must be flexible enough to allow for variation and experimentation while meeting the needs for standardization of educational requirements and service responsibilities.

To date, few nursing programs prepare graduates for ACNP roles other than neonatal NPs, pediatric NPs, and gerontological NPs. Most programs prepare adult or family primary care NPs, who then tailor their clinical experience to the specialty of interest. Educators must consider whether the trend to increase the numbers of ACNPs warrants recognition by offering the option of appropriate clinical and role content for in-patient practice within the curriculum.

In 1993, in the United States there were approximately 95,400 APNs with graduate education, with another 671,400 nurses certified in their specialty and holding baccalaureate degrees (National Council of State Boards of Nursing, 1993). Graduate preparation of the APN is a key criterion in the definition of advanced nursing practice (see Chapter 3). The National League for Nursing advocates graduate nursing education for the APN (National Council of State Boards of Nursing, 1993; National League for Nursing, 1994). This position is supported by the NANN, the professional organization that strives to represent the unique needs of the neonatal nursing specialty, which includes many APNs. It is the Association's belief that a common educational preparation, use of common advanced practice definitions, and clear ties to what roles APNs play in health-care delivery will increase the public's awareness of nursing's contribution to health care (NANN, 1994). NANN has established and published guidelines that address the entry level competencies of the NNP role, as well as general curriculum content guidelines for inclusion in an educational program that prepares NNPs (NANN, 1994). This information may be helpful to other ACNP programs as they develop. Chapter 4 discusses APN educational preparation in more detail.

CERTIFICATION REQUIREMENTS FOR ACNPs

Certification is provided by a non-governmental agency or association (National Council of State Boards of Nursing, 1993). It is a method of measuring and recognizing that an individual meets or exceeds minimal criteria designated for a specialty nurse. (For more discussion, see Chapters 3 and 22.) For the ACNP, however, there have been few avenues for certification. For the NNP specifically, the NCC Corporation in Chicago was the first agency to provide an examination designed for this specialty. It was available in the early 1980s. Almost a decade later the AACN identified a need for certification for ACNPs, especially pediatric and neonatal nurses. This examination was offered for the first time in 1993. The two examinations, although similar in scope (acute care), have different foci: the NCC examination is specific to the neonatal area, whereas the AACN examination tends to have more global concepts of critical care. Which is better? This choice is really up to the individual seeking certification, because this is still a voluntary process. This "voluntary" process, however, is a term of employment in some institutions. It is the position of the authors that certification in the appropriate specialty must be an integral part of the preparation for the ACNP, as it is for any APN role (see Chapter 3).

ORGANIZATIONAL PLACEMENT: SUPERVISION VERSUS COLLABORATION

The ACNP is often referred to by state practice guidelines as functioning under the "direct supervision" of physicians. As Safriet (1992) stated in her discussion about regulatory practices, this "old terminology" is a restriction on advanced practice. As the degree of responsibility and accountability for ACNPs and physicians increases, and as the management protocols of both professions overlap and broaden, ACNPs must gain uncontested authority to practice nursing in their advanced role within the professional domain of nursing (Steel, 1992). This change requires that the ACNP enter into an explicit collaborative practice with physician colleagues. ACNPs should collaborate with the physician in charge and ultimately be responsible for their own actions. ACNPs should not be put in the position of working under the supervision of a resident, because ACNPs are not part of the house staff. In setting up a model for how ACNPs will function in any given institution, it is of the utmost importance for the physician-ACNP relationship to be at the highest professional level of collegiality and for the ACNP to be a separate entity from the house staff. This collegiality can be facilitated by strong support and clear leadership from the nursing department, clear expectations from all parties, good communication skills between the ACNP and physician in charge, and mutual respect. Part of this collegiality can be built through the changes that are occurring within the health-care delivery environment.

The ACNP may be part of a joint professional practice with hospital privileges and report directly to the partners in the practice plan, or ACNPs may be hired by the hospital and report to the nursing executive or chief of a medical service.

The perceived lack of understanding of the ACNP role by nursing administration has been the primary rationale for placing ACNPs within a medical department. However, this is not the optimal resolution to the placement dilemma; it precludes the development of the relationship with nursing and creates some problems of its own. For instance, ACNPs can be easily overlooked within the medical department's decision-making process if they are not considered to be partners within the practice plan. There is potential for them to be dictated to rather than to be part of the decisions that affect them.

The authors believe that the preferred ACNP placement is within the nursing department, with an explicit collaborative relationship with the medical service. This is extremely important to the success of the role. It is vital that ACNPs have nursing support, especially if they are to participate in nursing endeavors. ACNPs, with their advanced education and advanced nursing skills, should be instrumental in influencing policy within the nursing hierarchy. ACNPs are capable of providing education, support, and mentorship to other nursing professionals on the health-care team. If ACNPs are hired by medicine they may not be encouraged to participate in nursing department activities, but ACNPs should insist on some relationship. There is a potential for the loss of a valuable nursing resource if nursing administrators do not embrace and foster ACNPs in their advanced nursing role. There is also a real danger that individual ACNPs will lose their identity as nurses and begin to identify entirely with medicine. This "medical identity" is particularly problematic when ACNPs are placed in house staff substitute positions.

Whether ACNPs are housed in nursing or not, effective relationships with nursing administration are important. There have been cases in which ACNPs found it difficult to function in their jobs with a reporting relationship to nursing. Depending on how nursing administration conceptualizes advanced nursing practice, nursing can be a great support or a formidable barrier to practice (see Chapter 24). Unfortunately, some nurse administrators view ACNPs as physician extenders only. Thus, when faced with budgetary or financial concerns, nursing administrators may see the ACNPs as a continual drain on nursing's budget and believe that they should be paid by medicine. Part of the problem is related to the unfortunate use in some institutions of ACNPs as resident substitutes only. In these cases nursing administration really does not have the potential benefit of the nurse's holistic care management but does bear the financial burden of the "medical coverage" problem. It is imperative that nursing professionals and educators speak about the advantages of the ACNP role to nursing administrators and that ACNPs refuse to function exclusively as physician substitutes. They must clearly demonstrate the advanced nursing aspects of their role if they are hired into a "substitute" position.

Some of the institutional regulations that pertain to general nursing staff may not be beneficial to APNs, who need autonomy to resolve issues creatively, flexibly, and without restriction. For example, scheduling needs and demands should serve the ACNP group, even though they may differ markedly from other nursing groups. ACNPs need to work closely with nursing administrators to facilitate understanding and appreciation of their role, thus enhancing their position within nursing.

Collaboration between physicians and ACNPs (see Chapter 11) is particularly essential to the continued development of the ACNP role. As the ACNP's scope of practice is delineated, collaboration will be a cornerstone of care management because no one specialty or discipline can meet all of the increasingly complex patient care needs. Other areas of collaboration will evolve through institutionally based practice opportunities; quality assurance activities, including published data on hospital's morbidity and mortality; and regulatory language that crosses disciplinary lines (McGivern, 1992). ACNPs may have particular difficulty claiming their clinical authority given the social structures of hospitals and the history of nurse-physician relationships. In many practices the physician has the ultimate authority regarding which approach to management will be taken. There is still an overall acceptance of this concept; the move to full collaboration is not completed. The ACNP who collaborates skillfully with physicians and other colleagues can help change the culture in hospitals so that a collaborative mode of practice prevails.

Social, legal, ethical, and economic reasons dictate the need for sound and effective collaborative relationships between ACNPs and physicians. Although it is feasible that experienced ACNPs will achieve a high degree of autonomy in their practice, the nature of acute care makes collaboration essential. Because patients often have complex health problems and constantly changing health-care needs, they provide a unique challenge to the members of the health-care team. Although ACNPs are adept at managing acutely ill patients, they need to be able to consult and collaborate with readily available physicians on a frequent "as needed" basis.

ECONOMIC AND MARKETABILITY ISSUES

The hiring and management of NPs in the acute care hospital is often a controversial and politically hot issue. There may be turf issues between nursing and medicine, and the kind of care the NP delivers may depend on who controls the economic pursestrings and who conducts the performance appraisals. Some economic disadvantages are attached to being hired by nursing administration in some instances. In today's environment the ACNP can be particularly vulnerable if nursing departments do not accept that ACNPs provide nursing care at an advanced level. Conversely, medical services often do not want to absorb the overhead associated with payment of ACNPs. ACNP fees for service may not be reimbursable from some third-party payers and there is often a misconception about what percentage of the ACNP's role is considered to be medically oriented versus nursing oriented.

ACNPs must understand the economic forces that influence their marketability. Although it is important for ACNPs to be as cost-effective as possible, it is also vital that they work toward being visible partners who can make significant economic contributions that serve to meet the fiscal demands of their health-care institution. This means that ACNPs must learn from and work with other APNs toward seeking nationwide reimbursement. Currently, many ACNPs are not reimbursed, although some states do allow some type of reimbursement for services provided by ACNPs. ACNPs must be politically astute and familiarize themselves with their state regulations regarding reimbursement, as well as continue to work with nursing organizations to optimize the status of all APNs. If they are eligible for reimbursement they must work with their administrators and with physicians to bring in revenue for their institutions. By doing this, ACNPs may enhance their ability to remain viable in a fickle health-care market (see Chapters 22 and 25).

STAFFING OR SCHEDULING

Most often, several ACNPs come together to form a team and utilize a team approach to provide services in their particular setting. Because acute care is provided on a 24-hour basis, an ACNP must be in-house at all times. Full-time coverage can be provided in a variety of ways. Many ACNP groups manage themselves autonomously, which includes making their own schedules. This allows the members of the group to maintain some flexibility in scheduling and control in self-governing. Many practice plans do not dictate how coverage is provided as long as it is done safely, equitably, and as cost-effectively as possible. To meet the workforce needs, different members of the team may choose to work 8-, 12-, 16-, or 24-hour shifts. Members of the team negotiate scheduling themselves in order to cover days or nights as needed.

In many settings, ACNPs provide management for an established caseload of patients and oversee certain aspects of patient management for the rest of their units. In some settings, however, the ACNPs "split" the workload with physicians and do not manage the same patients each day. This approach to care may be mandated because of the high acuity level of the patients. It is not the ideal way to provide patient care coverage, however. This method results in two undesirable effects: decreased continuity of care and fragmentation of the ACNP role. As noted earlier, one of the major satisfactions of the ACNP role is the ongoing relationship with the patient and family during the illness. If the ACNP does not follow the same patients on a daily basis, this relationship cannot develop to its fullest. More importantly, patient care can be compromised by the absence of a constant care provider who knows all aspects of the patient's condition, previous management strategies, and current and future health-care plans. Minor details are much more likely to be missed if the patient's care is managed by a different care provider every day. Also, important changes in the patient's condition or response to therapy may be missed when the care provider is not consistent. The fragmentation of patient care often leaves the ACNP relegated to doing the undesirable or less-satisfying portion of the workload. The inability to develop a care plan, implement it, and evaluate the patient's response to the plan decreases the opportunity for knowledge and skill development. Splitting the workload with physicians may also prevent the ACNP from having the opportunity to work with the most interesting or critical cases and reinforce the erroneous perception that the ACNP is simply a physician extender.

QUALITY IMPROVEMENT AND EVALUATION OF EFFECTIVENESS

It will take time for ACNPs to prove that they are cost-effective. Although NPs in primary care settings have compiled evidence to support their ability to provide quality, cost-effective care (Mundinger 1994; see Chapter 26), ACNPs must start to address these same issues and adequately prove their cost-effectiveness based on patient outcomes. Cost-effectiveness of primary care NPs cannot be routinely extrapolated to ACNPs working with hospitalized populations. There are few data at this point to substantiate claims of cost-effectiveness because of the relative newness of the ACNP role. How well ACNPs meet this challenge will determine the future of this role.

Because the NNP role is over 20 years old, more is known about this role than about other ACNP roles. However, despite the 20-year headstart, some important pieces of information are still missing. Interestingly, the one variable that is most often used to justify the existence of the NNP role—namely, cost-effectiveness—has not been thoroughly studied (Sims, Jasani, Yan, & Hodgman, 1987). The lack of studies of cost-effectiveness is probably due to the difficulty in identifying and quantifying all variables involved in health-care delivery. One recent study compared NNPs to pediatric house staff and showed that NNPs reduced costs by reducing the amount of ancillary charges and the number of days of hospitalization for their patients (Schultz, Liptak, & Fioravanti, 1994). Further studies must be undertaken with a focus on patient outcomes and economic outcomes to fully show the effectiveness of the ACNP role.

Although difficult to conduct, long- and short-term outcome studies will be necessary. It will be important not only to document accuracy and safety of treatment but also to note the effect of the ACNP role on patients' functional abilities, quality of life, and morbidity and mortality rates. Particular aspects to measure will be care related to patient education, counseling, and health promotion and maintenance. The impact of ACNP-delivered care on cost issues also should be studied. Does the care delivered by the ACNP affect length of stay, utilization of costly services such as ancillary testing and laboratory tests, or rehospitalization? How does the care provided by ACNPs compare with that provided by physicians? Further investigation is needed to determine characteristics that are unique to the ACNP role. Descriptive studies examining the domains of NP activities would define autonomous activities, delegated actions, and collaborative practice. What components of the care delivered are unique to the NP role in the acute care setting? Studies will be necessary to identify health-care subspecialties needing providers in the acute care setting as well as practice setting characteristics in which the ACNP can effectively deliver care. Finally, it will be helpful to identify current conditions that enhance or impede the ACNP in delivery of health care as the ACNP role continues to evolve. Barriers to practice in the ambulatory setting have been well documented. Little has been addressed in the acute care setting.

Ingersoll (1995) proposed that existing data sources are available to monitor ACNP performance and impact over time. Sources identified included consumers, peers, medical records, consultation notes (internal and external), daily or weekly process logs, quarterly reports, solicited and unsolicited letters, meeting minutes, hospital quality improvement data, publications (frequency, content, and type of journal), presentations (frequency, content, and location), and grant proposals (quality of proposal and revenue generated). Some of these data sources could be used for both process and outcome purposes. Ingersoll also pointed out that an important issue in the evaluation of NPs is the tendency to compare NP practice with physician practice. ACNPs bring additional aspects to their interactions with patients, families, and staff. It is not appropriate to only compare ACNP productivity with physician productivity in terms of numbers of patients covered or time spent with patients. NPs frequently spend more time with patients, and the patients assigned are often high-risk, elderly, or chronically ill; as a consequence, NPs may see fewer patients than physicians do.

Ostrea and Schuman (1975) examined quality of care provided by NPs practicing in an NICU. This study was conducted before certification or regulation of advanced practice occurred. They compared accuracy of the physical examination between NPs and physicians. The NP's examination was the same as the physician's 72% of the time. Minor differences in the remaining 28% related to the timing of the examination. NPs tended to spend more time actually conducting the examination, but the "content" of the examination was similar to that of the physicians' examinations. Mothers utilizing the NP service reported increased education about their own or their baby's care. The NP's patients were also more likely to return for clinic appointments.

Liljeblad (1993) noted improved family and staff satisfaction with the addition of NNPs to the NICU. The health-care team found it easier to establish trust and rapport with the parents of patients because there was consistent communication between the NNPs and the families, which increased the family's involvement in decision-making about the care of their infant.

Mitchell et al. (1991) compared 10 new NNP graduates and 13 second-year pediatric residents. NNPs showed knowledge and problem-solving, communication, and clinical skills equivalent to those of a second-year pediatric resident. Spisso et al. (1990) studied the effectiveness of trauma NPs. They stated that although NP positions were more costly than house staff in relation to annual salary and actual hours worked, the positions remained cost-effective, evidenced by a mean reduction in the patient length of stay of 1.05 days. The amount billed and the revenue generated for procedures and assessments performed by NPs increased substantially. Costs were offset by reduction of out-patient clinic waiting times and reduction of patient complaints. They concluded that the ACNPs saved the house staff an average of 352 minutes per day. Nursing staff (93%) felt that the role was effective in discharging patients, and 97% listed the role as effective in interacting with patients and families and in providing a liaison between RNs and physician staff.

ADVANCED CLINICAL DIAGNOSTIC AND THERAPEUTIC INTERVENTIONS

Acquisition of advanced technical skills is a large and essential component of the ACNP's education and subsequent clinical responsibilities. Skills that were previously performed solely by a physician are now routinely performed by ACNPs. These procedures can include chest tube insertion, umbilical arterial and venous catheterization, suprapubic bladder tap, percutaneous central venous line insertion, peripheral artery line insertion, intubation, bone marrow aspiration, lumbar punctures, circumcision, thoracentesis, and aspiration of cerebrospinal fluid through a ventricular reservoir. It is important that these skills be gained under appropriate conditions, with adequate supervision and direction during the educational program. In addition, because these skills are an integral component of the nursing care provided by ACNPs, a method for maintaining and demonstrating continuing competence must be established. Methods of demonstrating quality improvement and maintaining competence in infrequently performed procedures must be identified. Another important issue is the structure of the ACNP's position. These procedures are important and required for total patient management; however, they should not be the primary focus of the position. ACNPs need to ensure that sufficient time is available for the advanced nursing aspects of their role as well. This issue should be integral in the planning and implementation of the role, position descriptions, number of patients in the ACNP's caseload, and number of budgeted positions.

BARRIERS TO THE ACNP ROLE

Despite a long history of advanced nursing practice with much success, there are still many barriers to successful implementation of APN roles. For the ACNP, barriers include prescriptive authority, funding for education, salary, and reimbursement for services. ACNPs need to be aware of these barriers and unite with other APNs within and outside their setting to address them. Because the focus of the ACNP is acute care, it is important that ACNPs evaluate all potential strategies and legislative efforts to ensure that the practice of ACNPs will be appropriately addressed in these efforts. These major barriers are discussed in this section, followed by discussion of strategies to alleviate the barriers.

PRESCRIPTIVE AUTHORITY

Thus far, 43 states have legislation authorizing NPs to prescribe or dispense medications. The requirements, limitations, scope, and regulation of prescriptive authority varies widely from state to state (see Chapter 22). Mahoney (1995) did a pilot study of adult NPs in Massachusetts and found that 67% of those eligible for prescriptive authority had not applied for it because their employers would not permit NPs to prescribe, regardless of enabling legislation. The greatest support for prescriptive authority as evidenced by the fastest adoption of NP prescriptive authority occurred among smaller, private practices with physician employers. By contrast, the slowest adoption appeared to be among large organizations, especially teaching hospitals. Complex bureaucratic structures requiring approval by multiple committees composed mainly of physicians and administrators appeared to be the greatest problem.

FUNDING FOR EDUCATION

Federal funding for ACNP education programs is currently limited. In many states, legislation addressing advanced nursing practice uses the provision of primary care as part of the definition of the NP, thus imposing a barrier to ACNPs. Currently, most funding for NP programs is targeted at those providing primary care NPs. More of the pending legislation, however, is using a broader definition of "primary care," defining it as the first contact with the health-care system rather than preventative services in the restrictive sense. This shift toward defining primary care as a patient's first contact with the health system coupled with the support of continuous versus episodic care may help promote advanced practice educational opportunities, particularly those that are not specific to setting or type of care. Increasingly, care is population- and specialty-focused. The authors hope that ACNPs will be recognized as providers of care to many people formerly cared for by physicians in subspecialities and that ACNP education warrants federal support through graduate medical/nursing funds.

SALARY

ACNPs have widely varying salary ranges. NNPs have reported salary ranges from $19,000 to $150,000! The salary range is based not only on position responsibility but on geography and the perceived need for the role (Smithing & Wiley, 1995). As other ACNP specialties develop, salary issues may become more important. Salaries that are too low may preclude the development of potentially effective ACNP roles; however, salaries that are too high may also preclude the development of ACNP roles, because institutions may decide that it is more cost-effective to hire physicians.

REIMBURSEMENT FOR SERVICES

Reimbursement for services has been a historical barrier to the NP, especially the primary care NP. Direct economic competition between physician and NP may not be an obstacle in hospital-based practice situations, in which both groups are salaried or responsibilities are disparate. Medicare, Medicaid, and most other third-party payers pay hospitals for total operating costs, and most hospital accounting systems simply lump the costs of NP services together with other types of operating costs (Office of Technology Assessment, 1986). The hospitals are then responsible for paying salaried employees. Parrinello (1995) stated that there are no existing mechanisms for direct reimbursement for ACNPs who provide care to hospitalized patients. Although the federal government provides for reimbursement of all health-care providers in its programs (Medicare, Medicaid), individual states control what providers are eligible for reimbursement. Many states do not allow reimbursement for services not provided directly by physicians. Some states allow reimbursement for NP services as being "indirectly" provided by the physician. This issue is extremely important for ACNPs as well as for other hospital-based APNs.

The threat of government-mandated health-care reform triggered industry-driven health-care changes. One significant change that will affect the reimbursement issue is the capitation reimbursement system. In capitated systems, a specified amount of money is paid for health care regardless of how much it actually costs the system to provide that care. Thus, the fewer tests and interventions and the shorter the hospital stay, the healthier the system is financially. In this system, it doesn't matter who does the test, sees the patient, or delivers the care, as long as the quality is satisfactory. NPs may gain an edge from this system, because they are generally less expensive than specialist physicians, order fewer tests, and send patients home earlier (Parrinello, 1995).

STRATEGIES FOR ELIMINATING BARRIERS

Barriers to the ACNP role must be addressed by the individuals in the role, the educational programs that prepare them, the institutions that employ them, and the professional organizations that represent them. Some of the strategies recommended by the AACN specific to the ACNP role are discussed in this section (ANA/AACN, 1995) (see Table 16–2).

ACNPs should develop relationships with committee members, chairpersons,

TABLE 16–2. STRATEGIES FOR ELIMINATING BARRIERS TO PRACTICE
FOR ADVANCED PRACTICE NURSING

Be visible.

Articulate clear messages.

Know your opposition.

Include specific acknowledgment of advanced practice nursing and a basic definition of advanced practice nursing in legislative efforts.

Vest sole governmental authority over advanced practice nursing in the state board of nursing.

Eliminate statutory requirements for formalized APN-physician collaboration or practice agreements or requirements for physician supervision or direction of advanced practice nursing.

Include language that provides "plenary" prescriptive authority.

Include the definition of collaborative practice in legislative reports that accompany state statutes.

Modify statutory definitions of the practice of registered or professional nurses to include those acts authorized by the state board of nursing for advanced practice.

Expand reimbursement to include all services provided by APNs within their scope of practice.

Eliminate eligibility coverage requirements that depend on physician collaboration or supervision.

Eliminate restrictions on geographic or practice settings for services provided by APNs that are covered by federal regulations.

Eliminate payment differentiation between and among specialty categories of APNs.

Extend Medicaid regulations to reimburse APN services.

Include nondiscrimination requirements for health insurance, health-care service plans or contracts

Adapted with permission from ANA/AACN. (1995). *Standards of clinical practice and scope of practice for the acute care nurse practitioner.* Washington, D. C.: American Nurses Publishing.

assembly, congressional and senate leaders, and other health-care providers. In their own institutions, ACNPs should be active and involved in the leadership of nursing. Participation in local, state, and national professional organizations is a key activity to enhance visibility and understanding of the ACNP role.

ACNPs must be able to accurately describe their role and disseminate information about their role to other health-care providers, agencies, administrators, consumers, and other key people involved in decision-making. ACNPs must be able to educate others about their role and the benefits they provide.

APNs must know who the opposition is and take action to remove specific barriers to their practice. ACNPs should identify the people or groups who oppose the role and prepare appropriate data to dispute their claims.

Legislation in relationship to advanced practice should include a definition that will not limit or restrict the ability of APNs to practice within their scope of practice. Nor should such legislation mandate that practice be predicated on direct physician supervision. For example, plenary prescriptive authority is the least restrictive form of prescriptive authority, allowing APNs to administer, dispense, and prescribe controlled substances without the supervision, control, or oversight of another professional. When revisions of an individual state's nurse practice acts are being considered, language should be included that will allow other care providers to carry out orders written by all APNs. This language should also include nondiscrimination requirements for hospitals and other health-care agencies to grant clinical and admitting privileges to APNs.

SUMMARY

Health care has changed dramatically in organization and structure in response to internal and external demands. Nursing is a profession that strives to meet society's demand for nursing care. As a result, nursing continues to change and evolve as a profession. The ACNP role was developed in response to a perceived need for NPs in the critical care area. The NNP role has the longest history, because it was developed in the 1970s in response to a need for health-care providers in the NICU. This clinical role has remained relatively constant, with the NNP providing care for pre-term and critically ill newborns in the NICU. However, educational preparation for the role has progressed through several stages, from strictly hospital-based training programs, through certificate programs, to graduate education. Other ACNP roles, such as pediatric critical care, adult health, burn patient care, oncology patient care, and emergency department care, may benefit from the NNP experience in role development and design of educational curricula. Further development of the ACNP role should be based on an orderly, systematic evaluation of the need for the role, the critical content needed for successful practice in the role, and successful integration with other members of the health-care team. The ACNP role must be consistent with other APN roles, although the practice area may be different. ACNPs must be involved in the development of course curricula, development of role components, and evaluation of the role. Because this is a relatively new role, the ACNP must participate in efforts by nursing organizations to grant full recognition, reimbursement privileges, and prescriptive authority for APNs in order to make sure that the roles are based on appropriate definitions that include the acute care activities of the ACNP.

REFERENCES

American Association of Critical Care Nurses (1995). *Advanced nursing practice: Facts and strategies for regulation, reimbursement and prescriptive authority.* Washington, D. C.: American Association of Critical-Care Nurses.

American Nurses Association (1995). *Social policy statement.* Washington DC: American Nurses Publishing.

American Nurses Association. (in press). Scope and standards of advanced practice nursing. Washington, D. C.: American Nurses Publishing.

American Nurses Association and American Association of Critical-Care Nurses (1995). *Standards of clinical practice and scope of practice for the acute care nurse practitioner.* Washington, D. C.: American Nurses Publishing.

Clancy, G.T., & Maguire, D. (1995). APN in the neonatal intensive care unit. *Critical Care Nursing Clinics of North America, 7*(1), 71–76.

Clochesy, J. M., Daly, B. J., Idemoto, B. K., Steel, J., & Fitzpatrick, J. J. (1994). Preparing APNs for acute care. *American Journal of Critical Care, 3*(4), 255–259.

Dale, J. C. (1991). New role for PNPs in an inpatient setting. *Journal of Pediatric Health Care, 5*(6), 336–337.

Gleeson, R. M., McIlvain-Simpson, G., Boos, M. L., Sweet, E., Trzcinski, K. M., Solberg, C. A., & Doughty, R. A. (1990). APN: A model of collaborative care. *Maternal Child Nursing, 15*(1), 9–12.

Harrigan, R. C., & Perez, D. (in press). Neonatal nursing and its role in comprehensive care. In C. Kenner, J. W. Lott, & A. Flandermeyer (Eds.), *Comprehensive neonatal care: A physiologic perspective* (2nd ed.). Philadelphia: W. B. Saunders.

Ingersoll, G. L. (1995). Evaluation of the APN role in acute and specialty care. *Critical Care Nursing Clinics of North America, 7*(1), 25–33.

Keane, A., & Richmond, T. (1993). Tertiary NPs. *Image: Journal of Nursing Scholarship, 25*(4), 281–284.

King, K. B., & Ackerman, M. H. (1995). An educational model for the acute care nurse practitioner. *Critical Care Nursing Clinics of North America, 7*(1), 1–7.

Kubala, S., & Clever, L. H. (1974). Acceptance of the nurse practitioner. *American Journal of Nursing, 74*(3), 452–453.

Liljeblad, C. Y. (1993). Neonatal nurse practitioners: Paving the way for case management of chronically ill infants and their families. *Journal of Perinatal & Neonatal Nursing, 7*(3), 49–58.

Mahoney, D. F. (1995). Employer resistance to state authorized prescriptive authority for NPs: Results of a pilot study. *Nurse Practitioner, 20*(1), 58–61.

McGivern, D. O. (1992). The role of the nurse on the interdisciplinary treatment team. *NLN Publications*, 15-2464, 183–210.

Mitchell, A., Watts, J., Whyte, R., Blatz, S., Norman, G. R., Guyatt, G. H., Southwell, D., Hunsberger, M., & Paes, B. (1991). Evaluation of graduating neonatal nurse practitioners. *Pediatrics, 88*(4), 789–794.

Mundinger, M. O. (1994). Sounding board: Advanced-practice nursing—good medicine for physicians. *New England Journal of Medicine, 330*(3), 211–214.

Murphy, M. A., Gitterman, B. A., & Silver, H. K. (1985). Hospital nurse practitioners: A trial approach. *Pediatric Nursing, 11*(4), 269–273.

National Association of Neonatal Nurses (1994). *Program guidelines for neonatal nurse practitioner educational preparation.* Petaluma, CA: NANN.

National Council of State Boards of Nursing (1993). *Position paper on the regulation of nursing practice.* Chicago: NCSBN.

National League for Nursing (1994). *NLN Health Care Update, 1*,4, 1–4.

Office of Technology Assessment (1986). NPs, physician assistants, and certified nurse-midwives: A policy analysis (OTA Study). Washington, D. C.: U. S. Government Printing Office.

Ostrea, E. M., Jr., & Schuman, H. (1975). The role of the pediatric nurse practitioner in a neonatal unit. *Journal of Pediatrics, 86*(4), 628–631.

Parrinello, K. M. (1995). APN: An administrative perspective. *Critical Care Nursing Clinics of North America, 7*(1), 9–16.

Prescott, P. A., & Driscoll, L. (1980). Evaluating nurse practitioner performance. *Nurse Practitioner, 5*(4), 28–29, 31–32.

Richmond, T. S. & Keane, A. (1992). The tertiary care nurse practitioner. *Journal of Nursing Administration, 22*(11), 11–12.

Safriet, B. J. (1992). Health care dollars and regulatory sense: The role of APN. *Yale Journal on Regulation, 9*(2), 417–488.

Schultz, J. M., Liptak, G. S., & Fioravanti, J. (1994). Nurse practitioners effectiveness in NICU. *Nursing Management, 25*(10), 50–53.

Silver, H. K., & McAtee, P. (1988). Speaking out: Should nurses substitute for house staff? *American Journal of Nursing, 88*(12), 1671–1673.

Sims, M. E., Jasani, N., Yan, J., & Hodgman, J. E. (1987). Care of very low birth weight infants by neonatal nurse clinicians. *Journal of Perinatology, 7*(1), 55–57.

Smithing, R. T., & Wiley, M. D. (1995). Nurse practitioner salary survey results. *Nurse Practitioner, 20*(1), 78.

Spisso, J., O'Callahan, C., McKennan, M., & Holcroft, J. W. (1990). Improved quality of care and reduction of house staff workload using trauma NPs. *Journal of Trauma, 30*(6), 660–665.

Spitzer, W. O., Sockett, D. L., Sibley, J. C., Roberts,

R. S., Gent, M., Kergen, D. J., Hackett, B. C., &
Olynich, A. (1974). The Burlington randomized
trial of the nurse practitioner. *New England Journal of Medicine, 290*(5), 251–256.

Steel, J. E. (1992). High-tech RN emerges in acute
care: As I see it. *American Nurse, 3,* 4.

Swan, B. A. (1993). Nurse practitioners and anesthesiologists: A collaborative practice model.
Nurse Practitioner, 18(1), 10, 13.

Watkins, S., Kirchoff, K. T., Hartigan, E. G., & Karp,
T. (1992). Development of a program for neonatal intensive care units managed by neonatal
nurse practitioners. *Nursing Clinics of North
America, 27*(1), 87–97.

CHAPTER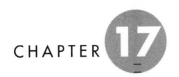

The Blended Role of the Clinical Nurse Specialist and the Nurse Practitioner

Allison Weber Shuren

INTRODUCTION

This chapter describes the evolution and operationalization of blended-role advanced nursing practice (ANP). The blended-role advanced practice nurse (APN) is defined as a graduate of a master's degree program in nursing that provides didactic and clinical preparation in both the clinical nurse specialist (CNS) and nurse practitioner (NP) concentrations and who is eligible for certification in a specialty area as well as certification as an NP. The blended-role APN demonstrates the eight core ANP competencies through the provision of comprehensive primary and specialty care to a defined population across settings from primary through tertiary care. In practice, blended-role preparation combines the strengths of two traditional roles—the primary health-care skills of NPs and the in-depth, specialty knowledge of CNSs—maximizing expertise and enabling the APN to assume expanded responsibilities for the more complex health problems experienced by patients today (Hockenberry-Eaton & Powell, 1991).

EVOLUTION OF THE BLENDED ROLE

The development of an ANP role that blends the practice of the CNS and NP cannot be traced to any particular event. Some authors believed that the skills and strengths of NP and CNS roles should or would be combined to meet projected health-care needs (Kitzman, 1989; Spross & Hamric, 1983). Instead, the blended role seems to be a natural evolution of two ANP roles that have expanded and matured, yet it is an ANP role distinct from either CNS or NP. Kitzman (1989) pointed out that CNSs and NPs have contributed significantly to the growth of the other's practice. CNSs have been credited with cultivating a climate within nursing open to expanded nursing practice (Kitzman, 1989), for developing theory-based practice, and for establishing the behavioral expectations of a nurse in advanced practice (Hanson & Martin, 1990). NPs can take credit for expanding practice beyond traditional nursing boundaries (Mauksch, 1978), developing collegial relationships with physicians (Kitzman, 1989), fostering lay recognition of APNs, and promoting consumer acceptance of advanced nursing practice (Hanson & Martin, 1990). As both CNS and NP roles develop, patient populations are being identified whose needs can be met by an APN with dual preparation as a CNS/NP.

Historically, the CNS has been viewed as a specialist in nursing care who provides direct and indirect nursing care for a specific patient population in secondary and tertiary in-patient care settings. In contrast, NPs have been viewed as generalists who provide primary and preventative care and treatment of illnesses for a broad patient population in out-patient care settings. However, the current reality is that CNSs can be found in outpatient settings providing extensive primary and preventative services and assessment and management of illness (Brooten et al., 1991; Damato et al., 1993; Sawyers, 1993), and NPs are practicing in tertiary care centers managing acute and chronic illnesses for specific patient populations and improving nursing care through education, consultation, and research (Dale, 1991; Davitt & Jensen, 1981; Gleeson et al., 1990; Hunsberger et al., 1992; Keane & Richmond, 1993; Nemes et al., 1992; Weinberg et al., 1983).

Despite this crossover of the CNS and NP roles and the societal needs that could be met by a blended-role APN, merged roles and reconceptualized ANP educational models have and continue to be much-debated topics among nursing leaders, educators, and APNs. Even a brief review of the nursing literature elicits numerous articles and editorials both in support of and in opposition to merging APN roles (Keane & Richmond, 1993; King & Ackerman, 1995; McGivern, 1993; Page & Arena, 1994; Snyder & Mirr, 1995). Some authors believe that the debate is more theoretical and based on minimal research (Fenton & Brykczynski, 1993). Others suggest that the merger is inevitable and believe that blending the roles would be advantageous for health-care organizations, patient care, and graduate nursing education (Cooper, 1990; Elder & Bullough, 1990; Wright, 1990; McGivern, 1993). Yet others assert that the roles are distinctly different in scope of practice and setting and should be maintained as such (Beecroft, 1994; King & Ackerman, 1995; Page & Arena, 1994; Zimmer et al., 1990). Some authors support separate CNS and NP scopes of practice but suggest uniting all APNs under singular titling (Galassi & Wheeler, 1994). However, most nursing leaders and APNs themselves agree that a common core of knowledge, skills and competencies, and professional attributes exists that should be required of both the CNS and NP and that differences between the two are largely based on focus of service (Forbes et al., 1990; Jackson, 1995; Pearson, 1990; Sawyers, 1993).

TRENDS IN HEALTH CARE AND OPPORTUNITIES FOR APNs

Until recently, the health-care industry in the United States has been driven by the medical model of disease diagnosis and treatment. Consequently, society has come to expect that quality health care is achieved through expensive, specialized, high-technology treatment of disease with little attention paid to prevention of illness. This philosophy has not resulted in a healthier population (Allan & Hall, 1988) but rather in uncontrollable expenditures and a propensity to seek health care only when a problem exists. As the United States moves into the 21st century, the burden of an illness-driven health care system on the country's economy has reached crisis proportions. Escalating costs, decreasing economic and human resources, shifting patterns of disease and demographics, changing political forces, and more ardent consumerism have led to scrutiny of the current delivery systems. The existing infrastructure is unable to provide cost-efficient, easily accessible, quality health care to all citizens of this country. This new concern has resulted in some radical shifts in traditional medical care and has provided new opportunities for innovation in health-care delivery.

The most significant change is directly related to managed care and capitated reimbursement strategies (see Chapter 22). Simply put, these strategies try to ensure cost-containment through limited, efficient use of resources and standardization of reimbursement paid for health-care services. Managed care is the driving force behind several other shifts in the delivery of health care. Specialty in-patient services are being downsized or abandoned in favor of out-patient management of disease. This shift has led to shortened hospital stays (Shugars et al., 1991) and an increase in the acuity of patients in hospitals and other settings. As a result, there is a need for more comprehensive ambulatory and home-care services to care for out-patients with conditions of increasing complexity.

Managed care is also driving the medical community to reexamine physician training and workforce needs. Current projections suggest greater demands for general practitioners to manage overall patient care and act as "gatekeepers" to costly specialty care. To meet this need, the Council on Graduate Medical Education is advocating a decrease in specialty residency programs and a restructuring of medical training to attract more physicians to primary care; the goal for the future is to have a more even distribution of physician expertise, with 50% of physicians being generalists and 50% being specialists (Kindig et al., 1993). This change will dramatically reduce available hospital resident coverage and has already left some institutions in a quandary as to how they will meet patient care needs.

Managed care is not the only pressure forcing reorganization of the current health-care system. Shifting patterns of disease and demographics in this country as a result of advanced life-saving medical technology has, in part, increased the elderly and chronically ill populations. Today, consumers are more sophisticated and have higher expectations of providers and payers of health care. People are unwilling to, nor should they, accept lack of continuity of care, difficult access to health-care providers, or limitations on their decision-making power. These trends further burden a system unprepared to provide adequate preventive health care or to provide rehabilitation, coordination of services, and continuity of care for those in need of specialized long-term follow-up.

Forces and counterforces are increasing the pace of change in today's health-care system. The apparent paradigm shift from an illness-driven health-care industry to one emphasizing primary health care and prevention means that organizations and individuals struggle to accommodate multiple, simultaneous changes. Cost-effective health care to prevent disease and provide quality care to those who are acutely and chronically ill are the bottom lines. Reengineering, redesign, and restructuring (i.e., redefinition of roles and of work and the use of less expensive care providers) are the focus of many institutional initiatives designed to respond to these pressures. Efforts to control costs and to forge a new balance between primary care and illness services are driving changes in the availability and types of positions in health care.

From the chaos of numerous health-care reform initiatives, consensus is emerging on three key issues: more primary health-care clinicians are needed to provide essential services; alternatives to deal with anticipated residency shortages in acute care must be established; and health-care delivery systems must be coordinated and comprehensive to manage patients with highly complex conditions and with both acute and chronic illnesses. These issues present opportunities for APNs to reach beyond established boundaries, to be responsive to the changing health-care needs of patients and society, and to become a greater presence in the health-care system.

Blended-role APNs are uniquely prepared to address these three issues. The incorporation of the primary health-care expertise of a traditional NP with the clinical and leadership skills of the traditional CNS distinctly prepares the blended-role APN to expand and extend the boundaries of advanced nursing practice. A full range of health and illness services can be provided for a defined patient population while minimizing discontinuity in care. For example, the child with leukemia can receive health and illness services from the pediatric NP with a clinical specialization in oncology; the adult with chronic obstructive pulmonary disease would receive similar services from the adult NP who has specialized in pulmonary nursing. The blended-role APN can bridge gaps between in-patient and out-patient settings and between medicine and nursing to provide holistic and continuous care to a specific population. In addition, the blended-role APN possesses the NP competencies that have been associated with quality, cost-effective care, and favorable patient outcomes (Office of Technology Assessment, 1986; Safriet, 1992), attributes the health delivery system desperately needs.

LITERATURE REVIEW

Constrained by controversy, past descriptions of the blended role of the CNS and NP were more ideological than operational. Davitt and Jensen (1981) provided one of the earliest job descriptions in the literature that parallels the blended-role APN practice described in this chapter. These authors described the role of an APN, titled an acute care nurse practitioner (ACNP), with a cardiac surgery team. The scope of practice of this innovative position was based on the premise that collaboration between nursing and medicine leads to improved patient management. The ACNP's responsibilities included direct care activities, such as daily management of in-patient preoperative and postoperative patients and short-term out-patient follow-up, and indirect care activities, such as patient, student, and resident teaching; surgical nursing staff development; research; and consultation services.

According to Davitt and Jensen, the ACNP was viewed as an integral part of the cardiac surgery team by both medical and nursing colleagues. The ACNP was particularly valued for the continuity in patient care, because the ACNP was the consistent member of a team whose surgical residents rotated off the service frequently. However, the most important contribution of the ACNP was the ability to bring expert patient assessment and clinical management skills together with knowledge gained from extensive nursing experience to all aspects of specialty patient care. For example, the ACNP's preoperative evaluation included not only a standard history and physical examination but a review of psychosocial concerns, in-depth patient and family education, and assessment of discharge needs.

Spross and Hamric (1983) proposed a model describing future CNS practice. According to their projections, a time would come when there would be a need for a nurse with a master's degree who had the clinical and scholarly skills of both the NP and the CNS (Spross & Hamric, 1983). At the time, advanced registered nurse practitioner (ARNP) was proposed as the title for the CNS of the future. This title, in use in some statutes, would reflect the role that emerged from combining NP and CNS preparation and practice. The practice of this future APN combined the domains of service and scopes of practice of NPs and CNSs (Spross & Hamric, 1983). The ARNP was seen as a practitioner who would be client-based rather than setting-based, providing care in primary, secondary, and tertiary settings to ensure continuity of services to a specialty-based patient population. Through independent and interdependent practice with physicians, the ARNP would deliver direct care, such as advanced clinical assessment, management of acute and chronic problems associated with a specific patient population, and ongoing anticipatory guidance about potential diagnosis-specific problems as well as generic primary prevention education. The ARNP would also provide vital indirect patient care through activities such as expert clinical consultation, coordination and facilitation of services, and promotion of improved nursing practice.

Gleeson and coworkers (1990) reported a model of collaborative practice that suggests how and why a blended-role APN may be the right "APN solution" for a defined population and one that is different from either a CNS or a NP. When an institution expanded from a pediatric orthopedic facility to a multispecialty children's hospital, its leaders identified a need for clinicians capable of managing a growing patient population and of ensuring continuity of care. These clinicians were called APNs and functioned as both CNSs and pediatric NPs in daily practice. The APNs in this model functioned in both in-patient and out-patient settings. They provided such traditional NP services as histories and physical examinations, assessment and treatment of common chronic illnesses in collaboration with physicians, interpretation of diagnostic data, prevention of potential health problems, and extensive patient and family teaching. By virtue of their specialty knowledge in neurology or rheumatology, they also could manage clinical issues specific to their specialties. Like a traditional CNS, this APN also had responsibilities for nursing staff and community development by providing educational programs, participating in committee work, preparing professional materials for publication, and providing expert consultation. Although they did not use objective measures, Gleeson and colleagues hypothesized that their model would improve the quality of patient care by increasing continuity and coordination of services; providing closer, ongoing monitoring; increasing patient teaching; fostering greater emphasis on health and the prevention of problems; and providing cost-effective care.

At the time of their projections, Spross and Hamric (1983) were suggesting one ANP role. As this textbook indicates, advanced nursing practice has evolved differently. Core competencies of advanced nursing practice can be described, but they are operationalized differently depending on the types of APN's practice. Despite the descriptions of what the author considers a blended-role APN, roles that fully operationalize both CNS and NP skills have been slow to develop. This may be due to unanswered questions regarding educational preparation, statutory and regulatory issues concerning advanced nursing practice, reimbursement structures, and the absence of opportunities to institute this type of APN position. The debate on merging CNS and NP curricula and skills to prepare one type of APN has overshadowed discussion and conceptualization of an APN who is jointly prepared as both a CNS and an NP. However, the early descriptions of a combined CNS/NP role are consistent with the definition and practice characteristics of a blended-role APN as described in this chapter. Some of the literature on APNs who use both CNS and NP skills, but not in a blended role as described here, is incorporated later in discussions of the differentiation of APN positions and issues in implementation of blended-role advanced nursing practice.

SCOPE OF PRACTICE OF BLENDED-ROLE APNs

The blended-role practice described in this chapter is similar to the description of ACNP practice described by Davitt and Jensen (1981) but also aims to push the current boundaries of advanced nursing practice. It is based on the literature described earlier, a definition of advanced nursing practice developed by the American Nurses' Association (ANA) and being reviewed by its constituents (Cronenwett, 1995), the definition of advanced nursing practice described in this text (see Chapter 3), and the author's experience in a blended-role APN position.

The scope of practice of a blended-role APN spans traditional NP and CNS practice and integrates both medical and nursing paradigms and perspectives to benefit patient care. Blended-role practice includes direct and indirect medical and nursing care. The blended-role APN requires extensive knowledge related to assessment, diagnosis, and clinical management. This knowledge must draw from the biopsychosocial sciences that are basic to both medical and nursing practices as well the knowledge developed within each discipline. Thus, blended-role APNs are as skilled at diagnosing and treating a life-threatening illness as they are at diagnosing and treating the uncertainty, anxiety, and caregiver burdens associated with the illness. These APNs also demonstrate the eight core competencies described in this text (see Chapters 6 through 13). As a member of a nursing department and of a medical team, the blended-role APN has to meet expectations from both. Therefore, this APN does need clearly delineated practice objectives, accountability, and boundaries.

Although the blended-role APN prepares separately as both an NP and a CNS, the unique quality of this blended position is the opportunity to bring the in-depth knowledge learned from both curricula to every interaction with patients, families, and colleagues. To try to divide the blended-role APN's daily activities into clearly defined subroles of either the NP or CNS or to do an activity breakdown would diminish the integration of practice that is this APN's greatest asset. The best, most efficient method to explain the APN's scope of practice is to describe direct and indirect patient care and organizational responsibilities separately.

DIRECT PATIENT CARE

The most visible direct patient care activities are the APN's clinical responsibilities. This includes ongoing and comprehensive health assessment, diagnosis, and treatment of complex responses to actual and potential health problems, management of acute and chronic illnesses, promotion of wellness and preventative care, and identification of nursing care needs for a specific patient population. The blended-role APN integrates the CNS skill of in-depth assessment and the interpersonal, coaching, and teaching expertise of both CNSs and NPs into clinical problem-solving and decision-making. As a result, apparently traditional medical evaluations and treatments are transformed, reflecting a synthesis of medicine and advanced nursing practice (see Chapter 6).

As integral members of health-care teams, blended-role APNs must delineate the expanded scope of their practice and negotiate patient coverage during off time in collaboration with physician colleagues. Criteria should be agreed on to guide the selection of the in-patients and out-patients whose care will be the APN's responsibility. To avoid overextension of the APN and to enable the APN to provide the range of services that he or she can offer, a maximum caseload of patients must be agreed on. In addition, time and activities relating to ambulatory patient care should be stipulated. Specifically, the APN should have a standard clinic schedule, limitations on numbers of patients seen per clinic, and guidelines for decision-making, as well as criteria for patient phone call triage. Human and other resources such as clinical assistants and computers to address clerical functions associated with patient care in this APN practice need to be negotiated during the hiring process. Ignoring this aspect of providing care may mean that the APN performs these functions by default, compromising productivity and cost-effectiveness. Other personal and political consequences may ensue, such as APN job dissatisfaction and devaluation of APN contributions.

Direct Patient Care Vignette

R.S. is a 6-month-old white male born at 36 weeks' gestation to a 36-year-old gravida 2, para 2, white female. During his first day of life R.S. was noted to have excessive drooling, difficulty feeding with associated coughing, sputtering, and circumoral cyanosis. At 12 hours of age he was transferred from the local community hospital to the children's hospital level-three nursery for a surgical consultation to rule out esophageal malformations. The APN's initial contact with R.S. and his father was on the baby's arrival to the nursery.

Over the ensuing hours R.S. underwent various radiographic studies that revealed esophageal atresia and tracheoesophageal fistula, dextrocardia with normal intracardiac structure, patent urachus, and vesicoureteral reflux. Once the diagnosis had been established and the decision was made to bring R.S. to the operating room within the following 24 hours, the attending surgeon and the APN met with the new father to explain his son's congenital anomalies and the surgery needed to correct the malformation of the baby's esophagus. After answering all the father's questions and obtaining informed consent for the upcoming procedure, the surgeon left. The APN remained with R.S.'s dad to ensure that he understood the information he was just given and to offer him another opportunity to ask questions. During this time the APN also offered assistance to Mr. S. in explaining the news to his wife, who was still a patient at the local community hospital. Without hesitation he accepted and dialed the phone.

On day two of life R.S. was taken to the operating room for repair of his esophageal malformation. However, once in the operating room it was discovered that only the tracheoesophageal fistula could be repaired. The esophageal atresia was not correctable at this time because of the distance between the proximal and distal esophageal buds. Therefore, the decision was made to allow the esophageal buds to grow and to attempt repair when R.S. was older. Before leaving the operating room to speak with Mr. & Mrs. S., the surgeon contacted the APN so they could meet with the new parents together. Postoperatively, R.S.'s surgeon and the APN collaboratively decided that the APN should care for R.S. instead of a rotating surgical resident because R.S. would require continuity of care during his hospitalization and frequent long-term follow-up.

Each morning the APN was responsible to present the infant's physical examination, diagnostic data, and plan of care for the day on surgical rounds. The remainder of the day was spent carrying out those plans agreed on by the surgeon, ongoing assessment, and planning for discharge. On the APN's days off, arrangements were made for the on-call resident team to cover the care of the infant. However, the APN was expected to leave a clear plan of care for this time.

The days that followed were difficult for the parents and child. Mrs. S. wept many tears onto the isolette that kept her infant son warm and safe. Every day her list of questions seemed to grow longer and longer, but each day the APN and she worked through the lengthy list until Mrs. S again felt secure that she had answers to each one of them. The APN also connected Mrs. S. with a mother of a child with similar anomalies to give her other sources of emotional support and guidance.

Over the next several weeks R.S. stabilized. The APN initiated an enteral feeding plan, initiated prophylactic antibiotic therapy secondary to the infant's vesicoureteral reflux, and implemented a safe method to provide control of the baby's oral secretions through continuous nasal esophageal pouch suction. Throughout this period of recovery the APN cared not only for this infant's daily physical needs but also coordinated referrals to consulting specialty services and had ongoing contact with the primary care pediatrician. The APN also worked closely with the in-patient nursing staff, home health-care nursing team, and family, providing education on the child's congenital anomalies, surgical needs, and daily care needs as well as organizing this complex discharge.

After 32 days in the hospital R.S. was discharged. The APN now became responsible for R.S.'s out-patient follow-up. He was monitored by the APN every other week in the multidisciplinary surgery clinic and biweekly by telephone follow-up. The surgeon and APN would routinely review R.S.'s progress and collaboratively revise his plan of care. Clinic visits incorporated not only clinical assessment of R.S. but also assessment of his nutritional status, development, preventative health-care needs, and his family's coping. Due to the complexity of R.S.'s care and need for frequent follow-up with the surgical team, his contact with his primary care pediatrician was infrequent, limited to some routine well-child care (i.e., immunizations). The APN became the person Mrs. S. depended on to assess her child or to answer any questions regarding R.S.'s health or general infant growth and development. In fact, whenever she brought R.S. to the emergency room she would request that the APN be called even though a resident was attending to R.S.'s needs.

Despite continuous nasal esophageal suction, R.S. had ongoing difficulty controlling his oral secretions. He presented frequently with symptoms of upper respiratory infections and increased work of breathing, which raised considerable suspicion that the infant was microaspirating. He required several short-stay admissions to the hospital for pulmonary toilet. Because of this change in his progress, R.S. was prepared for the final repair of his esophageal atresia. He was admitted to his attending surgeon, but the APN assumed daily clinical care of the child in collaboration with the surgeon as with every previous admission.

Unfortunately, R.S.'s hospitalization was again lengthy and his discharge complicated by home care needs and limited insurance coverage. However, the transition home was eased by the relationship that had developed between the APN, the home care primary nurse, the medical equipment company, and the family throughout the many months they worked together to care for R.S. R.S. has been home now for several months; he is still enterally fed but is beginning to learn how to orally feed. The APN continues to see him in clinic every 2 to 3 weeks and remains in routine contact with his pediatrician. As R.S. continues to improve, his surgical follow-up will decrease, but the APN will continue to have some ongoing contact with his family to observe R.S.'s growth and development and work in conjunction with his primary care physician to ensure that he is referred to appropriate specialists (i.e., occupational therapy) as needed. In addition, the APN is available to Mr. and Mrs. S. for support and answering questions.

INDIRECT PATIENT CARE

The APN's indirect patient care activities have three foci: the specific patients with whom the APN works, patients not directly managed by the APN (i.e., patients who are covered by a resident), and the patient population within the APN's specialty as a whole. Examples of indirect patient care activities include providing and soliciting consultations regarding clinical management, teaching, counseling, and discharge planning; participating in patient care conferences and team meetings; offering formal and informal educational presentations for nursing and medical personnel who work with the APN's specialty population; and participating in continuous quality improvement initiatives and research projects related to the APN's specialty population or nursing practice.

Unlike the need to specifically negotiate direct patient care responsibilities with collaborating physicians, control of indirect patient care activities must be within the purview of the APN. Some administrators, who are uncomfortable with granting the APN the autonomy necessary to execute this role, may try to establish specific percentages of time spent in each indirect patient care activity. This is counterproductive. Instead, the APN and administrators should mutually agree on short and long-term goals for the APN that support both the nursing mission and the medical mission of an institution. The exact percentage of time the APN spends preparing and executing indirect patient care responsibilities will depend on the demands of the APN's direct patient care activities, requests from other health care professionals, the availability of the APN, the priority of an activity, and the APN's personal ability to set limits on projects undertaken.

Unlike a CNS or NP who works in a specific practice setting, the blended-role APN moves freely between in-patient and out-patient care areas and has a unique opportunity to affect the quality of patient care not only in an isolated setting but throughout the continuum of care. Some of an APN's indirect patient care activities may include developing and directing process improvement projects with health-care team members from both environments. Consider the following example.

Indirect Patient Care Vignette

When reviewing her patient telephone log book the APN noticed an increasing number of phone calls from parents regarding gastrostomies and enteral feeding. Though the trend was interesting, the APN put it out of mind. Several weeks later the APN and surgical nutritionist were discussing a patient receiving gastrostomy tube feedings. In the course of the conversation the nutritionist mentioned that the parents of this particular patient expressed concern that they were discharged from the hospital without clear knowledge of how to properly care for their daughter's gastrostomy tube or how to trouble-shoot the feeding pump. In fact, over one weekend the parents had to call the hospital four times, including once in the middle of the night for advice on a leaking gastrostomy tube and pump difficulty.

After this conversation the APN decided to investigate these parents' concerns. The APN found that their child had been discharged from the hospital on postoperative day two and that formal gastrostomy education was not documented in the patient medical record. Next, the APN asked several surgery clinic nurses whether they were experiencing inconsistencies in parent knowledge of gastrostomies and enteral feeding. They were readily able to give several recent case scenarios of parents who felt uncomfortable with the care of their child's gastrostomy.

The APN believed there could be numerous reasons for the decline in the quality of patient-parent education, but the most likely problems were shorter lengths of hospitalizations and decreases in the ratio of professional nursing staff to patients, making it difficult for an RN to block out time for teaching. With these thoughts in mind the APN assembled and chaired a task force of nurses and a nutritionist representing several in-patient units, out-patient clinics, and the home health-care department and charged the group to brainstorm for new methods to standardize parent education about gastrostomy tube care and enteral feeding to ensure that all bedside caregivers responsible for teaching were competent and comfortable with the material.

The group prepared an easy-to-follow teaching manual. The APN was responsible for preparing and editing the manuscript, providing more in-depth information when necessary, distributing the material, and being accessible to all nursing staff for questions. To further supplement the written information, the APN and two members of the task force held informal question-and-answer in-services for nursing staff to clarify any information.

ORGANIZATIONAL RESPONSIBILITIES AND ACTIVITIES

Depending on the position of the APN within the organization, the APN may have significant leadership opportunities. As a member of the nursing organization the APN may influence the direction of nursing within the institution by participating in the development of department policies, standards of care, and research objectives. Within the medical community the blended-role APN regarded as a colleague can be an integral participant in medical committees, education, and resident training. In addition, APNs' experiences in collaborating with other health-care professionals and as change agents make them excellent candidates to participate in or chair interdisciplinary groups or task forces that address interdisciplinary and interdepartmental issues. This is particularly relevant in the current environment of managed care and efforts to standardize care using critical paths and practice guidelines. The APN as both a bedside clinician and champion for quality, cost-efficient patient care is especially poised to lead critical path design teams.

DIFFERENTIATING BLENDED-ROLE PRACTICE FROM OTHER APN ROLES

While the debate continues over titling and scopes of practice (Galassi & Wheeler, 1994; Hanson & Martin, 1990; Schroer, 1991; Sparacino, 1993), APNs are meeting the challenges of the changing health-care environment by expanding their knowledge and continuing to extend the boundaries of advanced nursing practice. While the profession attempts to resolve questions regarding titling and scopes of practice, individual APNs must be clear on how their practices differ from and complement one another in order to remain viable resources to patients and to avoid becoming victims of reengineering. The blended-role APN described in this chapter incorporates competencies and knowledge that would also be found in the practices of a primary care NP, a tertiary care CNS, and a tertiary care NP. This blended-role APN differs from a primary care NP because the APN works with a specialty population and provides primary health care and specialized clinical management to patients across primary, secondary, and tertiary care settings. Compared with tertiary care NPs (at least as these positions are currently evolving), the blended-role APN's scope of practice differs in the amount of out-patient follow-up that is incorporated into clinical responsibilities. Unlike the tertiary care NP, who is responsible for a variety of acutely or critically ill patients and for limited ambulatory care activities (if any), the blended-role APN is responsible for ongoing follow-up of a circumscribed patient population. The APN described in this chapter also has explicit responsibility for executing traditional CNS subroles. The blended-role APN provides direct care and facilitates continuity of care for specialty patient populations that frequently move in and out of acute and chronic illness states. Therefore, this APN role requires a strong theoretical and clinical knowledge base in acute care as well as preventative and primary care.

The blended-role APN differs the most from the APN case manager. Both are educationally prepared for the role of primary coordinator of care by virtue of their master's degrees and share some role overlap (Papenhausen, 1990). The APN case manager (see Chapter 20) is accountable for clinical and fiscal outcomes; the blended-role APN cannot afford to be oblivious to fiscal outcomes, but primary responsibility will fall to someone else. With APN case managers there is greater emphasis on organization, coordination, and monitoring of patient care (Smith, 1994) and on system-level interventions (see Chapter 20) to enhance quality of care and contain costs. The most notable difference in practice is evident in the level of direct tertiary clinical management of patients. Most APN case management models (Schroer, 1991) include elements of direct patient assessment and clinical decision-making in ambulatory care settings but end there. Although APN case managers closely follow established patients when they are admitted to the hospital, they typically relinquish direct patient management to the hospital-based team.

ISSUES IN IMPLEMENTATION AND DEVELOPMENT OF THE BLENDED ROLE

ORGANIZATIONAL PLACEMENT

Several patterns of organizational placement for hospital-based APNs have been described (El-Sherif, 1995; Richmond & Keane, 1992) (see Chapter 24). The difference among them lies in the reporting relationship of the APN to nursing and medicine. The success or failure of one option over another depends on the philosophies and politics of the institution, the existing relationships between physicians and nurses at the institution (both at the medical and nursing director level and at the individual level), and the opinion of the individual APN. One alternative is a dual reporting relationship (El-Sherif, 1995) in which the APN has appointments and responsibilities in departments of nursing and medicine. Depending on the degree of involvement of each department head, this option can provide a strong sense of interdisciplinary teamwork or prohibit the professional growth of the APN. With this type of organizational placement, the APN should ensure that expectations for APN practice of both individuals are clear and documented. The APN should also expect at least one yearly meeting, attended by both advisors, to review past goals and set reasonable objectives for each new year of employment.

A second alternative is for the APN to be placed solely within the nursing department. Some authors suggest that this model allows the greatest opportunity for leadership activities within nursing and reflects the autonomous nature of APN practice (El-Sherif; Richmond & Keane, 1992). Even in this type of arrangement, good communication and collaborative relationships with physician colleagues who have clinical and administrative responsibilities are essential to success in the blended role. Although such a structure may serve to strengthen nursing within an organization, it can be a barrier to role implementation and interdisciplinary teamwork if the organizational climate is one of "us versus them."

A third option is for the APN to report solely to the medical director of the specialty practice (Richmond & Keane, 1992). This relationship can help build mutual respect between APNs and physician colleagues if each member of the team is considered equally important to the patient outcome. If, however, the relationship is one of superior and inferior roles, the APN is unlikely to grow as an autonomous practitioner, and collaborative, interdisciplinary care most likely will go unsupported.

APNs may also find themselves faced with inter- or intra-departmental issues regarding financial compensation. Whether an APN has a singular or dual reporting relationship may or may not influence an APN's salary and benefits. The department paying the APN may feel more entitled to the practitioner's time. Thus an APN should be clear on the financial arrangements of any position prior to accepting the role. For example, nursing may pay an APN's salary but bill the specialty medical service for the medical aspects of the blended-role APN's practice (Malone, 1989). This is particularly important when the medical service collects fees from third-party payers for the services actually provided by the APN (Griffith & Robinson, 1993).

NEGOTIATING RELATIONSHIPS AND ACCOUNTABILITY

The blended-role APN can be in a powerful or precarious position within the hospital environment. Depending on the circumstances that led to the creation of the position, the APN may be viewed by different health-care team members as either a godsend, a threat, or both. Within the nursing organization the APN should be an active member of the APN group whether or not management reporting relationships include a line to nursing. This group will be indispensable for insight into the official and "unofficial" institutional structure, strategies for incorporating oneself and one's practice into that structure, and helping to identify important clinical issues that are common to many ANP roles. If the institution separates APNs into separate associations of CNSs and NPs, the blended-role APN should find a way to participate in the charters of each (e.g., alternate attendance at the meetings of each). This situation not only can be time-consuming but also a bit uncomfortable. The APN may be viewed by both groups as a an outsider, despite the APN's qualifications to be titled as either a CNS or an NP. The APN should look on this predicament as an opportunity to cross new boundaries and represent the commonalities between all APNs and to facilitate communication that could lead to some exciting collaborative projects.

Teamwork and collaboration are also absolutely necessary between the APN and the specialty physician group. Ideally, APNs are viewed as essential members of the professional team who have authority and accountability for their practice and offer unique nursing knowledge and perspectives on patient care. If this is not the case, the APN may be resented by some physicians who feel that their territory has been invaded, especially if the APN has replaced a position that was once filled by a resident. Whether explicit or implicit, some APNs may feel pressured to outperform medical resident counterparts or withstand a trial of "proving" one's ability to provide safe, quality patient care. The issue of establishing credibility is not a new one for APNs—CNSs have had to demonstrate it to nursing staff, and NPs have had to demonstrate it to physicians. Establishing credibility is often a matter of time, patience, and the development of mutual respect, which evolves as new team members share common patient-related experiences. However, in the acute setting the pressure to prove oneself may include challenges to APNs to eliminate clinical nursing activities from patient care, such as health education, psychosocial support, and preventative services (Mundinger, 1994). One strategy to minimize this obstacle is to ask the medical director of the specialty team to send a letter of introduction that describes the APN's role and credentials to departments and individuals likely to be affected by this role. Such a letter explicitly sponsors and supports the APN's practice. If the environment does not improve with time, the APN should collaborate with nursing and medical colleagues to assertively seek additional approaches to clarify roles (see Chapters 11 and 24).

The APN's relationships with staff nurses and other health-care professionals will vary. The power and gender issues that can dominate physician-nurse communications (see Chapter 11) are less likely to be a barrier to establishing working relationships with staff. The ability of the APN to relate to staff nurses' work experiences, including workload issues and intuitive judgments about patient conditions, is often beneficial in establishing effective collaboration with other nurses. Staff may feel more comfortable relaying clinical information to the APN. Blended-role APNs may find some of the suggestions from the CNS literature helpful in forging positive relationships with staff nurses (Koetters, 1989). On the other hand, nurses may be unclear as to the difference between the blended-role APN and other APNs, perceive the APN as elitist, and question the abilities of the APN out of unfamiliarity and concern for their patient. Because APNs have responsibilities formerly held by physicians exclusively, staff nurses may expect blended-role APNs to be more like physicians in their clinical management of patients. Staff nurses may be uncomfortable with any expression of uncertainty by the APN, however warranted, especially if they are looking for certainty or comfort with a patient's changing condition. Staff nurses may also feel threatened by another new position in an atmosphere of work redesign and job eliminations. However, the APN's ability to cross boundaries can present exciting new chances for staff nurses to become involved in activities once perceived as out of their area of practice.

EVALUATION OF PRACTICE

As direct patient care providers, blended-role APNs should determine a method of evaluating their patient outcomes as well as a self-evaluation tool. Hamric (1989) offers several strategies that the blended-role APN may find useful (see also Chapter 26). The APN may be included in the medical department's performance improvement/quality assurance program and morbidity and mortality reviews. This should be decided on when negotiating the terms of the APN's practice within the medical team. Depending on the APN's patient population one may also choose to monitor specific patient outcome measures, such as lengths of stay, complications, readmissions to the hospital, visits to the emergency room, or patient satisfaction. This information is important for evaluating the effectiveness of the blended-role APN and for establishing credibility among nursing and medical peers. During these cost-conscious times, the APN should also be prepared to collect data reflecting cost savings related to APN practice. These might include increases in patient referrals due to the APN's community outreach, more effective use of resources associated with appropriate and timely referrals initiated by APNs, or decreased use of the health-care system due to improved patient adherence to medical and nursing regimens.

APNs should do a self-evaluation, analyzing annual goals and objectives and formally reporting accomplishments. Peer evaluation from selected colleagues in nursing and medicine is also important for the professional growth of the APN and should be a part of at least a yearly review.

ROLE DEVELOPMENT

The concept of role development has been examined for both the CNS (Hamric & Taylor, 1989; Holt, 1987) and the NP (Busen & Jones, 1995; Malkemes, 1974; Thibodeau & Hawkins, 1994). Like most professionals, all APNs move through phases of role development as they mature in their practices. The blended-role APN is no different, except that unlike a CNS or NP the blended-role APN must master the four subroles of CNS practice and incorporate each into an active practice of direct patient clinical management. Some feel that this task is impossible, but this actually evolves naturally if the APN has been educationally prepared to understand both roles.

In actual practice, the APN is unlikely to develop each subrole simultaneously. Rather, role development will occur on a continuum as the position evolves. Depending on the APN's confidence level with the clinical management of both in-patients and out-patients within his or her specialty patient population, the APN initially may focus on this aspect of blended-role practice. Much like the novice NP, the blended-role APN must become comfortable with blending aspects of medicine and nursing through a nursing perspective (Fenton & Brykczynski, 1993) and concentrate on developing support from physician and nursing colleagues.

Ideally, while the APN focuses on becoming proficient in direct patient care activities, the APN should also be assessing overall patient care, nursing staff competency, and organizational structures in order to identify goals for indirect care activities. Unlike the CNS, whose role might develop in isolation from physicians in the clinical setting, blended-role APNs are in a position to incorporate physicians more easily into their project planning. This makes gaining medical support for the blended-role APN's CNS activities easier and offers an exceptional opportunity to help medical colleagues understand this contribution to patient care.

EDUCATIONAL PREPARATION, CERTIFICATION, AND CREDIBILITY

A brief review of any nursing journal provides evidence of the transitional state of advanced nursing practice and the numerous and variable graduate education programs preparing these professionals (Burns et al., 1993). Changing, expanding, and emerging APN roles are in part responsible for this state of flux as organized nursing and educators attempt to catch up and respond to the many factors shaping contemporary advanced nursing practice. There is clearly a need for common core curricula standards for all APN students to build professional credibility and to ensure quality, safety, and efficiency of the care provided to clients. However, role-specific didactic content and clinical practica are needed within programs to nurture established and emerging differentiated APN practices. This is particularly true for the student wishing to practice as a blended-role APN. The following discussion on preparation for the blended role is meant to provide a way of thinking about how to provide or acquire the knowledge and skills needed. The author had a clear vision of what she wanted to do and deliberately sought dual preparation.

In order to integrate NP and CNS practices, the blended-role APN must reach competency in the practice of each of these traditional roles. Competency in primary care is crucial for the blended-role APN, more so than the tertiary care NP because the APN will be responsible for long-term out-patient management of patients. As envisioned, the blended-role APN may in fact work closely with or temporarily replace a patient's primary care provider, depending on the community practitioner's level of comfort with the patient's specialty illness. So, the APN should be prepared to provide primary, preventative health care. With the emergence of ACNP curricula and depending on the specialty area in which the blended-role APN chooses to practice, blended-role APN students may need to complete courses in ACNP tracks (Hravnak et al., 1995). King and Ackerman (1995) suggest that curricular content for NP practice in acute care can be analyzed along four dimensions: patient vulnerability, intensity of the environment, complexity of clinical management, and immediacy of intervention required. Types of content needed to acquire competency in the care of an acutely ill specialty population would include physical assessment, complex clinical decision-making, pharmacology and therapeutic management, organization of health service, ethics, and legal aspects of advanced nursing practice (Keane and Richmond, 1993; Keane, Richmond, & Kaiser, 1994). For example, a blended-role APN desiring to work with surgeons who admit patients to intensive care settings would need to be comfortable with the care of critically ill patients.

Blended-role APN students must also acquire the in-depth knowledge of the nursing care of the specialty population of interest and sufficient preparation in theoretical and practical content related to the traditional subroles of the CNS (e.g., organizational psychology, change theory, consultations processes). The clinical knowledge of the CNS typically involves an in-depth understanding of the health phenomena (e.g., child development) or illness phenomena within a specialty and how patients experience these phenomena. Thus, pediatric oncology CNSs understand the biological behavior of tumors, the scientific basis for treatment, the types and patterns of responses of children and their parents to diagnosis and treatment, and a range of interpersonal, pharmacological, and non-pharmacological therapies to manage predictable and less common responses and symptoms. This knowledge informs the CNS's direct care (preparing patients for treatment, administering treatment, consulting with others to manage complex problems). This knowledge also guides other activities (e.g., program development, deepening the knowledge of other staff caring for the patient).

Factors that might influence the choice of a blended-role APN might include populations whose problems are complex and unusual, a desire to work as part of a clinical service that is small or not widely available (e.g., a blended-role APN in oncology might enable patients in rural areas to remain in their communities for routine chemotherapy treatments), or the APN's own desire to maximize marketability. Credibility of blended-role advanced nursing practice is based, in part, on educational preparation. As graduate nursing education is currently structured, the course of study for a blended-role APN would be longer than for the student wishing to pursue traditional CNS or NP training. The student will need to seek out flexible, visionary schools of nursing that will allow some individualized program development, but the student must complete both courses of study. Each of these areas is important to the blended-role APN and should be incorporated into a program of study after the foundation of primary care is completed. APNs who are CNSs or NPs and who wish to practice in a blended role should look for post-master's programs that will enable them to acquire the knowledge and skills needed to assume this position.

As graduate programs reorganize to teach all APNs the core competencies and ensure greater consistency in core curricula for APNs, preparation for the blended role should not be quite so arduous and complicated. As new, enterprising ANP roles are emerging it is evident that graduate nursing education must keep pace with health trends (de Tornyay, 1992). All APNs need to be prepared in the eight core competencies. However, there is a need to analyze existing and emerging APN jobs to identify the emphasis given the core competencies within specific APN roles and any additional competencies needed to practice in particular APN jobs. Then, general and specific educational programs can be designed to help students accomplish their professional goals as well as meet the expectations of prospective employers.

Like any profession, nursing is responsible to prepare qualified practitioners or accept skepticism from critics. APNs' greatest defense against roadblocks to advanced nursing practice is to obtain the education and experience that will best prepare us. As Chinn (1991, p. 253) stated, "control of knowledge is the most powerful tool sustaining oppressive relationships."

In addition to education, credibility in the world of health care is also a function of credentials. Thus, the blended-role APN must be certified as an NP by a professional organization in the area of practice. The APN should also become specialty-certified if an examination exists. Other credentials required of the individual practitioner, such as state licensure or prescriptive authority, must also be considered (see Chapter 22).

TITLING OF BLENDED-ROLE APNs

Difficulties with APN titling (Sparacino, 1993) and a summary of efforts to build consensus around the meaning of advanced nursing practice (Cronenwett, 1995) have been described. However, it must be acknowledged that if and when *advanced practice nurse* is accepted by the profession and policymakers as a term that embraces a variety of APN positions, the issue of titling the blended-role APN remains difficult. Spross and Hamric (1983) proposed the ARNP title for the role described in this chapter. Since that time, the ARNP title has been increasingly used in state regulations to refer to the NP. Consequently, it has significant problems as a title that would readily convey that the APN possesses blended-role skills.

Some authors have implied that the ACNP combines the skills of the CNS and NP. However, as discussed in this chapter under differentiation of APN roles, the ACNP role does not represent blended-role skills but rather NP skills that focus on patients in acute care settings (see Chapter 16). ACNP roles as they are being described and operationalized are not congruent with the blended-role practice described here.

Some leaders are advocating the generic title of APN for the blended role (Snyder & Mirr, 1995). This stance supports the merging of CNS and NP roles into one APN role. Combining the skills and competencies of the CNS and NP has been the focus of this chapter, and is an important trend in the continuing evolution of advanced nursing practice. But the title APN is more appropriately used as an umbrella term to describe all ANP roles, including CNS, CNM, CRNA, NP, ACNP, AP case manager, and the blended-role CNS/NP (see Chapter 3). Restricting the APN title to only the blended role does not seem feasible or desirable. But the contention here is that the title should reflect the actual practice and should be discrete if the practice is discrete. Because the blended-role APN is a distinct ANP role, it needs a distinct title.

This leaves the possibilities of "blended-role APN"*—the title used throughout this chapter—or "CNS/NP." In practice, the author has chosen to use NP when introducing herself to clients because laypersons are more likely to be familiar with this term. In the position description, in interactions with colleagues, and in other work situations, the author endeavors to explain and clarify the similarities and differences between her practice and the practices of CNSs and NPs. As more APNs are prepared for, and function in, blended CNS/NP roles, CNS/NP may come to be a position title that is widely understood.

CONCLUSION

The future of health care is uncharted. Changes in reimbursement strategies, legislation, the professional workforce, and societal health-care needs represent opportunities that can support the continued growth of advanced nursing practice. APNs have demonstrated their ability to provide cost-efficient, quality, health care to a wide range of patient groups. The current challenge in this evolving, competitive environment is to ensure a role for advanced nursing practice within any future health-care system. The blended-role APN, by virtue of preparation as both CNS and NP, is uniquely qualified to provide a range of services throughout the continuum of care, ensuring continuity for patients. The most exciting opportunity the blended role offers is to provide expanded services to patients, some traditionally considered within medicine's purview but now offered by APNs who bring a nursing perspective. The challenge to the health-care system and to APNs in the blended role is to identify the populations of patients who will benefit most from this type of provider and the cost savings associated with such care.

APNs must join together to share experiences and knowledge in order to continually improve the services provided to society and to confront existing barriers to practice, such as disparate reimbursement mechanisms and prescriptive authority and the efforts of organized medicine to constrain advanced nursing practice. To ensure a future for advanced nursing practice, APNs must never stop planning for the future.

---

*The word *blended* was deliberately chosen rather than merged, mixed, or combined because of connotations related to purposefulness, shading, and harmony.

REFERENCES

Allan, J. D., & Hall, B. A. (1988). Challenging the focus on technology: A critique of the medical model in a changing health care system. *Advances in Nursing Science*, *10*(3), 22-34.

Beecroft, P. C. (1994). CNS: Thriving or heading for extinction? *Clinical Nurse Specialist*, *8*(2), 63.

Brooten, D., Gennaro, S., Knapp, H., Jovene, N., Brown, L., & York, R. (1991). Functions of the CNS in early discharge and home follow-up of very low birthweight infants. *Clinical Nurse Specialist*, *5*(4), 196-201.

Burns, P. G., Nishikawa, H. A., Weatherby, F., Forni, P. R., Moran, M., Allen, M. E., Baker, C. B., & Booten, D. A. (1993). Master's degree nurs-ing education: State of the art. *Journal of Professional Nursing*, *9*(5), 267-277.

Busen, N. H., & Jones, M. E. (1995). Leadership development: Educating nurse practitioners for the future. *Journal of the American Academy of Nurse Practitioners*, *7*(3), 111-117.

Chinn, P. L. (1991). Looking into the crystal ball: Positioning ourselves for the year 2000. *Nursing Outlook*, *39*(6), 251-256.

Cooper, D. (1990). Today-assessments and intuitions: Tomorrow-projections. In P. S. Sparacino, D. M. Cooper, & P. A. Minarik (Eds.), *The Clinical Nurse Specialist Implementation and Impact* (pp. 285-311). Norwalk, CT: Appleton & Lange.

Cronenwett, L. R. (1995). Molding the future of advanced practice nursing. *Nursing Outlook, 43,* 112-118.

Dale, J. C. (1991). New role for pediatric nurse practitioners in an in-patient setting. *Journal of Pediatric Health Care, 5*(6), 336-337.

Damato, E. G., Dill, P. Z., Gennaro, S., Brown, L. P., York, R., & Brooten, D. (1993). The association between CNS direct care time and total time and very low birth weight infant outcomes. *Clinical Nurse Specialist, 7*(2), 75-79.

Davitt, P. A., & Jensen, L. A. (1981). The role of the acute care nurse practitioner in cardiac surgery. *Nursing Administration Quarterly, 3,* 16-19.

de Tornyay, R. (1992). Reconsidering nursing education: The report of the Pew Health Professions Commissions. *Journal of Nursing Education, 31*(7), 296-301.

Elder, R. G., & Bullough, B. (1990). Nurse practitioner and clinical nurse specialists: Are the roles merging? *Clinical Nurse Specialist, 4*(2), 78-84.

El-Sherif, C. (1995). Nurse practitioners—Where do they belong within the organizational structure of the acute care setting? *Nurse Practitioner, 20*(1), 62-65.

Fenton, M. V., & Brykczynski, K. A. (1993). Qualitative distinctions and similarities in the practice of clinical nurse specialists and nurse practitioners. *Journal of Professional Nursing, 9*(6), 313-326.

Forbes, K. E., Rafson, J., Spross, J. A., & Kozlowski, D. (1990). The clinical nurse specialist and nurse practitioner: Core curriculum survey results. *Clinical Nurse Specialist, 4*(2), 63-66.

Galassi, A., & Wheeler, V. (1994). Advanced practice nursing: History and future trends. In S. M. Hubbard, P. E. Greene, & M. T. Knobf (Eds.), *Oncology Nursing* (pp. 1-10). Philadelphia: J. B. Lippincott.

Gleeson, R. M., McIlvain-Simpson, G., Boos, M. L., Sweet, E., Trzcinski, K. M., Solberg, C. A., & Doughty, R. A. (1990). Advanced practice nursing: A model of collaborative care. *MCN, 15*(1), 9-12.

Griffith, H. M., & Robinson, K. R. (1993). Current procedural terminology (CPT) coded services provided by nurse specialists. *Image, 25*(3), 179-186.

Hamric, A. B., & Taylor, J. W. (1989). Role development of the CNS. In A. B. Hamric & J. A. Spross (Eds.), *The Clinical Nurse Specialist in Theory and Practice* (2nd ed., pp. 41-82). Philadelphia: W. B. Saunders.

Hamric, A. B. (1989). A model for CNS evaluation. In A. B. Hamric & J. A. Spross (Eds.), *The clinical nurse specialist in theory and practice* (2nd ed., pp. 83-106). Philadelphia: W. B. Saunders.

Hanson, C., & Martin, L. L. (1990). The nurse practitioner and clinical specialist: Should the roles be merged? *Journal of the American Academy of Nurse Practitioners, 2*(1), 2-9.

Hockenberry-Eaton, M., & Powell, M. L. (1991). Merging advanced practice roles: The CNS and NP. *Journal of Pediatric Health Care, 5,* 158-159.

Holt, F. M. (1987). Developmental stages of the clinical nurse specialist role. *Clinical Nurse Specialist, 1,* 116-118.

Hravnak, M., Kobert, S. N., Risco, K. G., Baldisseri, M., Hoffman, L. A., Clochesy, J. M., Eudy, E. B., & Snyder, J. V. (1995). Acute care nurse practitioner curriculum: Content and development process. *American Journal of Critical Care, 4*(3), 179-188.

Hunsberger, M., Mitchell, A., Blatz, P., Paes, B., Pinelli, J., Southwell, D., French, S., & Soluk, R. (1992). Definition of an advanced nursing role in the NICU: The clinical nurse specialist/nurse practitioner. *Clinical Nurse Specialist, 6*(2), 91-96.

Jackson, P. L. (1995). Opportunities and challenges for PNPs. *Pediatric Nursing, 21*(1), 43-46.

Keane, A., & Richmond, T. (1993). Tertiary nurse practitioners. *Image, 25*(4), 281-293.

Keane, A., Richmond, T., & Kaiser, L. (1994). Critical care nurse practitioners: Evolution of the advanced practice nursing role. *American Journal of Critical Care, 3,* 232-237.

King, K. B. & Ackerman, M. H. (1995). An educational model for the acute care nurse practitioner. *Critical Care Nursing Clinics of North America, 7,* 1-8.

Kitzman, H. J. (1989). The CNS and nurse practitioner. In A. B. Hamric & J. A. Spross (Eds.), *The Clinical Nurse Specialist* (2nd ed., pp. 379-394). Philadelphia: W. B. Saunders.

Kindig, D., Cultice, J., & Mullen, F. (1993). The elusive generalist physician: Can we reach a 50% goal? *Journal of the American Medical Association, 270*(9), 1069-1073.

Koetters, T. L. (1989). Clinical practice and direct patient care. In A. B. Hamric & J. A. Spross (Eds.) *The clinical nurse specialist in theory and practice* (2nd ed., pp. 107-124). Philadelphia: W. B. Saunders.

Malkemes, L. (1974). Resocialization: A model for nurse practitioner preparation. *Nursing Outlook, 22*(2), 90-94.

Malone, B. L. (1989). The CNS in a consultation department. In A. B. Hamric & J. A. Spross (Eds.), *The clinical nurse specialist in theory and practice* (2nd ed., pp. 397-413). Philadelphia: W. B. Saunders.

Mauksch, I. (1978). The nurse practitioner movement—Where does it go from here? *American Journal of Public Health, 68,* 1074-1075.

McGivern, D. O. (1993). The evolution to advanced nursing practice. In M. D. Mezey & D. O. McGivern (Eds.), *Nurses, nurse practioners: Evolution to advanced practice* (pp. 3-30). New York: Springer.

Mundinger, M. O. (1994). Advanced practice

nursing—Good medicine for physicians? *New England Journal of Medicine, 330,* 211-213.

Nemes, J., Barnaby, K., & Shamberger, R. C. (1992). Experience with a nurse practitioner program in the surgical department of a children's hospital. *Journal of Pediatric Surgery, 27*(8), 1038-1042.

Office of Technology Assessment, U.S. Congress (1986). *Nurse practitioners, physicians assistants, and certified nurse midwives: A policy analysis* (Health Technology Case Study 37, OTA-HCS-37). Washington, D. C.: U.S. Government Printing Office.

Page, N. E., & Arena, D. M. (1994). Rethinking the merger of the clinical nurse specialist and the nurse practitioner roles. *Image, 26*(4), 315-318.

Papenhausen, J. L. (1990). Case management: A model of advanced practice? *Clinical Nurse Specialist, 4*(4), 169-170.

Pearson, L. J. (1990). 25 years later 25 exceptional NPs look at the movement's evolution and consider future challenges for the role. *Nurse Practitioner: The American Journal of Primary Health Care, 15*(9), 9-31.

Richmond, T. S., & Keane, A. (1992). The NP in tertiary care. *Journal of Nursing Administration, 22*(11), 11-12.

Safriet, B. J. (1992). Health care dollars and regulatory sense: The role of the advanced practice nurse. *Yale Journal on Regulation, 9*(2), 417-487.

Sawyers, J. E. (1993). Defining your role in ambulatory care: Clinical nurse specialist or nurse practitioner? *Clinical Nurse Specialist, 7*(1), 4-7.

Schroer, K. (1991). Case management: Clinical nurse specialist and nurse practitioner, converging roles. *Clinical Nurse Specialist, 5*(4), 189-194.

Shugars, D. A., O'Neil, E. H., & Bader, J. D. (Eds.) (1991). *Healthy America: Practitioners for 2005, an agenda for action for the U.S. health profession schools.* Durham, N. C.: The PEW Health Professions Commission.

Smith, L. D. (1994). Continuity of care through nursing case management of the chronically ill child. *Clinical Nurse Specialist, 8*(2), 65-68.

Snyder, M., & Mirr, M. P. (Eds.) (1995). *Advance practice nursing: Guide to professional development.* New York: Springer.

Sparacino, P. S. (1993). The advanced practice nurse: Is the time right for a singular title? *Clinical Nurse Specialist, 7*(1), 3.

Spross, J., & Hamric, A. B. (1983). A model for future clinical specialist practice. In A. B. Hamric & J. Spross (Eds.), *The clinical nurse specialist in theory and practice.* New York: Grune & Stratton.

Thibodeau, J. A., & Hawkins, J. W. (1994). Moving towards a nursing model in advanced practice. *Western Journal of Nursing Research, 16*(2), 205-218.

Weinberg, R. M., Likestrand, J. S., & Moore, S. (1983). In-patient management by a nurse practitioner: Effectiveness in a rehabilitation setting. *Archives of Physical Medicine and Rehabilitation, 64,* 588-590.

Wright, J. E. (1990). Joining forces for the good of our clients. *Clinical Nurse Specialist, 4*(2), 76-77.

Zimmer, P., Brykczynski, K., Martin, A. C., Newberry, Y. G., Price, M. J., & Warren, B. (1990). *Advanced nursing practice: Nurse practitioner curriculum guidelines* (Final Report: NONPF Education Committee). Washington, D. C.: National Organization of Nurse Practitioner Faculties.

CHAPTER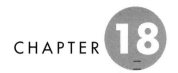

The Certified Nurse-Midwife

Margaret Dorroh
Sheila F. Norton

INTRODUCTION

Nurse-midwifery has made many contributions that have paved the way for advanced nursing practice (ANP) to flourish. These efforts have included the development of standards and core clinical competencies and successful legislative and regulatory initiatives. These activities were instrumental in securing prescriptive authority and direct reimbursement by insurers for certified nurse-midwives (CNMs). Despite these contributions, the specialty of nurse-midwifery has not joined forces with the nursing profession's efforts to organize and align all advanced practice roles. Several factors may account for this, including competing professional priorities related to availability of and access to midwifery services, which are discussed later in the chapter. Paradoxically, availability and access have been central arguments for health-care reform initiatives that promote ANP roles. To general readers of this text as well as to CNMs themselves, it may seem that CNMs do not quite fit in the movement to bring APNs together. Although we support all of the criteria for ANP practice put forth in this text, the authors are mindful and respectful of the many initiatives and risks CNMs have taken to cultivate a clinical and political environment that seems ready to accept them, clinical nurse specialists (CNSs), certified registered nurse anesthetists (CRNAs), and nurse practitioners (NPs) as legitimate and visible providers of care across all settings. Therefore, we describe nurse-midwifery practice so that the reader can appreciate why it is seen as an ANP role. We offer our own perspectives on the issues that prevent full integration of nurse-midwifery into advanced nursing practice. Even though the move toward advanced practice has not fully engaged nurse-midwifery and all CNMs, nurses and nurse-midwives alike are stakeholders in issues related to this level of professional practice. The reflections offered in this chapter are meant to foster dialogue, understanding, and wisdom as nurses and nurse-midwives work to accomplish their goals related to practice. It is our hope that as stakeholders, nurses and nurse-midwives will continue to work productively and collaboratively on activities that promote advanced nursing practice.

HISTORICAL PERSPECTIVE

The word *midwife* has had the same meaning in all times and in all cultures. In Biblical times, the midwife assisted a woman in labor, helped with the delivery, and provided aftercare for the mother and child. Novice midwives acquired knowledge and skill from practical training with experienced midwives and through their own observation and experience. Skilled midwives provided emergency medical or surgical assistance as needed and, in recognition of their importance, were exempted from injunctions against work on the Sabbath when performing their duties. Present-day midwives are granted the same privilege!

In colonial times, midwives were an integral part of community life and were highly respected. By the early 1900s, a number of developments had considerably diminished that respect and led to an ebb in the practice of midwifery. A key factor was the medicalization of childbirth. By the early 1900s, the medical field had become highly competitive; attending labor and delivery was a way physicians could establish a practice. Families pleased with the medical care provided at childbirth would return to the same physician for other care. This phenomenon combined with women's low social status made it difficult for midwives to compete against physicians. Although the arrival of physicians on the childbearing scene was late, this accident of history continues to influence the regulation and practice of nurse-midwifery.

The renaissance of midwifery in the United States was not to occur for more than two decades, although it remained part of mainstream health care in many European, Asian, and African countries. Like the emergence of other forms of advanced nursing practice, the resurgence of midwifery and the evolution of nurse-midwifery occurred in response to the need for care by the underserved. By the late 1960s, the contributions of nurse-midwifery were accepted and recognized. The profession was inundated with requests for nurse-midwives and was criticized for not having enough CNMs trained to meet the needs of women in this country. This led to a proliferation of nurse-midwifery educational programs and the development of more nurse-midwifery practices. Table 18–1 presents a timeline of key events that influenced the development of modern nurse-midwifery as described by Varney (1987).

THE NURSE-MIDWIFERY PROFESSION IN THE UNITED STATES TODAY

STATISTICAL OVERVIEW

The American College of Nurse-Midwives (ACNM) defines a CNM as an individual educated in the two disciplines of nursing and midwifery. There are more than 5,000 active and student members of the ACNM (Nitzsche, 1995). In 1994, 72.6% of CNMs had master's degrees (57% of which were in nursing), and 3.8% had doctoral degrees (D. Williams, CNM, MS, Professional Affairs Liaison, ACNM, personal communication, October 12, 1995). Approximately 2% of nurse-midwives are men (ACNM Public Relations Department, personal communication, October 3, 1995). In 1992, 185,000 births were attended by CNMs, and it has been estimated that by 2000, 10% of all births in the U.S. will be attended by CNMs (Nitzsche, 1995).

EDUCATION

The qualified CNM has completed an educational program approved by the ACNM Division of Accreditation and has ACNM certification. The DOA is responsible for overseeing programs preparing nurse-midwives. An accredited program is one that has been recognized as carrying out the philosophy, purpose, and objectives set forth by its faculty and as having met the standards established by the ACNM for the preparation of competent nurse-midwives. There are 43 nurse-midwifery educational programs (Nitzsche, 1995). Although the majority of programs prepare students at the master's level, certificate programs continue to exist. This is in keeping with the ACNM position that two educational tracks should be available. This official stance conflicts directly with the criterion of graduate education for advanced practice nursing adopted by many nursing organizations (see Chapter 3) and supported by this book; however, it is consistent with the ACNM's commitment to ensure access to nurse-midwifery services. This complex issue is examined in more detail in the Professional Issues section.

TABLE 18–1. THE EVOLUTION OF NURSE-MIDWIFERY: A TIMELINE OF CRITICAL EVENTS

Year	Event	Significance
Colonial times to early 1900s	Midwives traveled to the colonies. They were respected in communities and trained in apprenticeships. Practices were often handed down from mother to daughter.	Midwifery had a strong basis in service to others—went beyond an occupation—often seen as a "calling"—the women who practiced midwifery tended to be rich in life experience if not in formal education.
Early 1900s	Midwifery was co-opted by organized medicine.	Decreased number and experience of practitioners effectively put midwives "in the closet."
1925	Frontier Nursing Service was founded in Hyden, Kentucky.	Imported British-trained midwives utilized the nursing model. Designed to meet the specific needs in an underserved area. Births took place in homes. Neonatal mortality rate 9.1/1000 births from 1925 to 1951 (not matched by U.S. at large until 1990s).
1931	The Maternity Center Association, in New York, opened the Lobenstine Clinic.	Provided care for immigrant families in upper Manhattan tenements.
1932	The first nurse-midwifery education program was developed at the Lobenstine Clinic.	Offered advanced preparation in midwifery to public health nurses. Acknowledged relationship of nursing and midwifery.
1941	The Tuskegee School of Nurse-Midwifery opened in Alabama.	Access to nurse-midwifery education for minorities
1943	The Catholic Maternity Institute was founded in Santa Fe, New Mexico.	
Mid-1940s	The National Organization of Public Health Nurses (later absorbed into the American Nurses' Association) was established for nurse-midwives.	Recognition of midwifery as having a foundation in nursing.
1955	The American College of Nurse-Midwives was founded.	Began formalizing standards for education, certification, and practice. The basic certificate program was the norm—also provided a formal voice for nurse-midwives.
Early 1960s	A certified nurse-midwife pilot project was conducted in Madera County, California.	
Late 1960s and 1970s	Nurse-midwifery services and educational progams (mostly certificates) proliferated, free-standing birth centers were developed.	Increased utilization of and demand for CNMs in a variety of settings
1980s	Malpractice crisis arose.	Closed some practices and threatened closure at some programs until issue resolved.
1980s and 1990s	Certified nurse-midwives moved to graduate level education.	Majority of progams now prepare students at master's level
1990s	The milieu for health-care practice is changing; certified nurse-midwives are moving toward primary care of women.	CNMs adapting to environment in which quality, access, and cost must all be addressed.

LEGAL REQUIREMENTS FOR PRACTICE

CNMs must comply with the legal requirements for the practice of nurse-midwifery in the jurisdiction in which they practice. (The term *jurisdiction* reflects the inclusion of the District of Columbia, the Virgin Islands, and Puerto Rico as well as the 50 states.) The practice of nurse-midwifery differs in the various jurisdictions because of legal, regulatory, and other influences. Such influences include statutes, rules and regulations, opinions of the state attorney general, court decisions, licensure, registration, and certification. The political climate affects nurse-midwifery practice and can promote or restrain the practice of CNMs. For example, the relative power of constituencies such as medical and nursing organizations and consumer groups and the relationships among them can shape legislation and patterns of referral to CNMs. Laws and other ordinances that regulate CNM practice should ensure that all practitioners are qualified to practice nurse-midwifery. The ACNM recently reaffirmed the autonomy with which the CNM practices. The ACNM's official clinical practice statement on independent nurse-midwifery practice is presented in Box 18–1.

CONTINUING EDUCATION

In addition to obtaining initial certification through examination and licensing, CNMs must demonstrate evidence of continuing competency by means of continu-

---

BOX 18–1 CLINICAL PRACTICE STATEMENT ON INDEPENDENT NURSE-MIDWIFERY PRACTICE
(American College of Nurse-Midwives, 1995)

It is the position of the ACNM that nurse-midwifery practice is the independent management of women's health care, focusing particularly on pregnancy, childbirth, the postpartum period, care of the newborn, and the family planning and gynecologic needs of women. This practice occurs within a health care system that provides for consultation, collaborative management or referral as indicated by the health status of the client.

Independent nurse-midwifery practice enables CNMs to utilize knowledge, skills, judgment and authority in the provision of primary women's health services while maintaining accountability for the management of patient care in accordance with the ACNM *Standards for the Practice of Nurse-Midwifery*.

The ACNM believes that independent practice is not defined by the place of employment, the employee-employer relationship, requirements for physician co-signature or the method of reimbursement for services. Nor should *independent* be interpreted to mean *alone*, as there are clinical situations where any prudent practitioner would seek the assistance of another qualified practitioner.

The ACNM also believes that collaboration is the process whereby health care professionals jointly manage care. The goal of collaboration is to share authority while providing quality care within each individual's professional scope of practice. Successful collaboration is a way of thinking and relating that requires knowledge, open communication, mutual respect, a commitment to providing quality care, trust, and the ability to share responsibility.

ing education and peer review through the ACNM's Continuing Competency Assessment program. To maintain their certification, all CNMs must enroll in and complete a cycle every 5 years that consists of 50 or more hours of continuing education relevant to nurse-midwifery. In addition, most state and/or regional divisions of ACNM have in place sophisticated programs of peer review in which all practitioners are encouraged to participate.

THE ACNM

The growth and development of American nurse-midwifery owe much to the ACNM, founded in 1955. As noted earlier, the ACNM accredits nurse-midwifery programs and has structures in place to ensure continuing competency in nurse-midwifery practice. The philosophy promulgated by the ACNM informs the education and practice of all nurse-midwives (Box 18–2).

The Code of Ethics of the ACNM (Ad Hoc Committee on Code of Ethics, 1990) aligns with the American Nurses' Association's (ANA's) Code of Ethics. A CNM has professional moral obligations. The code identifies the obligations that guide the CNM in the practice of nurse-midwifery and clarifies what consumers, the public, other professionals, and potential practitioners can expect of the profession. Nurse-midwifery exists for the good of women and their families; this good is safeguarded

---

BOX 18–2 ACNM PHILOSOPHY
(American College of Nurse-Midwives, 1989)

Nurse-midwives believe that every individual has the right to safe, satisfying health care with respect for human dignity and cultural variations. We further support each person's right to self-determination, to complete information and to active participation in all aspects of care. We believe the normal processes of pregnancy and birth can be enhanced through education, health care and supportive intervention.

Nurse-midwifery care is focused on the needs of the individual and family for physical care, emotional and social support and active involvement of significant others according to cultural values and personal preferences. The practice of nurse-midwifery encourages continuity of care; emphasizes safe, competent clinical management; advocates non-intervention in normal processes; and promotes health education for women throughout the childbearing cycle. This practice may be extended to include gynecological care of well women throughout the life cycle. Such comprehensive health care is most effectively and efficiently provided by nurse-midwives in collaboration with other members of an interdependent health care team.

The ACNM assumes a leadership role in the development and promotion of high quality health care for women and infants both nationally and internationally. The profession of nurse-midwifery is committed to ensuring certified nurse-midwives are provided with sound educational preparation, to expanding knowledge through research and to evaluating and revising care through quality assurance. The profession further ensures that its members adhere to the *Standards for the Practice of Nurse-Midwifery* in accordance with the *ACNM Philosophy*.

by practice that is consistent with the *ACNM Philosophy* (ACNM, 1989) and *ACNM Standards for the Practice of Nurse-Midwifery* (ACNM, 1993). The belief that pregnancy and childbirth are normal life processes is at the heart of nurse-midwifery practice. The nurse-midwife learns to be "with woman" (the original meaning of *midwife*) without having to "manage" pregnancy, labor, or delivery. The patience to allow normal processes to proceed at an unhurried pace is one of the nurse-midwife's skills. This is one of the key differences between nurse-midwifery and medical approaches to the care of women. Adherents of the medical model tend to intervene even when things are proceeding normally. In nurse-midwifery, when intervention is indicated, CNMs ensure that it is integrated into care in a way that preserves the dignity of the woman and her family. The Code of Ethics further describes expectations regarding practice competence, nurse-midwife/client relationships, ethical responsibilities, collegial practice, and nondiscrimination. Responsibilities for conducting research in nurse-midwifery and for supporting community and political activities that promote access to health care are also delineated.

Preparation for nurse-midwifery draws on certain concepts and skills from nursing, the social sciences, and public health. The core competencies for basic nurse-midwifery practice (ACNM, 1993) reflect the philosophy and values advanced by the ACNM and provide the basis for accrediting educational programs and certifying nurse-midwives. These competencies are the fundamental skills and behaviors expected of the new graduate (ACNM, 1993). The core competencies include the components of nurse-midwifery care and nurse-midwifery management processes, both of which are further described later.

Through its standards, position statements, and other documents, the ACNM continues to shape nurse-midwifery practice. Among ANP organizations (with the exception of nurse anesthetists, perhaps), the ACNM and its affiliated organizations are unique in the scope of their activities, which include establishing core competencies and practice standards, accrediting educational programs, and establishing mechanisms for initial certification and assurance of continued competency in nurse-midwifery. An understanding of the role of the ACNM in shaping practice and familiarity with the documents cited or reproduced here will help the reader appreciate the similarities and differences between CNMs and other APNs.

ADVOCACY AND CLIENT EDUCATION: CORNERSTONES OF NURSE-MIDWIFERY PRACTICE

Nurse-midwifery is multifaceted, constantly evolving, and broader in scope than it was first envisioned by its pioneers. Nurse-midwives have in common with all APNs the characteristics of using a holistic perspective, establishing a partnership with the client, involving significant others and family members in care, using clinical reasoning, managing health and illnesses, and using processes to perform self-evaluation. To further understand nurse-midwifery practice, it is helpful to take a close look at the core competencies related to advocacy and client education.

ADVOCACY

Advocacy is central to nurse-midwifery practice. Client education and support of clients' rights and self-determination inform every aspect of nurse-midwifery care.

These values have been challenged by the burgeoning growth of medical technology in the last two decades. The availability of highly technical interventions for many aspects of childbearing, such as infertility, monitoring pregnancies, and delivery conflicts with the traditionally low-technology, low-interventionist approach of CNMs. Vulnerable populations (e.g., women who have not had access to early prenatal care or low-income women receiving care at a teaching hospital clinic) are more likely to be exposed to high-technology interventions. This presents CNMs with several challenges: to evaluate technologies to determine whether and how they can be incorporated into nurse-midwifery care, to incorporate such therapies into practice in ways that are consistent with nurse-midwifery's values, to explain technology in a way that empowers women to make informed decisions, and to provide equal access to the technology.

CLIENT EDUCATION

Client education is another cornerstone of nurse-midwifery practice and is integral to the CNM's advocacy role. CNMs fulfill the role of advocate best when they have invested time, effort, and caring in establishing a partnership with the client and providing her with the teaching and counseling that is characteristic of nurse-midwifery practice. A recent study of 1,181 women suggests that this emphasis on education explains some differences between nurse-midwives' and obstetricians' care processes (Oakley et al., 1995). Although many processes were similar, the nurse-midwives emphasized educational/psychosocial care and restrained use of technology tailored to the individual, whereas the obstetricians' practice reflected routine use of state-of-the-art technology. CNMs' emphasis on education enables women to participate knowledgeably and fully in their care. The value of a partnership that has been built over the course of the pregnancy becomes eminently clear during labor, when decisions have to be made. CNMs understand that a woman in the midst of labor may not be in the best position to make good, coherent decisions. The CNM and informed significant others can act in the client's best interests at this time, because the woman's goals and her contingency plans for events that might interfere with them have been jointly determined by the time labor begins.

Client education, never an easy task, is made even more daunting by the rapidity with which new technologies are developed, tested, and offered to women. Many women make decisions about their care without adequate information and are then left to suffer any consequences (Franklin, 1994). The CNM is often a woman's best hope of receiving adequate information and of ensuring she is not left bewildered and alone. Nurse-midwives bring the gifts of skill, knowledge, and love to a health-care setting that can be devoid of human warmth, all the more so as the technological aspect of care becomes more and more complex. There can be few more noble tasks than providing every woman a safer passage to motherhood and a better future for her children and family (Hsia, 1991).

THE CURRENT PRACTICE OF NURSE-MIDWIFERY

SCOPE OF PRACTICE

Originally, midwifery practice was limited to prenatal, intrapartum, postpartum, and newborn care. Today, while some CNMs limit their practice or are limited by their practice settings to pregnancy care alone, nurse-midwifery care has expanded to include the primary care of women, preconception, gynecological, contraceptive, and infertility care. Nurse-midwives care for teenage women, women in their childbearing years, and women in midlife or those who are elderly. This expansion is due largely to consumer demand and the need for greater access to these services. Interestingly, in many other countries midwifery practice continues to be somewhat restricted to care related to childbirth only.

Scope of practice refers to what CNMs are actually doing in practice once the core competencies have been met. The ACNM (1992) provides a guide for the evaluation and addition of other skills and procedures to nurse-midwifery practice. Thus, procedures such as circumcision, vacuum extraction delivery, endometrial biopsy, colposcopy, and elective termination of pregnancy can be included in some CNMs' practice. The term *scope of practice* is also used to differentiate nurse-midwifery practice that is office-based, providing no labor and delivery care, from full-scope practice, which includes labor and delivery care. Both types of practice may or may not include the additional procedures previously mentioned.

The ACNM Core Competencies (1993) codify knowledge and practice expectations of the graduate CNM, serve as a guide for educational programs, and represent basic CNM practice to other organizations, health-care professionals, and practice settings. Table 18–2 offers an overview of nurse-midwifery practice, including the knowledge needed and the processes used to provide care. Care of women at other developmental stages or with other health-care needs follows similar guidelines. Nurse-midwifery practice incorporates knowledge of the following: normal human physical and psychological development; anatomy and physiology; physiological and psychological deviations from normal; embryology and genetics; reproduction; sexuality; and pharmacology. CNMs recognize indicators of developmental changes throughout women's life cycles and can counsel women regarding health promotion measures specific to these changes. They know indicators of problems with sexuality and can provide counseling or initiate consultation or referral for problems outside the scope of nurse-midwifery practice. Like all APNs, CNMs are familiar with deviations from normal, risk factors, appropriate preventive measures, and interventions for selected pathology. Whatever a woman's developmental stage or health-care concern, CNMs are expected to teach and counsel clients regarding self-care practices, health promotion, nutritional issues, emotional concerns, and sexuality. Nurse-midwifery practice includes well-defined processes for interacting with physicians and other colleagues to ensure high-quality care. The core competencies, practice guidelines, and agency- or practice-specific policies establish the standards of care within the scope of practice for a particular agency or practice setting. Readers will also recognize many similarities in the values and philosophy guiding CNM practice to those guiding care in other advanced practice roles, especially OB-GYN NPs.

Although nurse-midwifery practice overlaps with aspects of care provided by other health professionals, elements of care provided by CNMs are unique to this group of health-care providers. CNMs are not limited to modern allopathic (medical) approaches and may advise clients to use measures from older traditions that women have found comforting and effective. Such treatments may include acupressure, herbals, homeopathics, sea bands, healing touch, positioning, and nutritional interventions. These complementary interventions are most likely to be used for the common discomforts of pregnancy, during labor, for premenstrual problems, or for menopausal symptoms.

TABLE 18–2. OVERVIEW OF NURSE-MIDWIFERY PRACTICE

	General Women's Health	Pregnancy	Intrapartum	Postpartum	Care of the Newborn
Knowledge needed	Bioethics Interpersonal communication Culture and community resources Counseling Normal reproductive biology Scientific bases of prescriptions to prevent or facilitate pregnancy	Genetics Physiology of normal pregnancy Embryology Pathophysiology Risks Clinical indicators for complications Pharmacokinetics of medications commonly used in pregnancy	Anatomy of normal and abnormal labor in all stages Anatomy of fetal skull and its landmarks Prescription of medications and solutions	A&P of the puerperium involutional process Lactation and methods for facilitation or suppression Recognition of deviations from normal	A&P and indicators of normal adaptation to extrauterine life Stabilization of the neonate
Assessment and diagnosis	History, physical, lab data, and health risks	Parameters and methods for assessing progress of pregnancy and fetal well-being	Progress of labor Maternal and fetal status	Emotional, psychosocial, and sexual factors	Neonatal physical assessment Neonatal gestational age assessment
Teaching	Health promotion Preventative self-care	Childbirth education Parenting Nutritional education	Reinforcing labor comfort measures taught in childbirth classes Hygiene	Anticipatory guidance re: self-care, infant care, family planning, family relationships	Infant care Nutritional needs of the infant

Comforting	Drug and nondrug measures for discomforts related to menstruation and menopause Information on coping with stress	Drug and nondrug measures for the discomforts of pregnancy	Sensitivity to emotional changes Hands-on-care Drug and nondrug measures for pain Local and pudendal anesthesia administration	Managing discomforts of puerperium	Enhancing bonding
Supporting	Active listening	Assists and supports the woman in decision making	Physical and emotional support	Supports woman in breastfeeding and self- and infant care	Support for the changes in family structure with a new member
Treatment and management	Promotion of family-centered care	Monitoring progress of pregnancy	Monitoring progress of labor Managing abnormal birth events Placental expulsion Repair of lacerations or episiotomy	Appropriate interventions for any deviation from normal	Facilitates adaptation of newborn to extrauterine life
Coordination and complex management	Collaboration, referral Practice/business management Promotion of the continuity of care Consultation and co-management	Advocacy Care jointly planned with woman Develop a birth plan Manage deviations from normal	Back-up plans for emergencies in place Promotion of continuity of care	Provides for continuity of care for the woman and neonate	Resuscitation and emergency care when needed Referrals as necessary

NURSE-MIDWIFERY MANAGEMENT PROCESSES

Regardless of practice setting, the process of nurse-midwifery management has four aspects: independent management, consultation, co-management (collaborative management), and referral (ACNM, 1993). Implicit in the process are timely action and documentation of the three aspects other than independent management (Avery, 1993). The key differences among these aspects of management relate to accountability.

INDEPENDENT MANAGEMENT. CNMs are responsible and accountable for the management decisions they make in caring for clients. CNMs provide *independent management* when they systematically obtain or update a complete and relevant database for assessment of the client's health status. This includes the history, the results of the physical examination, and laboratory data. On the basis of these findings and the interpretation of them, CNMs accurately identify problems and diagnoses. They delineate health-care goals and formulate and communicate a complete needs/problem list in collaboration with the woman. CNMs know when consultation, co-management, or referral is needed and initiate these interactions in a timely manner.

CONSULTATION. When CNMs identify problems or complications, they seek advice from another member of the health-care team, often a physician, but not always an obstetrician. When they retain independent management responsibility for the client while seeking advice, this is called *consultation* (ACNM, 1992). A consultation may center around an ongoing health problem (e.g., hypothyroidism); a nonobstetrical, time-limited problem that arises during pregnancy (e.g., bronchitis or food poisoning), or an obstetrical complication (e.g., size/date discrepancy). After consultation, the CNM and the woman discuss the recommendations, if any, and modify the plan of care accordingly. In the process of consultation, CNMs do not abdicate responsibility for decisions. If they seek consultation from another professional and the suggestions the other professional makes do not seem to be in the client's best interests, they will not be used. Thus, the process of consultation used by CNMs is consistent with the consultation process described in Chapter 8. It is fair to say that novice CNMs are likely to consult often and to use most of the recommendations they receive until they acquire more experience. Consulting is one way of continuing to learn. The experienced CNM is likely to have a tentative plan in mind when consulting and uses consultation to verify the approach or to seek alternatives. It is important to emphasize that CNMs assume direct responsibility for implementing the plan of care in light of their independent management role.

CO-MANAGEMENT OR COLLABORATIVE CARE. One outcome of consultation may be the decision to shift to *co-management or collaborative care*. This usually occurs if part of the woman's care is an ongoing medical, gynecological, or obstetrical complication beyond the scope of the CNM's practice (ACNM, 1992). In this situation, the CNM and physician *collaboratively manage* the patient, with the CNM defining and retaining accountability for nurse-midwifery aspects of care (ACNM, 1993) (see Chapters 8 and 11 for further discussions of consultation and collaboration, respectively).

REFERRAL. When CNMs identify the need for comprehensive management and care outside the scope of nurse-midwifery practice, they direct the client to a physician or another professional for management of the particular problem (ACNM, 1993). *Referral* involves the transfer of some or all of the care and some or all accountability to another provider. This management aspect is usually temporary, and once the client's condition returns to that which is within the CNM's scope of practice, the CNM resumes independent management or co-management. For example, the CNM would refer a woman to an internist for hospitalization for pneumonia, to a surgeon for appendicitis, or to an obstetrician for a cesarean birth. Once the woman regained her health or recovered from surgery, she could return to the CNM's care.

The details of these aspects of management are developed by individual CNMs in concert with obstetrical consultants/backup and the practice settings in which nurse-midwifery practice takes place. In addition to these patterns of care, CNMs also serve as consultants to, or co-manager with, other providers including physicians, APN colleagues, registered nurses, physical therapists, and mental health colleagues.

PRACTICE SETTINGS

One soon learns that there are many different practice styles and roles in nurse-midwifery, from full-scope CNMs to office-based CNMs who are not on a call schedule and do not do deliveries. CNMs practice in urban, suburban, and rural areas in a variety of settings. They practice in tertiary and secondary hospitals, often as part of a group practice of CNMs or CNMs and OB-GYN or family practice physicians. CNMs are employed by health maintenance organizations and neighborhood health centers. Many CNMs are in private practice, either self-employed or employed by physicians or other CNMs. In some settings, the CNM is the primary care provider; in others, the CNM may have a much more circumscribed practice. The CNM's actual practice depends on the needs of the population being served, the CNM's willingness to undertake a variety of functions, the availability of educational resources for the many different functions a CNM performs in a specific setting, the particular needs and requests of clients, the availability of physician and CNM colleagues for backup and coverage, and other organizational variables.

Some of the settings in which nurse-midwives provide labor and delivery care are *clients' homes; free-standing birth centers; birth centers within hospitals; and traditional labor and delivery units of community, regional, and tertiary care hospitals.* For clients, the choice of setting may be a matter of philosophy, comfort, convenience, degree of medical risk, or a combination of these factors. Each setting has its unique set of advantages and disadvantages, and the ACNM has published a position statement on practice settings (ACNM, 1980).

Using the client's home as the setting for birth seems in many ways ideal. What could be more family centered? The CNM is in a position to evaluate the client's resources and help her prepare for childbirth and motherhood within her own setting. Any problems the client might have will be much more apparent if she is seen in her own home. Risks of iatrogenic complications or nosocomial infections are minimized. After the birth of the baby, the client can rest or sleep in her own bed, comfort and nurse the baby at will, and enjoy the attention and support of her loved ones. Birth at home certainly makes inclusion of family members in the birth (if the mother desires it) a simpler matter than in some other settings.

There are disadvantages to home birth, as well. The client's home may be too far away from emergency services. It might be difficult to have the degree of privacy needed for the birth if the house is crowded. Depending on the mother's other responsibilities and support system, her ability to rest may be promoted or compromised. The nurse-midwife's resources may be spread too thin, for instance, when two clients are in labor at the same time—on opposite sides of town. It can be difficult to get medical backup (either house calls or admitting privileges) for home births in some areas.

The *free-standing birth center* offers solutions to some of the problems with home births. It usually has homelike, attractive birth rooms. Selected emergency equipment is available, which can save crucial seconds that in a less controlled environment might be spent searching for such items. The CNMs and clients are at one location, and more than one client can be cared for at a time. The disadvantages of the free-standing birth center are similar to those of home birth. When an emergency exceeds the birth center's resources, the client must be transported to a hospital for care. Another important factor is that the client has to get up and take her baby home in a relatively short time, because birth centers do not generally have the ability to keep clients more than 24 hours.

The *birth center within the hospital* would seem to offer safety in emergencies as an advantage, but many believe that the simple proximity of epidural anesthesia, operating rooms, and other highly interventive technologies leads to their increased use. It is easy to lose sight of the "high-touch-low-tech" approach when one is located in the midst of multitudinous technical devices (Fullerton, 1994a). Being within the hospital setting does eliminate some of the problems nurse-midwives have encountered in obtaining medical backup when needed, however.

DIFFERENCES IN PRACTICE BETWEEN NURSE-MIDWIVES AND OTHER PROVIDERS

The most significant difference between CNMs and OB-GYN NPs and family NPs is in the area of delivery. OB-GYN and family NPs do not provide independent or co-management of care during labor and delivery. Some OB-GYN NPs and CNMs may have practices that are evenly divided between pregnancy-related and gynecological services. Others limit their practices to pregnancy-related care. Family NP practices are usually even more varied and include men's and children's care as well as women's health care.

The practices of maternal-child health CNSs and nurse-midwives also overlap in many ways. Like family or OB-GYN NPs, maternal-child health CNSs do not provide independent management of labor and delivery. However, they are likely to be involved with specific patients and programs related to mother-infant services. Brooten et al.'s (1986) study of CNS interventions with premature infants is an example of such intervention. The maternal-child health CNS often has more preparation in the care of older infants and children than does the CNM. Unlike the CNM or the OB-GYN NP or family NP, the maternal-child health CNS is also likely to be responsible for some staff development related to mother-infant care. He or she is more likely to practice in a hospital or community health or public health agency.

There are midwives who are not nurses. In the United States, they are known as professional midwives (preferred term), independent midwives, apprentice midwives, community midwives, or lay midwives. They are most likely to practice within their communities, providing care to pregnant women and attending home births. Their practices are determined partly by the degree to which a particular jurisdiction regulates midwifery and partly by what the prevailing consumer demand and level of medical support are for this type of care. CNMs and midwives relate to each other differently depending on the perceived quality of care provided by both groups, the ability to recognize mutual interest in providing high-quality women's health care, and the consumer demand and medical support for each group within a particular community. The debate over nonnurse midwifery is discussed further in the professional issues section.

Recent research suggests that CNMs and OB-GYN physicians differ most in the processes they use in providing care (Oakley et al., 1995). Many differences between CNMs and obstetricians can be explained by the differing values between medicine and nursing/midwifery. CNMs approach the care of women, particularly during pregnancy, with the expectation that all will occur normally until proven otherwise. OB-GYN physicians are trained to diagnose and treat abnormalities and approach the care of women with the expectation that problems commonly will occur. Each professional group has expertise of value to the other. Successfully meeting the challenges of working together with OB-GYN physicians is as essential to providing nurse-midwifery care as are the core competencies for practice.

SUMMARY

It should be evident from this discussion of nurse-midwifery care, scope of practice, management processes, and practice settings that CNMs have many opportunities to influence women's health care. Nurse-midwifery allows its practitioners to provide client-focused care that is both autonomous and collaborative within or across a variety of settings (Crofts, 1994). It offers a woman the opportunity to obtain, throughout her life as well as during her childbearing years, accessible, understandable high-quality care that will be safe, satisfying, and individualized to her and her family's needs and desires.

AN EXEMPLAR OF NURSE-MIDWIFERY PRACTICE

The day-to-day practice of midwifery is basically the same in all settings. In this section, I (Dorroh) describe my own practice in a free-standing birth center to illustrate how the components of nurse-midwifery care are put into practice.

The client education process often begins before a client is accepted into the practice. Weekly seminars are held to provide prospective clients with information to assist them in deciding where to have their babies. The seminars are held in the waiting area of the birth center so that we can give guided tours and point out the comfort measures (such as the whirlpool tub) and the equipment on hand to handle normal deliveries and emergencies. Finances are discussed. The fee is generally half that required for obstetric care in a hospital setting with a physician, or it may be even less. Most insurers and Medicaid will provide reimbursement.

Clinical documentation must be meticulous, and forms assuring that accurate, consistent, and complete information is obtained are used. Thorough health and family histories are taken. The questions asked elicit information about the woman's physical health and her psychological well-being. How does she feel about being pregnant? What kind of support system does she have in place? What resources might she have that are not currently being called upon? Was the pregnancy planned or a surprise? What are her family circumstances? Is there a stable relationship? Are there other children? I document both positive and negative influences that can have an impact on the client's health and the health of her baby. Once the assessment is complete, risk factors that would prevent us from being able to accept a client are reviewed; if we cannot accept a client, we make a referral. If no risk factors are identified, we schedule the client's first visit.

As soon as my partner and I accept a client into the practice, we emphasize to her the educational component of nurse-midwifery care. To be active participants in their care, clients are taught to obtain their own weight and do their own dipstick urine tests. They participate in charting the information and can watch the progress of the pregnancy firsthand. The program of care for pregnant clients at our birth center includes 10 to 15 prenatal visits, childbirth classes, labor and delivery in the birth center, a home visit within 72 hours, and two office follow-up visits for mother and baby.

Client visits are scheduled on a daily basis. My partner and I jointly make out a call schedule. She takes somewhat more on-call time in return for my doing most of the administrative duties. We see pregnant clients, postpartum clients with their babies, as well as gynecological clients during office hours. The amount of time scheduled for a visit is based on need. A first visit for a pregnant patient is an hour long. An established gynecological client who is coming for her contraceptive injection requires only a few minutes, long enough to be sure she's having no problems with the shot.

A pregnant client is given the CNM's pager number and instructions on how and when to use it. She is also given backup phone numbers for the rare occasion when the pager fails to work. When a client is in active labor or her membranes have ruptured, she calls the CNM on call. She is met at the birth center and examined. We do not admit clients to the birth center until they are in active labor, because we are restricted by law as to how long the stay can be. If a client lives far away, we can keep her around and not officially admit her until she is in active labor. We stay with our clients in the birth center while they labor. We always have an assistant, usually a registered nurse (RN), with us at each delivery. We call the RN in according to need. If the CNM attending the client is tiring from having been up for a long labor, or several labors, the RN can be called to come in early to care for the client while the CNM rests. Sometimes, the RN is not needed until nearly time for delivery.

The mother-to-be helps us to accommodate her wishes by preparing a birth plan. As her due date nears, one of her tasks, along with packing a bag to bring to the birth center and readying her home for a baby, is to write a birth plan. We give her a form that asks whom she wants to be with her, what she imagines labor will be like, what she *hopes* labor will be like, and what comfort measures she would like to use during labor. We use this tool in several ways. We evaluate the effectiveness of our teaching by reading what the woman thinks labor will be like. Fears not previously unearthed may be revealed. This gives us another chance to resolve any emotional factors that could hinder a successful labor. Knowing the person(s) the client wants with her during labor lets us, as the care managers, keep the client's birth supporters restricted to those she wants present. This is discussed ahead of time, because sometimes it happens that people want to be at the birth whom the client does not particularly want at that time. If we are aware of who these people are, we can prevent them from attending. It is important to do so, because too many people present at labor without specific functions to fulfill can sap the energy of the laboring woman. How many are too many is variable.

The list of comfort measures is mainly a reminder to us, though a key contribution from the client. In the thick of labor, a woman may forget that she was looking forward to the Jacuzzi for relaxation and pain relief. A glance at the birth plan helps us try the things the client has already identified as potentially helpful to her. The birth plan helps to emphasize to the client that this is *her* labor. She has responsibilities and rights. Her dignity and worth as a human being are underscored. We try to nourish the woman's self-esteem and strengths that help in all of life, and certainly during labor. The stronger the woman is in every way, the better her outcome is going to be.

The clients are given plenty of written material to help them remember everything. (If a client is unable to read, we spend extra time giving information verbally and making sure she understands.) For instance, to help the client assume responsibility for herself and her labor, we ask her to bring with her to the birth center the foods and drinks she would like while laboring and certain supplies, such as peri pads, bed pads, and diapers. Clients take their babies home dressed in their own clothes and wrapped in their own blankets. They take with them a booklet they were given in the postpartum classes. The booklet describes mother and baby care in detail for the first few days. Because mothers and babies go home quickly, often in about 4 hours, it is imperative that the mother is prepared for checking the baby's temperature and respirations, checking her own uterus, and recognizing signs of complications that require attention right away. These are all listed and there is room for notes and questions. Having a reference helps new moms feel more secure—if they feel something needs attention, they can just look in the booklet and see. If they don't find it there, they can always call the nurse-midwife. But they usually find what they need to know in the booklet. It often confirms what they sensed—either that everything was okay or that they need to get in touch with the nurse-midwife. Thus, we start them out reinforcing their faith in their own perceptions regarding their infants.

We work diligently to empower our clients, to enhance their decision-making abilities, to reinforce the mind-body connection, and to enhance family life by helping women find their personal power. When I think of the enormous effects of empowerment, two new moms come particularly to mind.

M.L.'s case is proof positive of the benefits of teaching new mothers to trust their feelings and make decisions based on them. On the third or fourth day, M.L.'s baby ceased nursing well. He had been nursing vigorously and now was not. Nursing poorly is one of the signs listed in our booklet as requiring professional help. M.L. insisted to her husband that they had to go to the emergency room immediately. (They lived a long distance from the birth center, and it had been decided earlier that if there should be a problem that seemed serious she should go to a nearby emergency room, rather than try to get to the CNM.) Initially, doctors could find nothing wrong, but M.L. insisted they keep looking. As it turned out, the baby had a congenital heart defect that does not show up on clinical examination until 3 or 4 days after birth. M.L. said she was glad she had been given the information at the birth center; it gave her the confidence to trust her feelings that something very serious was wrong. The baby had heart surgery and is doing well.

A woman with confidence and trust in herself can do almost anything, as the case of S.J. shows. S.J. was 26 years old and came to the birth center soon after it opened to have her fourth child. She had a high school education and was home with her children, all of whom were under the age of 5. Her self-esteem was negligible. Her husband came to a few of the prenatal classes but was sullen and unsupportive. S.J. seemed to droop. But she was an excellent mother and was an attentive and fast learner at everything to do with childbirth, childrearing, and health in general. Her interest and enthusiasm grew as we reinforced her abilities and strengths. By the time she gave birth to her son, she seemed a different person from the withdrawn, self-effacing young woman we'd met 7 months earlier. Two years after this baby's birth, S.J. paid a visit to the birth center. "I just wanted to thank you," she said. "Before I came here, I never felt I was any good at anything. You told me I was a good mother, you noticed how well cared for my children were, and you encouraged me to learn all about birth and even let me borrow books and tapes. Well, I learned I was good—at a lot of things! You all showed me that. And I wanted you to know I'm in nursing school now because I want to be able to do what you do—not just take care of people physically, but help people grow."

The ability to have such a positive impact on others is very satisfying for us. However, it is clear that being a nurse-midwife does not entail "doing it all" for our clients. It is far more important, and healthier for all concerned, to teach our clients so that they are empowered to provide themselves and their families with the best possible care for every situation. We cannot be there for every health difficulty our clients may have, but we can give them the confidence that they *know* when something is wrong and the knowledge of what to do in various situations. Nurse-midwives *give* from the core of their being. They listen, which is one of the crucial skills nurse-midwives bring to their practice. The listening is more than an auditory experience. Nurse-midwives listen observantly to hear clearly. They communicate confidence in and care of their clients in everyday matters. They hear clearly, and their clients respond.

The rewards of our practice are many, but we have faced some challenges, too. On the rare occasions that things go wrong, we are scrutinized intensely. Vacation coverage is difficult to find. Other challenges have been complying with regulations and legislation, finding appropriate resources for medical consultation and referral, and dealing with misperceptions of our practice within the larger health-care system. These issues are not unique to our practice, as the next section shows.

PROFESSIONAL ISSUES

IMAGE

The word *midwife* conjures up a variety of images, from the vague to the positively surreal. After their first encounter with a nurse-midwife, many people comment that they are "surprised at how normal she was." But most people are unable to say just what they expected. Expectations that have been voiced about nurse-midwives, and shattered, include, "Old, stooped, with stringy gray hair," "Someone shuffling around in jeans and Birkenstocks," "A far-out radical with love beads," "Backward." These images are damaging and misleading.

Regardless of their appearance or political views, CNMs are professionals guided by the philosophy and code of ethics of the ACNM. Nurse-midwives hear the need for their practice—the need of women to reclaim their own strengths and abilities. Strengthening women is the way to strengthen families. But women's strength can die if not nurtured. And nurturing is what CNMs do as much as anything else.

In caring for women and families, it is imperative that CNMs also care for themselves. In the effort to meet the physical, cognitive, emotional, personal, and political challenges the practice of nurse-midwifery provides, individual CNMs and the profession as a whole must be cognizant of their own needs for nurturing and find sources from which to obtain it. The following are some of the challenges faced by nurse-midwives.

PROFESSIONAL DEVELOPMENT

H.O. Thompson & Thompson (1987) stated that if CNMs are to survive as professionals they need to practice competently, work cooperatively with other team members, maintain their commitment to high-quality care for all women and families, and continue their progress toward the attainment of professional accountability and maturity. Indeed, CNMs are expected to be leaders and change agents. Like other APNs, CNMs are responsible for evaluating their practice through self-evaluation, peer review, chart review, and other mechanisms. Using a Self-Reporting Form, CNMs must document their continuing competency for the ACNM. Acceptable evidence includes retaking the national examination or attending a number of continuing education programs. Publications, presentations, completion of a college level course, or participation in peer review can be used in lieu of a certain number of the required continuing education units.

Like other APNs, as CNMs become more experienced, they often extend the depth and breadth of their care. Options for professional growth include developing a specialty or subspecialty, acquiring additional primary care skills, learning additional procedures, combining teaching with clinical practice, and embarking on a collaborative or independent practice.

NURSE-MIDWIFERY EDUCATION

The official position of the ACNM has been that two educational tracks should continue to be available for individuals who wish to become nurse-midwives—the master's degree and the certificate program. This conflicts with the consensus of most of the nursing profession that a master's degree in nursing be required for advanced nursing practice, which is also the premise of this book. Why is this so? First, the ACNM maintains that no demonstrable difference can be ascertained by examination or in clinical practice between certificate-prepared and master's-prepared CNMs. There is no evidence that nurse-midwives with a master's degree in nursing are safer or more effective practitioners than those who graduate from certificate programs. Furthermore, the ACNM believes that the quality of the individual nurse-midwife at entry into practice is assured by the ACNM's Division of Accreditation. The second and more compelling (or more understandable) argument has to do with several organizational and professional commitments and initiatives of the ACNM, which are described below.

The assertion of no difference can be challenged on grounds other than safety and efficacy. Although there may not yet be discernible differences in clinical outcomes and certification examination scores, it is possible that the questions that would uncover differences have not yet been asked. Clinically, differences may be more apparent in the processes of care and the range and type of problems that can be solved. Also, APNs bring more than their clinical competence to the practice setting. Questions regarding type and complexity of consultations sought and offered by CNMs might uncover differences between master's- and certificate-prepared CNMs.

Barron McBride (1995) has proposed differentiated practice as a solution to the variation of educational levels within the nursing profession as a whole. She suggested that all nurses are knowledge workers and that the range and type of knowledge used in practice vary on the basis of education. Such a solution might also be appropriate and more acceptable within nurse-midwifery and midwifery, particularly when one considers the issues discussed below. More research on the issue of differences in practice based on education will be needed to derive differentiated practice patterns within midwifery. An additional factor to consider regarding differences in practice is the issue of leadership. Perusal of several volumes of the *Journal of Nurse Midwifery,* the official journal of the ACNM, indicates that CNMs prepared at the graduate level are more visible and involved in professional leadership activities, such as writing for publication and holding national office in the ACNM, than are certificate-prepared CNMs.

Priority commitments of the nurse-midwifery organization may also interfere with taking a stand on education for advanced nursing practice in midwifery. There are too few CNMs to meet the health-care needs of pregnant women, and the ACNM has undertaken an initiative to narrow the gap between the numbers of CNMs available and the numbers needed by 2000. Nurse-midwifery attracts a variety of adult learners from various backgrounds: foreign-trained nurses and nurse-midwives; RNs with diplomas, associate degrees, and bachelor's degrees in nursing and other fields; and professional (community or lay) midwives. The rigors of the accreditation and certification processes are designed to ensure that both master's programs and certificate programs produce graduates who possess the core competencies. To make more nurse-midwives available to address the needs of pregnant women, nurse-midwifery education must be accessible and affordable. There is also an effort to recruit potential students from the communities where nurse-midwives are most needed—in underserved communities. Members of some of these communities have few financial resources. Master's programs are often longer, more expensive, and less accessible than certificate programs. Some influential consumer leaders in the women's health movement maintain that nurse-midwives are so badly needed that to require a master's degree is a disservice to the women and communities who need midwifery services.

In addition to meeting the need for CNMs, the ACNM has embarked on two other initiatives that complicate the issue of its taking a stand on the master's degree in nursing for nurse-midwifery: It is collaborating with the Midwives Association of North America to develop accreditation and certification processes for the preparation and certification of midwives who are not nurses or other health professionals, and it is exploring mechanisms to enable other health professionals, such as dietitians and physical therapists, to enter midwifery.

These developments may be viewed in two ways. One perspective is that these initiatives further obscure advanced nursing practice and make it even more difficult for APNs to attain some of the regulatory and legislative supports they seek. On the other hand, the ACNM may be at the cutting edge of developing a transdisciplinary workforce, a legion of people with different backgrounds but the same core set of midwifery competencies. It is difficult to predict where this type of cross-training will go. It is interesting to speculate on the combined talents of a midwifery practice whose members include certified midwives who are APNs, physical therapists, and dietitians. Such a group does seem consistent with projections regarding the type of workforce needed in the future (Senge, 1994).

In our opinion, the ACNM's commitments to expand the pool of available nurse-midwives and ensure a diverse nurse-midwifery workforce make it difficult for the organization to advocate master's level preparation for all CNMs. Several observations can be made, however, that suggest that the mainstreaming of nurse-midwifery within advanced nursing practice may be inevitable. Despite the fact that they are not officially associated with advanced nursing practice, CNMs are developing in ways congruent with the vision that is bringing together CNSs, CRNAs, NPs, and other APNs. The core competencies defined by the ACNM and their operationalization are consistent with the core competencies of advanced practice described in Chapter 3. Most nurse-midwifery education is delivered in master's level programs. Clinical and regulatory issues such as access to and availability of services as well as second licensure for APNs are likely to engage CNMs in collaborative efforts to promote the values and vision driving advanced practice. Some states already require a master's degree for licensing as an APN (including CNM) and/or for prescriptive authority; others have established a date by which a master's degree will be required. These precedents could well affect federal funding for nurse-midwifery education. It is unlikely that nurse-midwives will risk the legal privileges for which they fought so hard by resisting efforts to ensure a common definition of advanced nursing practice across state and federal laws and regulations. Appeals to the ACNM have been made by CNMs in states that have passed the requirement for a master's degree. The ACNM Board of Directors has responded by reaffirming support for certificate programs and referring members to other resources and offering specific strategic suggestions. Safriet (1992), an attorney, has argued that consistency in the definition of advanced nursing practice and in the criteria for being licensed as an APN is needed if APNs are to be able to practice with the autonomy that other professionals enjoy. In the current climate, however, it is difficult to anticipate how nurse-midwifery will address the regulatory complexity that is likely to result from the entry of nonnurses into midwifery. Whether the regulatory climate will be more or less open to innovative programs such as those contemplated by the ACNM is not clear.

These are the driving forces that are likely to carry CNMs and nurse-midwifery along in their currents or wake as ANP roles are defined and regulated at federal and state levels. Failure to be involved or opposition to the changes will undermine nurse-midwifery's efforts to secure accessible health care for individuals and may well undo its historical legislative achievements, which have enabled CNMs to practice autonomously.

COLLEGIAL RELATIONSHIPS AND AUTONOMY

It will come as no surprise to the reader that the factors that have been associated with job satisfaction are often the areas in which barriers to nurse-midwifery practice exist. These factors include working with competent personnel, having high-quality client interactions, having the time to provide a preferred style of care, being involved with clients' care plans and decision making, having good interpersonal relationships with other CNMs and with backup physicians, having professional autonomy, experiencing feelings of personal worth, and participating in teamwork (Collins, 1990). Although nurse-midwives can enjoy many of these rewards, as the earlier description of practice at the birth center shows, they often encounter difficulties in securing them, especially with regard to relationships with physicians, professional autonomy, and workload. For both the nurse-midwifery profession and individual CNMs, the goal is to pursue productive, collaborative relationships with all involved.

Physicians

Individual CNMs and individual physicians often get along and develop the kind of mature collaborative relationships described in Chapter 11. The current health-care environment, in which organizations and providers are scrambling to cut costs and services, is not conducive to building the kind of CNM-physician rapport that has made so many CNM-run practices successful, however. Barriers to effective working relationships between CNMs and physicians often arise within organizations, and they affect CNMs' ability to work autonomously. Although there may be individual members of organized medical groups with whom CNMs work well, the organizations themselves often spend time and money on efforts to restrict APNs' ability to practice autonomously. These efforts include lobbying against federal and state laws and regulations that are favorable to CNMs and other APNs. In Chapter 23, Doughty describes the American Medical Association's recent public relations campaign to convince the public that APNs and other non-physician providers are quacks. In a recent document, the American Medical Association described "integrated" practice with APNs, declaring that the physician is still "Captain of the Ship." Some state medical and nursing associations have found common ground on which to base organizational collaboration. However, CNMs who enjoy excellent collaborative relationships with individual physicians should be alert to the activities of organized medical groups both nationally and within their jurisdictions, so that they can protect their rights to practice nurse-midwifery and encourage their physician colleagues to speak out against limitations on CNM practice.

In hospitals and communities in which physicians continue to have (or are seen as having) power over who can and cannot practice, entrepreneurial CNMs may have more difficulty gaining clinical privileges or medical backup. Often, CNMs need to apply to a hospital's medical board if they wish to be able to attend laboring women in that hospital. CNMs who are the first APN to apply for these privileges in that hospital must be prepared to blaze a trail in everything, from attempting to change hospital bylaws and educating labor and delivery nursing staff regarding CNM practice, to obtaining a chart box in medical records, to negotiating for a locker in a changing room!

Whether they need clinical privileges or not, CNMs must have medical consultation and backup available. This requirement may be incorporated into a state practice act, but even if it is not, clinical practice and ACNM standards demand it. For the CNM working in an agency, formal and informal structures to ensure physician availability are likely to be established. If the CNM is the first one to practice in the organization, these structures will have to be developed. Regardless of practice setting, CNMs need to have a physician with whom they can consult or to whom they can make a referral when needed. Entrepreneurial CNMs will find physicians who are quite willing to be available and welcome the opportunity to collaborate. However, one may find oneself in the position of negotiating for such backup with physicians who are reluctant at best and actively hostile at worst. Many times, it is a matter of education, public relations (see Chapter 23), and consumer demand. Just seeing the care provided at a CNM-run birth center can diminish resistance and elicit support. A combination of interpersonal skills, business savvy, and marketing strategies can help CNMs overcome barriers that arise from lack of knowledge, lack of trust, and power imbalances.

Lay Midwives

With the increase in demand for midwifery services comes renewed discussion on the topic of nonnurse midwives. The combination of nursing and midwifery has provided a strong base for professional midwifery in the United States. But this is not the case in other countries where midwifery has a long history. Briefly, modern lay midwifery in the United States originated in the feminist and women's health movements of the 1960s and 1970s, not from the community midwives of earlier times (Ventre, Spindel, & Bowland, 1995). Lay midwives were described as an "underground" network that arose when physicians and CNMs were unwilling or unable to respond to some women's preference to deliver their babies at home. Initially, practice was based on experience and self- and group study. In the late 1970s, apprenticeship training and schools to prepare professional midwives emerged. MANA was founded in the early 1980s. This organization incorporates both non-CNM members with diverse midwifery educations and CNMs and has initiated discussion with the ACNM on such issues as education, core competencies, certification, and licensing.

In 1994, the ACNM Board of Directors, with support from the majority of ACNM members, voted to have the ACNM's Division of Accreditation explore accreditation of nonnurse midwifery educational programs and to have the ACNM Certification Council develop a certification examination (Ulrich, 1995). The ACNM has a strategic plan regarding the needs of certified midwives. The plan addresses consumer education, reimbursement, and legal authority to practice, the last is to be pursued and secured on a state-by-state basis (Ulrich, 1995). This is a major undertaking, one that may be hard for the APN who is not a CNM to understand or support but that is consistent with the ACNM's commitment to narrowing the gap between the services needed and the number of providers available. On the basis of a review of the strategic plan, we believe the ACNM considered every conceivable barrier to this initiative. What is not clear is how a nonnurse can be prepared to have "the same core competencies as a nurse-midwife" and "be expected to practice according to the ACNM Standards and Code of Ethics" without being a nurse. It would seem that some modification must be made in the core competencies for nurse-midwifery so that a certified midwife could not be construed as practicing nursing.

This description of ACNM initiatives and plans is intended to help the reader understand why CNMs do not fit smoothly in advanced nursing practice. True to its history, nurse-midwifery is blazing an unprecedented and risky trail that will elicit various reactions such as rejection, curiosity, disapproval, and encouragement from the nursing profession. In the past, this pulling away from the crowd has led to changes that have benefited the nursing profession at large. The ACNM initiative addresses many of the reasons lay midwives gave for returning to school to become CNMs: leadership skills, legal issues, and expanded practice skills (Ventre et al., 1995).

BARRIERS TO PRACTICE

Legislative, Regulatory, and Financial Barriers

Last but not least, there continue to exist barriers to full-scope nurse-midwifery practice. Restrictions to practice can be found at the local, state, and federal levels. If interpersonal, marketing, and public relations efforts fail to secure admitting and clinical privileges for CNMs, legislation that ensures CNMs and other APNs access to these privileges will be needed. Inequitable reimbursement for their services remains a problem for CNMs in many states. Legislation and regulations that mandate reimbursement equitable to the value of CNMs' work, practice costs, and malpractice expenses must be enacted. Nurse-midwifery care should be an option in managed care systems, but it may not be if APNs and consumers do not make their voices heard. Nurse-midwives must have prescriptive authority, and greater uniformity and consistency of regulations at the federal and state levels for prescribing and dispensing medications are needed. Nurse-midwives must be assured of a continuing source of professional liability insurance. Allocations for nurse-midwifery education from federal and state funding agencies are at risk in the current political climate, in which many politicians are seeking to minimize government initiatives that promote health and education. Medicare and Medicaid must ensure facility fee payment for birth centers.

Workload

When there is a full complement of CNMs to share the work of night call (e.g., being on call one or two nights a week), clinics, and other responsibilities, the unpredictable timing of labor and delivery and the erratic sleep patterns that result are manageable. For many CNMs, especially those in solo or independent practices, however, a full complement of staff is a luxury. To give their best to their clients and to stay healthy, CNMs with a heavy on-call schedule need to develop self-care strategies that enable them to balance work with personal responsibilities and relationships. The sabbatical has been proposed as one way to promote professional development while decreasing the demands of full-scope practice. This is likely to work only in large, well-funded practices. In addition, finding other CNMs who can cover for vacation and sick time can become a minor crisis. The physical and emotional demands of "catching" babies, in addition to the long hours and periods of sleep deprivation, mean that nurse-midwifery is not for everyone. For those who love it, the satisfaction of watching pregnancy progress, the physical and mental demands of labor and delivery, the element of unpredictability in the timing of birth, and the joy of birth make nurse-midwifery fascinating, exciting, and personally rewarding.

CONCLUSION

In spite of the resistance from the established medical community, there is a growing demand and need for nurse-midwives' unique services. Nurse-midwives are woman centered and family centered. They have been thinking globally and acting locally long before it became trendy to do so. They are called to do what they do. As long as there is a woman carrying a baby within her body who wishes to give birth in a loving and natural fashion, there will be a need for nurse-midwives.

Nurse-midwifery, advanced nursing practice, and the profession of nursing in general are at a critical juncture. Although nurse-midwifery is standing somewhat apart from advanced practice efforts, it seems clear that there is a need to recognize the interdependence of advanced practice and nurse-midwifery. By examining the separate yet related courses being charted by the nursing profession (related to ANP) and by nurse-midwives (to meet demands for midwifery services) one sees that there is great potential for divisiveness at a time in our history when we need to be unified. The directions nurse-midwives are pursuing may seem unfathomable to those outside nurse-midwifery. The authors have each been involved in political battles for the right to practice and have watched nurse-midwifery evolve from different regions of the U.S. We believe there is vision and wisdom in the ACNM's initiatives that will benefit advanced nursing practice and APNs in the long run. However, there appear to be many forces driving the nursing profession toward requiring a master's degree for second licensing, and to mount an opposition to this requirement is unlikely to be successful. It will drain energy away from CNMs and all APNs whose main goals are to improve access to health care and to provide that care. More important, it could undermine every hard-won political and legislative victory. All CNMs need to give serious consideration to the insights of Safriet, who maintains that APNs will only be able to practice autonomously when there is a uniform definition of ANP on which laws and regulations are based (1992).

CNMs have often led the nursing profession into the future, and many of the initiatives mentioned in this chapter indicate that the profession continues to move forward. It may now be time for CNMs to join forces *with* the nursing profession, which is investing its energy and resources in preserving and expanding the climate for autonomous nursing practice that CNMs helped create.

REFERENCES

Ad Hoc Committee on Code of Ethics. (1990). *Code of ethics for certified nurse-midwives.* Washington, DC: ACNM.

American College of Nurse-Midwives. (1993). *Core competencies for basic nurse-midwifery practice.* Washington, DC: ACNM.

American College of Nurse-Midwives. (1993). *Standards for the practice of nurse-midwifery.* Washington, DC: ACNM.

American College of Nurse-Midwives. (1992). *Expansion of nurse-midwifery practice and skills beyond basic care competencies.* Washington, DC: ACNM.

American College of Nurse-Midwives. (1992). *Collaborative management in nurse-midwifery practice for medical, gynecological, and obstetrical conditions.* Washington, DC: ACNM.

American College of Nurse-Midwives. (1989). *Philosophy of the American College of Nurse-Midwives.* Washington, DC: ACNM.

American College of Nurse-Midwives. (1980). *ACNM statement on practice settings.* Washington, DC: ACNM.

Avery, M. D. (1992). Advanced nurse-midwifery practice. *Journal of Nurse-Midwifery, 37,* 150–154.

Barron McBride, A. (1995, September). A "20/20" Vision of Nursing's Future. Address presented at the 25th Anniversary of Alpha Chi Chapter, Sigma Theta Tau, Boston College, Boston, MA.

Brooten, D., Kumar, S., Brown, L. P., Butts, P., Finkler, S. A., Bakewell-Sachs, S., Gibbons, A., & Delivoria-Papadopoulos, M. (1986). A randomized clinical trial of early hospital discharge and home follow-up of very-low-birth-weight infants. *The New England Journal of Medicine, 315*(15), 934–939.

Collins C. (1990). CNM job satisfaction: Luxury or necessity? Presented at the ACNM Convention, Atlanta, GA.

Crofts, A. J. (1994). Entrepreneurship—the realities of today. *Journal of Nurse-Midwifery, 39,* 39–42.

Flanagan, J. (1993). Speaking up and talking out—barriers to nurse-midwifery practice. *Journal of Nurse-Midwifery, 38,* 246–251.

Franklin, M. (1994). The nurse-midwifery challenge. *Journal of Nurse-Midwifery, 39,* 110–111.

Fullerton, J. T. (1994a). Reflections on nurse-midwifery role and functions. *Journal of Nurse-Midwifery, 39,* 107–109.

Fullerton, J. T. (1994b). Task analysis of American certified nurse-midwifery. *Journal of Nurse-Midwifery, 39,* 348–357.

Fullerton, J. T., & Wingard, D. (1990). Methodological problems in the assessment of nurse-midwifery practice. *Applied Nursing Research, 3,* 153–159.

Heaphy, K. H. (1987). Nurse-midwifery practice and undergraduate nursing education: A unique model. *Journal of Nurse-Midwifery, 32,* 98–100.

Hsia, L. (1991). Midwives and the empowerment of women. *Journal of Nurse-Midwifery, 36,* 85–87.

Hunter, L. P., & Lops, V. R. (1994). Critical thinking and the nurse-midwifery management process. *Journal of Nurse-Midwifery, 39,* 43–46.

Jenkins, S. M. (1994). The myth of vicarious liability. *Journal of Nurse-Midwifery, 39,* 98–105.

Keleher, K. C. (1993). Sabbatical leaves for nurse-midwives in clinical practice. *Journal of Nurse-Midwifery, 38,* 165–167.

Nitzche, R. E. (1995). 40 years old and still growing. *Quickening, 26*(2):2.

Oakley, D., Murtland, T., Mayes, F., Hayashi, R., Petersen, B. A., Rorie, C., & Andersen, F. (1995). Processes of care: Comparisons of certified nurse-midwives and obstetricians. *Journal of Nurse-Midwifery, 40,* 399–403.

Rooks, J. P., Carr, C. C., & Sandvold, I. (1991). The importance of non-master's degree options in nurse-midwifery education. *Journal of Nurse-Midwifery, 36,* 124–130.

Safriet, B. (1992). Health care dollars and regulatory sense: The role of advanced practice nursing. *Yale Journal of Regulation, 9,* 417–488.

Scupholme, A., Paine, L. L., Lang, J. M., Kumar, S., & DeJoseph, J. F. (1994). Time associated with components of clinical services rendered by nurse-midwives. *Journal of Nurse-Midwifery, 39,* 5–10.

Scupholme, A., & Walsh, L. (1994). Home-based services by nurse-midwives. *Journal of Nurse-Midwifery, 39,* 358–362.

Senge, P. M. (1990). *The fifth discipline: The art and practice of the learning organization.* New York: Doubleday Currency.

Smithing, R. S., & Wiley, M. D. (1994). Most prenatal care meets ACOG standards. *Nurse Practitioner, 19*(12), 7.

Thompson, H. O., & Thompson, J. E. (1987). Toward a professional ethic. *Journal of Nurse-Midwifery, 32,* 105–109.

Thompson, J. (1993). The ACNM's visionary planning. *Journal of Nurse-Midwifery, 38,* 283–284.

Ulrich, S. (1995). Strategic plan for certified midwives. *Quickening, 26,* 29.

Varney, H. (1987). *Nurse-midwifery* (2nd ed.). Boston: Blackwell Scientific Publications.

Ventre, F., Spindel, P. G., & Bowland, K. (1995). The transition from lay midwife to certified nurse-midwife in the United States. *Journal of Nurse-Midwifery, 40,* 428–432.

Whitfill, K. A., & Burst, H. V. (1994). ACNM accredited and pre-accredited nurse-midwifery education programs. *Journal of Nurse-Midwifery, 39,* 221–236.

Wingeier, R., Bloch, S., & Kvale, J. K. (1988). A description of a CNM-family physician joint practice in a rural setting. *Journal of Nurse-Midwifery, 33,* 86–92.

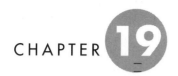

CHAPTER 19

The Certified Registered Nurse Anesthetist

Margaret Faut-Callahan
Michael Kremer

INTRODUCTION

Nurse anesthesia is the oldest organized specialty in nursing. Standardized postgraduate education, credentialing, and continuing education were all areas pioneered by certified registered nurse anesthetists (CRNAs). CRNAs were among the first nurse specialists to receive direct reimbursement for their services, and they have a history of activism in legislative and regulatory matters, such as prescriptive authority. This chapter discusses professional definitions of nurse anesthesia practice and the history of nurse anesthesia as it relates to nursing. The American Association of Nurse Anesthetists (AANA) is described, and its model of professional competence for CRNAs is presented. Nurse anesthesia education, credentialing, certification, and recertification processes are all explored. A profile of current CRNA practice is described, reimbursement mechanisms are described, and projections for future trends are provided.

HISTORY OF NURSE ANESTHESIA

Nurse anesthesia became formalized as a clinical nursing specialty during the first two decades of the 20th century. Nurse anesthetists pioneered new anesthetic developments, such as early techniques for trauma anesthesia during World War I. CRNAs collaborated with physicians and engineers to develop new and better anesthesia equipment. There is evidence that nurses were involved with administering anesthesia during the American Civil War and the Franco-Prussian War in Europe (Garde, 1988).

High surgical mortality in the late 19th century caused surgeons such as the Mayo brothers to seek and train nurses as anesthesia providers. Several compelling reasons led to this decision. In this era, medical students, interns, or laypersons administered anesthesia. Education was limited for these early anesthesia providers. Medical students and interns frequently were more interested in the surgical procedure itself than in providing anesthesia care (Thatcher, 1953). This interest in surgery superseded the development of essential clinical anesthesia traits such as vigilance and expertise in the management of anesthetized patients.

Also in the late 19th century, Catholic sisters who had been trained by surgeons provided the impetus for anesthesia care by nurses. Thatcher (1953) chronicles the careers of many pioneering religious and lay nurse anesthetists. Missionary nuns, such as the German Hospital Sisters of the Third Order of Saint Francis, established hospitals and settlements along railroad lines (Kelly, 1994). In 1912, one of the first standardized educational programs in nurse anesthesia was located at St. John's Hospital in Springfield, Illinois, operated by the Franciscan nuns.

Alice Magaw, a pioneering nurse anesthetist, was initially trained in anesthesia by surgeon William Mayo. Magaw had a reputation for impeccable anesthesia care. She is credited with providing early leadership in anesthesia at the Mayo Clinic (Bankert, 1989). In contrast with less well-trained providers, Magaw believed in and practiced rapid identification of and response to changes in the condition of anesthetized patients.

Magaw was an early contributor in the areas of nursing research and leadership. She published a paper in a medical journal, the *Northwestern Lancet*, describing how she had safely anesthetized 3,000 patients. By 1906, Magaw had provided a series of 14,000 anesthetics without a mortality (Bankert, 1989). This is especially noteworthy at a time when surgical mortality was markedly higher than it is today.

British physician anesthetists visiting the Mayo Clinic were impressed with Magaw's skill and noted differences in her practice of clinical anesthesia versus theirs. These physicians noted that Magaw's use of lower levels of anesthesia (ether) reflected what they perceived as her concern for patient safety. This anesthetic technique involved less physiological trespass than the then-current British practice of maintaining deep planes of surgical anesthesia with chloroform (Bankert, 1989; Thatcher, 1953).

During World War I, another pioneering nurse anesthetist, Sophie Winton, provided battlefront anesthesia care. Winton was awarded the Croix de Guerre for her service as a nurse anesthetist in Mobile Hospital Number One in the Chateau-Thierry area of France. Further, AANA founder Agatha Hodgins served with surgeon George Crile and others from the Lakeside Hospital in Cleveland during the First World War.

The leadership of Hodgins in nurse anesthesia did not end at the battlefield. Hodgins spearheaded development of the AANA when social and economic forces caused nurse anesthetists to organize nationally. The collapse of the national economy in 1929 revived physician interest in anesthesia, along with a desire to eliminate economic competition from nurse anesthetists (Thatcher, 1953).

At the same time, the American Nurses' Association (ANA) sponsored a movement to consolidate nurse anesthesia with nursing service in hospitals. Hodgins had experience in attempting to deal with the ANA about the relationship of nurse anesthetists and nursing. Hodgins had been coolly received when speaking before a 1909 ANA meeting and again before the Cleveland division of the League of Nursing Education in 1921 (Thatcher, 1953). ANA delegates proposed to combine office nurses and nurse anesthetists as a special section at an ANA sectional meeting held in Birmingham in 1930 where Anne Beddow presided. She was a leader in the attempt to combine the interests of office nurses and nurse anesthetists. Since Beddow was from the South, where the work of office nurse and nurse anesthetist was often combined, this sectional combination of the two groups seemed a logical development. A resolution was prepared for presentation: "Resolved: that it is the purpose of this meeting that a section be organized for the development and future growth of office nurses, which should be requested of the official board of the American Nurses' Association" (Thatcher, 1953, p. 182).

After discussion, the resolution was revised to read that a request be made for a place on the programs of state and district meetings of the ANA for the discussion of the problems of nurse anesthetists and office nurses. From there on the idea was aborted. The ANA president recommended to state presidents that a forum for nurse anesthetists be provided at state and district meetings. In 1931, a summary of replies was presented to the association's board of directors, at which time no action was taken. The matter of forming special sections was referred to the special committee on Sections, which subsequently recommended that further organization of sections be discouraged (Thatcher, 1953). This was not congruent with Hodgins' goals for her specialty area. Hodgins' vision was for a separate, distinct organization for nurse anesthetists. No one had been so bold and visionary about a nursing specialty in the sense that the specialist had the right to renounce the parent organization and set up standards for the perpetuation of the specialty per se. No nurse had so tested the flexibility of the nursing profession and the relation of nurse specialists to the whole group (Thatcher, 1953).

Hodgins synthesized her thinking about the profession of nurse anesthesia in a speech before a group of anesthetists at a 1932 Pittsburgh meeting: "It is also a basic principle that the development of any field of endeavor is best obtained by organizing in a coherent group, those most familiar with its needs and most concerned about its continuance and progress. This basic reason for a separate organization must be kept in mind to avoid confusion of purpose" (Thatcher, 1953, p. 198).

Although a separate nursing specialty organization in anesthesia may be needed to advance knowledge specific to that specialty, current practice in nurse anesthesia reflects collaboration with mainstream nursing. The AANA has liaison activity with nursing organizations such as the Federation of Nursing Specialty Organizations (NFSNO) and the Nursing Organizations Liason Forum (NOLF), and the AANA works with the ANA on areas of mutual legislative and regulatory concern. Some additional remarks of Agatha Hodgins on the affiliation of nurse anesthetists with other professional groups follow.

> *Applied to this immediate problem it means a clear acceptance of the*
> *fact that anesthesia, by its very nature, impinges closely on surgery*
> *and less closely on nursing, it is entitled to a place as a separate*
> *division of hospital service, its study being considered a distinct art*
> *and science. The administration of anesthetic drugs touches so closely*
> *on the protection of human life that a lesser valuation of its*
> *importance is deplorable and serious. It is our contention that the vital*
> *character of the work makes imperative not only the establishment of*
> *educational standards, but recognition of the fact that a graduate*
> *nurse, before administering anesthetics, should hold a certificate from*
> *a recognized school of anesthesia. . . .*
>
> (Thatcher, 1953, p. 198)

Hodgins next discussed the difficulties nurse anesthesia had with professional identity and establishment of liaisons with organized nursing and medicine:

> *. . . [A]lthough doing a work of immense and real importance, there*
> *is at present no place for our group as such. We must therefore create*
> *this place and the sooner done, the better. We have equal rights with*
> *other groups, to our distinct place, not as a side issue of other larger*
> *groups but as an organization concerned with the carrying on of a*
> *vital work.*
>
> (Thatcher, 1953, p. 198)

As more nurses entered the specialty of nurse anesthesia, it was apparent that standardized education and credentialing were necessary. Thus, nurse anesthesia became the first clinical specialty to incorporate these measures. Although courses in nurse anesthesia were developed in the early 1900s, the formation of the National Association of Nurse Anesthetists, later the AANA, in 1931, provided an organization for educators and practitioners to address concerns for the specialty.

PROFESSIONAL DEFINITIONS

A certified registered nurse anesthetist (CRNA) is a registered nurse who is educationally prepared for and competent to engage in the practice of nurse anesthesiology. CRNAs are both responsible and accountable for their individual professional practices. Nurse anesthetists are capable of exercising independent professional judgment within their scopes of competence and licensure (Jordan, 1994).

Nurse anesthesia is not a medically delegated act (Jordan, 1994). The practice of anesthesia is not exclusively the practice of medicine or the practice of nursing. It has been said that if anesthesia is administered by a nurse, it is the practice of nursing, whereas physician-administered anesthesia is the practice of medicine (Gunn, 1991).

Licensure for CRNAs and other advanced practice nurses (APNs) varies by state, as discussed elsewhere in the text (See Chapter 22). No states require that nurse anesthetists be supervised by anesthesiologists. CRNAs work in collaboration with providers from a variety of backgrounds: surgeons, dentists, podiatrists, and anesthesiologists. The degree to which CRNA practice is addressed in state nurse practice acts is not consistent, with states such as New Jersey prescriptively legislating nurse anesthesia practice to a higher degree. For example, legislated prescriptive authority for APNs exists in over 40 states at this writing, but the degree to which these laws affect CRNA practice varies. Debate continues as to whether CRNAs need prescriptive authority to work in most settings. Conventional wisdom holds that CRNAs do not require prescriptive authority protection because CRNAs are most commonly institutionally based and administer, but do not independently prescribe, medications. Federal law indicates that nurse anesthesia practice and related drug administration is not prescriptive but is rather a request for anesthesia services. Selecting anesthesia techniques and selecting and ordering drugs by nurse anesthetists are not construed as prescriptive behavior by the federal courts (Tobin, M., personal communication, 1995).

Nurse anesthesia practice is, by both historical and legal precedent, part of nursing practice. Two precedent-setting cases were *Frank v. Smith*, 175 Ky. 416, 194 S.W. 375 (1917, cited in Thatcher, 1953) and *Chalmers-Francis v. Nelson*, 6 Cal.2d 402, 57 P.2d (1936, cited in Thatcher, 1953). The latter case involved Dagmar Nelson, a California nurse anesthetist. Legal challenges to Nelson's right to provide anesthesia came from local anesthesiologists, with resulting litigation, eventually going to the United States Supreme Court. The professional organization representing CRNAs at that time, the National Association of Nurse Anesthetists, filed an amicus curiae brief with the Supreme Court. The case was a watershed in deciding the legality of nurse anesthesia (Bankert, 1989). Case law is replete with other examples of successful challenges by nurse anesthetists for their right to practice.

The question of which professional group CRNAs should be aligned with has been a topic explored legally, ethically, and educationally since the inception of the practice of nurse anesthesia. Some courts of law have held that nurse anesthesia is not the practice of medicine, but it is by virtue of their nursing licenses that CRNAs are enabled to practice anesthesia legally. Other courts have found that anesthesiology cannot be easily classified within either the discipline of nursing or the discipline of medicine (Waugaman, 1991).

The roles of physicians and nurses in anesthesia overlap. The components of this overlap include a similar educational heritage, comparable socialization into the specialty, constant time and space in the operating room environment, and the same relationships and therapeutic interventions with patients. The non-curative nature of surgical anesthesia is more similar to the practice of nursing than it is to medicine (Faut, 1984).

Callahan (1995) reports that there is an 88% role overlap in the practice of nurse anesthetists and anesthesiologists as evaluated by experts in both fields. The findings of Callahan mirror those of Cromwell and Rosenbach (1988), health-care economists who extensively studied economics in anesthesiology and cost-effective anesthesia provider mixes. These investigators found that CRNAs were under-utilized close substitutes for anesthesiologists and that full utilization of CRNAs would result in significant savings on health-care expenditures.

Acknowledging that the practices of nurse anesthetists and anesthesiologists are similar, the courts had to decide if nurse anesthetists and anesthesiologists indeed compete in practice settings (*Oltz v. St. Peter's Community Hospital*, 861 F.2d 1440, 1443 [9th Cir. 1988, cited in Bankert, 1989]; *Bahn v. NME Hospitals, Inc.*, 772 F.2d 1467, 1471 [9th Cir. 1975, cited in Bankert, 1989]). There is no other area of health care in which a provider can substitute for a physician as completely as does the CRNA in the provision of anesthesia services. Institutional credentialing may limit the ability of CRNAs to perform functions such as discharging patients from the facility or in components of prescription. However, strategies have been developed to overcome these barriers in various settings.

SCOPE OF PRACTICE

Anesthesiology is the art and science of rendering a patient insensible to pain by administration of anesthetic agents and related drugs and procedures. Anesthesia and anesthesia-related care are those services which anesthesia professionals provide on request, assignment, or referral by the patient's physician (or other health-care professional authorized by law), most often to facilitate diagnostic, therapeutic, or surgical procedures. In other instances, the referral or request for consultation or assistance may be for management of pain associated with obstetrical labor and delivery, management of acute or chronic ventilatory problems, or management of acute or chronic pain through the performance of selected diagnostic or therapeutic blocks or other forms of pain management (American Association of Nurse Anesthetists, 1992a).

The scope of practice of the CRNA encompasses the professional functions, privileges, and responsibilities associated with nurse anesthesia practice. These activities are performed in collaboration with qualified and legally authorized professional health-care providers. CRNAs are prepared to recognize situations in which care requirements are beyond their individual competencies and to seek consultation or referral when such situations arise (American Association of Nurse Anesthetists, 1992a).

Anesthesia care is provided by CRNAs in four general categories: (1) pre-anesthetic evaluation and preparation, (2) anesthesia induction, maintenance, and emergence, (3) post-anesthesia care, and (4) peri-anesthetic and clinical support functions. Parallels between nursing and nurse anesthesia can be seen. CRNAs perform pre-anesthetic assessments, plan appropriate anesthetic interventions, implement planned anesthetic care, and evaluate patients postoperatively to determine the efficacy of their interventions.

CRNAs working alone routinely perform all these aspects of clinical practice. When CRNAs and anesthesiologists work together in "team" anesthesia, a variety of factors, such as local anesthesia practice patterns, determine to what extent each practitioner is involved in these anesthesia care areas.

Nurse anesthetists frequently work with anesthesiologists. With continued debate about the "anesthesia care team," e.g., CRNAs practicing with anesthesiologists, some of the principles elucidated by Dripps (1977) place this discussion in a constructive perspective. This pioneering academic anesthesiologist described his perception of CRNA capabilities and working relationships with CRNAs and anesthesiologists:

> *It is apparent that the physician anesthesiologist offers greater depth of training than the nurse anesthetist, but this does not necessarily qualify the physician as a better anesthetist. By achieving the technical skills and the appropriate experience and knowledge, a conscientious nurse can easily surmount the gap in training. An anesthesiologist, acting as a technician, who fails to keep abreast of advances in medicine soon loses the advantage. In most large hospital departments, nurse and physician anesthetists and technicians work in harmony . . . Considering the extensive national demands for anesthesia care it is unlikely that all anesthetics will ever be given solely by physicians. As paralleled by the trend toward midwifery in obstetrics, there is and always will be a need for nurse anesthetists.*

(Dripps, 1977, p 3)

Since the time of these thoughts by Dr. Dripps, nurse anesthesia education has advanced tremendously, and although anesthesiology residency programs take longer, educational requirements are similar.

It is clear that preoperative evaluation has become more complex with the increasing acuity of hospitalized patients. Thorough pre-anesthetic assessments, in concert with further assessment specialists as indicated, are essential activities at which nurse anesthetists must be proficient. Other aspects of pre-anesthetic patient preparation are requesting indicated diagnostic studies; selecting, obtaining, ordering, or administering preanesthetic medications and fluids; and obtaining informed consent for anesthesia (American Association of Nurse Anesthetists, 1992a).

CRNAs in states with legislated prescriptive authority for APNs have prescriptive authority encompassing legend, and in some cases Schedules II–V controlled substances, in addition to their previously mentioned ability to select, obtain, or administer anesthetics and adjuvant drugs. Federal law has held that selecting and administering anesthetics does not constitute prescription. Rather, these practices are viewed as parts of performing anesthesia services (M. Tobin, personal communication, 1995). Whether a CRNA is in solo practice or working with anesthesiologists, the legally defined scope of CRNA practice allows for selecting, obtaining, ordering, or administering pre-anesthetic medications and fluids as part of providing the requested anesthesia services.

Developing and implementing an anesthetic care plan is another aspect of

CRNA practice. This care plan is formulated with input from the patient, the surgeon, and in team anesthesia settings with the collaborating anesthesiologist. Similarly, the choice of administering regional or general anesthesia is not solely the province of any one of the aforementioned participants. Input from the patient, the surgeon, and the anesthetist is relevant in the important decision about which type of anesthetic to administer in a given situation. Compromise and flexibility may be necessary to achieve the goals of surgery and anesthesia without incident.

CRNAs select, obtain, or administer the anesthetics, adjuvant drugs, accessory drugs, and fluids necessary to manage the anesthetic, to maintain the patient's physiological homeostasis, and to correct abnormal responses to anesthesia or surgery (American Association of Nurse Anesthetists, 1992a). When CRNAs perform these activities, they are recognized legally to be providing anesthesia services on request and thus not to be prescribing as defined by federal law.

Monitoring is another vital area in which CRNAs participate. Nurse anesthetists select, apply, and insert appropriate non-invasive and invasive monitoring modalities for collecting and interpreting patients' physiological data. These activities are all recognized components of anesthesia services performed on request by CRNAs and are not prescriptive. Criteria for the use of invasive monitors and who places them vary by institution and geographical region. Professional fees associated with the placement of devices such as pulmonary artery catheters at times leads to conflict over which practitioner, e.g., anesthetist or surgeon, will place invasive monitors and thus receive the reimbursement.

Nurse anesthesia practice also includes airway management using endotracheal intubation, mechanical ventilation, and pharmacological support both within and outside the operating room. In some settings, CRNAs are the sole providers of this service. A combination of technical skills required for airway management utilizing a variety of instruments, knowledge of respiratory anatomy and physiology, and pharmacology is important. For example, indiscriminant use of muscle relaxants in critically ill, ventilator-dependent patients can occur (Loper, Butler, Nessly, & Wild, 1989). CRNAs need to remind clinicians caring for ventilator-dependent patients that sedative/amnestic drugs and analgesics need to be included when critically ill patients are mechanically ventilated.

Nurse anesthetists manage emergence and recovery from anesthesia by selecting, obtaining, ordering, or administering medications, fluids, or ventilatory support in order to maintain homeostasis, to provide relief from pain and anesthesia side effects, and/or to prevent or manage complications (American Association of Nurse Anesthetists, 1992a). These activities also fall within the scope of providing anesthesia services and are not prescriptive in the traditional sense, i.e., where a practitioner would write a prescription that any pharmacist would fill.

Releasing or discharging patients from a post-anesthesia care area and providing post-anesthesia follow-up evaluation and care related to anesthesia side effects or complications are other CRNA functions.

Regional anesthesia is used by many CRNAs in the management of surgical anesthesia, labor pain, and postoperative pain. CRNAs are increasingly involved with pain management services. The use of epidural analgesic infusions and patient-controlled analgesia has greatly contributed to the effective treatment of preventable pain. Nurse anesthetists should have a role in the formulation of protocols and staff education when acute pain protocols are introduced.

Nurse anesthetists respond to emergency situations by providing airway management skills and by implementing basic and advanced life-support techniques.

CRNAs can provide leadership in these settings, away from the operating room, reinforcing the need for nationally promulgated standards of anesthesia care. One of these standards of care, for example, is the use of capnography (CO_2 monitoring) to rule out esophageal intubation (American Association of Nurse Anesthetists, 1992a).

CRNAs are legally liable for the quality of the services they render. They make independent judgments and decisions as to the appropriateness of their professional service and its probable effect on the patient. A CRNA who believes that the health-care plan as it relates to anesthesia for a particular patient is inappropriate should seek consultation for more appropriate direction. CRNAs should serve as patient advocates and always seek resolution to these issues. If reasonable doubt continues, it is the responsibility of the CRNA to consider withdrawal from rendering the service, provided that the well-being of the patient is not jeopardized (American Association of Nurse Anesthetists, 1992a).

With more surgery conducted on an out-patient or same-day-admission basis—approximately 65% (Micek, 1993)—patients may not meet their anesthetist personally until shortly before surgery. Multiple mechanisms, such as telephone interviews or pre-anesthesia clinics, can be used to conduct pre-anesthesia assessment and allow anesthesia providers to discuss care options, procedures, and risks with patients. Patients and health-care providers continue to adjust to this reimbursement-driven shift in services. Clinical information obtained through telephone interviews is confirmed when patients arrive on the day of surgery. Detailed physical assessment and establishing rapport are activities conducted on the day of surgery.

Anesthesia services can facilitate diagnosis, as in the case of the "curare test" for myasthenia gravis. Anesthesia as a therapeutic modality is seen in the treatment of acute and chronic pain and has even been used in psychiatry for conducting patient interviews under the influence of ultra-short-acting intravenous barbiturates. However, the most common use of anesthesia resources is in the administration of surgical anesthesia.

Anesthesia is frequently used in obstetrics, providing labor and delivery analgesia. Regional anesthesia and applied pharmacology have greatly advanced obstetrical anesthesia. Epidural analgesia has become increasingly common for vaginal and cesarean section delivery, often obviating the need for general anesthesia and its attendant risks in the parturient (Bader & Datta, 1994). In addition to utilizing regional anesthesia in obstetrics and post-partum settings, CRNAs work collaboratively with other providers in these areas to manage intra- and post-partum pain with a variety of pharmacological and non-pharmacological modalities (Faut-Callahan & Paice, 1990).

CRNAs practice according to their expertise, state statutes or regulations, and local institutional policy. Nurse anesthesia is practiced in collaboration with legally authorized professional health-care providers. Institutional credentialing procedures may require additional evidence of clinical and didactic education in areas such as cardiothoracic or regional anesthesia. State nurse practice acts and practice patterns in the anesthesia community contribute to variability in the scope of nurse anesthesia practice in various settings.

Nurse anesthetists are bound by the standards of practice adopted by the profession (Table 19–1).

TABLE 19–1. STANDARDS FOR NURSE ANESTHESIA PRACTICE

Standard I
A thorough and complete preanesthetic assessment shall be performed.

Standard II
Informed consent for the planned anesthetic intervention shall be obtained from the patient or legal guardian.

Standard III
A patient-specific plan for anesthesia care shall be formulated.

Standard IV
The anesthesia care plan shall be skillfully implemented and the plan of care adjusted as needed to adapt to the patient's response to the anesthetic. Vigilance shall be maintained for untoward identifiable reactions and corrective actions initiated as required.

Standard V
The patient's physiological condition shall be monitored in a manner consistent with both the type of anesthesia care and specific patient needs.

Standard VI
There shall be prompt, complete, and accurate documenting of pertinent information on the patient's record.

Standard VII
The responsibility for the care of the patient shall be transferred to other qualified providers in a manner that assures continuity of care and patient safety.

Standard VIII
Appropriate safety precautions shall be taken to minimize the risks of fire, explosion, electrical shock, and equipment malfunction.

Standard IX
Appropriate safety precautions shall be taken to minimize the risk of infection for the patient, CRNA, and other staff.

Standard X
Anesthesia care shall be assessed to assure its quality.

Standard XI
The CRNA shall participate in a continual process of self-evaluation and strive for excellence in anesthesia practice.

Standard XII
The CRNA shall respect and maintain the basic rights of patients, demonstrating concern for personal dignity and human relationships.

From American Association of Nurse Anesthetists. (1992). *Guidelines and standards for nurse anesthesia practice.* Park Ridge, IL: American Association of Nurse Anesthetists.

CREDENTIALING OF CRNAs

To be a nurse anesthetist, one must meet four requirements: (1) graduating from an approved nursing school and holding a current state RN license, (2) graduating from a nurse anesthesia educational program accredited by the Council on Accreditation of Nurse Anesthesia Educational programs or its predecessor, (3) successfully completing the certification examination administered by the Council on Certification of Nurse Anesthetists or its predecessor, (4) complying with criteria for biennial recertification. These criteria are defined by the Council on Recertification of Nurse Anesthetists (American Association of Nurse Anesthetists, 1992b).

Competence can be partially assured through institutional credentialing processes. A hospital may delineate procedures that the CRNA is authorized to perform by the authority of the governing board. Guidelines for granting CRNAs clinical privileges are found in the *Guidelines and Standards for Nurse Anesthesia Practice* (American Association of Nurse Anesthetists, 1992a). Recommended clinical privileges for CRNAs are in the areas of pre-anesthetic preparation and evaluation; anesthesia induction, maintenance, and emergence; post-anesthetic care; and perianesthetic and clinical support functions.

ROLE DEVELOPMENT AND MEASURES OF COMPETENCE

The role of the nurse anesthetist encompasses many facets. Callahan (1994) described a competency-based model for nurse anesthesia practice that demonstrates the areas in which nurse anesthetists must strive to achieve competence (Fig. 19–1). The unifying themes of caring, collaboration, communication, and technology are defined in Table 19–2. Many of the characteristics of advanced nursing practice described in Chapter 3 are found in this model.

Although this model is in its infancy and further research with its use is in progress, it clearly depicts the many facets of the role of the CRNA. Munguia-Biddle and associates (1990) defined components of the model and suggested that the

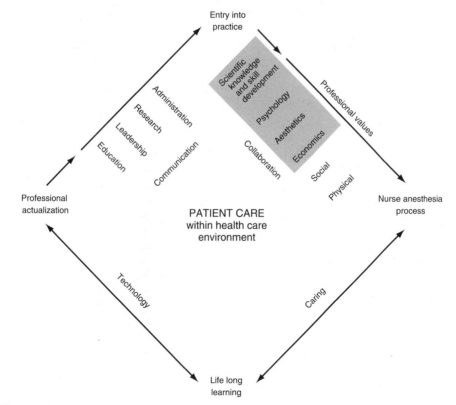

Figure 19–1. Nurse anesthesia practice model. (From Munguia-Biddle, F., Maree, S., Klein, E., Callahan, L., & Gilles, B. (1990). Nurse anesthesiology competence evaluation: Mechanism for accountability. Unpublished document. Park Ridge, IL: American Association of Nurse Anesthetists.)

TABLE 19–2. NURSE ANESTHESIA PRACTICE MODEL

The advanced practice of nursing in the specialty of nurse anesthesia has special attributes that speak to the strength and uniqueness of our role in the provision of anesthesia care in the health environment.

Caring for the patient as a holistic being is an important tenet of our professional behavior. We strive to be altruistic human beings, believing that caring is essential to one's personal development.

Collaboration between the nurse anesthetist and other members of the health-care team takes place in separate and joined activities and responsibilities that are directed at attaining mutual goals of excellence in patient care.

Communication is sharing information to achieve mutual understanding. Communication skills are a cornerstone of patient interviews, imparting information to other health professionals, documentation of practice, and participation as a contributory member in meeting society's health needs.

Technology denotes an area rich in technological advances and scientific content that requires strengthening and updating through the professional life. Practitioners have the ability to apply the nursing process to complex problems at a high level of competence.

From Munguia-Biddle, F., et al. (1990). Nurse anesthesiology competence evaluation: Mechanism for accountability. Unpublished document. Park Ridge, IL: American Association of Nurse Anesthetists.

nurse anesthesia process is a problem-solving model that utilizes assessment, analysis, planning, implementation, and evaluation in the complex decision-making and actions that exemplify practice within the health-care environment. They further define lifelong learning as a part of the nurse anesthesia process. This essential process function is in concert with the changing characteristics of nurse anesthesia practice.

Additional clarification of the components of the model is found in Table 19–3. It is clear that the nurse anesthesia process is in close alignment with the nursing process and emphasizes the importance of this approach to comprehensive anesthesia care.

NURSE ANESTHESIA EDUCATION

Nurse anesthesia education occurs in diverse settings. This is demonstrated by the many academic units that house nurse anesthesia educational programs. Educators in nurse anesthesia are proud of the educational diversity of their graduates. The relative value of this diversity has never been quantified in terms of an academic power base or educational credibility. This diversity exists because the nurse anesthesia educational community values various undergraduate degrees for entrance into nurse anesthesia programs and because of the initial difficulty nurse anesthesia educators met when trying to move certificate nurse anesthesia programs into schools of nursing. The AANA further promotes graduate education for entrance into practice, and by 1998 all nurse anesthesia programs must be at the graduate level. This requirement does not dictate the movement of programs into one academic discipline. This may stem from those programs that in the 1970s established relationships with whichever academic unit was open to affiliating with a nurse anesthesia program. The first four graduate programs in nurse anesthesia all had different academic affiliations: medicine, nursing, allied health, and education. These programs that pioneered nurse anesthesia education at the graduate level established relationships with those departments in colleges and universities that were willing to take risks with the small numbers of students in nurse anesthesia

TABLE 19–3. DEFINITION OF NURSE ANESTHESIA PRACTICE MODEL COMPONENTS

Professional Actualization

Professional actualization is a dynamic, ongoing endeavor to realize maximum development of professional potential.

Education. Provides an environment that allows for exploration and application of strategies to facilitate the preparation of future practitioners, thereby assuring continuance.

Leadership. Demonstrates the ability to define reality, set goals, communicate a vision, and influence the willing participation of others in purposeful action that is directed to goal achievement.

Research. Encourages active involvement in scientific inquiry as a consumer, participant, or contributor. It is the driving force of actualization that validates our role in the provision of anesthesia services, enhances growth for the nurse anesthetist and the profession, and leads to new knowledge and improved safety in patient care.

Administration. Provides the interface between people, groups, departments, organizations, professions, and society that enhances individual and collective professional growth.

Professional Values

A **profession** may be defined in terms of the dormains of human endeavor valued by the members of the profession. Such are the following domains within the profession of nurse anesthesia practice.

Intellectual. Integral concepts within this domain are based on advanced knowledge in the fields of anatomy, physiology, pathophysiology, technology, and pharmacology as applied to anesthetic practice. The continued development of technical expertise and competence in practice are inherent in this area of concern.

Psychological. The professional nurse anesthetist is concerned with enhancement of the patient's coping skills in a time of possible physical and emotional disruption produced by the perioperative experience. Recognition of the needs of the practitioner are expressed as concern with issues such as communication, autonomy, counseling, and impairment or incompetent practice within the workplace and the profession as a whole.

Aesthetics. Spiritual growth and religious preferences are recognized and respected as inherent to full development of human potential within the patient and the nurse anesthetist. Ethical development and involvement within the political realm encompassing the nurse anesthetist as a member of society is held to be a continual and necessary growth process.

Economics. We place great value on the historical role of the nurse anesthesia profession in providing continuity of anesthesia care that supports an economically viable health-care industry. The exploration of strategies leading to resolution of liability issues as well as mechanisms to increase feelings of potential job security are recognized as valuable to continued professional and personal growth and well-being.

Social. Valued concepts within this domain include enhancement and preservation of the professional role of nurse anesthetists in the societal health-care delivery system, legal and legislative responsibility for competent patient care, constant development of improved standards of care, patient education, and continued liaison with other health-care providers.

Physical. Patient safety and the interface between technology and humankind or machines and the patient are of paramount concern. The appropriateness of physical work that considers the impact of schedules, stress, fatigue, and vigilance must be demonstrated in the clinical setting as important factors in securing the patient care environment.

From Munguia-Biddle, F., et al. (1990). Nurse anesthesiology competence evaluation: Mechanism for accountability. Unpublished document. Park Ridge, IL: American Association of Nurse Anesthetists.

programs. This diversified model of nurse anesthesia education has proliferated in the last 15 years, and many of these long-established programs would find it difficult to change their academic affiliations (Waugaman, 1991).

As previously stated, the Catholic Franciscan sisters offered one of the first organized nurse anesthesia courses at St. John's Hospital in Springfield, Illinois, in 1912. Although other nurse anesthesia programs opened in the early 20th century, curricula and clinical experiences were not standardized. At the first meeting of the National Association of Nurse Anesthetists, educational standards for the specialty were discussed by founding members. Nurse anesthesia educators agreed that the minimum length of academic programs in the specialty would be six months. Formal accreditation of nurse anesthesia programs began in 1952 (Bankert, 1989; Thatcher, 1953).

In the mid-1970s, over 170 nurse anesthesia educational programs existed. Currently, over 90 CRNA educational programs operate in the United States. Of these 90 programs, more than 80% are affiliated with colleges or universities and offer master's degrees (Fig. 19–2). The rapid decline in the numbers of nurse anesthesia programs was a great concern to the specialty. The closures are attributed variously to physician pressure and declining support, the inability of hospitals to continue to financially support small programs, and lack of a geographically accessible university with which a nurse anesthesia program could affiliate. Those who argue that nurse anesthesia programs closed solely because of the graduate degree mandate offer little evidence to support this claim. Further, one can surmise that if this were the only reason, those programs would have remained in existence until 1998, when the master's degree will be required, and then closed. The external pressures on the academic program within nurse anesthesia cannot be minimized.

Despite the decline in the overall numbers of nurse anesthesia programs, many of which were certificate programs that had enrollments of less than five students, the level of educational programs changed dramatically. Further, overall numbers of graduates have steadied (Fig. 19–3).

After an initial decline in graduates, the newer graduate programs increased their admissions. To accomplish this, programs had to increase the numbers of clinical training sites (Fig. 19–4). The result has been a strengthened educational system, deeply entrenched in an academic model.

Colleges of nursing are more frequently becoming the sites for nurse anesthesia programs as nurse anesthesia and other advanced nursing practice (ANP) groups increasingly collaborate on legislative, policy, and educational matters. Agatha Hodgins' expressed desire for a separate professional organization and education process for nurse anesthesia has been partially supplanted by the rapprochement between nursing and nurse anesthesia. Coalitions of APNs have been effectively working together in Washington, D.C. during the recent debates on health-care reform. APNs have also been working in regions such as the northwestern United States, with regard to such things as achieving legislated prescriptive authority for advanced practice nurses.

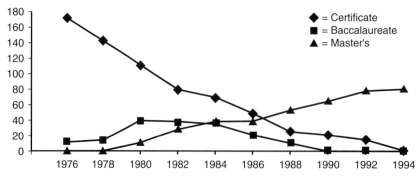

Figure 19–2. Numbers and types of nurse anesthesia programs, 1976–1994. (Used with permission of the Council on Certification of Nurse Anesthetists.)

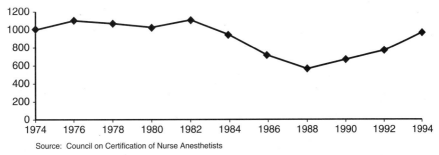

Source: Council on Certification of Nurse Anesthetists

Figure 19–3. Nurse anesthesia graduates, 1974–1994. (From the Council on Certification of Nurse Anesthetists.)

The minimum length of nurse anesthesia programs currently is 24 months. However, because of the combination of didactic and clinical time requirements, many programs are 27 to 36 months in length. Nurse anesthesia curricular requirements can overload the typical master's curricula. Because of the time commitment and academic rigor necessary for this specialty area, there is increasing interest in a clinical doctoral degree as the exit degree in nurse anesthesia. The vision of nursing leader Luther Christman, RN, PhD, for nurses to be prepared with advanced degrees both in their discipline and in a basic science could be a further extension of the thrust toward preparation beyond a master's degree for entry into this and other advanced practice specialty areas (Christman, 1977). Doctoral programs in nurse anesthesia are being developed. Further, many nurse anesthetists have pursued doctoral preparation in areas of pharmacology and physiology.

Nurse anesthesia educational curricula include time requirements for both didactic and clinical activities that reflect minimum standards for entry into practice. Academic content areas are crucial to prepare practitioners for beginning-level competence in a highly demanding, rapidly changing specialty. Various colleges and schools that administratively house nurse anesthesia programs may have additional academic requirements. Nurse anesthesia programs in colleges of nursing include core graduate-level courses taken by all graduate nursing students. These courses include graduate-level nursing theory, nursing research, advanced physical assessment, and pharmacology. The content areas and mandated time allocations for the nurse anesthesia core are listed in Table 19–4. These course requirements constitute 330 didactic hours.

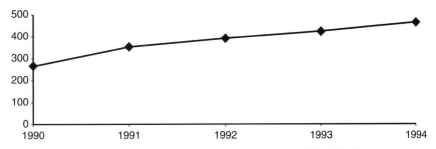

Figure 19–4. Number of clinical sites for nurse anesthesia programs, 1990–1994. (Used with permission of the Council on Certification of Nurse Anesthetists.)

TABLE 19–4. ACADEMIC COURSE REQUIREMENTS

Topic	Required Contact Hours
Professional aspects of nurse anesthesia practice	45
Advanced anatomy, physiology, and pathophysiology	135
Chemistry and physics of anesthesia	45
Advanced pharmacology	90
Principles of anesthesia practice	90
Clinical and literature review conferences	45

The clinical component requires that the student administer a minimum of 450 anesthetics, or 800 hours of actual anesthesia administration time. An external agency, the Council on Certification of Nurse Anesthetists, requires that students complete given numbers of surgical procedures and anesthetic techniques, e.g., all students must administer at least 45 general anesthetics using a mask airway (versus endotracheal intubation). Similarly, a required number of endotracheal intubations or thoracic surgical cases must be met for nurse anesthesia graduates to be eligible to take the national certification examination.

Most programs exceed these minimum requirements. In addition, many require study in methods of scientific inquiry and statistics, as well as active participation in student-generated and faculty-sponsored research (American Association of Nurse Anesthetists, 1992b).

The Council on Accreditation of Nurse Anesthesia Programs accredits nurse anesthesia educational programs. Programs must comply with written standards and guidelines. This council is composed of members from a variety of disciplines, including CRNAs, physicians, and other members of the professional community. The Council on Accreditation conducts mandatory, on-site program reviews at least once every six years. Nurse anesthesia educators and the Council on Accreditation of Nurse Anesthesia Programs have found that retaining a prescriptive curriculum in terms of hours and types of clinical experiences has helped the survival of educational programs. That is, when documented deviations from established standards for nurse anesthesia educational programs occur—e.g., physicians restricting clinical access—program directors can cite Council on Accreditation standards mandating these experiences.

Nurse anesthesia was the first nursing specialty to have mandatory certification. This process began in 1945, when the first certification examination in nurse anesthesia was given. The Council on Certification, like other AANA councils, is administratively independent of the AANA. The mission of the certification council is to certify nurse anesthesia graduates by examination, thus protecting and assuring the public regarding CRNA competency. The Council on Certification utilizes psychometricians, an academy of test-item writers, and computer-adaptive testing to assess beginning-level competence in nurse anesthesia graduates (Healey, I., personal communication, 1994).

Another AANA council, the Council on Recertification, was developed in the late 1960s. The impetus for its development was the need to document, for the public, continued professional excellence for practicing CRNAs. The recertification period for CRNAs is every two years and renewable. Documentation of anesthesia practice and continuing education activities is required for recertification. Continuing education must be approved by this council to meet requirements for recertification (American Association of Nurse Anesthetists, 1992b).

These three councils, plus the Council for Public Interest in Anesthesia, endeavor to assure the public that the education and practice of CRNAs is more than adequate for the demands of the specialty. Nurse anesthesia education continues to evolve along with education in other ANP areas.

NURSE ANESTHETISTS AND ACCESS TO CARE

Nurse anesthetists administer 65% of the 26 million anesthetics given in this country each year. Further, nurse anesthetists provide approximately 85% of anesthesia given in rural settings (Revak, G., personal communication, 1995). CRNAs collaborate closely with other providers, such as surgeons and primary care practitioners, in all settings. Without the services of CRNAs in these communities, many small hospitals would close, leaving few alternatives for health care. Some rural CRNAs have completed additional training in the management of acute and chronic pain and offer services such as pain clinics, so that patients do not have to travel to distant centers for pain treatment.

CRNAs have traditionally been represented in other underserved population setting areas. Urban and county hospitals frequently use CRNAs. Nurse anesthetists are actively involved in anesthesia care in settings such as Bellevue Hospital in New York, the Maryland Shock-Trauma Institute, Chicago's Cook County Hospital, and San Francisco General Hospital. Many CRNAs practice in the Veterans Administration hospital system, dealing with complex surgical patients. The military heavily relies on and actively recruits nurse anesthetists. A CRNA may be the only anesthesia provider on a Navy vessel. In such a situation, knowledge of regional anesthesia and the ability to practice independently enable the CRNA to capably respond to mass casualty situations, in which many trauma victims simultaneously require anesthesia.

CRNA PRACTICE PROFILES

Ninety-six percent (26,530) of practicing American nurse anesthetists are members of the AANA. The AANA surveys its members annually. For fiscal year 1994, AANA survey data revealed that 41% of CRNAs were hospital-employed, 34% worked in groups composed of both CRNAs and anesthesiologists, 12% were self-employed or CRNA-group-employed, and 13% were in other types of practices. These data reflected a trend away from hospital employment (AANA, 1995).

With increased managed-care market penetration in some geographical regions, hospitals have sought to decrease their fixed costs. These costs, such as payroll, have become increasingly important as the fiscal status of hospitals changes from a profit to a cost-center orientation (Kongstvedt, 1994). Many urban areas have excess licensed hospital-bed capacity, with decreased utilization of in-patient facilities due to managed care. These economic considerations have caused hospital employment for CRNAs and other APNs to be less common as cost-shifting of these providers out of hospitals occurs. This cost-shifting should lead to managing caseloads with fewer practitioners who may be group-employed or independent contractors.

Regarding practice locations, 66% of AANA members are employed in urban settings. In smaller localities, 30% of CRNAs work in towns with fewer than 50,000 residents, and 4% of CRNAs practice in rural areas (*AANA News Bulletin*, January, 1995). These rural CRNAs significantly increase access to health care for rural citizens.

The CRNA Manpower Study from the National Center for Nursing Research, United States Office of Health and Human Services (1991) projected a need for over 35,000 CRNAs by the year 2010. These findings were based on the demand for CRNAs in the late 1980s that exceeded the available supply. This demand was fueled by the closure of a number of nurse anesthesia educational programs and the removal of existing financial disincentives for the utilization of CRNAs (Faut-Callahan, 1991).

The anesthesia provider employment marketplace will be dynamic for the near future because of the impact of managed care and job displacement on both CRNAs and anesthesiologists. Multiple variables affect anesthesia provider mixes in various settings. The term provider mix refers to the following variations in anesthesia practice. Physicians may practice anesthesia without nurse anesthetists, in team anesthesia, or supervising one or more CRNAs, or CRNAs may practice anesthesia without physician-anesthesiologist collaboration. It is difficult to predict nurse anesthesia practice sites and the number of nurse anesthetists who will be clinically active in the year 2000.

Additionally, an Emory University program prepares anesthesia assistants, who work under physician supervision providing clinical anesthesia services. Practice privileges of anesthesia assistants, like those of physician assistants, are linked to a sponsoring physician. These clinicians are found in the southeastern and midwestern United States.

The impact of these additional providers, coupled with anticipated decreases in graduate medical education funding in specialty areas, further complicates the prediction of human resource requirements in anesthesia. In addition, a federal emphasis for training more primary health-care providers, at this writing, is causing shifts in funding from specialty to primary care areas in medicine.

Nurse anesthesia was originally an entirely female discipline. Following the decision to admit male nurses to the specialty in 1947 (Thatcher, 1953), nurse anesthesia became a popular career choice for many male nurses. The 1994 AANA member survey data demonstrated that 58% of CRNAs were women; the remaining 42% were men. This large number of men in the specialty is thought to be due to the large use of nurse anesthetists in the military during the earlier part of this century and to the higher-than-usual compensation for this type of nursing career.

Nurse anesthesia is known as a specialty in which practitioners are well compensated financially. CRNA salaries rose 54% between the years of 1987 and 1992. The average CRNA salary in 1992 was $82,700. However, the impact of managed care, with fewer surgical cases at lower rates of reimbursement, is expected to cause the salaries of CRNAs and other anesthesia providers to remain the same or to fall below current rates.

REIMBURSEMENT FOR CLINICAL SERVICES

In the early years of this century and through the 1950s, CRNAs were usually paid employees of either the surgeon or the hospital for whom they worked. In rural areas, CRNAs often contracted with hospitals to provide services based on fee-for-service structures—that is, a set amount of compensation per case as opposed to a straight salary for hours worked (Simonson & Garde, 1994).

With the advent of private payers such as Blue Cross/Blue Shield, only physician providers and hospitals were paid by the plan. Other health-care providers, such as CRNAs, psychologists, and physical therapists, would submit charges to the hospital or treating physician. The hospital or physician would then obtain reimbursement for services as "incident to" their own and pass the money on to the nonreimbursed provider (Simonson & Garde, 1994).

Because of escalating health-care costs in the 1970s and 1980s, Medicare instituted a Prospective Payment System (PPS) in 1983. Although initially this legislation affected only Medicare Part A (hospital costs), it ultimately affected Medicare Part B (physician and non-physician costs). PPS legislation mandated a fixed payment rate for all hospital care, covering all Part A services, paid to hospitals based on a patient's diagnostic-related classification group (DRG). This fixed rate was to cover all costs associated with hospital admission, including services provided by non-physician health providers. CRNAs were in great jeopardy under this system, for in their effort to cut costs, hospitals had no incentive to hire CRNAs, because their cost would come directly from the hospital DRG payment. Congress inadvertently created reimbursement disincentives for the use of CRNAs while bolstering incentives for the use of anesthesiologists. AANA lobbying efforts caused the Health Care Financing Administration (HCFA) to rewrite portions of this legislation, enabling all CRNAs to obtain direct Medicare reimbursement or to sign over their billing rights to their employer (Simonson & Garde, 1994).

Historically, anesthesia charges have been based on direct time involvement, either as a charge for simple time or as a charge based on a combination of time and the complexity of the anesthetic. The Relative Value Scale (RVS), developed in the 1960s, is used to determine anesthesia charges based on the complexity of the surgical procedure. The result is charges for "base units," or surgical procedures described by anatomical or functional units. Additional "modifier units" can be added to base units for factors such as emergency procedures, extremes of age, or anesthetic risk. After adding base and modifier units, time units are calculated at one unit per 15 minutes. Value of time units is determined by the payer, e.g., Medicare or Blue Cross/Blue Shield, and the market. One unit of anesthesia time may be billed at from $15 to over $60. The total of base, modifier, and time units determines the professional fee for the administration of anesthesia. Many third-party payers, such as Medicare and some Blue Cross insurers, completely ignore the practitioner's charges and base payments on their own fee schedule. These payments are often determined by what providers charge "on average" for their services (Simonson & Garde, 1994).

Attempts to control spiraling health-care costs and improve access to care have resulted in the proliferation of managed-care contracts and a resurgence of interest in health maintenance organizations (HMOs). CRNAs can expect that reimbursement rates will generally decrease in the near future. This decrease will affect anesthetists in any practice setting—self-, group-, or hospital-employed. Fee-for-service reimbursement structures, as described earlier, may become a thing of the past as managed care increasingly penetrates health-care markets. All providers, including physicians, may eventually be salaried. Despite the trend of increased managed care, organized medicine continues to advocate the fee-for-service system as the only means to maintain the integrity of the physician-client relationship and fights vigorously to maintain the status quo (Simonson & Garde, 1994). The economics of managed care do not ensure APNs access to clients based on their cost-effectiveness. Because of the desire to maintain fee-for-service payment in some settings, the most cost-effective provider may not be the one chosen for participation in managed care. Transitional mechanisms in vertical integration strategy (e.g., combining payers, providers, and a wide spectrum of services in the same network, such as physician hospital organizations [PHOs] still focus on physicians and hospitals as principal health-care resources. Some sources consider this a stop-gap measure, not addressing all players, such as insurance providers, in the system. Cost-effectiveness and provider practice profiles are increasingly considered in managed-care contracting, but there may be a reticence to disrupt traditional local practice patterns as managed care increasingly influences some markets (Kongstvedt, 1994).

AMERICAN ASSOCIATION OF NURSE ANESTHETISTS

Since its organization in 1931, the AANA has placed its responsibilities to the public above or at the same level as its responsibilities to its membership. The association has produced education and practice standards, implemented a recertification process for nurse anesthetists (1945), and developed an accreditation program for nurse anesthesia education (1952). It was a leader in forming multidisciplinary councils with public representation to fulfill the profession's autonomous credentialing functions (American Association of Nurse Anesthetists, 1992b).

When founder Agatha Hodgins became ill, Gertrude Fife, who provided anesthesia for pioneering heart surgeon Claude Beck, assumed the burden of developing the young National Association of Nurse Anesthetists (NANA) (Thatcher, 1953). The Association's name was changed to the American Association of Nurse Anesthetists in 1939. Helen Lamb, who served two terms as AANA president (1940–1942), worked exclusively with Dr. Evarts Graham, one of the first modern thoracic surgeons (Bankert, 1989). The first anesthesia administered for correction of tetralogy of Fallot was given by a nurse anesthetist. It is clear that early CRNA leaders were involved in dynamic practice settings with surgeons who were also leaders in their fields.

In addition to developing a professional identity for nurse anesthesia, early CRNA leaders developed educational standards for nurse anesthesia educational programs. These standards included a minimum program length of six months and, later, institution of mandatory certification and recertification policies.

The AANA was among the first nursing specialty organizations. Early affiliation with the ANA did not occur, as previously noted, because each organization had different ideas of what such an affiliation would entail (Gunn, 1991; Thatcher, 1953).

At a 1931 regional nurse anesthesia meeting, Agatha Hodgins put forth the essentials for a national organization of nurse anesthetists as she saw them:

> *Improvement of the present situation is in the hands of the nurse anesthetists themselves. If the work is to be properly safeguarded and hoped-for progress attained, it is necessary that remedies be applied to certain detrimental conditions now acknowledgly existing. It would*

> *seem that the first step should be the awakening of deeper interest*
> *and the development of constructive leadership. Following in logical*
> *order would be: self-organization as a special division of hospital*
> *service . . .; educational standards; postgraduate schools of*
> *anesthesia . . . required to conform to an accepted criteria of*
> *education; state registration, putting the right of the nurse anesthetist*
> *to practice her vocation beyond criticism; constant effort toward*
> *improving the quality of the work by means of study and research,*
> *thus affording still greater protection to the patient; [and]*
> *dissemination of information gained through proper channels.*
>
> (Thatcher, 1953)

The division between nurse anesthesia and nursing service has occurred in many practice settings in which CRNAs are responsible to the hospital rather than to the nursing administration.

With time, the breach between nursing and nurse anesthesia has narrowed considerably. Legislative and regulatory advances for APNs, such as direct reimbursement, prescriptive authority, and expanded scope of practice, have involved coalitions of APNs. As more nurse anesthesia programs have moved into schools of nursing, shared values have readily been identified by nurse anesthesia educators and nursing educators. These values include concepts such as ensuring access for 39 million Americans without health-care insurance to primary and specialty, cost-effective health care that can be provided by APNs.

The AANA represents 96% of the practicing CRNAs in this country (American Association of Nurse Anesthetists, 1995). This is an unusually high percentage of members for any professional organization. It is believed that this is due to the fact that the AANA endeavors to be responsive to member concerns. The AANA allows multiple venues for direct member input rather than relying on a delegate system for member feedback to leadership (Foster & Garde, 1994).

The AANA has steadily grown, responding to member needs and legislative, regulatory, practice, and educational concerns. The organization has 10 major departments at its Park Ridge, Illinois headquarters and in a Washington, D. C. office (Fig. 19–5).

AANA affairs are handled by an elected board of directors in conjunction with AANA staff members. More than 20 committees and subcommittees conduct activities directed by the board. Annually, the AANA conducts business at six national meetings held at various sites. Additionally, four autonomous councils function independently of the executive office. These councils have been developed autonomously of the AANA to avoid potential conflicts of interest in the areas of accreditation, certification, recertification, and public interest.

INTERNATIONAL NURSE ANESTHESIA PRACTICE

Internationally, nurse anesthesia practice exists in western Europe, portions of eastern Europe, Scandinavia, and parts of Africa and Asia. The International Federation of Nurse Anesthetists (IFNA) was chartered in 1989 with 11 founding member countries, and has grown to 20 member countries representing over 30,000 nurse

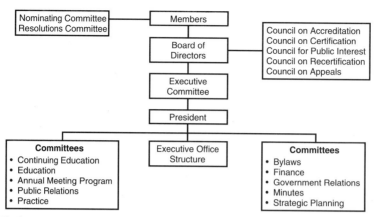

Figure 19–5. AANA organizational chart—communities of interest. (Used with permission of the American Association of Nurse Anesthetists.)

anesthetists worldwide. The AANA, under the leadership of past president and IFNA Executive Director Ronald Caulk, has spearheaded this fledgling organization. The IFNA meets every three years to discuss issues related to practice and education. Although the practice of nurse anesthesia reaches around the globe, the scope of practice and educational processes for nurse anesthetists varies from one country to another (Kelly, 1994). CRNA volunteers participate in charitable surgical services throughout the third world through services such as Operation Smile and the Orbis Project. These volunteer surgeons, nurses, and CRNAs provide services such as cleft lip and palate repair for children in underserved areas. Health Volunteers Overseas also provides voluntary anesthesia and surgical services in addition to teaching clinical anesthesia in third-world countries (Catchpole, M., personal communication, 1995).

FUTURE TRENDS: IMPACT OF MANAGED CARE AND HMOs

Historically, APNs and physician assistants have practiced collaboratively with physicians in HMOs, providing both primary and specialty care. HMO physicians acknowledge the continued role for APNs in HMOs (Bowser, 1994).

The increasing penetration of managed care into major health-care marketplaces results in fewer surgical cases being performed at lower rates of reimbursement. When surgery is done less frequently, a concomitant fall in demand for anesthesia services occurs, and competing institutions vie for managed-care contracts. Many major metropolitan areas have an oversupply of in-patient hospital beds. A paradigm shift in acute care has occurred, wherein hospitals are no longer financial profit centers but are now recognized as cost centers. Critical pathways and other utilization review mechanisms are used to minimize the average length of hospital stay (Sinioris, M., personal communication, 1994). A proliferation of out-patient and home health-care services has occurred and can be expected to continue. CRNAs and other APNs can play significant roles in this process.

Regarding the future of nurse anesthesia practice, it seems likely that hospital employment will be less common as hospitals decrease their fixed costs, such as payroll. Whether CRNAs will be self-employed, employed by CRNA groups, or employed by physician-CRNA groups will depend on local market dynamics. Independent contracting by CRNAs for their professional services will increase. It will be imperative for CRNAs and other APNs to know their worth in terms of billable revenue and quality of care provided for contract negotiation and public relations purposes.

In the future, each CRNA may practice in multiple settings with individually negotiated contracts. Home health services such as parenteral infusion therapy and management of chronic pain might be directed by CRNAs, as is already the case in some areas. These areas are natural extensions of anesthesia pharmacology and clinical skills. Myriad opportunities will exist for CRNAs and other APNs to collaborate in the management of acute and chronic pain and the treatment of respiratory and nutritional disorders.

To decrease the costs of providing surgical anesthesia when both physician anesthesiologists and nurse anesthetists collaborate, staffing ratios in team anesthesia, e.g., MDs and CRNAs working together, may change. In recent years, there has been one physician for every two CRNAs in many settings. This relationship is typically a collaborative one in which the anesthesiologist provides consultation when needed. This ratio has been determined more by the overabundance of anesthesiologists and barriers established by reimbursement methodology and is less likely due to a quality-of-care issue. Previous abuses in this area led to federally mandated anesthesia payment reform, the Tax Equity and Fiscal Reform Act (TEFRA) requirements. The ratio will most certainly change to a physician consultant for every three or four experienced CRNAs in the operating room.

The future of nurse anesthesia education and research is promising. With more CRNAs holding graduate degrees, there is more potential for basic and applied research by CRNAs. More graduate education in nursing, the basic sciences, and business will better enable CRNAs to collaborate with other investigators in the arenas of clinical and bench research; practice, legislation, and policy formulation will also be enhanced by this additional educational preparation. A greater nurse anesthesia voice in policy formulation has already been felt, with CRNA members sitting on state boards of nursing and in other governmental positions.

SUMMARY

Nurse anesthesia was the earliest nursing specialty. Nurse anesthesia was the first nursing specialty to have standardized educational programs, a certification process, mandatory continuing education, and recertification. Nurse anesthetists have been involved in the development of anesthetic techniques and equipment along with physicians and engineers. Nurse anesthetists have been nursing leaders in obtaining third-party reimbursement for professional services, in coping with challenges such as the PPS, and managed care.

CRNAs provide surgical and nonsurgical anesthesia services in a variety of settings both in the United States and in other parts of the world. CRNAs work independently or with physician collaboration and are capable of providing the full spectrum of anesthesia services.

Activism in the state and federal legislative and regulatory arenas is a recognized CRNA activity. Increasing coalition-building between nurse anesthetists, other APNs, and nursing educators is congruent with a shared nursing vision. This vision values health care for all Americans provided in a safe and cost-effective manner by APNs collaborating with other health-care professionals.

REFERENCES

American Association of Nurse Anesthetists (1992a). *Guidelines and standards for nurse anesthesia practice.* Park Ridge, IL: American Association of Nurse Anesthetists.

American Association of Nurse Anesthetists (1992b). *Qualifications and capabilities of the CRNA.* Park Ridge, IL: American Association of Anesthetists.

American Association of Nurse Anesthetists (January 1995). *AANA News Bulletin.* Park Ridge, IL: AANA.

American Association of Nurse Anesthetists (1995). *Report of fiscal year 1995 member survey data.* Park Ridge, Illinois: American Association of Nurse Anesthetists.

Bader, A., & Datta, S. (1994). Obstetric anesthesia. In Rogers et al. (Eds.), *Principles and practice of Anesthesiology.* (pp. 2065–2104). St. Louis: C. V. Mosby.

Bankert, M. (1989). *Watchful care: A history of America's nurse anesthetists.* New York: Continuum.

Bowser, R. (1994). Lecture from HMO physician administrator. Managed Care Course in Health Systems Management. Chicago: Rush University.

Callahan, L. (1994). Establishing measures of competence. In S. Foster, & L. Jordan (Eds.), *Professional aspects of nurse anesthesia practice* (pp. 275–290). Philadelphia: F. A. Davis.

Callahan, L. (1995). Unpublished doctoral dissertation. Tallahassee: Florida State University.

Christman, L. (1977). Doctoral education: A shot in the arm for the nursing professor. *Health Services Manager, 10* (5), 6–7.

Christman, L. (1980). Cited in clinical defense of Faut, MM. (1984). (pp. 14, 15). Chicago: Rush University.

Cromwell, J., & Rosenbach, M. (1988). The economics of anesthesia delivery. *Health Affairs, 7* (4) 118–131.

Dripps, R. (1977). Preface. In Dripps, et al. (Eds.), *Introduction to anesthesia* (5th ed., pp. 1–11). Philadelphia: W. B. Saunders.

Faut, M. (1984). *Doctoral education for nurse anesthesia practice. Unpublished Clinical Defense Paper.* Chicago: Rush University.

Faut-Callahan, M., & Paice, J. (1990). Post-operative pain control for the parturient. *Journal of Perinatal and Neonatal Nursing, 4,* (1), 27–41.

Faut-Callahan, M. (1991). Graduate education for nurse anesthetists: Master's versus a clinical doctorate. *National Commission on Nurse Anesthesia Education Report* (pp. 110–115). Park Ridge, IL: American Association of Nurse Anesthetists.

Foster, S., & Garde, J. (1994). The American Association of Nurse Anesthetists: The role of the professional organization. In S. Foster, & L. Jordan. (Eds.), *Professional aspects of nurse anesthesia practice.* Philadelphia: F. A. Davis.

Garde, J. (1988). Preface. In W. Waugaman, S. Foster, B. Rigor (Eds.), *Principles and practice of nurse anesthesia.* Norwalk, CT: Appleton & Lange.

Gunn, I. (1991). The history of nurse anesthesia education: Highlights and influences. *National Commission on Nurse Anesthesia Education Report,* (pp. 33–41). Park Ridge, IL: American Association of Nurse Anesthetists.

Jordan, L. (1994). Qualifications and capabilities of the certified registered nurse anesthetist. In S. Foster, & L. Jordan, (Eds.), *Professional aspects of nurse anesthesia practice* (pp. 3–10). Philadelphia: F. A. Davis.

Kelly, J. (1994). An international study of educational programs for nurses providing anesthesia care. *AANA Journal, 62* (6), 484–495.

Kongstvedt, P. (1994). *The managed health care handbook* (2nd ed.). Gaithersburg, MD: Aspen.

Loper, K., Butler, S., Nessly, M., & Wild, L. (1989). Paralyzed with pain: The need for education. *Pain, 37:* 315–316.

Micek, W. (1993). *Components of patient-centered care: Implications for surgical outpatient nursing practice.* Doctoral dissertation. Chicago: Rush University.

Munguia-Biddle, F., Maree, S., Klein, E., Callahan, L., & Gilles, B. (1990). *Nurse anesthesiology competence evaluation: Mechanism for accountability.* Unpublished document. Park Ridge, IL: American Association of Nurse Anesthetists.

Simonson, D., & Garde, J. (1994). Reimbursement for clinical services. In S. Foster, & L. Jordan (Eds.), *Professional aspects of nurse anesthesia practice* (pp. 129–142). Philadelphia: F. A. Davis.

Thatcher, V. (1953). *History of anesthesia with emphasis on the nurse specialist.* Philadelphia: J. B. Lippincott.

Waugaman, W. (1991). Nurse anesthesia: The practice of nursing, medicine or something else? *Nurse Anesthesia, 2* (4), 157–159.

CHAPTER 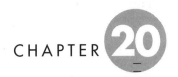 20

Nurse Case Management as an Advanced Practice Role

Vicky A. Mahn
Judith A. Spross

INTRODUCTION

Despite the fact that the much-needed reform of the health-care system that was debated in the early 1990s has not yet come to pass, marketplace reform *has* occurred (Baird, 1995). Increasing marketplace regulation affects delivery of care at every level. Managed care and case management (CM) are seen as ways of bringing some order to the chaos that exists in health care today. Although CM may appear to be a new concept, it has been recognized as an important part of the care continuum for nearly three decades. Contemporary nurse CM (NCM) reflects a natural evolution from nursing's history of client advocacy, social service, and public health. One could consider the private duty and public health nurses of earlier eras the forerunners of modern nurse case managers. Nurse practitioners and certified nurse-midwives also provide care that is congruent with CM concepts; their care results, for example, in improved access to health-care services and better care coordination between providers and continuity across settings (Newman, 1990; U.S. Congress, 1986). NCM is seen as a means of improving access to care in a timely manner.

NCM has been viewed as a way of enhancing the visibility of advanced nursing practice (ANP) (Cooper, 1990; Hamric, 1992). Many arguments have been made for having NCM done by advanced practice nurses (APNs) (Connors, 1993; Fralic, 1992; Hamric, 1992). Although the focus of this chapter is on the ANP case manager, at this stage of development NCM may be more similar to nurse-midwifery (see Chapter 18) than to other ANP roles. At the present time, it is not feasible for all nurse case managers to be APNs, because the need for nurse case managers is much greater than the supply of APNs (Connors, 1993). In this chapter, overviews of managed care, CM, and NCM are offered; ANP CM within the context of managed care and CM is described; the core skills, competencies, and accountabilities of ANP CM are identified; and issues related to ANP CM are discussed. It is hoped that this chapter will contribute to the evolution of ANP CM by stimulating further critical thinking and research on the contributions of ANP CM to the clinical and fiscal goals of managed care.

OVERVIEWS OF MANAGED CARE, CM, AND NCM

MANAGED CARE

Managed care is an integrated network that combines the financing and delivery of health-care services to covered individuals. Through arrangements with selected providers in the network, health services are furnished to members of the plan. Managed care systems are expected to have explicit standards for selection of the care providers and formal programs of quality improvement and utilization review. In managed care, financial incentives exist to encourage members to use providers associated with the plan and to follow procedures that help the plan to control costs. Financial incentives also encourage providers to control expenditures. Thus, managed care is a system of resource use and coordination of care that may be applied to *all* clients within a delivery system in order to optimize quality and cost-effective care. All managed care methods must address continuity of care and a continuous provider or group of providers (Zander, 1993). Managed care can be considered the structure under which health care is delivered and CM or NCM as the process by which managed care goals are often accomplished.

CM

CM is a process of resource management and patient outcome determination that focuses on the clinical production process and fiscal productivity (Pierog, 1991). This may be regarded as a conceptual definition, but CM may be operationalized differently. For example, CM can be a brokerage service for health-care resources provided on behalf of a payer or provider; it can be a discrete job or role; or it can be a system of care delivery in which specific attention is directed to the care of an individual for the purposes of identifying the most cost-effective treatments for resource-intensive conditions such as major trauma, AIDs, cancer, prematurity, and strokes. It is conceivable that such monitoring and coordination could be achieved without the patient's ever being seen by the case manager. Rather, the care is "managed" simply through the use of authorization procedures and the scrutiny of medical records. Regardless of how the term is used, the goals of CM are similar: to integrate quality, productivity, and costs by addressing systems, procedures, and roles to achieve desired patient and organizational outcomes (Zander, 1988). In this chapter, only clinical or direct care CM is discussed.

CM is a practice framework that has been implemented in a variety of settings by nurses, social workers, and other health-care providers. To foster a common understanding of the work done by professional case managers, the interdisciplinary Case Management Society of America (CMSA, 1994) has defined CM as "*A collaborative process which assesses, plans, implements, coordinates, monitors and evaluates options and services to meet an individual's health needs through communications and available resources to promote quality cost-effective outcomes*" (p. 60). This definition incorporates the system, clinical, and fiscal aspects that are central to CM approaches to providing care.

The CMSA's definition applies to all disciplines that practice CM; it is not specific to nurses. An interdisciplinary definition is useful, because it crosses a range of health-care systems and service settings. Some patient populations, such as indigent patients, may be best served by social work case managers. Other populations, such as patients with mild head injuries, may be best served by rehabilitation counselors. Although the definition of CM is consistent with the nursing process framework, it does not address the specialized clinical nursing expertise that seems essential to achieve optimal cost and quality outcomes in certain patients who require health promotion or illness management.

NCM

The American Nurses' Association (ANA, 1988) defined NCM as a health-care delivery process that aims to provide quality health care, enhance quality of life, diminish fragmentation, and contain costs. More recently, NCM has been characterized as a set of "goal-oriented activities that organize, coordinate, and monitor health care delivery based on measurable objectives designed to meet the needs" of chronically ill or complex patients (Doell Smith, 1994, p. 65). The primary reasons for using NCM to deliver care are to control costs, enhance quality of care, decrease fragmentation and duplication of services, and ensure accountability for achieving cost and quality outcomes through nursing interventions that are based on holism, scientific and experiential knowledge, and partnership with the patient. Other benefits of NCM have also been identified. It can increase provider control over the practice, enhance provider satisfaction, improve standards of care, promote interdisciplinary communication and collaboration, and increase the volume of cases and market share (Zander, 1993). Acute, primary, and community care settings are implementing innovative NCM programs as a way to promote quality outcomes in a cost-effective manner. Despite this growth, there is still considerable confusion about the definition and practice of NCM (Lyon, 1993). Although there are differences between ANP CM and NCM that are discussed later in Issues in ANP CM, this chapter is based on the following definitions of NCM and ANP CM:

> **Nurse Case Manager:** A nurse case manager is an experienced, bachelor's-prepared registered nurse (RN) who is accountable for managing a defined group of patients in order to optimize clinical and cost outcomes. Outcomes are achieved through clinical practice and partnership with patients and families over time and across settings, as well as through the coordination of services, expert communication and collaborative skills, and the use of population-specific guidelines.

> **ANP Case Manager:** An ANP case manager has graduate preparation in nursing and is accountable for managing a group of clinically complex or resource-intensive patients in order to optimize clinical and cost outcomes. Outcomes are achieved through the same processes used by the nurse case manager. In addition, the ANP case manager assesses the need for system or process improvements along the continuum of care and designs, facilitates, and monitors improvement initiatives.

NURSE CASE MANAGERS

PROFILE OF PRACTICE

Profiles of existing NCM practice are difficult to obtain, due to wide variation in job titles, work settings, and backgrounds of nurse case managers. In addition, lack of NCM-specific certification and the interdisciplinary nature of contemporary CM make it difficult to provide an accurate, descriptive profile. However, some inferences about NCM can be derived from what is known about CM generally.

Currently, the CMSA endorses the minimal requirement of a baccalaureate degree for certification as a case manager. Since 1993, case managers have had the option to become certified by taking a national CM examination offered by the Certification for Case Management organization. This examination tests a broad, interdisciplinary knowledge base and the credential offered is Certified Case Manager. The development of the certification examination was the result of collaboration among rehabilitation specialists, educators, nurses, social workers, and research professionals (Leahy, 1994). During the first year in which certification was available, a total of 14,078 individual practitioners applied to take the test. The work settings most frequently reported by these applicants were independent CM companies (23.8%), hospitals (11.7%), independent rehabilitation/insurance affiliates (11.0%), and health insurance companies (8%). The job titles most frequently named by these applicants included case manager (45.9%), RN (19.8%), rehabilitation counselor (10.9%), and administrator/manager (7.6%). It was not clear what percentage of applicants with the title "case manager" were RNs. A mean of 6.8 years of work experience providing CM services was reported; the mean age of applicants was 43.2 years (Leahy, 1994). The educational preparation of individuals taking the test was not reported. From the reported age and work experience, it seems that experience in a discipline precedes the assumption of a CM role.

It is likely that nurses are practicing CM in far greater numbers than these statistics suggest. Also, the distribution of work settings would probably have been quite different had a more homogeneous group of nurse case managers been surveyed. The literature on NCM indicates that nurse case managers (basic and advanced) are found in hospitals, community agencies, schools, and other settings.

TYPES OF NCM

Current models of NCM fall into two categories: NCM type models and organizational models. Two types of NCM have been identified (Brubakken, Janssen, & Ruppel, 1994; Zander, 1995). Zander (1995) compared "utilization review NCM" with "clinical NCM." In utilization review NCM, daily chart review is completed on all patients in the setting, to ensure that medical appropriateness, length of stay, and payer-based criteria are met. This is NCM by oversight. Patient contact is generally not required. Rather, the focus is on appropriate use of medical services, and the process of CM occurs behind the clinical scene through preapproval mechanisms, chart review, and monitoring of claims. This position helps reduce avoidable or nonreimbursable services or hospital days. Utilization review NCM positions are generally filled by RNs with various backgrounds.

Clinical nurse case managers have a relationship with patients and families, often provide direct care, and are accountable for overseeing the coordination of care (Brubakken et al., 1994; Zander, 1995); direct patient care is a critically important NCM activity. Clinical nurse case managers use their clinical expertise to influence the care of high-volume or high-risk groups of patients. They are likely to be employed in traditional settings, including hospitals, ambulatory surgery centers, primary care clinics, community health centers, and home health agencies. Generally, caseloads are determined by case type, diagnostic-related group, or service or product line. In some models, payer group may also be a determining factor of the nurse case manager's caseload. Clinical nurse case managers focus their expertise and coordinating efforts on a subgroup of patients within a health-care system who either are at risk for medical instability or place the providing health-care system at fiscal risk because of their high resource consumption. The clinical nurse case manager's caseload is likely to be smaller than that of the utilization review nurse case manager.

In addition to types of NCM, several organizational models of NCM have been used in both acute care and community agencies. NCM models may be health or illness focused. Although community and acute care models differ in terms of practice setting, target populations, and span of accountability, the success of NCM interventions relies on the nurse's clinical knowledge and expertise. Some populations for which NCM has been used include the chronically mentally ill (Bryson, Naqvi, Callahan, & Fontenot, 1990); HIV-positive women (Riley, 1992); perinatal clients (Ladden, 1991); clients in rural settings (Parker, et al., 1990); trauma patients (Daleiden, 1993); and community health centers for health assessment, counseling, education, and screening (Ethridge, 1991). Which NCM model a health-care agency chooses depends on the agency's goals and the creativity of the nurse case managers. Common organizational goals that justify the use of NCM include reducing lengths of acute care stay, readmissions, resource use and costs; increasing access to services and market share; and becoming a recognized center of excellence for a particular product line.

The Carondelet model of NCM is used to illustrate NCM in this chapter, because it is the setting of the exemplar ANP CM position described later. Readers are referred to other models, including the pioneering work in NCM done by Zander and her colleagues at New England Medical Center (Zander, 1988, 1990a). Figure 20–1 illustrates the operationalization of NCM at the Carondelet Health Care Corporation. A staff nurse in an acute care or primary care setting is accountable for outcomes of care within a condensed time frame, such as a shift, clinic visit, or unit-based episode. In contrast, the accountability held by the nurse case manager extends beyond such time frames and geographical boundaries. Other NCM programs within the system support single episodes of care (clinical CM) or long-term client relationships (community CM). An example of episodic clinical CM is the NCM program for open heart surgery patients; the nurse case manager's accountability extends from preadmission to postdischarge, after which NCM responsibilities revert back to the community nurse CM as needed (Mahn, 1993). In episodic NCM, the nurse case manager maintains a relationship with the patient, assesses the patient's daily progress, and provides patient and family education and discharge planning services, but the direct clinical care is provided by the staff RN. In community NCM, nurses with varying clinical backgrounds are employed to partner with a wide range of patients with chronic disease over time and across settings, in order to promote greater self-care (Ethridge & Lamb, 1989). In the community NCM model, the nurse-patient relationship and NCM activities extend from the time the client is enrolled into the NCM program to the termination of the relationship (Ethridge & Lamb, 1989). Community nurse case managers follow patients with chronic illnesses, such as those with end-stage pulmonary disease, multiple sclerosis, congestive heart failure, and atrial fibrillation.

Regardless of the type of NCM or the organizational model of NCM used, nurses who provide CM bring an understanding of disease processes, therapies, and responses to illness and treatment that other disciplines may not offer. The

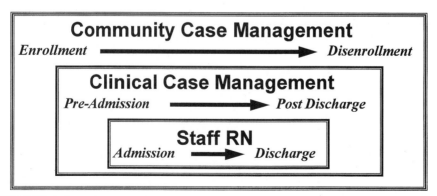

FIGURE 20–1. Span of accountability for nursing case management roles. (Reprinted with permission from Carondelet Health Care Corporation, 1995.)

goal of both NCM and CM is to accomplish the quality and fiscal outcomes sought by managed care systems. However, in NCM the methods for accomplishing quality and cost outcomes rely on a nursing perspective: advocacy for access, holistic assessment, partnership with patients and families over time, interventions related to health promotion and self-care skills, and coordination of care across settings (Smith, 1993). Increasingly, one finds that nurse case managers are sharing direct and indirect fiscal risk with their sponsoring organizations. In some organizations, continued employment of the nurse case manager is contingent upon the person's ability to demonstrate a cost savings of at least his or her annual salary.

NCM AND ADVANCED NURSING PRACTICE

OVERVIEW OF NCM FUNCTIONS

Despite the lack of sufficient research on NCM, some generalizations about its activities and functions may be made (Table 20–1). The nurse case manager must have sufficient clinical expertise to understand the needs and clinical management of specific patient populations. The nurse case manager's clinical interventions are often directed toward enhancing patients' and their families' self-care skills by helping them access appropriate health-care services and community resources. Prior clinical experience is critical for (1) anticipating the likely trajectory of certain illnesses; (2) understanding and making choices among alternative interventions; (3) analyzing variances from standards of care and critical pathways; (4) understanding the clinical judgments of other providers; and (5) negotiating among patients, providers, and payers. The nurse case manager must also be able to influence the delivery system in which the care is provided; this is essential. The interpersonal skills nurses bring to their care of patients are just as important in their relationships with other parties within CM systems. Those that are particularly important to the NCM role at the system level of intervention are collaboration, communication, and conflict resolution (Connors, 1993). The reader must realize

TABLE 20–1. ACTIVITIES OF NURSE CASE MANAGERS

*Collaboration with administrative, management, and clinical staff who are responsible for specified patient groups

*Assessment, planning, implementation, coordination, referral, and evaluation of patients and families in assigned target populations

*Provision of internal consultation to other disciplines and departments with the goal of managing care of patients and families expeditiously

*Participation in the development of documentation systems and tools (i.e., critical pathways or practice guidelines) to monitor clinical and fiscal outcomes

*Collecting, analyzing, and sharing of data and information in order to influence process improvements and support integration of core systems and processes within the care environment

*Development of partnerships with physicians in order to achieve clinical and fiscal outcomes

*Teaching and coaching other caregivers on the health-care team regarding clinical, fiscal, and system processes related to patient care management

*Role-modeling of professional nursing practice

that in contemporary NCM practice, these activities are carried out by nurse case managers with varying levels and types of preparation and experience; current practice does not routinely require the nurse case manager to have advanced nursing education. Given this book's focus on advanced nursing practice, NCM activities and functions are described and illustrated using the ANP competencies described in Chapters 6–13.

CONGRUENCE OF NCM WITH ANP COMPETENCIES

In health-care settings where high-tech, sophisticated medical care is provided, APNs have been valued for their specialized knowledge and their training in complex decision making (Madden & Reid Ponte, 1994). Some authors have noted that NCM practice is consistent with the expectations of APNs (Connors, 1993; Fralic, 1992; Hamric, 1992; Newman, cited in Smith, 1993). Hamric (1992) analyzed the NCM literature and suggested that the NCM role be viewed as an ANP role. She exhorted APNs to "confront the challenge of case management forcefully and articulate their role to this practice modality" (Hamric, p. 13). Interestingly, NCM functions (see Table 20–1) closely align with the traditional subroles of the clinical nurse specialist (clinical practice, consultation, education, and research) (Hamric, 1989) and incorporate the clinical nurse specialist's change agent, management, and leadership skills (Gournic, 1989).

The parallels between ANP CM and the traditional clinical nurse specialist role are also reflected in the number of NCM articles published by clinical nurse specialists (e.g., Cronin & Maklebust, 1989; Flynn & Kilgallen, 1993; Lynn-McHale, Fitzpatrick, & Shaller, 1993; Nugent, 1992; Sherman & Johnson, 1994; Strong, 1992; Trinidad, 1993; Wagner & Menke, 1992). Patient populations who have been cared for by clinical nurse specialists include multisystem failure patients in critical care (Strong, 1991), long-term care patients (Schroer, 1991), trauma patients (Daleiden, 1993; Rotz, Yates, & Schare, 1994), pediatric patients with cardiac defects or chronic illness (Doell Smith, 1994; Gaedeke-Norris & Hill, 1991), and patients who have undergone coronary artery bypass graft (Tidwell, 1994). Tidwell (1994) also described three different ways in which clinical nurse specialists are used in NCM.

Jenkins and Sullivan-Marx (1994) proposed a primary care delivery model in which nurse practitioners would practice as nurse case managers in community health settings, childbirth centers, home settings, skilled nursing facilities, and acute care settings. In this model, ANP case managers would oversee a caseload of clients and their families. Expert physical and emotional assessment skills, independent decision making, and interdisciplinary collaboration are essential for the effective management of patients. To promote health and prevent illness, the program goals would be to promote exercise, appropriate use of assistive devices, stress management, and symptom control. Areas for program development might include activities such as water aerobics, Tai Chi, biofeedback training, and nutritional counseling. The ANP case manager would be accountable for evaluating the clinical and fiscal outcomes related to the interventions and resources expended on the patient population.

Because the ANP case manager is an emerging ANP role, the eight ANP competencies are used here to help the reader see how the ANP case manager is likely to be different from more established ANP roles. Table 20–2 demonstrates that NCM functions are congruent with the ANP competencies described in Chapters 6–13.

TABLE 20–2. ADVANCED NURSING PRACTICE (ANP) COMPETENCIES AND NURSE CASE MANAGEMENT (NCM) SKILLS AND FUNCTIONS

ANP Competency	NCM Knowledge/Skill	NCM Function
Direct care	*In-depth, specialized assessment skills *Expert, clinically relevant technical skills *Establishment of patient outcomes	*Find and screen cases *Conduct health assessments *Develop and review critical pathways *Coordinate interventions of other providers *Link patient with appropriate resources *Monitor patient's progress toward goals *Evaluate effects of interventions
Expert guidance and coaching	*Education of patient, family, and other providers	*Educate staff nurses and other providers about clinical, fiscal, and system processes *Coach patients and families through developmental, health, and illness transitions
Consultation	*Provision of case consultation *Securing of consultation to enhance care and NCM	*Participate in work redesign *Initiate systemwide process improvements (e.g., documentation tools)
Research interpretation and use	*Collection, analysis, and synthesis of data	*Evaluate program outcomes such as quality and costs of care
Collaboration	*Communication, coordination, and negotiation	*Monitor service plan regarding quality, timeliness, quantity, costs of services, and effectiveness *Develop critical pathways and other clinical guidelines
Change agency	*Assessment of systems and organizations	*Initiate systemwide improvements *Identify needs for new services/programs
Ethical decision making	*Recognition and raising of ethical dilemmas	*Meet both system/fiscal and client goals

Sources: Hamric (1992), Connors (1993), and chapter narrative

Direct Care, Expert Coaching, and Ethical Decision Making

In Chapter 6, Brown notes that establishment of partnerships with patients, holistic assessment, and diverse management approaches are among the key components of the direct care provided by APNs. These aspects of direct care also underlie the effectiveness of NCM. The nurse case manager's ability to help patients achieve their health-care goals is thought to be closely related to the nurse-patient relationship. The NCM literature consistently advocates a relationship focus (Fralic, 1992; Lamb & Stempel, 1994; Newman, Lamb, & Michaels, 1989). Qualitative research in which patients experiencing NCM were interviewed suggested that the process used in NCM practice is one in which the nurse case manager becomes a "trusted insider" to the client. As the process unfolds, patients integrate the nurse's teaching and coaching so that they become their own "insider experts," able to make judgments about their need for care (Lamb & Stempel, 1994). Until the nurse case manager becomes a trusted insider, interventions to optimize wellness or foster self-care skills may have limited impact. Within the partnership context, patient and family values and health perceptions must be honored. Trust may initially be created through clinical credibility and expert power, but it must be sustained by the authenticity of the relationship. Lamb and Stempel (1994) suggested that successful outcomes such as fewer days in the hospital and critical care unit, fewer readmissions, and reduced use of emergency room services are related to "monitoring and teaching activities of the nurse case managers, which occur in the context of a caring nurse-client relationship" (p. 9). This understanding of why NCM works has theoretical support (Newman, 1994). Thus, the expert coaching and guidance described by Clarke and Spross in Chapter 7 are central to ANP CM practice. With regard to holistic assessment and the use of diverse management approaches, the ANP case manager might be more likely than other APNs to perform more detailed assessment of environmental, organizational, and contextual factors that affect *individual* patients because of the emphasis on achieving both clinical and fiscal outcomes.

Embedded in the concept of partnership with patients and families is the APN's role as client advocate. In NCM, the ANP case manager is often able to advocate more effectively for clients than is possible in other systems. If the organization is truly committed to quality and customer satisfaction, the barriers to effective advocacy are fewer. The ANP case manager's dual accountability for patient and organizational outcomes may give rise to ethical dilemmas with somewhat different features. For example, patient and organizational outcomes can come into conflict, and these conflicts are likely to be more visible because the costs of clinical decisions are monitored. The ANP case manager must be able to articulate the decision options' risks and benefits for the patient and organization. Within the NCM process, APNs have opportunities to apply "preventive ethics" (see Chapter 13). For example, a well-designed critical pathway (which incorporates expert clinical judgment) may indicate that a particular patient population can be discharged to home within a week of admission. However, if successful discharge depends on adequate social supports and a patient does not have these, the pathway and the data used to develop it can provide the justification for deviating from the pathway. Knowledge of fiscal variables and costs of services also enables ANP case managers to articulate the costs of *not* pursuing a decision that is in the patient's best interests, in order to persuade others to do what is best for the patient.

Collaboration, Consultation, Change Agency, and Leadership

The ANP case manager's accountability for accomplishing clinical, fiscal, and organizational outcomes significantly influences the expression of these particular competencies. This accountability is probably one of the key differences between the ANP case manager and other APNs. The responsibilities of ANP case managers require simultaneous and synchronous use of these ANP competencies. One of the advantages of being a nurse case manager is that the APN has clear authority and accountability for the clinical care delivered and for making the system work. This may be one of the reasons so many clinical nurse specialists have moved into ANP CM roles; this position directly links the APN to outcomes. Another advantage is that the ANP case manager can have considerable influence in shaping an environment that promotes collaboration within and across disciplines. These competencies are operationalized in such activities as the development and implementation of standards, guidelines, and other tools, such as critical pathways. Such tools balance costs, processes, and outcomes by organizing the care: Who should deliver the care? In what sequence? What outcomes are to be achieved? Within what time frame? (Nugent, 1992; Zander, 1993). How guidelines are derived is beyond the scope of this chapter, but the nature of the questions indicates the importance of leadership, consultation, and interdisciplinary collaboration if the work is to be done well, cost-effectively, and efficiently.

Figure 20–2 illustrates that the nurse case manager influences individual patients and families as well as other disciplines and providers who are associated with the process of delivering clinical care in order to achieve improved outcomes. Nurse case managers must therefore have enough autonomy and control over their daily work and time schedule to be able to shift back and forth between involvement with direct care and with system issues in order to achieve desired outcomes for individual patients and the aggregate population. The nurse case manager is the "glue" that provides continuity for both individual patients and providers across the continuum of settings in which care is provided. The relationship process is intentionally placed centrally and prominently to emphasize the importance of relationships with patients and their families and with other providers to accomplish individual and collective outcomes.

Work redesign and process improvements within clinical services or the care setting are also strategies for achieving quality and cost outcomes in health delivery systems (Baird, 1995). Because ANP case managers are members of a team that is economically accountable for treating, comforting, and administering care within specified time frames, they can become champions for continuous quality improvement within their areas of clinical accountability. Their high level of involvement in providing care, analyzing the care delivery system for costly inefficiencies and inconveniences, and initiating process improvements legitimizes ANP case

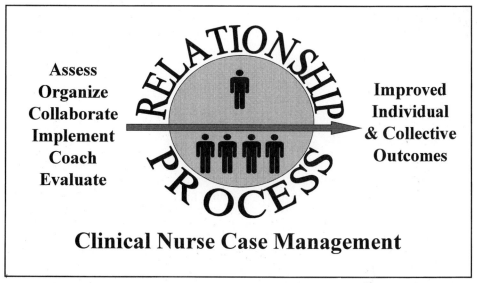

FIGURE 20–2. Conceptualization of clinical nurse case management role, with focus on clinical practice and systems improvement. (Reprinted with permission from Carondelet Health Care Corporation, 1995.)

managers' change agent skills, which should be well polished (see Chapter 12). The ANP case manager also pursues economy of effort: the development of CM strategies for one population may benefit other patient groups. An example is the nurse case manager who cared for a population of open heart surgery patients. In an effort to reduce postoperative pulmonary complications in this population, the ANP case manager collaborated with others on the team to develop guidelines for evaluation of preoperative pulmonary functioning and effective weaning of patients from the respirator after open heart surgery. When these protocols were found to be effective in open heart surgery patients, they were quickly adapted to guide the care of thoracotomy patients, resulting in improved clinical outcomes for this population as well.

Research Interpretation and Use

Much of NCM is data driven. The advanced education, research skills, and specialized knowledge base of ANP case managers enable them to apply research methodologies and continuous quality improvement principles into NCM practice. NCM and continuous quality improvement are linked in philosophy and process (Cesta, 1993). It is essential that the ANP case manager be able to lead an interdisciplinary team toward data-based conclusions and process improvements. He or she must be able to influence practice patterns and develop meaningful standards, practice protocols, and clinical pathways that promote teamwork, improve customer satisfaction and clinical outcomes, and reduce costs. For example, a nurse case manager may evaluate blood use practices for open heart surgery patients. On the basis of current use patterns and associated clinical outcomes, the nurse case manager may recommend a reduction in blood-ordering practices from six to two units of packed red blood cells with no adverse clinical outcomes and a resultant cost savings to the organization. Such recommendations are more readily implemented in the practice setting when a meaningful data analysis is completed and presented by a recognized clinical expert who is part of the health-care team. The ANP case manager must be able to influence the activities of both individual patients and groups of health-care providers within the delivery system toward goal setting and achievement. The APN's skill in evaluating NCM programs using research approaches will contribute to a better understanding of the role of the nurse case manager in health care.

OUTCOMES OF ANP CM

Clinical and other outcomes of ANP care in general are discussed in Chapter 26. Such information is useful to APNs and administrators who are considering an ANP CM model of health-care delivery. Studies and reports of ANP CM suggest that such models result in several outcomes. Patient-related outcomes include reductions in length of stay (Ling, 1993; Rudisill, Phillips, & Payne, 1993; Tidwell, 1994), improved collaboration among disciplines (Ling, 1993; Rudisill et al., 1993), and increased reimbursement for services or decreased costs (Gibson, Martin, Johnson, Blue, & Miller, 1994; Ling, 1993; Rudisill et al., 1993; Tidwell, 1994). Although this is not an exhaustive review, these data together with Girouard's review of research on APNs in Chapter 26 indicate that APNs are well positioned to play leading roles in accomplishing the goals of managed care through NCM.

EXEMPLAR OF ANP CM

The ongoing development of an open heart surgery program illustrates the functions of ANP CM. A nonprofit, community hospital faced with a rapidly growing capitated payer mix experienced a high rate of readmissions after coronary artery bypass graft (CABG) surgery. An ANP case manager was hired to coordinate the interdisciplinary team and assist in the development of practice protocols that would improve both clinical and fiscal outcomes for CABG patients. In addition, the ANP case manager would partner with all patients undergoing CABG surgery and their families to ensure that patient education, proper clinical management, and appropriate transfer and discharge took place along all points of service within the health-care network.

Beginning with a comprehensive analysis of current care processes, the ANP case manager reported that the preoperative management of CABG patients was fragmented and cumbersome when viewed from the patient's perspective. Patients underwent a preadmission testing process that took 3 hours; traveled to six different departments within the hospital; and were interviewed by eight different health-care providers, often being asked for the same information several times. The ANP case manager collaborated with these providers so that at each point in the preadmission process, bits of information were given to patients in an attempt to provide some preoperative instruction. This was a stopgap approach while the ANP case manager continued to problem-solve. Although patients received more education, the fragmentation persisted: the lab technician drew preoperative blood samples or drew blood for preoperative tests and instructed patients not to remove the wristband needed for type and cross-match. The preadmissions nurse told patients when to withhold food and fluids. The respiratory therapist instructed patients in the use of the incentive spirometer, and the cardiac rehabilitation nurse instructed the patient in coughing and deep-breathing exercises. At each stop, patients were asked for their names, allergies, and current medications. Finally, multiple documents and forms were generated by each provider, information that ended up in their departments for later referral, rather than in the patient's medical record.

The ANP case manager brought the team together and told them the story of the current process. Unanimously, the team recommended the creation of a "one person, one place" preoperative program for all CABG patients. It was decided that the ANP case manager would coordinate all preoperative lab work, electrocardiogram testing, and preoperative teaching. In addition, surgical permits; advanced directives; and a comprehensive patient assessment, including physical, emotional, functional, and social assessments, would take place to prepare each patient for surgery. Before each patient's preoperative visit, the ANP case manager reviewed his or her medical history, prior lab results, electrocardiogram, and radiology reports. In this manner, the case manager was able to eliminate redundant questioning of the patient and family and avoid unnecessary duplication of costly preoperative tests required for CABG patients. Within 6 months, the ANP case manager reported to the team a resultant cost savings of 11% associated with preoperative testing; complete elimination of last-minute surgical cancellations for all open heart patients; and a high degree of patient, staff, and physician satisfaction with the program.

The ANP case manager made daily rounds on all CABG patients as they transitioned from the intensive care unit to the step-down unit. Patients and families expressed appreciation for the continuity and partnership offered by the ANP case manager. Because the case manager had seen patients before they underwent surgery, she often identified subtle changes from patients' preoperative baseline physical and emotional status, resulting in earlier identification of complications, which were immediately communicated to other members of the health-care team. The ANP case manager evaluated each patient for response to medications, therapies, and mobility. Recommendations for altering patients' plan of care were communicated to the appropriate team member. Assessment findings and recommendations were recorded in the interdisciplinary progress notes. The ANP case manager also coordinated patient care conferences for patients who required more aggressive management postoperatively and became the "driver" to implement the resultant recommendations in a timely manner.

As the program matured, partnership with the hospital's key cardiothoracic surgeons developed. As the ANP case manager continued to demonstrate her competency in physical assessment and interpretation of lab findings, surgeons and other members of the health-care team began to value her as an expert coordinator and patient advocate. Not only did the ANP case manager establish herself as a trusted insider with patients and families, she established herself as a trusted insider with members of the health-care team.

The ANP case manager's ability to influence patient care outcomes quickly expanded into the ability to influence hospital systems that affected the care of open heart surgery patients. She facilitated the work of an interdisciplinary continuous quality improvement (CQI) team, which resulted in the development of standards and protocols that promoted timely and appropriate patient care management. Critical pathways were developed and quickly recognized as a valuable tool to guide the patient through the health-care system. The ANP case manager was consulted by other departments to assist in establishing process improvements and programs for staff development. Protocols for the appropriate use of postoperative respiratory therapy treatments were established with the Respiratory Care Department. Standing protocols for preoperative administration of cardiac medications and prophylactic antibiotics were developed in the Pharmacy Department. Routine initiation of cardiac rehabilitation was established, and aggressive postoperative mobilization procedures were initiated in collaboration with the intensive care and step-down units. Finally, protocols for identifying preoperative risk and fast-tracking open heart patients off the ventilator postoperatively using shorter acting anesthetics and more appropriate analgesics were developed through collaboration with the surgical and anesthesia departments.

Recognizing the need to ensure adequate home follow-up for CABG patients as an essential part of reducing readmissions, the ANP case manager developed standard protocols for initiating home health care after discharge. In collaboration with the Utilization Management Department, referral processes to the authorized agencies were developed. Some patients did not meet payer-dependent criteria for home health care but still required continued monitoring and reinforcement of education and support; the ANP case manager established a routine for seeing these patients in their homes 2 to 3 days after discharge.

Equipped with a stethoscope, blood pressure cuff, and pulse oximeter during the home visit, the ANP case manager performed a physical examination, paying particular attention to wound status, pulmonary function, and hemodynamic response to activity. The relationship she had established with the patient and family in the hospital became the ANP case manager's most effective tool for supporting the patient in making the challenging lifestyle changes required postoperatively. This included proper administration of medications, diet modification, smoking cessation, and entry into a regular exercise routine. The ANP case manager identified patients who required immediate medical evaluation or adjustment of medications and, in an effort to minimize time constraints and obtain necessary medical support, placed a call to the surgeon's office from the patient's home to inform him of her findings and obtain the necessary orders. Calls to the surgeon's office from the ANP case manager when she was in the field received high priority and were immediately dispatched, so that the surgeon would contact the ANP case manager before she left the patient's home. Upon returning to the hospital, the ANP case manager used the transcription service to document her findings and record any medical orders she received to adjust medications or treatment plans. Copies of this record were forwarded to the patient's surgeon, cardiologist, and primary care physician by the Medical Records Department. Finally, patients who required more than two home visits by the ANP case manager either were reevaluated for their ability to meet home health care criteria or were referred to a community-based nurse case manager for longer follow-up in the community.

The ANP case manager developed an extensive evaluation plan to monitor clinical and fiscal outcomes associated with the program. Through collaboration with the Quality Management Department and cost accounting, data were obtained to evaluate lengths of stay, readmission rates, adverse medical outcomes, and costs. An executive summary provided to the hospital administration team revealed that the NCM program had contributed to a decrease in length of stay from 9 to 6 days, a reduction in readmission rate from 30 to 3%, a 56% reduction in adverse medical outcomes, and an 11% reduction in total cost the first year of the program.*

CREDENTIALING, EDUCATION, AND EXPERIENCE: PREPARING FOR ANP CM

ANP case managers should meet the requirements for ANP licensure in their jurisdictions. If certification in one's practice area or specialty is not yet a requirement for ANP licensure, the ANP case manager should be certified in a specialty (e.g., gerontology, rehabilitation, oncology, and critical care) at the ANP level, if it is available. Certification as a case manager may or may not give the APN interested in being a case manager an edge when seeking a job. This is likely to depend on the particular job as well as the job market and the availability of case managers.

To meet the growing need for nurse case managers, many schools of nursing are now providing graduate curricula with a specialty in NCM. A few recommendations about the educational preparation of APNs for NCM can be made. Fralic (1992) observed that the successful nurse case manager is able to operate in an unstructured environment and has a high tolerance for ambiguity, uncertainty, and change. The nurse case manager is "required to bring innovation, enthusiasm, and confidence to the role" (Fralic, 1992, p. 14). ANP graduate education fosters these qualities through its emphasis on socialization, self-learning, and self-direction, as

---

*This vignette is based largely on the clinical practice of the author, who wishes to acknowledge Carondelet St. Joseph's Hospital's administrative leadership, surgeons, and stafff, who collectively made the clinical NCM program a success.

well as content on change theory. In addition, advanced clinical and leadership skills help students develop these characteristics.

Nugent (1992) identified the broad supportive theoretical background required by the ANP case manager in the development of clinical, collaborative, and management skills. This background must include nursing theory, developmental theory, stress theory, crisis theory, conflict management, role negotiation, consultation theory, motivation, ethics, change theory, quality improvement, teaching/learning, and organizational and cost analysis. In addition to a strong theoretical base, an understanding of managed care, capitated markets, changing reimbursement structures, and integrated delivery networks must be part of ANP case managers' knowledge base, so that they can keep pace with the changing healthcare system.

Master's level coursework should include core courses in conceptual models and nursing theory, the conduct and use of research, role development for advanced nursing practice, as well as advanced nursing theory within a clinical specialty. Content may include skill development related to communication, interdisciplinary collaboration and health-care management, health-care financing, risk analysis, statistics, and family and community assessment (Table 20–3). Just as role socialization and mentoring are critical to the development of the clinical nurse specialist (Hamric & Taylor, 1989), students in ANP CM curricula must experience the NCM role during clinical experiences with practicing APNs. Given ANP CM's similarity to the traditional clinical nurse specialist role, it is reasonable to assume that a developmental process exists in which the ANP case manager experiences the phases of role development as described by Hamric and Taylor (1989) (see also Chapter 5). The authority to change the system inherent in the ANP CM role may modulate some aspects of role development (e.g., frustration).

ISSUES IN ANP CM

DIFFERENTIATING ANP CM FROM OTHER ANP ROLES

The ANP case manager has much in common with the traditional clinical nurse specialist, in that both clinical and system level interventions are a job expectation.

TABLE 20–3. CONTENT FOR GRADUATE EDUCATION FOR ADVANCED NURSING PRACTICE (ANP) CASE MANAGERS

Theoretical*	Clinical and Practical Experiences
*Midrange nursing theories	*Comprehensive health assessments
*Stress	*Specialty-related assessments and interventions
*Crisis	*Family assessment
*Human development	*Community assessment
*Motivation	*Clinical practice with ANP case managers
*Organizational psychology	*Risk analysis
*Change and innovation	*Collection, analysis, and reporting of case management program data
*Conflict negotiation	*Case-based analyses of nurse case management (NCM) coordination and
*Teaching/learning	interventions
*Health-care financing and economics	*Multiple opportunities to collaborate and negotiate with providers and payers

*This content is in addition to what would be needed for preparation for the ANP competencies described in Chapter 3 or would require special emphasis because of the nature of NCM practice.

Most of the literature on ANP CM is based on the experiences of clinical nurse specialists. In the same way that the clinical nurse specialist considers organizational goals and implements and evaluates systemwide projects and programs (Gournic, 1989), the ANP case manager promotes process improvements and a better understanding of how nonroutine, complex patient populations are cared for within existing systems. Like clinical nurse specialists, ANP case managers must be prepared to justify the value of their work to the health-care organization in terms of quality and cost outcomes. ANP case managers differ most from other ANP roles in being responsible for fiscal as well as clinical outcomes. The ANP case manager's accountability for clinical, system, and fiscal outcomes is likely to lead to complex ethical dilemmas in which all of these responsibilities must be weighed. Because NCM is a service to both patients and the organization, conflicts can arise when choices for individuals must be weighed against system level goals. Nurse case managers must be mindful of balancing the mission and values of their sponsoring organization with the obligations inherent in the professional nurse-client relationship. Client advocacy is just as important in this ANP role. However, the ANP case manager is likely to have to be more creative or more explicit regarding why some system or fiscal outcome is being compromised or sacrificed in the interests of patient care. The ANP case manager must be articulate about exceptions and the short- and long-term benefits of pursuing a course of action that does not balance (or appear to balance) all three responsibilities.

Finally, a broader span of accountability is an important dimension that differentiates ANP CM from basic NCM. APNs who are authorized to diagnose, treat, and prescribe are likely to assume CM responsibilities. The ability to measure the effectiveness of the role so that it is "value added" to the organization is a key component of the ANP case manager's accountability (Fralic, 1992).

DIFFERENTIATING ANP CM FROM NCM

Although descriptions of NCM are most consistent with ANP competencies and the APN is viewed by many as the ideal nurse case manager (Connors, 1993; Cronin & Maklebust 1989; Hamric, 1992; Zander, 1990), this approach is not yet feasible; the supply of APNs is insufficient to meet the health-care system's needs for effective care coordination and case management (Connors, 1993; Zander, 1990). Given the rapidity with which NCM is taking hold as a system for delivering care, what kinds of analysis might ensure that patients who need ANP CM get it? Research (Ethridge & Lamb, 1989; Lamb & Stempel, 1994) and anecdotal reports (Connors, 1993) suggest that there are some patients whose care can be managed and coordinated by nurses who are not APNs. However, research also indicates that nurse case managers require a minimum of a baccalaureate education to be successful at predicting and documenting measurable outcomes (Ethridge & Lamb, 1989). The volume of literature on APNs in CM also indicates that there are patients who require ANP CM. Two discussions in the literature offer some approaches that may help to differentiate basic NCM from ANP CM.

Calkin (1984) differentiated advanced nursing practice from basic nursing practice on three dimensions: education, experience, and patient complexity. She used a bell curve as a way of understanding the different problem-solving skills of novices; experts by experience; and APNs, specifically clinical nurse specialists. She postulated that nurses deal with a range of human responses that exist in a normal distribution. Calkin described the knowledge and skills of the novice nurse as best suited to managing a narrow range of typical and predictable human responses to health and illness. Experts by experience demonstrate skills superior to novices when dealing with the same situations that the novice is able to handle (e.g., earlier recognition of problems and faster problem solving). In addition, they are capable of assessing and intervening in a broader range of human responses than the novice. When compared with APNs, experts by experience are more likely to describe their expert interventions in terms of intuition. Calkin characterized the clinical nurse specialist as academically and clinically prepared to intervene effectively for a full range of human responses to actual or potential problems. Thus, in addition to education and experience, basic NCM could be differentiated from ANP CM along the dimensions of patient complexity (physical, emotional, or social) and predictability of clinical course.

In her consideration of some of these issues, Connors (1993) suggested that care management could be conceptualized as a continuum anchored by care coordination on one end and case management on the other. She asserted that every patient needs care coordination but not all patients need case management. "Case management, in its most limited application, is usually reserved for patients or clients with more complex health care needs, that is, high-risk, high-volume, high-costs patients and those with catastrophic illnesses" (Connors, p. 192). In the continuum description, care coordination is linked with health and CM with illness. In our opinion, this is a limitation of the continuum she described. As an example, a mother and baby who are healthy but live in a crime-ridden area may be considered high-risk clients because of limited social supports and a risk of exposure to violence. Nevertheless, the continuum may provide a tool for analyzing and differentiating basic NCM from ANP CM.

On the basis of the contributions of Calkin (1984) and Connors (1993), we suggest that basic and advanced NCM could be differentiated along several dimensions. Research is needed to validate these ideas. First, it seems important to describe and differentiate care coordination from case management. As the preceding discussion suggests, care coordination (or NCM practiced by experts by experience) may best describe the processes used to achieve clinical and fiscal outcomes when clinical situations are simple, common, time limited, predictable, or require few and inexpensive resources. Clinically, patients with novel or uncommon diagnoses and patients whose care is complex, resource intensive, or unpredictable are likely to need an APN. High-volume patients may need ANP CM initially so that the systems, critical pathways, and standards of care that ensure achievement of clinical and fiscal outcomes can be analyzed and developed; as experience with such patients accumulates, their care, while complex, may become more routine and no longer require ANP CM. Organizationally, the type of NCM needed could depend on several variables: the numbers and types of clinicians involved in the network (the more clinicians there are, the less predictable behaviors and interactions will be), the status of guideline use and development (the greater the number of people who need to be brought together to learn to use existing guidelines or developing new guidelines, the more complex the scenario), the degree to which existing practices must be changed to ensure that clinical and fiscal outcomes are reached or the need for concurrent program development as NCM is implemented (the more change needed, the more organizationally and interpersonally complex the scenario). The more complex and uncertain the organizational variables, the more an organization needs APNs practicing within their CM systems. Research that tests these ideas would determine whether NCM is only an ANP role or whether, as an application of Calkin's analysis might suggest, some NCM can be done by experts by experience whereas other NCM must be done by APNs. These deliberations informed the definitions of the ANP case manager and nurse case manager presented at the beginning of this chapter.

At this stage in the evolution of NCM, health-care agencies do employ experts by experience as nurse case managers to oversee care for patients who fit the preceding descriptions of populations needing ANP CM. This is particularly so when staff turnover is high or when primary staff nurses need ongoing education and support to manage these more complex case types. Moving experienced nurses into NCM roles is seen as a way to recognize and retain experienced nurses while promoting a successful, professional practice model (Zander, 1990a). As experience with NCM accumulates, the profession will be in a better position to determine what mix of APNs and experts by experience is needed to provide care coordination and CM services that ensure that clinical, fiscal, and system goals are met.

FUTURE DIRECTIONS

Diverse settings are incorporating the NCM role into their operations in order to address the complex economic and clinical demands placed on them by today's health-care system. Future trends will likely include employment of ANP case managers in primary care settings and physician offices. As medical practices become affiliated with physician-hospital organizations and enter into capitated managed care contracts with payers, patient volume per physician is likely to escalate, making it more feasible to provide health prevention and health maintenance through less expensive nursing resources. The assurance of appropriate patient and family education and the monitoring of physical, emotional, and functional health that nurse case managers provide will enable physician groups to manage more effectively larger caseloads of patients within a provider contract.

Continued initiatives in organizational restructuring and redesign offer ANP case managers numerous opportunities to improve core hospital/organizational processes to the benefit of consumers. As expert clinicians with system savvy, ANP case managers will serve as consultants to health-care providers and payers who wish to redesign and develop innovative health-care delivery systems over the next decades.

A needed national focus on primary care is placing new emphasis on preventive programs such as pediatric immunizations, mammography, eye examinations for diabetics, Pap smears, and prenatal care. As health-care delivery systems strive to create integrated services that emphasize disease prevention and early detection of serious and potentially costly conditions, nurse-midwives, clinical nurse specialists, nurse practitioners, and other APNs will find new opportunities for advanced nursing practice. These APNs are likely to assume ANP case manager roles. They will learn the additional CM-related knowledge and skills they need on the job and through continuing education. This trend is similar to the historical evolution of nurse practitioners. As NCM continues to evolve, more and more graduate programs are likely to offer courses specific to ANP CM.

It is likely that certification in NCM will become a reality; whether it will be specific to APNs remains to be seen. Given the breadth of knowledge and skills needed to do NCM effectively, it is hard to imagine such a certification not being in advanced nursing practice. As research on care coordination and CM by nurses and APNs becomes available, it should inform the decisions of the profession with regard to certification.

ANP case managers who practice in settings with advanced clinical accountability and autonomy may in the future require prescriptive privileges in order to provide the best, most cost-effective service within a managed care environment (L. Curtin, personal communication, 1995). It will be important to evaluate the impact on clinical and cost outcomes of ANP case managers who are authorized to diagnose, treat, and prescribe. One can imagine some time savings alone when one considers the number of calls made to physicians to get appropriate prescriptions or to determine the need for referrals.

Finally, although reimbursement for NCM service has traditionally taken the form of hourly or salaried pay associated with employment by a health-care organization, direct reimbursement for NCM services and inclusion in capitated contractual funds will become more widely available. Changing reimbursement structures will be open doors for independent NCM practice and consultation. Today the majority of nurse case managers in practice agree that their role is not the same as when they initially started and will certainly evolve further as the future unfolds. The shape of the nurse case manager role is dynamic and responsive to changes in the health care environment. The years ahead will be an exciting time for APNs and NCM.

REFERENCES

American Nurses' Association. (1988). *Nursing case management*. Kansas City, MO: Author.

Baird, S. (1995). The impact of changing health care delivery on oncology practice. *Oncology Nursing: Patient Treatment and Support, 2*(3), 1–13.

Brubakken, K., Janssen, W., & Ruppel, D. (1994). CNS roles in implementation of a differentiated case management model. *Clinical Nurse Specialist, 8,* 69–73.

Bryson, K., Naqvi, A., Callahan, P., & Fontenot, D. (1990). Brief admission program: An alliance of inpatient care and outpatient case management. *Journal of Psychosocial Nursing, 28*(12), 19–23.

Calkin, J. (1984). A model for advanced nursing practice. *Journal of Nursing Administration, 14*(1), 24–30.

Case Management Society of America. (1994). CMSA proposes standards of practice. *The Case Manager, 5*(1), 59–70.

Cesta, T. (1993). The link between continuous quality improvement and case management. *Journal of Nursing Administration, 23*(6), 55–61.

Connors, H. (1993). Impact of care management modalities on curricula. In K. Kelly & M. Maas (Eds.), *Managing nursing care: Promise and pitfalls* (pp. 190–207). St. Louis, MO: Mosby.

Cooper, D. M. (1990). Today—Assessment and intuition: Tomorrow—Projections. In D. M. Cooper, P. A. Minarik, & P. S. A. Sparacino (Eds.), *The Clinical Nurse Specialist: Implementation and Impact* (pp. 285–298). Norwalk, CT: Appleton & Lange.

Cronin, C., & Maklebust, J. (1989). Case-managed care: Capitalizing on the CNS. *Nursing Management, 20*(3), 38–47.

Daleiden, A. (1993). The CNS as trauma case manager. *Clinical Nurse Specialist, 7,* 295–298.

Doell Smith, L. (1994). Continuity of care through nursing case management of the chronically ill child. *Clinical Nurse Specialist, 8,* 65–68.

Ethridge, P. (1991). A nursing HMO: Carondelet St. Mary's experience. *Nursing Management, 22*(7), 22–27.

Ethridge, P., & Lamb, G. (1989). Professional nursing case management improves quality, access and costs. *Nursing Management, 20*(3), 30–35.

Flynn, A., & Kilgallen, M. (1993). Case management: A multidisciplinary approach to the evaluation of cost and quality standards. *Journal of Nursing Care Quality, 8,*(3), 58–66.

Fralic, M. (1992). The nurse case manager: Focus, selection, preparation, and measurement. *Journal of Nursing Administration, 22*(11), 13–14, 46.

Gaedeke-Norris, M., & Hill, C. (1991). The clinical nurse specialist: Developing the case manager role. *Dimensions of Critical Care, 10,* 346–352.

Gibson, S., Martin, S., Johnson, M., Blue, R., & Miller, D. (1994). CNS-directed case management: Cost and quality harmony. *Journal of Nursing Administration, 12*(6), 45–51.

Gournic, J. (1989). Clinical leadership, management, and the CNS. In A. B. Hamric & J. Spross (Eds.), *The clinical nurse specialist in theory and practice* (2nd ed., pp. 227–250). Philadelphia, PA: W. B. Saunders Company.

Hamric, A.B. (1989). History and overview of the CNS role. In A.B. Hamric & J.A. Spross (Eds.), *The clinical nurse specialist in theory and practice* (2nd ed., pp. 3–18). Philadelphia, PA: W. B. Saunders Company.

Hamric, A.B., & Taylor, J.W. (1989). Role development of the CNS. In A.B. Hamric & J.A. Spross (Eds.), *The clinical nurse specialist in theory and practice* (2nd ed., pp. 41–82). Philadelphia, PA: W. B. Saunders Company.

Hamric, A. (1992). Creating our future: Challenges and opportunities for the clinical nurse specialist. *Oncology Nursing Forum, 19*(1, Suppl.), 11–15.

Jenkins, M., & Sullivan-Marx, E. (1994). Nurse practitioners and community health nurses: Clinical partnerships and future visions. *Nursing Clinics of North America, 29,* 459–471.

Ladden, M. (1991). On-site perinatal case management: An HMO model. *Journal of Perinatal-Neonatal Nursing, 5*(1), 27–32.

Lamb, G., & Stempel, J. (1994). Nurse case management from the client's view: Growing as insider-expert. *Nursing Outlook, 42,* 7–13.

Leahy, M. (1994). *Validation of essential knowledge dimensions in case management* (Technical Report, Case Management Research Project. Rolling Meadows, IL: Foundation for Rehabilitation Certification, Education, and Research.

Ling, K. (1993). Initiation and evaluation of managed care at Johns Hopkins Hospital. *Nursing Administration Quarterly, 17*(3), 54–58.

Lynn-McHale, D., Fitzpatrick, E., & Shaller, R. (1993). Case management: Development of a model. *Clinical Nurse Specialist, 7,* 299–307.

Lyon, J. (1993). Models of nursing care delivery and case management. *Nursing Economics, 11,* 163–169.

Madden, M., & Reid Ponte, P. (1994). Advanced practice roles in the managed care environment. *Journal of Nursing Administration, 24,* 56–62.

Mahn, V. (1993). Clinical nurse case management: A service line approach. *Nursing Management, 24*(9), 48–50.

Newman, M. (1990). Toward an integrative model of professional practice. *Journal of Professional Nursing, 6,* 167–173.

Newman, M. (1994). *Health as expanding consciousness* (2nd ed.). New York: National League for Nursing Press.

Newman, M., Lamb, G., & Michaels, C. (1989). Nurse case management: The coming together of theory and practice. *Nursing & Health Care, 12,* 404–408.

Nugent, K. (1992). The clinical nurse specialist as case manager in a collaborative practice model: Bridging the gap between quality and cost of care. *Clinical Nurse Specialist, 6,* 106–111.

Parker, M., Quinn, J., Viehl, M., McKinley, A., Polich, C., Detzner, D., Hartwell, S., & Korn, K. (1990). Case management in rural areas: Defini-

tion, clients, financing, staffing, and service delivery issues. *Nursing Economics, 8*(2), 103–109.

Pierog, L. (1991). Case management: A product line. *Nursing Administration Quarterly, 15*(2), 16–20.

Riley, T. (1992). HIV-infected client care: Case management and the HIV team. *Clinical Nurse Specialist, 6,* 136–140.

Rotz, N., Yates, J., & Schare, B. (1994). Application of the case management model to a trauma patient. *Clinical Nurse Specialist, 8,* 180–186.

Rudisill, P., Phillips, M., & Payne, C. (1993). Clinical paths for cardiac surgery patients: A multidisciplinary approach to quality improvement outcomes. *Journal of Nursing Care Quality, 8*(3), 27–33.

Schroer, K. (1991). Case management: Clinical nurse specialist and nurse practitioner, converging roles. *Clinical Nurse Specialist, 5,* 189–194.

Sherman, J., & Johnson, P. (1994). CNS as unit-based case manager. *Clinical Nurse Specialist, 8,* 76–80.

Smith, M. (1993). Case management and nursing theory-based practice. *Nursing Science Quarterly, 6*(1), 8–9.

Strong, A. (1991). Case management of a patient with multisystem failure. *Critical Care Quarterly, 11*(6), 10–18.

Strong, A. (1992). Case management and the CNS. *Clinical Nurse Specialist, 6,* 64.

Tidwell, S. (1994). The critical care clinical nurse specialist as case manager. In A. Gawlinski & L. Kern (Eds.), *The clinical nurse specialist in critical care* (pp. 62–79). Philadelphia, PA: W. B. Saunders Company.

Trinidad, E. (1993). Case management: A model of case management. *Clinical Nurse Specialist, 7,* 221–223.

Office of Technology Assessment. U.S. Congress. (1986). *Nurse practitioners, physician assistants, and certified nurse midwives: A policy analysis* (Health Care Technology Study No. OTA-HCS-37). Washington, DC: U.S. Government Printing Office.

Wagner, J., & Menke, E. (1992). Case management of homeless families. *Clinical Nurse Specialist, 6,* 65–71.

Zander, K. (1988). Nursing case management: Strategic management of cost and quality outcomes. *Journal of Nursing Administration, 18*(5), 23–30.

Zander, K. (1990). Case management: A golden opportunity for whom? In J. McCloskey & H. Grace (Eds.), *Current issues in nursing* (pp. 199–204). St. Louis, MO: Mosby.

Zander, K. (1993). The impact of managing care on the role of a nurse. In K. Kelly & M. Maas (Eds.), *Managing nursing care: Promise and pitfalls* (pp. 65–82). St. Louis, MO: Mosby.

Zander, K. (1995). A look to the future. In K. Zander (Ed.), *Managing outcomes through collaborative care* (pp. 195–207). Chicago, IL: American Hospital Association.

PART IV

ISSUES IN THE CONTINUING EVOLUTION OF ADVANCED NURSING PRACTICE

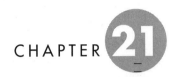

CHAPTER 21

Faculty Practice: Uniting Advanced Nursing Practice and Education

Diana L. Taylor

From the time that nursing education moved into the university setting, there has been a concern that education must be clearly linked with practice. Faculty practice, as a component of advanced nursing practice (ANP), is the link between education and practice. The challenge for advanced practice nurse (APN) faculty is to link scholarship with expert clinical practice. In the rapidly changing health-care environment, links between practice and education may provide ANP with the best approach to solutions for both practice and education. Faculty practice may reverse the trend of moving the most knowledgeable APNs away from the patient or the practice setting while providing opportunities for testing nursing theory, developing innovative practices, and exploring research questions.

This chapter summarizes the historical development of faculty practice, provides a definition of faculty practice based on existing research and practice, describes the current state of faculty practice by APN faculties, describes existing faculty practice models, and proposes future directions and strategies for partnerships between advanced nursing practice and education. Although this chapter is limited to the discussion of "practice" by APN faculty, the domain of faculty practice is clearly more than clinical practice by nurse educators. This chapter focuses on the multiple components of faculty practice by APNs—educational, research, administrative, and clinical practice—and the models developed by APN educators to link scholarship and practice in the preparation of future APNs.

HISTORICAL PERSPECTIVE ON FACULTY PRACTICE

Faculty practice was a non-issue in the early days of nursing education because the educator was the practitioner. During the era of diploma schools, nursing training was conducted in the hospital. Although theory classes may have been taught by nurses with specialized knowledge, most clinical expertise was gained from nurses who cared for patients. The head nurse usually functioned as the main source of clinical teaching.

Since the 1940s, nurse training has become nursing education. The teaching center has shifted from the hospital to educational institutions (Christy, 1980; Mauksch, 1980a). With the growth of baccalaureate programs, nursing faculty became increasingly focused on education for themselves and their students. Practice, though important, played a secondary role. In the world of academia, advanced degrees and research, not clinical proficiency, were of primary importance. Although educators were concerned about the declining influence of practice on nursing education and vice versa, the distance between education and service widened.

The expansion of clinical nurse specialist (CNS) roles in the 1960s and the advent of nurse practitioner (NP) roles in the 1970s may have stimulated nursing educators to re-examine more seriously the significance of practice. Much of the early clinical education for nurse anesthetists (CRNAs), nurse-midwives (CNMs), and NPs was supervised by physicians. As ANP education moved to the graduate level, there was a need for nurse educators to become expert practitioners. Advanced practice certification required a practice component, which also established practice as a legitimate faculty role. However, this clinical role developed slowly within graduate education (Table 21–1).

TABLE 21–1. HISTORY OF FACULTY PRACTICE DEVELOPMENT

Year	Historical Event
1956	First nursing education/service unification model at University of Florida
1961	Academic-Service Collaboration model at Case Western Reserve University
1970	Unification model expansion at Rush University and University of Rochester
1979	American Academy of Nursing (AAN) Resolution in support of faculty practice
1985	AAN/Robert Wood Johnson Foundation supported faculty practice symposium
1993	National Organization of Nurse Practitioner Faculties publication: *Faculty Practice-Models and Methods*
1993–1995	American Association of Colleges of Nursing symposium on advancing faculty practice

The first attempt to unite nursing service and nursing education, which provided the basis for the early faculty practice models, occurred in 1956. Dorothy Smith, Dean of the School of Nursing at the University of Florida and the Director of Nursing Service at the University Hospital, envisioned an education-service structure that would provide a demonstration of the intellectual nature of clinical nursing, support nursing education within nursing service, develop nursing systems that crossed education and service, and guarantee faculty practice (Fagin, 1986). With Dorothy Smith as the administrator of both nursing education and nursing service, the faculty taught students and provided patient care within their faculty role.

In 1961, Rozella Schlotfeldt, using a different model at Case Western Reserve University, developed an "academic-service collaboration" system for uniting education and service. This collaborative model formalized collaboration between faculty and clinicians through joint appointments. Instead of one person simultaneously holding positions at both the school and the clinical agency, a faculty member's prime responsibilities were with the school along with an appointment within the clinical area. Although the administrations of the school and the clinical area were separate, some of the salary costs were shared. Case Western Reserve University's standard of academic leadership and practice collaboration have influenced many current methods for faculty clinician appointments (Fagin, 1985).

In the early 1970s, Luther Christman, Dean of the College of Nursing at Rush-Presbyterian University, and Loretta Ford, Dean of the School of Nursing at the University of Rochester, developed an organizational structure, generally known as the "unification" model, that unified administration of the clinical agency and the school of nursing (Christman, 1982). The unification model of faculty practice was an organizational innovation whose primary purpose was to improve the relationship between nursing service and nursing education. In the unification model, all levels of faculty served jointly as clinicians and educators, and the Dean of the School of Nursing assumed authority and accountability in nursing education, nursing practice, and nursing research, demonstrating that clinical expertise by nursing faculty members can unite nursing service and nursing education (Grace, 1981).

These two examples of nursing education-service unification were important for providing legitimacy to faculty practice, demonstrating nursing autonomy as well as interdisciplinary collaboration, and attaining national and political support for nursing services (DeLeon, 1994; Fagin, 1986). Data show that although these models have not been widely replicated because of an overemphasis on merger and unification and too little focus on the practice partnerships, they have reduced the existing education-practice gap (Andreoli, 1993; Gresham-Kenton, 1989). More importantly, these early models provided the impetus for the development of a wide variety of faculty practice endeavors. Throughout the 1970s, nursing faculties attempted to institutionalize practice within the academic system using a variety of organizational structures (Barnard, 1983; Barnard & Smith, 1985).

In 1979, the American Academy of Nursing supported faculty practice through the passage of a resolution (American Academy of Nursing, 1980). With support from the Robert Wood Johnson Foundation, the Academy sponsored four symposia that have continued to provide the knowledge base for the development and implementation of faculty practice. In these symposia on faculty practice, nursing leaders provided important perspectives on the role of faculty practice in nursing education. Mauksch (1980a) proposed that nursing practice is an essential component of the role of the nurse educator if one is to keep the respect of other health professionals, improve communication with students, and increase realism in the classroom. According to Mauksch, nursing service also accrues benefits from faculty practice. Students are prepared to enter institutional practice, nursing staff profit from increased exposure to new knowledge and new ideas for patient care, educators have increased knowledge of the nursing care delivery system, and the potential exists for greater mutual respect between clinicians and educators. All of these factors contribute to the advancement of the nursing profession.

During the 1980s, nursing faculty experimented with multiple strategies for integrating practice and education roles. Collaborative arrangements developed between individual faculty and practitioners independent of structural or organizational changes (Fagin, 1986; Mauksch, 1980b). An "integrated model" in which faculty and graduate students shared patient care responsibilities was developed at Pennsylvania State University and the University of Wisconsin-Milwaukee (Stainton, 1989). At multiple locations nationwide, CNS faculty were influential in the development of "collaborative models" in which CNSs provided the links between hospital-based nursing service and nursing education. The focus was on collaboration at the level of the APN (communication, consultation) and at the level of the organization (organizational consent and policy) (Styles, 1984). Another example, a "partnership model" of faculty practice, was implemented at the University of Pennsylvania, incorporating clinical and educational excellence, research and scholarship, and professional empowerment as broadly defined faculty practice goals (Fagin, 1986). Structural changes within the School of Nursing allowed clinicians to advance within the academic system. The addition of a formalized academic appointment track for the clinical professor allowed for promotion and advancement for the clinically expert nurse educator. Common to these integrated or partnership models is the focus on redesigning faculty roles rather than redesigning the organization in order to link advanced nursing practice and education.

By the early 1990s, faculty practice became a widely written about and debated issue. In spite of a lack of consensus about its definition, purposes, or implementation, faculty practice remains the prevailing method for uniting practice and education. ANP faculty are searching for ways to integrate practice into their teaching and research roles because of ethical, professional, regulatory, and academic requirements. New partnerships and links with community agencies, church groups, school-based clinics, and health-care delivery systems have been formed for APN faculty research and practice. The latest model of linking practice and education was described as an "entrepreneurial model" (Potash & Taylor, 1993) in which faculty design their practice, determine their goals and objectives, and provide client services as part of their faculty duties. In the entrepreneurial model, faculty may utilize the practice as a teaching site, a research site, or both; frequently they are paid for their services for direct patient care, consultancy, or technical assistance. These arrangements permit many variations in services, client population, setting, business arrangements, and outcomes. A few schools of nursing have emerged as leaders in promoting this entrepreneurial model of faculty practice and are described later in this chapter (University of Tennessee-Memphis, Oregon Health Sciences University, University of California-San Francisco, University of Rochester, University of Texas-Houston, University of Utah, Vanderbilt University, to name just a few). An entrepreneurial approach to faculty practice shifts the focus from an education-service orientation to a business model in which resources are assessed, resources are matched to goals, and outcomes are evaluated (Walker, 1993). Business principles combined with educational goals can be directed toward advancing nursing education, nursing practice, and nursing research, especially those involved with health-related interventions, costs, and patient outcomes. Currently, the American Association of Colleges of Nursing continues to support the development of entrepreneurial faculty practice activities through annual symposia for faculty development.

By the year 2000, almost 50 years after Dean Dorothy Smith pioneered the first model to link nursing practice with nursing education, integration may occur through flexible partnerships that are based on population needs and health professional education planning. During the next decade, nursing education will continue to develop or expand faculty practice as an important component of both education and research missions. ANP faculty will continue to provide the leadership.

CURRENT STATUS AND DEFINITIONS OF FACULTY PRACTICE

In an applied discipline, faculty practice consists of doing what the teacher-practitioner teaches others to do. In the context of nursing, practice connotes the focus and intent to study, improve, and master both the substance and the process of delivering nursing care (McClure, 1987). Historically, definitions of faculty practice have been numerous and diverse. Durand claimed that "faculty practice means the practice of nursing as performed by faculty in the context of being faculty" (Durand, 1985, p. 38). Joel defined faculty practice as "direct or indirect involvement in provision of service [by nursing faculty] to the consumer" (Joel, 1983, p. 49). She believed that faculty practice must be scholarly and result in publication. Although provision of care to clients is often the central focus of faculty practice, moonlighting is not considered faculty practice by most schools of nursing (Nugent, Barger, & Bridges, 1993). In contrast, Anderson and Pierson maintained that faculty practice should be an addition to the expected teaching role accomplished through joint appointment, moonlighting, or summer employment (Anderson & Pierson, 1983, p. 9). A recent survey of selected members of the National Organization of Nurse Practitioner Faculties (Potash & Taylor, 1993) concluded that the definition of faculty practice should include multiple roles (consultant, researcher, administrator, and clinician), in multiple settings (clinics, hospitals, home care), and using multiple structural and economic models (entrepreneurial, volunteer, joint practice).

Faculty practice by APNs is scholarly based professional activity: the provision or facilitation of the delivery of nursing care through advanced behaviors of research, mentoring, leadership, collaboration, and direct patient care that encompasses patient outcomes as well as scholarship and student learning. On one level, faculty practice has the good of the faculty and its students as its prime concern, offering an area in which faculty members can maintain their clinical expertise and identity as nurses. On another level, faculty practice functions primarily for the good of the profession and of the recipients of nursing care; furthermore, activities resulting in research and publication both enhance the profession and ultimately improve patient care.

A review of faculty practice definitions from five schools of nursing* (at which most faculty practitioners function as APNs) might yield a composite definition of faculty practice that includes the following language:

> *Faculty practice includes all aspects of the delivery of health care through the roles of clinician, educator, researcher, consultant, and administrator. Faculty practice activities within this framework encompass direct nursing services to individuals and groups, as well as technical assistance and consultation to individuals, families, groups, and communities. In addition to the provision of service, practice provides opportunities for promotion, tenure, merit, and revenue generation. A distinguishing characteristic of faculty practice within the School of Nursing is the belief that teaching, research, practice, and service must be closely integrated to achieve excellence. Faculty practice provides the vehicle through which faculty implement these missions. There is an assumption that student practica and residencies as well as research opportunities for faculty and students are an established component of faculty practice.*

Clinical faculty practice by the APN is the direct (or indirect) nursing of individuals, groups, and families. Direct clinical practice includes services directed toward individuals, families, and groups whether in primary, secondary, or tertiary settings. Indirect clinical practice includes the provision of consultation services or technical assistance (e.g., a geriatric consultation service for elderly clients and their families, consultation for a pediatric pain management clinic, or a diabetes consultation service). The general faculty practice definition extends beyond APN practices. It encompasses other specialized roles as well, e.g., educator, administrator, or researcher. The practice role of the educator (other than student teaching) may be in curriculum consultation, program development and evaluation, or provision of continuing education activities (e.g., summer institutes, professional training). Administrative faculty practice may include the formation of a consultation practice in which faculty provide technical assistance to health-care organizations. The practice role of the nurse researcher, aside from direct scientific investigation, might include consultation to health-care organizations for the supervision of

---

*Faculty practice definitions from the following nursing schools were used in this definition: Oregon Health Sciences University, the University of California, San Francisco, the University of Colorado Health Sciences Center, the University of Oklahoma, and the University of Texas, Houston.

clinical nursing research projects. It is important to understand that these roles are not advanced nursing practice as defined in Chapter 3.

RESEARCH ON FACULTY PRACTICE

Regardless of how narrow or broad the definition of faculty practice, many schools of nursing have begun to institutionalize practice in education. Most studies of faculty practice have used clinical practice as the definition of practice in surveys of ANP educators. One survey, whose definition of faculty practice excluded care provided indirectly through students during clinical supervision, revealed that 40% of the 302 respondents (master's or doctoral-prepared faculty) were engaged in clinical practice (Steele, 1991). Choudry (1992) surveyed university-level nursing faculty and found that although 77% were teaching in a clinical area, only 59% were engaged in some form of clinical practice. A 1992 survey of NP faculty members attending a national meeting found that 90% (36) were engaged in practice activities (Potash & Taylor, 1993). The respondents' practices were described as providing direct care to diverse groups of clients in clinics or community settings in which the services were supported by direct and full reimbursement. These faculty held master's or doctoral degrees and incorporated teaching into their practices (35%) or both teaching and research into their practices (41%).

Just, Adams, and DeYoung (1989) surveyed 909 educators about how and why faculty were implementing practice. Of these university faculty, 94% reported "skill maintenance" as the primary reason for faculty practice; they also reported personal satisfaction, improved credibility, and financial reasons for developing practice as part of their educator role. Generally, studies of faculty practice by university nursing faculty suggest that practice is an important component of their educator role. Specific faculty practice competencies identified as important by university-level faculty include demonstration of an expertise in a specialized area of clinical nursing, use of research findings in the practice of nursing to improve client health, and provision of theory-based nursing practice.

In general, faculty practice has been found to enhance teaching, improve the quality of patient care, improve the credibility of nursing education, maintain clinical skills, and generate research opportunities. A study of 55 schools of nursing with active faculty practice programs described four major benefits. For the schools' surveyed, faculty practice benefits included (1) enhanced learning experiences for students, (2) initiation of clinical research projects, (3) higher faculty satisfaction, and (4) the ending of clinical learning site shortages (Maurin, 1986). Although most descriptive surveys report benefits from faculty practice activities, little objective evidence exists about patient, professional, or organizational outcomes related to faculty practice. When data from large samples demonstrate that measurable outcomes, such as improved curricula development, enhanced patient outcomes, or increased clinical research, are strongly correlated with practice, much of the current ambiguity surrounding benefits will be resolved.

Various authors discuss benefits assumed to be associated with faculty practice (Herr, 1989; Just et al., 1989; Kramer, Pollifroni, & Organek, 1986; Millonig, 1986). Benefits to the educator-practitioner are personal, such as keeping clinical skills current, serving as a role model for students, personal satisfaction, and supplemental income. Academic advantages of faculty practice include access to practice-relevant research, preparing relevant curricula and courses, and the generation of ideas for research and publication. At the level of the student, faculty practice provides students with competent clinical teaching and competent faculty. Nursing students who had been taught by faculty involved in practice scored higher on integration of theory into practice, realistic perception of the work environment, and use of nursing research (Kramer et al., 1986). At the level of the organization, faculty practice appears to improve the relationship between nursing service and nursing education.

Extending these benefits to the nursing profession, faculty practice contributes to the advancement of the profession by ensuring that highly prepared graduates enter the work force, by improving nursing practice through research, and by increasing mutual respect between educators and clinicians that contributes to the advancement of the profession. As the health-care system changes, nursing faculty practice provides models for nursing's role in managed care.

ADVANCED PRACTICE NURSING FACULTY PRACTICE MODELS

Since the inception of the "unification" model of faculty practice in which nursing educators linked with hospital-based nurses, new models of linking nursing practice and nursing education have been developed. Most of these faculty practice models have been developed by APN faculty and are vital to the education of APNs. Faculty practice models can be described by *structural types* (nursing centers, joint appointments, faculty development), by *faculty roles* (teacher, practitioner, administrator, consultant roles), by *specialty practice* (community health, elder care, primary care, school health, midwifery services, anesthesia services, symptom management), or by *administrative aspects* of faculty practice (volunteer model, collaborative arrangements, revenue generating, contractual model) (Table 21–2). Certainly, some of these typologies will overlap in any one faculty practice. For example, midwifery faculty may implement a birth center using a revenue-generating reimbursement system in their role of practitioner-educator. CNS faculty collaborate or contract with an oncology service to provide cancer treatment symptom management. Or, community health faculty and NP faculty collaborate to provide health services to a homeless shelter on a contractual or volunteer basis.

This section describes a variety of different types of faculty practices. All of these faculty practices are implemented by APNs (CNMs, CNSs, CRNAs, and NPs). Although the following examples represent multiple roles, types of practice arrangements, and practice specialties, there are similarities among all of them that demonstrate the importance of faculty practice in the development and education of APNs.

Discussion is limited to direct and indirect clinical practice by APN faculty, although faculty practice roles of educator, researcher, and administrator are also outlined in Table 21–2 (faculty development and technical assistance). Examples of a faculty development model have been described by Wandel (1991) and Turner and Pearson (1989). Faculty practice by researchers and administrators has been commonly implemented as technical assistance to health-care organizations (Campbell & King, 1992; Donnelly, Warfel, & Wolf, 1994; Potash & Taylor, 1993).

UNIFICATION MODEL OF FACULTY PRACTICE: IMPLEMENTING THE PRACTITIONER-TEACHER ROLE

Luther Christman's unification model of faculty practice has been modified (Andreoli, 1993) at Rush-Presbyterian University (Chicago), where one of the first

TABLE 21–2. FACULTY PRACTICE MODELS FOR ADVANCED NURSING PRACTICE

Structure Types	Faculty Roles	Specialty Practice	Administrative Type
Faculty development	APN, researcher, administrator	All specialties, all APN roles	Volunteer, contract, joint appointments
Unification model	Teacher-practitioner, administrator, researcher	Traditionally hospital-based specialties, includes ambulatory specialties; CNS, CNM, CRNA, some NP roles	Nursing dean/director develop institutional partnerships
Clinical consultancy	Clinician, educator	All specialties—usually hospital or institution-based; CNS, CRNA	Joint appointments, contracts
Clinical/summer camp health services	Clinician, educator, administrator, researcher	Child/adolescent health, rehabilitation, chronic disease; CNS, NP	Contracts, research grant support
Hospital-based services	Clinician, administrator, researcher	Midwifery, oncology, ambulatory care, anesthesia, child/adult chronic disease management; CNS, CNM, CRNA, some NPs	Contracts, joint appointments, other collaborative arrangements
Technical assistance and consultation	Administrator, researcher	Hospital, long-term care, community institutions; outcome research, research utilization; CNS, nurse administrators	Contracts, joint appointments, joint ventures, volunteer
Case-management services	Clinician	Home-health, community health, oncology, symptom management, perinatal, neonatal; CNS, some NPs	Contracts, nursing centers, joint ventures, joint appointments
Community-based services	Clinician, administrator, researcher	Community health, primary care, underserved populations, homeless health clinics; CNS, SNM, NP	Grant supported, contracts, volunteer
Nursing centers	Clinician, administrator, researcher	Wellness, geriatric, rural, student health, midwifery, community health; CNM, CNS, CRNA, NP	Contracts, school-owned, joint ventures, grant supported

models of merging service and education was implemented. Faculty are involved in patient care activities, staff development, consultation, patient education, hospital committees, clinical management, and clinical research. In this modified unification model, teacher-practitioners provide indirect patient care for 40 weeks of each year while supervising undergraduate students and direct care during school breaks, on holidays, and during nursing shortage periods. Faculty are active in patient-related clinical conferences and participate in team decision making about patient care. In their consultant role, the teacher-practitioner consults with staff nurses and physicians in their area of expertise (e.g., skin problems, incontinence, pain, ethical decision making, acquired immunodeficiency syndrome [AIDS] complications, breast-feeding mothers, pain management in cancer patients, enterostomy therapy, cardiac rehabilitation, bereavement counseling). Other consultation activities include the development of patient teaching aids; development of a new patient-centered model of care with associated technology and reorganization; and creating clinical pathways for decreasing length of stay, decreasing costs, and improving quality of care. The practitioner-teacher is also involved with management activities, such as working with unit leadership in staff meetings, chart audits, new staff orientation, and staff performance appraisals. Committee membership for the practitioner-teacher might also include review of accreditation criteria, standards of practice, nursing care evaluation, new products, and discharge planning procedures.

The multiple roles of the teacher-practitioner in the unification model suggests a high workload, no matter how integrated these roles. In addition, the non-clinical activities of the teacher-practitioner emphasize institutional service unrelated to education (staff development, medical center committees). It is unclear how educational issues, such as curriculum development, are managed by the teacher-practitioner in this unification model. However, this faculty practice model can inform education about ways to reduce unnecessary workload on the education side of the teacher-practitioner responsibility. Although an early model of faculty practice, the unification model may provide a model for faculty practice implementation in an integrated managed care environment of the future.

CLINICAL CONSULTANCY AS FACULTY PRACTICE

This model of faculty practice is most often implemented by CNS faculty through contractual arrangements or joint appointments to nursing staff or health-care agencies. CRNAs often assume the role of consultant to nursing staff for pain management support. Polifroni and Schmalenberg (1985) described activities of faculty clinical consultants as *direct patient care* (assumes responsibility for specific aspects of patient care), *role modeling* (paired with staff nurses to assess difficulties or demonstrate new or different ways of proceeding with care), *staff development* (patient assessment, problem-oriented records, peer review, teaching and learning projects), *administrative projects* (new forms, standards of care, flow sheets in critical care units), *information resource* (source of current information for staff), and *nurse manager support* (managerial and clinical matters). The faculty member functions as a resource person on the average of 1 day per week in giving nursing care and consulting with nursing staff or working collaboratively with nursing administration.

CLINICAL CAMPS OR SUMMER CAMP HEALTH SERVICES

Both NP-prepared and CNS-prepared faculty have developed faculty practices at clinical and summer camps for healthy children and adolescents, adolescents with chronic diseases, and adults with developmental disabilities and mental illness (Aroian & Rauckhorst, 1985; Arthur & Usher, 1994). The primary purpose of these faculty practices is the maintenance of clinical skills.

These faculty practices are often developed using contractual arrangements for summer funding for faculty on 9-month appointments. In addition to salary augmentation, these summer faculty practices provide autonomy, time flexibility, and the ability to develop nurse-initiated interventions. Some faculty have also included student participation and the development of research projects.

HOSPITAL-BASED FACULTY PRACTICE

Faculty at the University of Virginia School of Nursing developed an in-patient oncology and geriatric rehabilitation unit where they provided direct patient care as part of their faculty role (Lee, Levy, Dix, & Tatum, 1987). Noted benefits of this faculty practice to advanced nursing practice were described in a number of ways. First, this faculty practice served as an experimental model in an in-patient hospital. Second, it provided clinical experience for APN students in a nurse-directed environment. Third, the faculty practice provided an opportunity for collaborative clinical research between faculty and staff nurses. Administratively, this project was a joint venture between the school of nursing and nursing service. Faculty practitioners were in non-tenure track, 12-month positions that were funded jointly by the two institutions.

Gresham-Kenton (1989) described collaborative models of CNS practice that implemented a variety of collaborative methods between hospital-based nursing service and nursing education. These models illustrate a corporate approach in which initial decision-making occurs at the level of nursing dean, director, or vice-president. Successful implementation depends on the CNS in a practitioner-teacher role. Some of these arrangements have included an exchange of resources or shared funding. Examples of successful collaborative models include an in-patient and home-care pediatric service in Colorado and a Teaching Nursing Home Project in New Jersey.

Many nurse anesthesia faculty practices are integrated into hospital-based anesthesiology departments in which CRNA faculty contract to provide a portion of the anesthesia services along with supervision of students. Some CRNA faculty have joined together as small faculty practice groups and contract as a group; other CRNA faculty act as independent contractors in a part-time faculty-practitioner role. At the University of Tennessee-Memphis School of Nursing, CRNA faculty have full-time faculty appointments in the School of Nursing but the hospital reimburses the School for the CRNA faculty clinical services (R. Lester, personal communication, 1995). Because most CRNA training programs are situated in schools of medicine or schools of allied health, CRNA faculty practice development has been limited. However, a few CRNA faculty have included practice as a part of their faculty appointment. For example, at the University of Alabama-Birmingham, CRNA faculty practice in hospital sites for at least 1 day each week, and the hospital reimburses the CRNA program, which supplements the CRNA faculty salary (J. Williams, personal communication, May, 1995). Most CRNA faculty have part-time academic appointments and part-time clinical appointments, which allow CRNAs to supplement their academic salaries and combine their teaching role with their practice role.

Nurse-midwifery faculty have developed multiple arrangements within hospital settings. Some CNM faculty have developed independent birth centers or birth centers associated with medical centers (see the later section, "Nursing Centers"). Other examples of CNM faculty practices include contractual arrangements between the school of nursing and a hospital for specific nurse-midwifery services (intrapartum services, resident/medical student teaching, pregnancy/post-partum care services). Joint appointments of CNM faculty shared between schools of medicine and nursing provide another alternative to the contractual arrangements, but the nurse faculty may have dual institutional requirements (see the discussion of the Yale University model under "Business Arrangements for Faculty Practice Models"). Still another arrangement used by CNM faculty involves the CNM being employed by (or contracting with) an OB-GYN faculty practice within a school of medicine but providing education primarily to medical students and residents and secondarily to nurses (Davis & Zatuchni, 1993).

CASE MANAGEMENT AS FACULTY PRACTICE

The Loyola University Niehoff School of Nursing, in association with a University-affiliated home health agency, provides joint appointments to agency administrators and CNSs in the School of Nursing. APN students are assigned to the home health agency for learning experiences (Murray, Hackbarth, Sojka, & Swanston, 1987). In this joint venture, two faculty share a half-time CNS position at the home health agency, where 75% of their practice time is delegated for patient case management and 25% is delegated for administration, research, and fundraising.

Starck, Walker, and Bohannan (1991) described an oncology case management example of faculty practice at The University of Texas Health Science Center-Houston School of Nursing. Doctorally prepared faculty with specialization in clinical oncology nursing provide case management for a group of hospitalized cancer patients in a large teaching/research oncology center. Graduate nursing students work in collaboration with a faculty member who provides case management services, including symptom management during cancer treatments. Networking by the faculty member helps facilitate opportunities for student and staff nursing research. The School of Nursing provides all administrative and contracting services for the individual faculty member, in this case a contract with oncology medical faculty for 50% of the nurse faculty's salary.

There are few examples of case-management as faculty practices in the current literature; this area of advanced nursing practice is one of future development for nursing educators as well as an area that needs the attention of nursing centers operated by schools of nursing.

COMMUNITY-BASED FACULTY PRACTICES: HOMELESS SHELTER CLINICS

Kean College of New Jersey Department of Nursing developed a partnership with a homeless shelter in which faculty and students provide direct health and nursing services to homeless families (Campbell, 1993). The partnership allowed establishment of a site for interdisciplinary student learning and multidisciplinary faculty practice and research. Nursing faculty coordinated with other disciplines from Kean College such as medical record administration, social work, sociology, psychology, public administration, and early childhood education faculty. Specific services that faculty and students provide to homeless families include family assessment, planning, and implementation of interventions, such as traditional health-care services, parenting skills, how to access social service agencies, counseling to assist families in coping during the homeless crisis, and remediation or assistance with learning for children whose education has been interrupted. Unique to this faculty practice is the interdisciplinary student learning in which students help organize and administer the shelter, set up and maintain records, locate and obtain funds, or train personnel to work with shelter residents alongside other professional graduate students. Benefits of this faculty practice are not limited to student experiences. Nursing faculty and students have access to actual service situations that future APNs must be able to manage and opportunities to study and learn from actual service situations in order to remain current in practice. The faculty practice also benefits the homeless shelter by enabling the shelter to negotiate access to experts without incurring the expenses that usually accompany consultation. Collaboration in grant writing and access to the College Grants Office is another benefit.

Although the previous faculty practice was implemented by Community Health CNS faculty, two other faculty practices in homeless shelters have been implemented by NP faculty at State University of New York-Buffalo and the University of California, Los Angeles Schools of Nursing. In both of these settings, faculty and students provide primary care to homeless shelter residents. Funding for homeless shelter health services in these (and other) faculty practices is through public health contracts, university or federal grants, and faculty volunteers.

NURSING CENTERS

The previous examples of faculty practices were primarily models involving one to several faculty who have developed individual arrangements with an organization or agency external to the school of nursing. The nursing center owned or operated by a school of nursing is a more recent development of group faculty practice. Nursing centers are characterized by nurse management; nursing control of practice; direct access to nursing services; holistic, client-centered services; and reimbursement for services rendered (Riesch, 1992). Nursing centers may be community-based, affiliated with hospitals or schools of nursing, or free-standing entrepreneurial centers; most are sponsored by nursing schools. According to a 1991 study by Barger, 51 nursing centers have been developed since 1985 and provide a wide variety of health-related services.

Phillips and Steele (1994) described the roles of APN faculty in nursing centers. CNS faculty have developed nursing centers focused on specialty care such as cardiac care, oncology, premature birth prevention, and primary care or case management of persons with chronic diseases (multiple sclerosis, AIDS). Nursing services by CNS faculty include symptom and treatment management, prevention of complications, and disability limitation. CNSs have expanded both the boundary and the dimension of their scope of practice in nursing centers (Davis-Doughty, 1989). NP faculty in nursing centers also deliver a wide variety of primary and specialty care services. Many of the services developed by NP faculty overlap with those of primary care physicians, such as primary care services to adolescents in group homes, school health services, school and camp physical examinations, and acute and chronic disease management in ambulatory clinics in hospitals, student health centers, and mobile health units. However, other NP faculty practices in nursing centers involve independent nursing interventions such as school health educational services, spiritual counseling services, and health promotion interventions. Nurse-midwifery faculty have developed free-standing birth centers or midwifery services as part of an existing faculty group practice.

A few examples of nursing centers established by nursing faculty follow; they represent specialty or role-specific practice ventures as well as examples of innovative models of the integration of advanced nursing practice and education.

Nursing Center for Older Adults

School of nursing centers also provide for the integration of student learning experiences and research projects. Hawkins, Igou, Johnson, and Utley (1984) described the development of the Wellness Center located in a senior center building, a joint venture of the Boston College School of Nursing and a small local township. The nursing center provided preventive health maintenance, early detection of disease, health maintenance for chronic conditions, and coordination of care with other professionals. The School of Nursing originally provided a full-time NP (or a full-time equivalent) and established a community advisory board. Multiple research projects were generated from the center, such as measurement of the cost-effectiveness of care, measurement of outcomes from interventions, description of clinical phenomena (incontinence), and the study of interdisciplinary team function. A federal grant funded by the Division of Nursing to expand services combined with Medicare reimbursement supported additional faculty.

At the University of Washington School of Nursing, a joint venture with a local developer resulted in the establishment of a faculty-operated long-term care facility, the Ida Culver House. A local developer, working with the School of Nursing, built a state-of-the-art senior living center and health-care center. Faculty operate the health-care facility, which provides a living laboratory for nursing research and student education experiences.

Rural Nursing Centers

Nursing faculty have developed nursing centers in rural communities that are directed to special populations such as migrant health outreach services, multiphase health screening for the elderly, and long-term care for persons with hypertension. Many of these faculty practices are nursing centers without walls; faculty locate the centers in unique places such as grocery stores, laundromats, gas stations, cafes, churches, local school events, schools, and daycare centers.

A Community Nursing Center in a rural community was developed by faculty at the University of Texas-Galveston (Fenton, Rounds, & Iha, 1988). Community health nursing faculty and NP faculty jointly provide primary care and community nursing services in a rural Texas community. In addition to disease management and health promotion services, nursing faculty assess community needs, identify necessary resources, gain support of the community, and increase access to health-care services. Services are provided in non-traditional ways through outreach activities. The nursing center is also used as clearinghouse for government and private health organizations that can provide financial aid, assistance with disabilities and daily living, and transportation and case management. Faculty are also involved in fundraising activities. Funds come from a combination of state and federal grants, insurance reimbursement, private foundation support, community resources, and local fundraising.

Student Health Centers and School-Based Nursing Centers

A few nursing schools have begun operating student health services using a nursing center model. The faculty at the University of Tennessee-Memphis operate the campus student health service, where students pay an annual fee at the time of registration and receive all of their primary care from nursing faculty. In addition to providing health services for students at the Memphis campus, the faculty contract with other schools for student care. The student health center is used by other APN faculty to evaluate nursing therapeutics and nursing practice models (examples are also found at the Pace University and California State University-Sonoma Schools of Nursing).

Many faculties are establishing nursing centers in elementary and high schools, especially in rural and inner-city schools, where children and adolescents have special health-care needs. Similar to community nursing centers, these faculty practices are developed in collaboration with teachers and parents to meet the primary health-care needs of the school-age child and adolescent. Most of these school-based nursing centers are funded by state or federal grants and staffed by CNS and NP faculty. Two nursing schools have developed school-based services administered by faculty traveling to various sites in a mobile van. CNS and NP faculty from San Francisco State University School of Nursing provide primary health care to inner-city high school students. In rural Mississippi, CNS and NP faculty from Alcorn State University provide similar services modified for school-age children and adolescents in rural communities. Gladstone School Center, a primary care clinic operated by Xavier University School of Nursing faculty, is located in an inner-city Chicago elementary school. All of these faculty practices provide nursing services to ethnic populations who are traditionally medically underserved.

Midwifery/Birthing Centers

Rather than focusing on the boundaries of obstetrical nursing practice within the medical model, CNMs have successfully built on a core of practice established through a long tradition of midwifery. CNM faculty in a number of nursing schools have successfully developed birth centers based on the distinct philosophy that characterizes the dimensions of CNM practice. Many of these CNM faculty practices provide an interdisciplinary focus in which midwifery students are taught alongside medical and nursing students.

Most CNM faculty are involved in clinical practice as part of their faculty role. Administrative arrangements are usually contractual between the CNM faculty and a clinical agency external to the school of nursing. Another common arrangement includes the CNM faculty whose primary appointment is with a school of medicine, and faculty practice is similar to medical faculty arrangements. Although many midwifery/birth centers are in operation, only a few are functioning as faculty practices. However, some notable midwifery centers are thriving as school of nursing centers. For example, the University of Utah School of Nursing recently completed the construction of a Family Birth Center that is owned and operated by CNM faculty (Amos, 1995).

Community Nursing Centers

Hampton University School of Nursing in Virginia has operated a community health nursing center since 1984, providing primary care, health promotion, and family-centered care to a racially diverse patient population. Health promotion and wellness programs are provided at the nursing center and in the community.

Faculty at the center integrate practice, teaching, and research. Undergraduate students are involved in community health projects, and NP students provide care under the supervision of faculty practitioners. Other nursing schools contract with the center to provide clinical experience for their graduate students. Clinical research conducted at the center includes description of cardiac risk factors for African-American men and the impact of clinical interventions on patient outcomes. The center contracts with physicians and local laboratories for consultation and diagnostic services. The center provides health care to homeless shelter residents as well as family planning services through contractual arrangements with the local health department. Employee health services are provided to Hampton University employees through informal agreements established with university administration. Approximately 20% of the center budget is funded by patient revenues, with the remainder funded through grants and university resources.

NEW AND FUTURE FACULTY PRACTICE MODELS

The growth of nursing centers and the necessary testing of outcomes of nurse-managed care in community-based settings depends largely on collaborative efforts between research and practice faculty. Successful new faculty practice ventures are promoting nursing practice as a new, complementary, community-based alternative that is responsive to patient needs. This care by nurses is based on measured outcomes and not used simply as substitute care for other providers. Differentiating a distinct scope of nursing practice that is separate but complementary to medicine will establish nursing centers as critical to a reformed health-care system. These new models assume partnerships between education and service. New forms of research are being integrated into faculty practices, for the development of health policy research and for measurement of cost/quality outcomes.

New and future faculty practice models will depend on education-practice partnerships that link practice and research interests for faculty and enhance education of students while attending to the "business" of providing professional nursing services. Entrepreneurship may be one model of uniting education, service, and research in the future. The entrepreneur is broadly defined as one who organizes, manages, and assumes the risks of a business or enterprise. Another term, "intrapreneur," refers to an entrepreneur working within an organization and may be more suitable for faculty who practice within their faculty roles. In the entrepreneurial model, individual faculty use a practice as a teaching or research site and are usually paid for their services. At the level of nursing service and education organizations, an entrepreneurial faculty practice model may be a joint venture between service and education—a nursing center with or without walls—that has multiple outcomes related to education, research, and revenue generation. It is obvious that entrepreneurial arrangements permit many variations in services, client population, locale of care, business arrangements, and outcomes. An entrepreneurial model allows a variety of arrangements to develop between health-care services and nursing education. This arrangement is based on the needs of the school of nursing and the existing health-care systems environment.

Integrating administrative and business components within practice-education partnerships distinguishes some current and future directions for faculty practice.

A few of these models in which entrepreneurship and business approaches are integrated are highlighted to demonstrate the multiple models and strategies implemented by nursing faculty. One of the most simple models is a contracting model in which a nursing faculty group or a school of nursing contracts with one or more health-care agencies. The individual faculty member or faculty group provides nursing services, usually with students, for a fee as specified in a contract. Many schools of nursing have instituted a contracting mechanism in order to generate revenue for the school or to supplement faculty salaries. Student-faculty research projects usually are generated in these practices and provide a source of outcome data in order to demonstrate nursing service effectiveness.

One of the many benefits of faculty practice contracts has been the formalization and visibility of nursing services through business and organizational procedures. Prior to the development of faculty practice contracts, nursing educators would "moonlight" or volunteer their services. Informal arrangements, without reimbursement, kept these valuable nursing services unstructured, invisible, and outside of the organizational mainstream. Other positive results include the empowerment of nursing faculty as they negotiate intra-institutional policies and develop business plans. A description of some of these faculty practices along with the "how-to" of establishing a business plan can be found in *Nursing Faculty Practice: Models and Methods* by Potash and Taylor (1993). Some newer examples of faculty practices that use contracting can by found at the University of South Carolina, Vanderbilt University, and the University of Texas-Houston Schools of Nursing. Vanderbilt's contracting model, in which the School has contracted with the State of Tennessee for Medicaid managed-care contracts, may be one of the most innovative and will provide a model for the future of faculty practice in this area (Conway-Welch, 1995).

BUSINESS ARRANGEMENTS FOR FACULTY PRACTICE MODELS

The University of Tennessee College of Nursing in Memphis has widely instituted an entrepreneurial practice model using contracting and nursing center structures. All faculty, including the dean, are encouraged to have a faculty practice. One provides primary care and screening to residents of the Memphis Jewish Home. The College has an annual contract with the Memphis Jewish Home that reimburses the College on a per-capita basis. As noted previously, the School of Nursing also operates the University's Student Health Center, combining a managed care and a nursing center approach.

A Community Nursing Center established at the University of Rochester School of Nursing is now a professional corporation providing women's health, adolescent and child care, school health, care of the elderly, care of the disabled, wellness programs, and consultation (Walker, 1994). Operating as an entrepreneurial faculty practice, clusters of service exist under a Community Nursing Center corporate umbrella (center without walls). Future plans will facilitate collaboration among nursing professionals for group practice and research. Additional plans for this innovative faculty practice include marketing NP services across the age span, consultation services, education services, and research services for proposal writing and program evaluation. Future innovations for ensuring the economic stability of these faculty practices include gaining market position in the business and health-care community via new contracts for health promotion in the work place, interdisciplinary collaborative practice, co-managed care agreements, and HMO care contracts.

A joint practice model at Yale University School of Nursing exemplifies another way to implement an entrepreneurial faculty practice structure in which the School of Nursing generates over 1 million dollars in clinical revenues through joint appointments. Although a joint practice model of faculty practice has been in effect for over 30 years at Yale, the current faculty practices are now poised to take advantage of managed care as it emerges in Connecticut. The Yale Midwifery Center has reorganized under a subcontract with the Yale–New Haven Hospital, and faculty are providing care at the Community Mental Health Center through joint funding from Yale–New Haven Hospital, the state, and the School of Nursing. The faculty maintain a full-time appointment in the School of Nursing, conduct research at their practice sites, and maintain administrative and academic assignments at both institutions (Krauss, 1995).

The University of Utah School of Nursing, like the University of Rochester, is realigning their faculty practices with managed care. Their challenge is to create faculty practices within an integrated system. The School has had faculty practices since 1986 and for the past 3 years has functioned under a faculty practice plan that rewards teaching, research, and practice activities. The faculty practice program includes a birth center and a symptom management clinic and will soon add a family primary care center. Although the faculty practice programs are not capitated, the School has contracts with managed care systems, and the faculty clinicians are designated providers under those contracts (Amos, 1995).

The CRNA faculty at the University of Alabama School of Health Related Professions has developed a salary supplement arrangement that allows CRNA faculty to supplement salaries with clinical revenues in the same way that nonclinical faculty supplement salaries with research grants (J. Williams, personal communication, May 1995). CRNA faculty have full-time appointments in the University and as part of their academic contract are allowed 52 days per year for clinical practice. In addition, liberal vacation policies allow for additional clinical practice and approximately $20,000 per year of salary supplementation.

Multiple financial systems exist for faculty practice at the University of California, San Francisco School of Nursing, where faculty contract with agencies, negotiate joint practice agreements, and operate a school-owned nursing center. The nursing center, a child health clinic, located in a largely Hispanic neighborhood of San Francisco, is staffed by bilingual faculty and students. School of nursing faculty and graduate students are also involved in research, and future plans include forming managed care arrangements (Duderstadt, 1995).

As market forces drive the health-care system, nursing faculty practices are attending to the business aspects of health-care delivery. As illustrated, business arrangements may be simple or complex and involve contracts with a variety of health-care systems; partnership arrangements with physicians, nurses, or other health-care personnel; and joint practice arrangements with agencies or groups. Some faculty practices are broad enough to include other faculty, nurses, or health personnel within one structural arrangement. Although evaluation of faculty practice structures and implementation issues are beyond the scope of this chapter, the reader is referred to Potash and Taylor (1993) for a complete discussion of these issues. This publication, supported and published by the National Organization of Nurse Practitioner Faculties, presents a framework for starting a faculty practice and describes procedures for structuring, planning, and evaluating a practice at different stages of its development.

IMPLEMENTING FACULTY PRACTICE: ISSUES, CHALLENGES, AND STRATEGIES

The general dilemma for nursing education is expressed by Nugent and colleagues (1993): "Nursing is a practice profession, therefore, the addition of practice to the mission of teaching, research and service not only seems logical but necessary" (p. 299). However paradoxes exist in the implementation of the practice role within an academic system. Practice has been found to contribute to scholarship and could or should provide a vehicle for achieving the goals of academia and promotion within the academic system. On the other hand, role fragmentation and work overload result when faculty attempt to address each work role function separately within the different social and bureaucratic structures of the school and health-care delivery system.

Faculty practice by APNs will continue to evolve in concert with the implementation of managed care and integrated health systems. Although these issues are beyond the scope of this chapter, other issues facing APN faculty, such as overcoming barriers to faculty practice, integrating practice into advancement criteria, creating stable funding for faculty practice, and developing balanced workload criteria, are covered in the following sections. Furthermore, continuing questions about the scope and nature of practice within an academic environment must be addressed by individual faculty practitioners and nursing education leaders. Although approaches to these questions, challenges, and issues will vary among institutions, some general considerations and strategies are proposed.

BARRIERS TO FACULTY PRACTICE

Most authors and faculty surveys agree on three major barriers to faculty practice: (1) lack of time, (2) lack of support for faculty practice from administration (dean, chairperson) or faculty peers, and (3) too few academic or monetary rewards. A few studies of faculty practice report excessive workload as the primary barrier to practice by nursing faculties (Barger & Bridges, 1987; Ford & Kitzman, 1983; Joel, 1983; Nichols, 1985). Many academic institutions are unable to provide time for nurse educators to practice in addition to carrying out other academic tasks (Barger, Nugent, & Bridges, 1992; Lambert & Lambert, 1993). Others report resistance on the part of nurse educators to assume additional activities without increased financial reward as a critical barrier to faculty practice (Barger & Bridges, 1987; Barger et al., 1992; Spero, 1980). Although many APN faculty are compensated for clinical practice within their faculty role, few receive "credit" toward tenure or promotion.

"Lack of time" results from the addition of practice to the faculty's existing teaching and research roles. Traditionally, clinical practice has been viewed negatively as an additive model by nursing educators because it appears to add another role to the traditional faculty education-research roles. Although "support" is not defined in studies, it generally refers to the lack of support from the school's administration and too little support from clinical site administration. Lack of support from the school's administration is most often associated with inflexibility in faculty workload requirements and inadequate administrative support for integrating practice, research, and education responsibilities. Direct administrative support for clinical practice may also be lacking. Barger & Bridges (1987) challenged the idea that administrative support was a major barrier to faculty practice. After surveying 1,036 nurse educators, these authors found that administration policies did not significantly affect the extent of faculty practice. However, personal factors, such as age, marital status, and educational level, did affect faculty practice. An inverse relationship was found between age, an earned doctorate, and the extent of practice, suggesting that older, doctoral-prepared faculty members are practicing less or not at all compared with their younger, master's-prepared colleagues.

Faculty practitioners may feel that they have to "do it all"—administer the practice in addition to providing clinical services as well as fulfill teaching obligations. Academic rewards are lacking because most schools do not consider faculty practice as a criterion for achieving tenure. Because research, teaching, and community service are the usual success factors in academia, practice outside of community service seems of lesser value. Monetary rewards have traditionally been lacking for nursing faculty practice, and direct payment for client services is at best, fledgling.

FACILITATION AND INHIBITION OF FACULTY PRACTICE

A few studies have surveyed faculty and schools of nursing about the personal and organizational factors related to faculty practice. In general, personal factors have been more positively related to faculty practice compared with academic or organizational factors. However, academic-related advantages of faculty practice and benefits to the nursing profession have not been investigated in most of these studies. One study reported that the majority of respondents practiced for personal reasons and most were not engaged in research or publishing (Anderson and Pierson, 1983). When participants in another study rank-ordered their reasons for practice, skill maintenance, personal satisfaction, and earning extra money were the top three (Just et al., 1989). Academic reasons, such as to develop curricula, generate research, and gather data for publication, ranked considerably lower. Steele (1991) also found that the faculty practitioner's perception of rewards from practice were associated more substantially with personal satisfaction than with academic advancement.

Nugent and coworkers (1993), using a Delphi procedure, studied 299 practicing faculty representing 170 schools to identify the top five personal and organizational factors that facilitate and inhibit practice. Organizational facilitators of faculty practice included faculty workload that reflected faculty practice in the same way as other academic missions, flexibility by the agency in which the faculty practiced, administrative support and value for practice, and promotion criteria that address practice and that reflect both administrative support and value. Organizational inhibitors of faculty practice included professional traditions, institutional bureaucracies, lack of structure and support for practice activities, the perception of practice as an additive function or service to the community, and inconsistent organizational support. Personal facilitators of faculty practice included attributes of caring and commitment, essential competency and knowledge, organizational skills, positive reactions from colleagues, and a supportive collegial environment in relation to institutional collaboration. Personal inhibitors to faculty practice included multiple role demands, lack of confidence in knowledge and skills, and lack of drive or commitment to practice.

CONSIDERATIONS AND CHALLENGES FOR APN FACULTY PRACTICE

As faculty practice has developed as a recognized element of nursing education, questions have emerged to challenge existing definitions and models. These questions may be used by APN faculty as they consider the development or expansion of faculty practice.

- *Should nursing education accept the academic model or the professional model for promotion and advancement? Or, should nursing education combine portions of both models to create a model more appropriate to a practice profession? (Forni & Welch, 1987). If nursing combines the academic-professional model, which professional model will be adopted? Academic medicine, law, social work, etc.?*

To teach and do research is the definition given to any university professor who "practices his profession" (Council of the American Association of University Professors, 1984, p. 31). For *nurse* faculty to practice the profession, it is expected that the faculty member will be involved in the nursing arena as well.

- *How are efforts in the area of faculty practice judged for promotion and advancement?*

In a survey of nursing school deans, 97% rated service as the least important criterion for advancement, with deans from graduate programs rating research as the most important criteria (Messmer, 1989). Practice is usually considered within the general category of professional, community, or university "service" in academic advancement criteria. In a study of allied health faculty, 7 of 10 items essential to promotion were related to scholarly activities, and 3 of 10 were related to service to the institution. None of the items was related to teaching or clinical care, even though faculty believed these items to be essential (Conine, Shilling, & Pierce, 1985). In a survey of medical school deans, 78% had changed or were in process of changing academic advancement criteria to give more weight to clinical and educational contributions than to research productivity (Bickel, 1991).

- *Should APN educators function as expert clinicians, expert educators, or both?*

APN preparation at the master's or doctoral level requires teachers with subject matter expertise. Most APNs have little background in education. Knowing something is no guarantee that one has the ability to convey it or to teach it to others. APN educators need clinical expertise and a strong knowledge base as well as the ability to impart knowledge to others.

- *How will the roles of practitioner, teacher, and researcher be balanced? What factors help faculty to be effective in these roles?*

The size of an academic institution, rather than level of education, drives the importance placed on research, teaching, and practice or service. Large institutions and health science universities are more likely to have graduate programs emphasizing research than smaller colleges, most of which have undergraduate programs (Zenas, 1988). Making faculty practice an imperative for all nursing faculty members requires adding practice as a fifth area of faculty responsibility. Requiring faculty to achieve in all areas (teaching, scholarly activity, research, practice, service) dilutes contributions and accomplishments, creates excessive workload, and decreases doctoral-prepared faculty (Rodgers, 1986).

■ *How are faculty practice efforts being evaluated? What effect does faculty practice have on teaching, research, and patient care? How can the effect be measured?*

Some schools of nursing are now beginning to include clinical practice within the pervue of promotion and tenure. Joint appointments make it possible for evaluation of clinical components of APN faculty practice.

Although these are only a few of the questions and challenges facing APN faculty practitioners, they demonstrate the larger issues that must be considered by schools of nursing when integrating practice with education. A few strategies for implementing successful faculty practice are described in the next section.

STRATEGIES FOR SUCCESSFUL APN FACULTY PRACTICE

Integration of the roles of educator, researcher, and practitioner is a persistent theme among many successful faculty practice models. A typical example may be as follows: an APN faculty member provides nursing or health-care services to individuals, families, or groups, supervises students, and conducts clinical research at the faculty practice site. The practitioner-teacher, either directly or indirectly through other clinical colleagues, provides nursing or health-related services, and students assist with client care and clinical research. Thus, one clinic site or service directed to a client population assists the faculty member with all three roles. The faculty member manages the practice, teaching, and research but may collaborate with other faculty colleagues to assist with duties and tasks. Gresham-Kenton (1989) described Luther Christman's concept of "economy of effort." CNS faculty considered a series of questions that allowed them to maximize every clinical teaching situation. Balance among each area of scholarly activity (teaching, practice, and service) will help avert faculty burnout and role conflict.

APN faculty should collaborate to customize academic advancement criteria to reflect the need of the faculty. Wright (1993) suggests a set of general criteria: to improve teaching and develop nursing research, but to maintain expertise in nursing practice. Others believe that developing a tenure and non-tenure, or two-track, system may encourage those not interested in doctoral study to pursue faculty practice and to provide appropriate criteria to reward expert practitioners. The typical hierarchy of research, teaching, service is reversed in the practice-education track, with nursing services, patient care, and competent practice-related skills considered the highest criteria. Most APN faculty agree that faculty practice should not be another added criteria that must be met in addition to the others. Some schools have revised their advancement criteria in an algorithmic approach: all faculty are required to teach, with faculty choosing either research *or* practice as the next criterion on which promotion and tenure decisions are based. The individual faculty member can make the decision about which model fits best with his or her career goals. de Tornyay (1988), a former nursing school dean, suggested that each school should develop its own list of activities that would be counted toward promotion and tenure: new models for delivering nursing service, demonstration projects, school-run clinics, school-operated day-care centers, private and group practices, consultation for community agencies, and using findings of nursing research to improve patient care. Also, because part of scholarship is the transmission of knowledge, credit could be given for developing computer programs that aid students' development of critical thinking or clinical judgment skills.

Collaboration with nurses, faculty, and other practitioners is an important factor in helping the faculty practitioner to develop support networks. For instance, an NP faculty member who manages a teen mothers' program established a cooperative relationship with a psychiatric CNS faculty colleague to provide mental health services to selected teens as well as to supervise student experiences in psychiatric assessment and management (Potash & Taylor, 1993). Collaboration may also facilitate direct payment for client services because of group nursing contracts with third-party payers or billing through agencies or physician colleagues. Creativity is another theme that is incorporated in successful faculty practice models. APNs are creating new ways to deal with familiar problems by embracing opportunities and exhibiting a willingness to pursue solutions rather than problems.

As faculty practice moves from a volunteer or collaborative model without reimbursement to either the school of nursing or the individual faculty member, stable funding will become an important consideration for the establishment of new or expanded faculty practice ventures. Although early faculty practices did not generate revenue and were not supported by grants, reduced funding for nursing education will require new or expanded faculty practices to generate revenue. Furthermore, academic salaries have lagged behind community salaries for APNs, and faculty practice revenues are used for salary supplements in order to retain talented APNs. Administrators believe that practice revenues should provide some support to the school of nursing general funds in the same way that research grants have provided financial support. Many schools of nursing and APN faculty are forming new organizational structures to allow competition in the current managed care market. The "health-care delivery system as a business" has forced nursing to integrate business principles into faculty practice. However, nursing's tradition has been to meet the needs of underserved patients and communities. The challenge to future faculty practice development will be to balance high-revenue-generating practices with practices that are critical to community needs regardless of revenue generation.

Organizational support from administration as well as from faculty governance and individual colleagues is essential. Simple changes in advancement criteria to include faculty practice can be made by nursing faculty, usually without central university approval. Certain procedures must be considered, such as faculty bylaws, voting procedures, and the establishment of a faculty practice committee, to define faculty practice and establish practice-related policy. Depending on the size of the school or faculty, the faculty practice standing committee may be separately formed or be composed entirely of faculty. A recognized faculty practice committee provides quality assurance, professional guidance, and policy development for APNs who practice as part of their faculty role. This professional and policy oversight will become more and more important with the establishment of managed care arrangements.

Faculty practice plans have been developed by a number of schools of nursing to provide guidance for financial and workload considerations. Although each state or institution has different requirements for the establishment of faculty practice plans, there are some general considerations in the establishment of a practice plan.

1. A practice plan must be developed jointly by the administration and the faculty.
2. A practice plan should balance faculty practice philosophy with financial considerations.
3. Financial incentives and revenue distribution must be included in a formal practice plan to promote the development of faculty practice within the school of nursing.

Although some schools of nursing only include revenue generation and distribution policy and procedures within their faculty practice plan, other schools have elaborated on types of practice or workload issues related to faculty practice. However practice-related workload is codified in a school, joint decision-making among administrators and faculty about workload issues is crucial to the success of APN faculty practice. Although an average of 1 day per week of "clinical practice" has been a traditional expectation or allowance, new workload models should be considered that depend on each school's faculty practice program.

If practice is not required of all faculty, viable options for attaining career goals for faculty who do wish to practice need to be offered or included in academic workload. Faculty practice that requires faculty members to practice what they teach, at a scholarly level, should be encouraged; this should be done without excessive workload or to the detriment of other components of nursing education.

Further consideration of these issues can be found in *Faculty Practice: Models & Methods* by Potash and Taylor (1993) as well as the proceedings of the Faculty Practice Conferences convened by the AACN (1993, 1994, 1995).

CONCLUSION

Faculty practice, which became an important issue in nursing education during the 1980s, may be one way to unify the profession for the future. APN educators have demonstrated that they can be role models in innovative nursing practices. Faculty practice can provide revenue for an institution as well as establish models of nursing care based on research and advanced practice. APNs, nursing administrators, and nursing educators have demonstrated that the whole is greater than the sum of the parts through their efforts at unifying education, practice, and, now, health-care delivery systems through faculty practice programs. Future development of faculty practice will include integrating practice into traditional academic missions of teaching and research, the development of stable funding, workload considerations, and academic advancement standards.

REFERENCES

American Academy of Nursing (1980). Resolution on unification of nursing service and nursing education. *American Academy of Nursing Newsletter, 1*(4).

American Association of Colleges of Nursing (1993, 1994, 1995). Faculty Practice Conferences.

Amos, L. (1995). A School of Nursing-owned Family Nursing Center. *Faculty practice in a managed care environment.* Proceedings of the Second Annual Faculty Practice Conference. Tucson, AZ: American Association of Colleges of Nursing.

Anderson, E. R., & Pierson, P. (1983). An exploratory study of faculty practice: Views of those faculty engaged in practice who teach in an NLN accredited baccalaureate program. *Western Journal of Nursing Research, 5,* 129-143.

Andreoli, K. G. (1993). Faculty improve clinical operations. *Journal of Professional Nursing*, *9*(4), 194.

Aroian, J. F., & Rauckhorst, L. M. (1985). Summer camp: An overlooked site for faculty clinical practice? *Nurse Educator*, *10*(1), 32-35.

Arthur, D., & Usher, K. (1994). An application of nursing faculty practice: Clinical camps. *Journal of Advanced Nursing*, *19*, 680-684.

Barger, S. E. (1991). The nursing center: A model for rural nursing practice. *Nursing & Health Care*, *12*(6), 290-294.

Barger, S., & Bridges, W. C. (1987). Nursing faculty practice: institutional and individual facilitators and inhibitors. *Journal of Professional Nursing*, *3*, 338-346.

Barger, S. E., Nugent, K. E., & Bridges, W. C. (1992). Nursing faculty practice: An organizational perspective. *Journal of Professional Nursing*, *8*(5), 263-270.

Barnard, K. E. (1983). *Structure to outcome: Making it work*. Kansas City, MO: American Academy of Nursing.

Barnard, K. E., & Smith, G. R. (1985). *Faculty practice in action*. Kansas City, MO: American Academy of Nursing.

Bickel, J. (1991). The changing faces of promotion and tenure at U. S. medical schools. *Academic Medicine*, *66*(5), 249-256.

Campbell, M. (1993). Multidisciplinary faculty practice and community partnership. *Holistic Nursing Practice*, *7*(4), 20-27.

Campbell, B. F., & King J. B. (1992). Public health service administration and academia. *Journal of Nursing Administration*, *22*(12), 23-27.

Choudry, U. K. (1992). Faculty practice competencies: Nurse educators' perceptions. *The Canadian Journal of Nursing Research*, *24*(3), 5-17.

Christman, L. (1982). The unification model. In A. Marriner (Ed.), *Contemporary Nursing Management*. St. Louis, MO: C. V. Mosby.

Christy, T. E. (1980). Clinical practice as a function of nursing education: A historical analysis. *Nursing Outlook*, *28*, 492-496.

Conine, T. A., Shilling, L. M., & Pierce, E. R. (1985). The relative importance of supportive data for promotion and tenure reviews. *Journal of Allied Health*, *14*(2), 183-190.

Conway-Welch, C. (1995). Integration of faculty practice into a state managed care setting. *Faculty practice in a managed care environment*. Proceedings of the Second Annual Faculty Practice Conference. Tucson, AZ: American Association of Colleges of Nursing.

Council of the American Association of University Professors (1984). The standards for notice of non-reappointment. *Policy documents and reports*. Washington, DC: AAUP.

Davis-Doughty, S. E. (1989). The CNS in a nurse-managed center. In A. B. Hamric & J. A. Spross (Eds.), *The clinical nurse specialist in theory and practice* (2nd ed., pp. 415-434). Philadelphia: W. B. Saunders.

Davis, L., & Zatuchni, G. I. (1993). Nurse-midwifery within a faculty group practice. *Nurse Practitioner Journal*, *18*(10), 14-15.

DeLeon, P. (1994). Nursing school administered clinics: An important policy agenda for the future. *Nursing Economic$*, *10*, 137-158.

de Tornyay, R. (1988). What constitutes scholarly activities? *Journal of Nursing Education*, *27*(6), 245.

Donnelly, G. F., Warfel, W., & Wolf, Z. R. (1994). A faculty-practice program: Three perspectives. *Holistic Nursing Practice*, *8*(3), 71-80.

Duderstadt, K. (1995). *The Valencia pediatric practice*. San Francisco, CA: University of California, San Francisco School of Nursing.

Durand, B. A. (1985). Defining faculty practice: A Look at Theory-Practice Relationships. In K. E. Barnard & G. R. Smith (Eds.), *Faculty practice in action* (pp. 38-40). Kansas City, MO: American Academy of Nursing.

Fagin, C. M. (1985). Institutionalizing practice: Historical and future perspectives. In K. E. Barnard & G. R. Smith (Eds.), *Faculty practice in action* (pp. 1-17). Kansas City, MO: American Academy of Nursing.

Fagin, C. M. (1986). Institutionalizing faculty practice. *Nursing Outlook*, *34*(3), 140-144.

Fenton, M. V., Rounds, L., & Iha, S. (1988). The nursing center in a rural community: The promotion of family and community health. *Family and Community Health*, *11*(2), 14-24.

Ford, L., & Kitzman, H. (1983). Organization perspectives on faculty and practice: Issues and challenges. In K. Barnard (Ed.), *Structure to outcome: Making it work* (pp. 13-30). Kansas City, MO: American Academy of Nursing.

Forni, P. R., & Welch, M. J. (1987). The professional versus the academic model: A dilemma for nursing education. *Journal of Nursing Education*, *3*(5), 291-297.

Grace, H. K. (1981). Unification, re-unification: Reconciliation or collaboration–bridging the education-service gap. In J. C. McCloskey & H. K. Grace (Eds.), *Current issues in nursing*. Boston: Blackwell Scientific.

Gresham-Kenton, M. L. (1989). The CNS in collaborative relationships between nursing service and nursing education. In A. B. Hamric & J. Spross (Eds.), *The clinical nurse specialist in theory and practice*. Philadelphia: W. B. Saunders.

Hawkins, J. W., Igou, J. F., Johnson, E. E., & Utley, Q. E. (1984). A nursing center for ambulatory, well, older adults. *Nursing & Health Care*, *5*(4), 209-212.

Herr, K. A. (1989). Faculty practice as a requirement for promotion and tenure: Receptivity, risk and threats perceived. *Journal of Nursing Education*, *28*(8), 347-353.

Joel, L. A. (1983). Stepchildren in the family: Aiming toward synergy between nursing education and service—from the faculty perspective. In D. E. Barnard & G. R. Smith (Eds.), *Structure to outcome: Making it work* (pp. 43-57). Kansas City, MO: American Academy of Nursing.

Just, G., Adams, E., & DeYoung, S. (1989). Faculty practice: Nurse educators' views and proposed models. *Journal of Nursing Education, 28*(4), 161-168.

Kramer, M., Polifroni, E. C., & Organek, N. (1986). Effects of faculty practice on student learning outcomes. *Journal of Professional Nursing, 2*(5), 289-301.

Krauss, J. (1995). Joint appointments for faculty practice. *Faculty practice in a managed care environment.* Proceedings of the Second Annual Faculty Practice Conference. Tucson, AZ: American Association of Colleges of Nursing.

Lambert, C., & Lambert, V. A. (1993). Relationships among faculty practice involvement, perception of role stress, and psychological hardiness of nurse educators. *Journal of Nursing Education, 32*(4), 171-179.

Lee, V. K., Levy, E. Y., Dix, P. E., & Tatum, M. F. (1987). Faculty as primary nurses on a model inpatient unit. *Nurse Educator, 12*(5), 16-19.

Mauksch, I. (1980a). A rationale for the reunification of nursing service and nursing education. In L. Aiken (Ed.), *Health policy and nursing practice,* New York: McGraw-Hill, 211-217.

Mauksch, I. (1980b). Faculty practice: A professional imperative. *Nurse Educator, 5,* 21-24.

Maurin, J. T. (1986). An exploratory study of nursing services provided by schools of nursing. *Journal of Professional Nursing, 2,* 277-281.

McClure, M. (1987). Faculty practice: New definitions, new opportunities. *Nursing Outlook, 35,* 162-166.

Messmer, P. R. (1989). Academic tenure in schools of nursing. *Journal of Professional Nursing, 5*(1), 39-48.

Millonig, V. L. (1986). Faculty practice: A view of its development, current benefits, and barriers. *Journal of Professional Nursing, 2*(3), 166-172.

Murray, K. M., Hackbarth, D. P., Sojka, S. A., & Swanston, L. J. (1987). Faculty practice in home health care: A new education and service relationship in process. *QRB,* 42-44.

Nichols, C. (1985). Faculty practice: Something for everyone. *Nursing Outlook, 33*(2), 85-90.

Nugent, K. E., Barger, S. E., & Bridges, W. C. (1993). Facilitators and inhibitors of practice: A faculty perspective. *Journal of Nursing Education, 32*(7), 293-300.

Phillips, D. L., & Steel, J. E. (1994). Factors influencing scope of practice in nursing centers. *Journal of Professional Nursing, 10*(2), 84-90.

Polifroni, E. C., & Schmalenberg, C. (1985). Faculty practice that works: Two examples. *Nursing Outlook, 33*(5), 226-228.

Potash, M., & Taylor, D. (1993). *Nursing faculty practice: Models & methods.* Washington, DC: National Organization of Nurse Practitioner Faculties.

Riesch, S. K. (1992). Nursing centers: An analysis of the anecdotal literature. *Journal of Professional Nursing, 8*(1), 16-25.

Rodgers, M. W. (1986). Implementing faculty practice: A question of human and financial resources. *Journal of Advanced Nursing, 11,* 687-696.

Spero, J. (1980). Nursing: A professional practice discipline in academia. *Nursing and Health Care, 1,* 22-25.

Stainton, M. C. (1989). The development of a practicing nursing faculty. *Journal of Advanced Nursing, 14,* 20-26.

Stark, P. L., Walker, G. C., & Bohannan, P. A. (1991). Nursing faculty practice in the Houston linkage model: Administrative and faculty perspectives. *Nurse Educator, 16*(5), 23-28.

Steele, R. L. (1991). Attitudes about faculty practice, perceptions of role, and role strain. *Journal of Nursing Education, 30*(1), 15-22.

Styles, M. M. (1984). Reflections on collaboration and unification. *Image, 16,* 21-23.

Turner, D. M., & Pearson, L. M. (1989). The faculty fellowship program: Uniting service and education. *Journal of Nursing Administration, 19*(10), 18-22.

Walker, P. H. (1993). A comprehensive community nursing center model: Maximizing practice income—a challenge to educators. *Journal of Professional Nursing, 10*(3), 131-139.

Wandel, J. C. (1991). Education-practice partnerships: Faculty practice as faculty development. *Journal of Professional Nursing, 7*(5), 310-318.

Wright, D. J. (1993). Faculty practice: Criterion for academic advancement. *Nursing and Health Care, 14*(1), 18-21.

Zenas, C. S. (1988). Achieving promotion and tenure: A strategic perspective. *Nurse Educator, 13*(1), 8-13.

Additional Readings

American Nurses Association (1987). *The nursing center: Concept and design.* Kansas City, MO: American Nurses Association.

Baillie, L. (1994). Nurse teachers' feelings about participating in clinical practice: An exploratory study. *Journal of Advanced Nursing, 20,* 150-159.

Barger, S. E., Nugent, K. E., & Bridges, W. C. (1993). Schools with nursing centers: A 5-year follow-up study. *Journal of Professional Nursing, 9*(1), 7-13.

Batey, M. V. (1983). Structural consideration for the social integration of nursing. In Barnard, K. E. (Ed.), *Structure to outcome: Making it work.* Kansas City, MO: American Academy of Nursing.

Budden, L. (1994). Nursing faculty practice: Benefits vs costs. *Journal of Advanced Nursing, 19,* 1241-1246.

Collison, C. R., & Parsons, M. A. (1980). Is practice a viable faculty role? *Nursing Outlook, 28,* 677-679.

Council on Medical Education. (1990). Principles for graduate medical education. *Journal of the American Medical Association, 263*(21), 2917-2931.

Dickens, M. R. (1983). Faculty practice and social support. *Nursing Leadership, 6,* 121-127.

Duga, A. B. (1985). Expanding nursing's practice terrain: Imperatives for future viability. *Public Health Nursing, 2*(1), 23-32.

Gilson-Parkevich, T. (1983). Stepchildren in the family: Aiming toward synergy between nursing education and service—from the nursing service perspective. In Barnard, K. E. (Ed.), *Structure to outcome: Making it work.* Kansas City, MO: American Academy of Nursing.

Hunter, J. K., Crosby, F. E., Ventura, M. R., & Warkentin, L. (1991). National survey to identify evaluation criteria for programs of health care for homeless. *Nursing and Health Care, 12*(10), 536-542.

Kean College of New Jersey Department of Nursing (1990). *Learning center for health guidelines.* Union, NJ: Kean College of New Jersey.

Lassan, R. (1994). Nursing faculty practice: A valid sabbatical request? *Nursing Forum, 29*(2), 10-14.

Lindsay, A. M. (1989). Health care for the homeless. *Nursing Outlook, 37*(2), 78-81.

McClure, M. (1981). Promoting practice-based research: A critical need. *Journal of Nursing Administration, 7,* 66-70.

Mezey, M. D., Lynaugh, J. E., & Cartier, M. M. (1988). The teaching nursing home program, 1982-87: A report card. *Nursing Outlook, 36*(6), 285-288.

Napholz, L. (1993). An academic nursing center integrating education, role modeling, and research. *Nurse Educator, 18*(4), 3-5.

Rosswurm, M. A. (1981). Characteristics of 23 faculty group practices. *Nursing & Health Care, 2*(6), 327-330.

Shah, H. S., & Pennypacker, D. R. (1992). The clinical teaching partnership. *Nurse Educator, 17*(2), 10-12.

Williamson, N., McDonough, J. E., & Boettcher, J. H. (1990). Nurse faculty practice: From theory to reality. *Journal of Professional Nursing, 6*(1), 11-20.

Yarcheski, A., & Mahon, N. E. (1985). The unification model in nursing: A study of receptivity among nurse educators in the United States. *Nursing Research, 34,* 120-125.

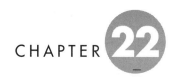

CHAPTER 22

Health Policy Issues: Dealing with the Realities and Constraints of Advanced Nursing Practice

Charlene M. Hanson

INTRODUCTION

Advanced practice nurses (APNs) have been on the cutting edge of health care for several decades, breaking new ground in order to care for high-risk and underserved populations across the country. Over the years, APNs have pushed at the outer limits of the domain of nursing in order to expand their scope of practice and to move into innovative practice arenas. Thus, any discussion of health policy or regulatory issues that deal with advanced nursing practice is, by definition, dynamic and subject to change from day to day. A constant ebb and flow of policy changes affects APNs at any given time. At both the federal and the state levels, this is a time of shifting sands and changing models for nursing practice in all settings. The unsettled congressional climate with regard to health care, and more specifically Medicare and Medicaid, influences the practice of all nurses. In addition, because the individual states regulate all health-care providers through statute and rules and regulations, the state of policy issues varies with each state's legislative agenda.

This chapter will help the reader acquire a sense of the health policy issues and regulatory realities that currently face nurse practitioners (NPs), certified nurse-midwives (CNMs), clinical nurse specialists (CNSs), and certified registered nurse anesthetists (CRNAs). Important aspects of "playing" in the political and legislative arena are also discussed. However, for specific questions about up-to-the-minute current rules and regulations, especially those that pertain to singular requirements for prescriptive authority and reimbursement, the reader is referred to individual local and state regulatory bodies for practice requirements.

EVOLUTION OF ADVANCED NURSING PRACTICE IN THE U.S. HEALTH-CARE SYSTEM

HISTORICAL PERSPECTIVE

APNs have made great strides in the expansion of their education and practice roles since the early days in each specialty. These accomplishments are well described in Chapter 1 and in the specific chapters about each advanced practice role. Nurse-midwives have made major strides in their practice area since nurse-midwifery was founded by Mary Breckinridge at the Frontier Nursing Service in the Appalachian Mountains of Kentucky in 1925 (Ernst, 1994). Furthermore, NPs in all specialties have moved from a predominantly medical model of short-term education to a broader scope of practice, serious political acumen, and strong professional thrust. Registered nurses were prepared to deliver primary health care to children in the first NP program at the University of Colorado School of Nursing in 1965. National certification for NPs was established in the 1970s. The modern CNS emerged in response to the recognized need to improve the quality of patient care and the clinical practice of professional nursing, primarily in the acute care setting (Hamric & Spross, 1989). CRNAs bring a rich history of anesthesia practice from before the turn of the century. This rich heritage of the evolution of advanced nursing practice (ANP) has involved serious policy and regulatory dilemmas that need to be well understood by all APNs so that acceptable policy decisions can be enacted.

CURRENT PRACTICE CLIMATE FOR APNs

Many positive and negative factors influence the education and practice arenas of APNs. The "fit" for APNs during an era of health-care reform is an important one that needs serious and thoughtful deliberation about the trends in practice and regulation into the next century. This fit requires an in-depth study of education, regulation, and policy issues that affect all of nursing but clearly have the most serious impact on APNs. The different education, certification, and individual scope-of-practice policies from one advanced nursing specialty to another complicates issues for policymakers and regulators. Also, social and economic factors, such as poverty, lack of insurance, family violence, and HIV status, directly affect the demand for, education of, and practice parameters of APNs. The climate of nursing practice is also influenced greatly by what is happening in other health-care disciplines. For example, the trend toward primary care physicians and away from specialty medical practice has definite implications for advanced nursing practice (Rentmeester & Kindig, 1994). Currently, the combined health-care needs of an aging population, a period of economic retrenchment, and the move toward a prepaid system of primary, community-based managed care have assured a positive trend for the enhancement of APN practice into the next century (Vector Research Inc., 1995).

HEALTH POLICY ISSUES AFFECTING APNs

Donna Shalala, U.S. Secretary of Health and Human Services, described trends into the 21st century. She suggested that Americans will receive health care in a broader health-care model based on primary care, prevention, and wellness. She predicted a highly collaborative, interdisciplinary system, one in which advanced nurse providers come into their own. This community-based health-care system will require all providers to work within a capitated structure that allows for predetermined payment structures to keep costs down (Jennings & Towers, 1994).

Aiken and Salmon (1994) identified five priority areas in which nursing can help to solve the problems driving the need for reform of the U.S. health-care system. These areas are restructuring hospitals, improving the accessibility of primary care, contributing to the viability of academic health centers, improving care to the underserved, and redesigning the role of public health in a reformed system. APNs can and should provide leadership to address each of these areas. APNs who serve both as excellent hospital-based caregivers and as quality community-based care providers will be competitive players during the reform era, in which access to primary health care—especially for rural, minority, and high-risk populations—will be given priority. One approach to increasing access is to increase the supply of APNs, who, with appropriate training in their areas of specialty and working in collaborative settings, can offer care similar in quality to that of physicians and at less cost (Brown and Grimes, 1993; Safriet, 1992).

MANPOWER PROVIDER ISSUES—THE NEED FOR APNs

There is an overwhelming need for APNs in a wide variety of settings within the current health-care environment (Vector Research Inc., 1995). Women's health NPs are the mainstay of contraceptive and well women's care for the women in lower socio-economic strata in the United States (Wysocki, 1995). Since the early days, APNs of all types have been the model of episodic and chronic caregivers in rural and underserved populations. Acute care NPs (ACNPs) are developing practices in acute care hospitals and out-patient departments. CRNAs provide the majority of the anesthesia (about 65%) for small rural hospitals and support anesthesiology teams in the large ones. They are the sole anesthesia provider in 30 to 35% of all hospitals, 85% of which are in rural areas (OTA, Health Care in Rural America, 1990). Increasing APN workforce needs are predicated on two major issues. First is the rapid movement toward managed care and the educational lag time predicted for physicians to get up to speed in primary care areas. Second are cost issues, for APNs are cheaper to train than physicians and they are cost-effective providers (Office of Technology Assessment, 1986; Vector Research Inc., 1995). Safriet (1992) emphasized the 1986 OTA study that showed that within their area of competence, APNs provide care that is safe, comparable, efficient, and cost-effective. APNs offer a genuine potential for immediate improvement in the delivery of health care in this country. Physicians have pursued specialty care while APNs have increased access to basic health-care services in a wide variety of geographic and practice settings.

There is concern, however, that although APNs have the education and experience to offer quality care, they will continue to be used as "shadow providers" who are holistically caring for patients within the shadow of the physician who has prescribing and reimbursement capabilities (Wilcox, 1995). This concern is perceived as the major constraint to advanced practice nursing in the United States today.

Issues related to the national workforce of APNs will take priority at the policy table into the year 2000. Breakthroughs in the health-care reform debate have brought about a re-examination of roles throughout the health-care system. The implications for direct caregivers, such as CNMs, CNSs, NPs, and other APNs cannot be overestimated. APNs will likely have a significant role as primary care providers in the proposed community-based health-care model—especially in rural and underserved populations with special needs.

In 1995 the U.S. Bureau of Health Professions convened the National Advisory Committee on Nursing Education and Practice (NACNEP) and the Council on Graduate Medical Education (COGME) for the first time ever to conduct a study on the integrated requirements for physicians, APNs, and physician assistants (PAs) for providing primary care services to the U.S. population. This landmark work, which provides a model for projecting needs and the mix of providers, clearly demonstrates the role of APNs in the workforce into the next century (Vector Research Inc., 1995). Promoting health and positive lifestyle strategies is an ideal fit for nurses, who generally have superior skills in these areas. In addition to the APNs who practice in primary care settings, the CNS and the nurse case manager can well address the specialized needs of persons with chronic illnesses, both at home and in hospital settings. Thus, APNs should have little difficulty in carving out an important role as the new system emerges, but they will need to carefully monitor and direct practice definition and regulation.

INFLUENCE OF THE MANAGED CARE SYSTEM

The national health-care reform debate that began with the Clinton administration has served as a catalyst for change at both the state and the local levels as well as in Congress. There is a definite movement toward capitated systems of care (providers are prepaid for caring for a population of patients) that will require that nurses understand, to a much higher degree, how much it costs to diagnose and manage a patient or family per visit. The onus will be on educators to prepare students who can clearly articulate to employers, partners, and insurers how much it costs them to provide care to a group of patients. An APN needs to clearly understand many issues. For example: how much does a well-child examination cost? Are there specific diagnostic tests that need to be done? What does a routine visit cost for an elderly diabetic with hypertension? —a new visit for a healthy prenatal client? —anesthesia for minor out-patient procedures? —particular nursing interventions for the chronically ill? These questions and a myriad of others about operational expenses and overhead costs are on the minds of all APNs as the system of care changes in the United States. The role of the APN in these policy discussions, which will shape health-care delivery and reimbursement, cannot be underestimated.

In 1994, Peter Buerhaus, Director of the Harvard Nursing Research Institute, outlined four critical issues that nurses facing managed competition need to address. First, APNs must realize the depth of opportunities for APNs in fee-for-service, prepaid markets and proceed appropriately into these markets. Second, as part of that effort, APNs must ensure that the minimum package of benefits includes APN services. Third, any managed care system must meet both the clinical and economic interests of APNs. Fourth, Buerhaus suggested that nurses must make sure that the turmoil does not detract from the value of nursing services (Buerhaus, 1994).

How APNs will fit into managed care systems is a critical issue for nurses. It will be incumbent upon APNs to know how to contract for their services at the individual level as they negotiate an employment package but, even more importantly, they need to be present at the negotiation table where the rules for managed care systems are made. This means that APNs must position themselves visibly on executive boards and committees and to be included as members of management teams who are setting the policies for managed care provider services.

The times have been positive for APNs to showcase their practices and to be seen as viable alternatives to physician-based health care. This increased visibility makes it imperative that APNs monitor the competencies of their own practices.

Recent acts of Congress that have cut federal programs for the poor will augment the need for APNs while they reduce funds for health care and increase the stress placed on the health problems of the underserved. The American Nurses Association's (ANA's) *Nursing's Agenda for Health Care Reform* (American Nurses Association, 1991) has lasted well in the health-care reform debate and continues to be an important reference for APNs who want to better understand how to improve access and reduce cost. Nursing's agenda is a prevention-driven, managed-care approach that conserves resources. It includes several themes: universal access to health care, emphasis on primary and preventive care, shared consumer and provider accountability for health-care decision-making, and holistic health-care services that emphasize affordable quality.

FUNDING FOR NURSING EDUCATION

The risk of lowering quality and competence as nursing struggles to prepare large numbers of APNs for the work force rapidly and with too few faculty is a serious concern. A recent survey by the National Organization of Nurse Practitioner Faculties (NONPF) showed that the number of institutions offering NP programs increased by 50% between 1992 and 1994. Additionally, the number of ANP tracks within graduate nursing programs has increased even faster, from 227 programs in 1992 to 370 in 1994. This unprecedented rise in ANP education puts a serious strain on funding, faculty, and clinical settings (Harper & Johnson, 1995).

Funding for all of nursing education continues to be a major issue for nurses at the policy table. In the past, nursing looked almost exclusively to the Health and Human Services (HHS) Division of Nursing for training dollars for nurse education rather than looking toward patient revenues, even though nurses are the largest group of health caregivers (Helms, Anderson, & Robnett, 1994). The current policy of funding graduate medical education with Medicare pass-through dollars to academic health centers and to community-based health facilities is critical to the education of APNs. Negotiation for funding that is already in the legislative framework as well as for new funding will be critical if APNs are to play a significant role in the provision of health care in the next decade (Towers, 1995). These issues are currently and continually before Congress, and it will fall to APNs to carry the banner for these initiatives at the policy table and in the legislative arena.

National health priorities, based on health-care reform principles and Healthy People 2000 objectives, include access to care for everyone, a healthier population, and a move to a community-based, prevention-driven system of health care—a less costly system that does not lessen quality. These priorities also include health care for special high-risk aggregates, including the homeless, victims of AIDS, pregnant teenagers, and the elderly poor. These priorities will be difficult to address. Because APNs play a major provider role for these special populations, APNs need to be active participants in policy initiatives.

APN POLICY ISSUES IN THE CURRENT HEALTH-CARE SYSTEM

COLLABORATION VERSUS AUTHORITY FOR NURSING PRACTICE

Nursing's earliest efforts to establish professional identity for APNs focused on advancing education as well as gaining independence over nursing practice and autonomy from the medical community. These efforts were critical to the evolution of advanced practice in nursing, and great strides have been made over the years. The reality of the complex health-care system and the needs of a patient population that requires a multifaceted approach to multiple problems stress interdisciplinary team-building. This does not imply "parallel play" or working side by side but requires a true blending of nursing and medical models to offer a comprehensive health-care approach. Larger teams of health-care providers will collaborate to provide comprehensive care to families and whole communities. However, to be able to move forward as full-fledged team members in cooperation with other interdisciplinary health-care providers, APNs will need to shift their practice ideal from one of complete autonomy to a truly collegial interdisciplinary paradigm. A change is necessary. Does any health-care professional, including the most renowned vascular surgeon, practice with full independence? Or does this surgeon call upon the internist, the CNS, and the physical therapist to assist with providing competent and expert care? Will APNs do themselves a disservice if they maintain an isolationist stance based on barriers and past professional turf issues? Have APNs reached a point in their evolution at which they can feel comfortable as peers and colleagues with providers in other disciplines?

The real issue is not that APNs see themselves as needing to practice in a vacuum of independence apart from the health-care team. It is the hard fact that APNs must have authority over their own practices and the decisions they make about patient care. Only in this way can APNs move out of the darkness of being, as Wilcox stated, a "shadow provider" (Wilcox, 1995). This is the challenge for APNs across the nation who are working to clarify statutory policies within state boards of nursing. It may be that APNs will feel comfortable only when their position within the health-care community is fully secure in all states, and this will require serious political and legislative work.

SCOPE OF PRACTICE FOR APNs

Scope-of-practice issues are key to the debate about how the U.S. health-care system uses APNs as health-care providers and are inextricably tied to issues of barriers to practice. The ability to diagnose and manage clients independently and in collaboration with a physician colleague is inherent to the role of the APN. Each ANP role has a defined scope of practice, which may be fluid and evolving. Accountability becomes a crucial factor as APNs move toward authority over their own practice. It is important that scope-of-practice statements, which are portrayed in the chapters on direct care, identify the scope of each ANP role. It is important that scope-of-practice statements that are presented by national certifying entities are carried through in scope-of-practice language in state statutes.

APNs owe Barbara Safriet, Associate Dean at Yale Law School, a debt of gratitude for her clear vision and clarity in helping APNs understand and strategize about scope-of-practice and regulatory issues. Safriet (1992) noted that APNs are unique in that there is a multiprofessional approach to their regulation—based on ignorance and the fallacy that medicine is all-knowing and knows all about advanced nursing practice. Restraints result from ignorance about APN abilities, rigid notions about professional roles, and turf protection.

> States have used a variety of approaches to extend the scope of practice of nursing. Some have revised their Nurse Practice Acts (NPAs) to delete the absolute prohibition on diagnosis and treatment, or to add "nursing diagnosis." Some have added an "additional acts" clause to the NPA, authorizing some specially trained nurses to "perform acts of medical diagnosis and treatment" as specified by rules of the state nursing and/or medical boards or as "agreed upon by the professions of nursing and medicine." Some have added a generic category, or specific categories, of advanced practice nurses and have either defined their scope of practice or have authorized state nursing and/or medical boards to promulgate rules that do so. Some have revised their Medical Practice Acts (MPAs) to authorize physicians to "delegate" diagnosis and treatment tasks to nurses who have the necessary additional training."

(Safriet, 1992, pp. 445–446)

Safriet makes the case for a single statutory designation of APN, leaving any subsequent regulation and professional designations to individual boards of nursing and the national nursing specialty associations. She likens this statutory definition of APN to the generic term of physician, which includes all doctors. Further, as interdisciplinary models for care develop, it will be clear that each profession must regulate its own practitioners.

Safriet's insightful monograph makes the point that if APNs are competent enough to serve unsupervised in rural and underserved areas, they are certainly competent to practice in urban areas while supervised. If licensure means minimum competence to perform licensed activity, it should mean the same thing throughout the geographic boundaries of the state, as is the case for physicians.

LEGAL CONCERNS SURROUNDING ADVANCED NURSING PRACTICE

There are several reasons why the multiplicity of titles and roles for APNs is a problem from a policy viewpoint. The first and foremost reason is that it is confusing to policymakers and regulators. It is especially a problem at agencies such as the Health Care Financing Agency (HCFA), where major designations for Medicare and Medicaid reimbursement set the standard for all reimbursement across the country. In addition, discrepancies among states make mobility difficult for APNs in terms of prescriptive authority and reimbursement.

APNs are primarily responsible to and are disciplined by individual state boards of nursing. One of the licensing and credentialing difficulties faced by APNs is the variance in board regulations from state to state. In some states APN practice is governed solely by the board of nursing; in others it is jointly administered by the boards of nursing and medicine; and in still others it is governed by the board of pharmacy. In many states CNMs are answerable to nurse-midwifery boards that are attached to boards of medicine. CNSs who are not in prescribing roles may be governed solely by the board of nursing. Although the written protocol delegating medical acts that is co-signed by a physician preceptor is not as prevalent as it was in the 1980s, it is still the norm in some states, predominantly in the South.

As APNs move in and out of what is considered the domain of medicine, serious thought must be given to the standard by which APNs will be judged if they are deemed to have made an error. Although there are not many documented cases citing APNs who have injured patients by wrongful actions, the question about whether APNs should be tried by the courts using medical standards or nursing standards is important and needs to be clarified. It is incumbent upon APNs to set clear standards for practice that are based on clinical competency. CNMs and CRNAs are currently furthest along in this process.

CREDENTIALING ISSUES IN ADVANCED NURSING PRACTICE

It is important to differentiate which master's-prepared and nationally certified nurses are included within the title of APN. The ANA's definition requires that the role be clinically focused and that the APN give direct clinical care to patients. Using this definition, four groups make up advanced practice nursing: NPs in primary and acute care, CNMs, CRNAs, and CNSs. APN case managers are in transition to be included in these groups. This designation is primarily driven by which nurses are reimbursable and which nurses desire prescriptive and admitting privileges. The reason for this clear definition is that there must be an efficacious way for state boards to monitor the prescribing and reimbursement patterns of APNs. There must be a "count" that can be validated in order to assure patient safety and to monitor proper certification and credentialing.

The issue surrounding the credentialing of APNs has been difficult since its inception. There is ongoing tension between national certifying bodies and state regulators, as well as among bodies who accredit educational programs. CRNA and CNM certification and credentialing have been the most clearly uniform and standardized from the start, and these groups have structures in place that make credentialing at the state level unclouded and understandable. Because NPs have been prepared at either the graduate or the certificate level, it is difficult to set an across-the-board standard for certifying and credentialing NPs. Also, the issues surrounding CNS credentialing are fraught with confusion, because currently advanced-level certification examinations do not exist in all CNS specialties and all CNSs do not desire prescriptive or admitting privileges (Table 22–1).

Currently, the certification and credentialing of NPs is undergoing serious perusal because of a request by the National Council of State Boards of Nursing (NCSBN). The member state boards of nursing find it difficult to determine NP eligibility for state recognition because of the varied educational and certification routes that NPs can take to become APNs. In August 1995, the NCSBN Delegate Forum and the national certifying groups agreed to a one-year time frame to review and standardize the examinations. At the same time, the NONPF and the National League for Nursing (NLN) were charged with the task of developing a model for NP education program approval that would be endorsed by NP educators and regulators and that could be used to establish nationwide eligibility to sit for national certification. This task included a consideration for the articulation of non-master's-degree NP programs within the model.

Graduate programs in nursing and related fields that prepare APNs must be accredited as educationally sound, with appropriate content for the specialty and adequate clinical hours. The NLN accredits graduate programs in the nursing major but currently does not deal with the approval of specialty ANP content. The NONPF

TABLE 22–1. ANP NATIONAL CERTIFICATION BODIES

ANP Group	
CRNA	American Association of Nurse Anesthetists Council on Certification
CNM	American College of Nurse-Midwives Certification Council (ACC)
NP	American Nurses Credentialing Center (ANCC)
	American Academy of Nurse Practitioners (AANP)
	National Certification Board of Pediatric Nurse Practitioners and Nurses (NCBPNP/N)
	National Certification Corporation for the Obstetric, Gynecologic and Neonatal Nursing Specialties (NCC)
CNS	American Nurses Credentialing Center (ANCC)*
	Oncology Nursing Society (ONS)
Case manager	Interim Commission for Certified Case Managers (ICCCM) inter-disciplinary credential†

*Each CNS specialty has its own certification; some are at the master's level.
†Discussion is underway at the American Nurses Credentialing Center for the development of a master's level nurse case manager certification examination.

provides curriculum guidelines, program standards, and competencies to assist NP programs in this task. Furthermore, the national bodies for CNMs and CRNAs publish standards for their specialty education. Given the increased numbers of ANP programs in a variety of nursing specialties, the work being done to standardize education for APNs is of major importance. The proposed standardization of certification examinations and the approval of the NP educational programs would greatly assist state boards of nursing in their role of recognizing and regulating NPs for practice.

From a legal and regulatory standpoint, clear statutes are needed that offer broad practice standards to allow for mobility across state lines. This change will require national standards of practice as well as certification and credentialing requirements that can satisfy many different jurisdictions—not an easy task! These standards will require diligent collaboration between educators, state boards of nursing, the specialty professional associations, and all practicing APNs (Hanson, 1993). Part of the professional agenda that APNs need to address is the need for accountability and responsibility for competence in practice. As a professional group, APNs must build strong national standards of practice, scope, and skills. Experienced practitioners need to help peers gain greater competence and new skills. It is important that APNs not lose sight of the need to support each other and to mentor colleagues as the practice arena broadens.

CONSTRAINTS ON ADVANCED NURSING PRACTICE

The issues surrounding reimbursement, including lockout from managed-care groups, prescriptive authority, and admitting privileges, are usually perceived as the major constraints to advanced nursing practice. The American College of Physicians (1994) agreed and cited three issues that are central to expanding the roles of APNs in the health-care system—prescriptive authority, reimbursement, and legal scope of professional practice. These barriers, along with physician resistance, preclude the freedom to practice one's trade. State legislation and regulation discourage APNs from seeking employment even if jobs are otherwise available. As long as APNs offer cost-effective alternative care, there will be increased competition between medicine and nursing (Hanson, 1993; Safriet, 1992).

According to Sekscenski and coworkers (1994), states such as Illinois, Ohio, and Oklahoma, which have less favorable practice environments, have fewer such practitioners. This study analyzed variation in the regulation of NPs, PAs, and CNMs in all 50 states and the District of Columbia. The initial constraints to nurse-midwives were based on safety concerns with midwives in terms of the delivery of healthy infants and on the notion that CNMs provided second-class care. These charges have clearly been refuted by research. However, invisible constraints continue, such as liability surcharges and the inability to obtain consultation and referral for clients—restraints built on perceived threats to physician practice (Ernst, 1995).

There are many clear and direct restrictions on the scope of practice for APNs. The ones that come to mind most often are those that require formal practice arrangements with physicians—for example, written protocols, collaboration guidelines, and agreements outlining physician supervision. Furthermore, any rules requiring that APNs be restricted to care for certain populations, such as homeless or rural persons, in order to prescribe or to be reimbursed are clearly constraints to practice to the fullest extent of one's capabilities. Safriet (1992) warned that bias occurs when one profession regulates another, for even if the legislature supports advanced nursing practice, restrictions in the form of narrow rules and regulations, such as direct supervision or geographic boundaries, limit APN practice. Safriet (1992, p. 452) proposed that

> *requiring ongoing supervision mandates life-long apprenticeship. No matter how skilled the APN or how unskilled the physician, oversight is statutorily imposed as a condition of competence for APN practice. It allows for another profession to assess competence for the licensed practice of a professional from another discipline.*

PRESCRIPTIVE AUTHORITY

NPs and CNMs have been allowed at least some limited form of prescriptive authority since the mid-1970s. The latest documentation about the status of prescriptive authority for APNs was presented in the January 1996 issue of *Nurse Practitioner*. Pearson's latest yearly synopsis of state-to-state advanced nursing prescribing patterns notes that 44 states have some level of prescribing capabilities, although the degree of authorization varies widely. Several types of restrictions based on setting, protocol, and restricted formularies continue to limit APNs from prescribing within their education and practice capabilities (Pearson, 1996). A recent American College of Physicians survey showed that in 43 states, NPs have some level of prescriptive authority, and that 22 states grant statutory independent prescribing authority to NPs, although 7 exclude controlled substances. In some states, such as Texas, prescribing permission is restricted to areas of health-care shortage. In 8 states NPs must seek additional training to gain prescriptive privileges (American College of Physicians, 1994). To drive the point home, Safriet (1992) challenged that the question is not whether APN providers can and do prescribe but rather whether the state will acknowledge and authorize the prescriptive privilege. Again, Safriet's work is of enormous help to APNs as she lays out straightforward policy questions that APNs need to answer when trying to resolve prescribing barriers (Table 22–2). These questions offer important insight to APNs who are planning to seek positive legislative and regulatory change in state prescribing laws for APNs.

As noted, a major concern relative to the prescribing practices of APNs is the wide variance in the way prescribing rules and regulations are promulgated from

TABLE 22–2. QUESTIONS FOR POLICY DECISION
TO DETERMINE WHO CAN PRESCRIBE . . .

Which providers will be authorized to prescribe?
What drugs and devices may they prescribe?
What extent of authority conferred—independent vs. supervision?
In what setting, geographically, must the individual prescribe?
Who regulates APN practice—which state agency?—board of nursing?
What qualifications are needed, in addition to RN licensure and certification?

From Safriet, B. J. (1992). Health care dollars and regulatory sense: The role of advanced practice nursing. *Yale Journal of Regulation, 9*(2), 417–487.

state to state. Some states use drug formularies, which define classification of drugs or specific drugs that nurses can legally prescribe; in other states APNs have complete prescriptive authority within their nursing licensure; still other states use a specific written protocol clearly outlining the drug- and setting-specific requirements; and still others use practice agreements. Many states limit prescriptive privilege to master's-degree-prepared nurses. State-to-state mobility is greatly affected by the differences and nuances of law in each case. It is important that APNs who are moving to a new state are well informed of the prescriptive authority guidelines for APNs in that given state. Chapter 25 offers further insight into prescriptive authority concerns for APNs seeking to practice in settings that require the ability to prescribe therapeutics.

REQUIRED PHARMACOLOGY EDUCATION

State boards of nursing need to clearly document the numbers of hours of pharmacology required for one to receive and maintain prescriptive privileges in terms of both educational programs and year-to-year continuing education. Advanced nursing programs, which previously integrated pharmacological content within clinical management courses, have moved toward separate defined pharmacology courses in order to comply with recent state requirements for a designated amount of pharmacology in advanced nursing education. Further, pharmacology content should be taught by faculty pharmacists or nurse/pharmacists who have an in-depth knowledge of therapeutic prescribing. Some states are currently requiring that specific course and content hours be verifiable in order to be used in an application for prescriptive authority. Furthermore, several states require documentation of the number of hours of continuing education for pharmacology per year or per cycle. The direction is clearly to require APNs to attend ongoing continuing education in pharmacology in order to maintain prescriptive privileges. Therefore, states will need to move toward contracting with universities or other educational providers to offer timely continuing educational offerings and over-distance learning modalities (e.g., interactive television) in order to meet the needs of isolated rural clinicians. Over time, the states will most likely move in the direction of interdisciplinary pharmacology education for both nurses and physicians.

REIMBURSEMENT ISSUES

On a par with the need to be able to prescribe medications for patients is the need to be appropriately reimbursed for care. Clearly, APNs must be paid for services rendered for health care whether they work independently, share a joint practice with a physician colleague, or are employed within a managed-care system or independent hospital. Although the individual states regulate the insurance industry, many of the private-pay insurance standards that are used to set payment mechanisms are modeled after federal Medicaid and Medicare policy. Federal mandates that encourage direct payment of non-physician health-care providers are often blocked at the state level by discriminating rules and regulations. Many third-party reimbursers, including some major insurance companies, are now reimbursing NPs directly. Others are not. As states move into managed care and large purchasing groups in which APNs are providing care as part of interdisciplinary teams, reimbursement is becoming more readily available. For a detailed description of specific reimbursers for health care see Chapter 25.

Federal policy via the Omnibus Budget Reconciliation Act (OBRA) 89 mandated Medicaid reimbursement for NPs. Pearson reported that by 1994 all states except the District of Columbia and Ohio reimbursed NPs for Medicaid patients (of these states, 37 reimburse at 80 to 100% of the physician Medicaid rate). These 37 states allow for third-party reimbursement that extends beyond Medicaid for APNs within state statute. It must be remembered that Medicaid is a shared program between federal and state government, and therefore the states individually determine reimbursement for APNs within state statute (Pearson, 1996).

CNMs succeeded much earlier than NPs did in getting third-party reimbursement, and by federal designation earn 65% of the physician fee. Medicaid funding for CNMs, which historically covered only obstetrical services, has recently been extended to cover gynecological services and family planning. CNMs were diligent in their legislative activism to achieve this Congressional policy change within the Medicaid system, which would expand their practice with women. CRNAs have carried out long-term legislative activity to receive equal payment for anesthesia services and should realize this goal in 1996. The reimbursement status for CNSs is setting- and task-specific. New legislation allows the CNS to reauthorize nursing home care and be reimbursed for care in rural areas; psychiatric/mental health CNSs can bill for mental health services. There has been a concerted effort by nurse lobbyists to include the CNS in legislative language that is proposed for APN reimbursement.

Medicare and Medicaid set the reimbursement standards for payment in this country. APNs have made great advances over the past 20 years in this area. The Omnibus Budget Reconciliation Act (OBRA) 90, the Rural Health Act, mandates payment directly to NPs, CNSs, and CNMs for their services in rural settings (see Chapter 25 for details). Expanding this coverage to include APNs in urban areas is a major thrust on the nursing policy agenda. Further, with regard to federal Medicaid policy, the HCFA recently extended to states the ability "to tailor the definitions to meet their individual needs," so that states control the level at which APNs are reimbursed. The federal requirement is that payment is consistent with economic indicators and quality of care. States have broad discretion in determining both fee levels and payment methodology for Medicaid. This is an important nuance and one that has caused vast discrepancy in reimbursement from state to state.

One of the ways that Medicare and Medicaid standards are set is through a Physician Payment Review Committee (PPRC), which uses a rating formula to place a value on physician tasks, overhead, and liability and malpractice costs. In 1992, Congress required the PPRC to review the tasks of non-physician providers, including APNs, in order to determine fair and equitable payment schemes. Interestingly, the PPRC chose to disregard educational costs when figuring payment schedules for physicians and then brought it back in when basing fees for non-physician providers. Safriet advised that without the differential for education built into the formula, there is not a need to differentiate payment and service; thus, there should be equal pay for equal service (Safriet, 1992).

Payment for APN services has long been controversial. The argument continues about whether nurses should be paid the same fee for service or be paid only a percentage of the physician payment. This is always a negotiable issue, and there is disagreement within medicine and nursing alike. It is difficult for nurse lobbyists who represent many types of APNs from several specialties to negotiate fair and equitable reimbursement that meets the needs of everyone. It has long been the norm for Medicare and Medicaid payers to only reimburse APNs who work with rural or high-risk underserved populations, not to reimburse all APNs. Reversing this inequity was a major effort at nursing policy tables during health-care reform and continues to be a priority policy issue.

The rules for Medicare are somewhat different from Medicaid rules and are more stringently tied to settings and special populations. In 1990 the HCFA extended payment for NP and CNS services in skilled nursing facilities. However, these payments are paid directly to employers with the stipulation that the APN work collaboratively with a physician. The Rural Nursing Incentive Act of 1991 went further by authorizing *direct* reimbursement to all NPs and CNSs practicing in designated rural areas. APNs employed in skilled nursing facilities and those under contract in HMOs are only paid incident to, i.e., as part of, physician services.

Payment by private insurers is contract-specific and varies with each state's insurance commission. The current climate of large-scale mergers between major private insurance companies to accommodate large managed-care structures has important relevance for APN reimbursement. It is critical that APNs position themselves to sit on policy-making boards for private enterprise. A prime example comes from the 1980s, a time when NPs lost their liability coverage nationally. NPs working through the National Alliance of Nurse Practitioners by negotiation and education gained access to the executive board at Mitchell, Cotterell, and Fifer as part of an advisement group. This activity cemented a long-term relationship that has brought a clear understanding about the practice of NPs and a newsletter for risk management with this major liability carrier (Hanson, 1985).

There is another key issue with regard to reimbursement for APNs. It should be noted that in managed-care contracts the level of reimbursement is immaterial. APNs and all other providers must deliver care at a fixed pre-set price; this can be an advantage if APNs are less costly to employ. Thus, it becomes critical for APNs to fully understand how much it costs them to provide care for patients with a variety of preventive, episodic, and chronic health problems and to be able to articulate to contractors that they are competitive in the marketplace.

Policy issues surrounding the reimbursement of APNs require careful reflection before strategies to remove constraints to payment are undertaken. Several important questions should be considered when shaping policy. For example, what services do APNs want to be paid for? Are they different from physician services or the same? Are there specific nursing services that need to be reimbursed? Is direct payment the issue or does it matter who gets the payment? Will the payment level be the same or lower than physicians receive for equivalent service? These are important questions because, in most states, APNs historically have been reimbursed indirectly, "incident to" physicians and at a considerably lower rate. It is advantageous for APNs who are planning to practice clinically, no matter what the setting or physician relationship, to seek counsel about the reimbursement realities in their state before beginning to care for patients.

PRACTICE PRIVILEGES

The need for hospital privileges for APNs varies according to the nurse's practice. For example, CNMs and many NPs cannot properly care for patients without the ability to admit to the hospital should the need arise. On the other hand, case managers are employed by the hospital and have no need for admitting privileges. CRNAs and some NPs have not needed to admit patients to the hospital independently in order to give comprehensive care but may need to see patients in the emergency room.

The rules for admitting patients to a hospital service are even more specific and variable than those for prescriptive authority and are bound to the local hospital or medical facility and the medical staff of the granting institution. APNs need to prepare their portfolio, gain the support of their collaborating physicians, and apply to the hospital or agency for privileges. Dialogue between the hospital administration, physician staff, and other stakeholders such as APN colleagues and other team members is necessary if admitting privileges are required for the desired practice role. Alliances with consumers offer added support to the application. In most hospitals, professional privileges are granted by a committee made up of physicians and administrators. An important step is to seek out the administrator responsible for the privileges committee and find out the procedure for application. Nursing administrators are often members of these committees, and the APN should meet with nurse colleagues for advice prior to the application process.

Some hospitals have specific guides and protocols for all non-physician providers; others do not. The determination of the specific privileges desired is critical to the process. For example, is it necessary to be able to admit or discharge patients; write orders; do particular procedures; visit in-hospital patients; or take an emergency room call? Many hospitals have different levels of hospital privilege, ranging from "full" to modified privilege, for specific functions. Asking for full privileges may not be prudent or useful in a particular setting.

It is important to remember that the attainment of hospital privileges is often a professional turf issue and fraught with political overtones. The task of overcoming this barrier to practice requires astute planning and careful attention to the "cast of characters" and set policies of the institution.

APN STRATEGIES FOR DEALING WITH LEGISLATIVE AND POLITICAL SYSTEMS

GENERAL POLITICAL STRATEGIES

In the current political climate it is critical that the professional posture of every APN be carefully thought out. It is imperative that APNs become unified as never before. APNs must develop a strategic plan for lasting unity that will provide political clout into the next century. APNs have come a long way in developing their political acumen at both state and national levels and have considerable power to achieve positive change if they capitalize on their newfound status and move forward in the right direction.

An important cohesiveness within nursing has emerged in response to health-care reform. The nursing profession, as a whole, is beginning to recognize its strength at the policy table. As far back as 1984, Nancy Milio cautioned that nurses must be prepared to forge alliances, do their homework, and bring their case before the public, and she predicted that it will be APNs who carry the message forward (Milio, 1984). More than 10 years later, Towers (1995, p. 44) cautioned the same thing. "It is clear that the contribution that nursing makes in the health-care arena must be brought forward. Nurses need to be heard, their data must be shared, their leadership enhanced. Nurses must take responsibility for education and communicating with legislators." Politics and ethics are inherent in relationships at all systems levels and most obviously in policy development. Therefore, nursing's ethical stance on social mandates that support poor and underserved populations needs to be clearly articulated (Aroskar, 1987). APNs have a responsibility to bring their views and perspectives to decision-making and policy forums. They need to turn competitors into partners to make change toward a more interdisciplinary system.

Professional turf issues have plagued APNs since the early days of their clinical practice. A lack of legal empowerment to practice to the fullest extent of knowledge and skills has been a dominant barrier to the optimal practice of NPs (Dempster, 1994). CNMs and CRNAs have the longest track record in dealing with these issues and have many successes to their credit. Health-care reform and managed-care dialogue have caused physicians and other important health-care stakeholders to retrench, which has heightened the perception of APNs as a threat. This has made the current political arena extremely sensitive.

BARRIER-SPECIFIC STRATEGIES

The political agenda that is carried out at the professional level (ANA/AMA) and between APN specialty organizations is much different from the agenda played out at the grass-roots level. There is strong evidence that locally practicing physicians and nurses have strong collaborative relationships and that they are frustrated by the lack of cohesion at the professional level at which policy is made. APNs must closely monitor policy issues through phone trees, newsletters, and regional meetings. There is no question that an important strategy for the removal of barriers is to enlist the grass-roots support of physician and nurse teams who are practicing successfully in a collegial manner.

APNs must launch strong grass-roots efforts to bring about positive policy changes in individual states. One strategy to assist in the improvement of practice environments for advanced practice is to create local networks of APNs within state structures that will help to remove barriers and develop workable practice guidelines. Close interaction with local collaborating physicians and leaders of local health-care entities is crucial. States that have made the greatest strides in removing practice barriers need to help states that have more serious constraints to advanced nursing practice.

Safriet's seminal monograph proposes several change directives that will require total commitment of all APN groups if present practice constraints are to be removed. Because many of the barriers facing APNs are embodied in statute and regulation, they are directly amenable to legislative reform. All of these directives require close interaction between state boards of nursing and the current regulators of APNs. Table 22–3 outlines changes needed in state statutes to remove constraints to advanced nursing practice.

There are a myriad of recent textbooks on the market, as well as a plethora of journal articles, that deal with the issue of grooming APNs with political savvy and know-how to circumvent the land mines of political and legislative action. Most of these resources are well-targeted toward helping the nurse gain confidence and expertise as a policymaker. The Additional Readings at the end of this chapter list some of these resources. It is recommended that all APNs, as part of their basic graduate program and through continued seminars and workshops, take advantage of these tools of the trade. Nurses have a formidable voting power base of over 2.2 million. This is an incredible strength for nurses but requires cohesiveness within the ranks in order to make positive change for advanced nursing practice. The notion that someone else will carry the flag is not realistic. Developing political

TABLE 22–3. CHANGES NEEDED IN STATE
STATUTES TO REMOVE PRACTICE CONSTRAINTS

- Eliminate all references to mixed regulator entities (i.e., regulation of APNs by more than one discipline)
- Vest sole governmental authority over APNs with the Board of Nursing
- Broaden Nurse Practice Acts to include specific knowledge about APNs and the basic definition of an APN but *not* specific categories of APN providers
- Use no qualifying language for diagnosis and treatment
- Empower boards of nursing to promulgate rules for APNs
- Eliminate statutory requirements for supervision
- Enact nondiscrimination clauses to reform Medicaid and Medicare
- Remove geographic and setting barriers to APN care

From Safriet, B. J. (1992). Health care dollars and regulatory sense: The role of advanced practice nursing. *Yale Journal or Regulation, 9*(2), 417–487.

acumen and competence is a required skill for all practicing APNs that is nurtured during graduate school under the direction of faculty policy advocates.

The following list offered by Lescavage (1995) is a good place for the individual APN to begin developing policy skills:

- Take part in the numerous fellowships and internships in Washington, D. C. and in one's own state
- Inform lawmakers of APNs' changing goals, ambitions, and needs
- Become a lobbyist—only 10 of 20,000 staffers are nurses
- Gain appointments to local, state, and national boards, commissions, task-forces, and cabinets
- Champion causes such as the elderly, teen pregnancy, violence, and AIDS
- Support nursing organizations and lobby for their interests
- Write letters and editorials
- Work on a campaign or, better still, become a candidate
- Be a strong voice in professional organizations
- *Most important*—develop political allies in Congress—move at once to address APN issues surrounding regulation, limitations on admitting privileges, limitations to prescriptive authority, and managed care

The need to be well educated and informed about issues is paramount to success. Furthermore, leaving behind clear and concise written material is a must. Legislators and their staff deal with many legislative issues concurrently, and it is critical to have any important documents at their disposal at all times. The information highway at the Capitol in Washington D. C. and each state house is developing rapidly. E-mail accounts are now the norm, and it is easy to FAX a one-page message within the hour. Voice mail makes it possible to leave a personal message with key staffers or the legislator. The Internet gives APNs the ability to track legislation within committees from hour to hour. This is an exciting time to be active in the policy arena, but the unbelievably fast pace requires a high level of commitment in order to stay informed.

The ANA devotes a great deal of effort in training nurses to become competent legislative activists, either through grass-roots lobbying within their home community or through direct face-to-face interaction with paid lobbyists on Capitol Hill. The *ANA Grassroots Lobbying Handbook* is useful in helping nurses to use their practice experience in the form of a story to legislators to make a request. There are also excellent data on the use of fact sheets, using statistics appropriately, and dealing with the media (deVries & Vanderbuilt, 1993). National APN organizations should follow the direction of the AMA public relations team and furnish state groups with position papers and talking points to be distributed by APNs throughout the state (Buppert, 1995).

Nurses have been criticized "on the Hill" for not being team players and for being self-serving in their quest for a piece of the action. It is important to be well informed about other issues that may affect health-care legislation or may be important to other stakeholders. Judi Buckalew, the first nurse to be appointed as a Special Assistant to the President of the United States, suggested that "the rule of thumb for having influence in Washington circles is to play both sides of the aisle. This is just smart politics. No matter who is currently in power, you should divide your energy and power evenly" (Pearson, 1987, p. 54). Playing a visible role in policy directives for the special populations that nurses serve is one way to do this. For example, working on policy agendas that support families, women, children, persons with AIDS, and rural elderly persons all indirectly offer an entrée into care given by nurses and APNs and thus into policy issues that deal with APN education and practice.

FUTURE-CASTING: WHERE DO APNs GO FROM HERE?

The current status of education and practice for APNs can really be voiced in a slight alteration of Dickens' words: "these are the best of times, these are the worst of times." APNs have realized their dream of providing care to diverse populations in a multitude of settings. The market for APN practice is generally favorable; jobs are plentiful; salaries are up. However, along with the good is the reality that nursing is in the spotlight. Other health-care stakeholders are following nursing's moves. It is an important time for competence and support for clear and useful regulation of advanced practice. It is also a time of partnerships. The whole persona of health care comes from a managed-care perspective, with team effort and interdisciplinary models the norm.

The future of APNs will be built on their ability to be even more politically astute and savvy into the 21st century. APNs will need to take an active role in their own destiny if barriers are to be removed. There will be an accelerated need for internal cohesion within advanced nursing practice, both at the grass-roots level and at the professional association level.

Health-care reform has served as a catalyst to move advanced nursing practice forward. The winners of the future are going to be cost-efficient systems of care that are driven by prevention. To this end, interdisciplinary health-care team practices will give APNs the supportive environment they need to practice at their highest level of excellence. Collaborative practice is one key to eradicating reimbursement and prescriptive authority barriers for APNs. A breakthrough in this area is the proposal by the American College of Physicians for programming that emphasizes team approaches to care (American College of Physicians, 1994). However, it is clear that APNs will need to closely monitor how collaboration is defined and implemented. APN leaders need to work closely with other disciplines and managed-care entities to develop new models for interdisciplinary practice.

As APNs move forward, it will be critically important that they be able to work collaboratively within the discipline of nursing to develop a gold standard of education and practice with standardized competencies and certifications based on clear education and practice outcomes. As new clinical roles emerge, it will of major importance to be able to embrace them within the structure of ever-evolving advanced practice.

The future will see collaboration and teamwork rather than competition. This will forge new partnerships and new alliances that have never before been considered. As expensive acute-care services begin to contract and consolidate, lower-cost community-based primary care and preventive services, including nurse-midwifery and birthing centers, will expand (Ernst, 1995).

Two things are certain: change will continue to come rapidly within health care at local, state, and federal levels, and APNs will be on the cutting edge of this change. The ability to work with policymakers and regulators will be key to the advancement of advanced nursing practice.

REFERENCES

Aiken, L. H., & Salmon, M. E. (1994). Health care workforce priorities: What should nursing do now? *Inquiry, 31* (fall), 318-328.

American College of Physicians (1994). Physician assistants and nurse practitioners. *Annals of Internal Medicine, 21,* 714-716.

American Nurses Association (1991). *Nursing's agenda for health care reform.* Washington, D. C.: American Nurses Association.

Aroskar, M. A. (1987). The interface of ethics and politics in nursing. *Nursing Outlook, 35,* 268-272.

Brown, S. A., & Grimes, D. E. (1993). Nurse practitioners and certified nurse midwives: A meta-analysis of studies on nurse primary care roles. Washington. D. C.: American Nurses Association.

Buerhaus, P. I. (1994). Managed competition and critical issues facing nurses. *Nursing and Health Care, 15,* 22-26.

Buppert, C. K. (1995). Justifying nurse practitioner existence: Hard facts to hard figures. *The Nurse Practitioner: The American Journal of Primary Health Care, 20*(8), 43-44, 46-48.

Dempster, J. S. (1994). Autonomy: A professional issue of concern for nurse practitioners. *Nurse Practitioner Forum, 5,* 227-232.

deVries, C. M., & Vanderbuilt, M. W. (1993). *The grassroots lobbying handbook: Empowering nurses through legislative and political action.* Washington, D. C.: American Nurses Association.

Ernst, E. K. (1995). Nurse midwifery: a nursing challenge. In J. C. McCloskey & H. K. Grace (Eds.), *Current issues in nursing* (pp. 241-247). St. Louis: C. V. Mosby.

Hamric, A. B., & Spross, J. A. (1989). *The clinical nurse specialist in theory and practice.* Philadelphia: W. B. Saunders.

Hanson, C. M. (1993). Our role in health care reform: Collegiality counts. *American Journal of Nursing, 93*(12), 16a-16e.

Hanson, C. M. (1985). *National Alliance of Nurse Practitioners.* Statesboro, GA: Personal Archives.

Harper, D. C., & Johnson, J. J. (1995). *NONPF workforce policy project: Trends in nurse practitioner programs.* W. K. Kellogg Foundation. NONPF Grant Office, George Mason University, Fairfax, VA.

Helms, L. B., Anderson, M. A., & Robnett, M. (1994). Funding for nursing education under Medicare: A window of opportunity. *Nursing & Health Care, 15,* 344-349.

Jennings, C., & Towers, J. (1994). Interview: Donna Shalala, Secretary, U.S. Department of Health and Human Services. *Journal of the American Academy of Nurse Practitioners, 6,* 409-412.

Lescavage, N. J. (1995). Nurses make your presence felt: Taking off the rose colored glasses. *Nursing Policy Forum, 1*(1), 18-21.

Milio, N. (1984). The realities of policymaking: Can nurses have an impact? *The Journal of Nursing Administration, 14*(3), 18-23.

Office of Technology Assessment, U.S. Congress, HCS37 (1986). *Nurse practitioners, physician assistants, and certified nurse midwives: A policy analysis.* OTA-HCS-37. Washington, D. C.: Government Printing Office.

Office of Technology Assessment, U.S. Congress, 483 (1990). *Health care in rural America.* OTA-H-434. Washington, D. C.: Government Printing Office.

Pearson, L. (1987). Judi Buckalew: Learning to play political hardball. *The Nurse Practitioner: The American Journal of Primary Health Care, 12*(1), 49-50, 52, 54.

Pearson, L. (1996). Annual update of how each state stands on legislative issues affecting advanced nursing practice: A survey of legal authority, reimbursement status, and prescriptive authority. *The Nurse Practitioner: The American Journal of Primary Health Care, 21,* 10–70.

Rentmeester, K., & Kindig, D. A. (1994). *Physician*

supply by specialty in managed care organizations. Madison, WI: School of Medicine, University of Wisconsin.

Safriet, B. J. (1992). Health care dollars and regulatory sense: The role of advanced practice nursing. *Yale Journal of Regulation, 9,* 417-487.

Sekscenski, E. S., Sansom, S., Bazell, C., Salmon, M. E., & Mullen, F., (1994). State practice environments and the supply of physician assistants, nurse practitioners, and certified nurse midwives. *The New England Journal of Medicine, 331,* 1266-1271.

Towers, J. (1995). A call to action: the GNE-GME-NEA debate. *Nursing Policy Forum, 1*(1), 40-45.

Vector Research Inc. (1995). Development of integrated requirements for PAs, NPs, CNMs, and physicians (MDs and DOs). HRSA Contract number 240-94-0033, U.S. Government, Bureau of Health Professions.

Wilcox, P. (1995, April). Advanced practice model response to needs of women at risk for female malignancies (Abstract Presentation), Oncology Nurses Society National Conference, Anaheim, CA.

Wysocki, S. (1995). *NANFPRH fact sheet.* Washington, D. C.: National Association of Nurses in Family Planning and Reproductive Health.

Additional Readings in Health Policy and Politics

Aiken, T. D. (1994). *Legal, ethical, and political issues in nursing.* Philadelphia: F. A. Davis.

Bagwell, M., & Clements, S. (1985). *A political handbook for health professionals.* Boston: Little, Brown.

Foster, S. D., & Jordan, L. M. (1994). *Professional aspects of nurse anesthesia practice.* Philadelphia: F. A. Davis.

Goldwater, M., & Zusy, M. J. (1990). *Prescription for nurses: Effective political action.* St. Louis: C. V. Mosby.

Harrington, C., & Estes, C. L. (Eds.) (1994). *Health policy and nursing: Crisis and reform in the U.S. health care delivery system.* Boston: Jones & Bartlett.

Johnstone, M. J. (1994). *Nursing and the injustices of the law.* Philadelphia: W. B. Saunders/Baillière Tindall.

Lee, P. R., & Estes, C. L. (Eds.) (1994). *The nation's health* (4th ed.). Boston: Jones & Bartlett.

Mason, D. J., & Talbott, S. W. (1985). *Political action handbook for nurses: Changing the workplace, government, organizations, and community.* Menlo Park, CA: Addison-Wesley.

Sharp, N. (1993). The path of legislation: best opportunities for nurses' input. *Nursing Management, 24*(9), 28, 30, 32.

Starfield, B. (1992). *Primary care: Concept, evaluation, and policy.* New York: Oxford University Press.

Strickland, O. L., & Fishman, D. J. (1994). *Nursing issues in the 90's.* Albany, NY: Delmar Publishers.

Wood, S. H., & Ransom, V. J. (1994). The 1990's, a decade of change in women's health care policy. *Journal of Obstetric, Gynecologic, and Neonatal Nursing, 23*(2), 139-143.

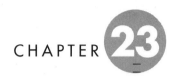

CHAPTER 23

Developing Markets for Advanced Nursing Practice

Susan E. Davis Doughty

HEALTH CARE AS A BUSINESS: A CALL TO ACTION FOR ADVANCED PRACTICE NURSES

Advanced nursing practice has roots in response to consumer demand. Nurse-midwives (CNMs) answered a call for safe birthing. Nurse anesthetists (CRNAs) practiced long before the field of anesthesiology evolved. Clinical nurse specialists (CNSs) responded to a need for expert practitioners at the nurse-patient interface. And nurse practitioners (NPs) grew out of the health-care crisis of the 1960s to provide increased access to patient care services. Today, health care and illness care are driven by market forces, and it is a serious problem that many Americans cannot access or afford health services. Advanced practice nurses (APNs) can help solve this problem if they understand marketing concepts and use marketing strategies. APNs who cannot get beyond an aversion toward marketing will be left behind. This chapter outlines marketing concepts and strategies, delineates marketable properties of APNs, itemizes barriers to effective marketing, and helps the APN to develop a personal market portfolio.

KEY MARKETING CONCEPTS

Marketing is anything and everything APNs do to promote their practice. Marketing differs from advertising in that advertising is a small part of marketing. Advertising has a bad reputation that it is focused, often in an annoying way, on materialism. Almost no one believes advertising's claims, yet it persists because it works. Curtin (1985) says, "Information is the coin to the realm, media its trading place, and advertising its medium." She suggests that nurses must let go of the notion that advertising is not done by respectable health-care professionals and recognize that it can be done honestly if incorporated into a marketing strategy that allows both the nurse and the consumer to win.

Good marketing is designed to educate others about nursing and sell a service from a position of strength (Caveen, Cheshire, Power, and Woolley, 1992). Johnson (1985) defines marketing as "professionally presenting the positive image you would like to convey to the other person or group." It is important for APNs to take a position regarding marketing as it relates to the provision of health care today. APNs cannot afford to be passive. Nursing values and information oriented toward the well-being and goals of the client can support ethical marketing. Responses to competition for finite health-care resources include the myriad of health-care marketing seminars advertised, hiring of health-care marketing consultants by agencies, and the development of marketing positions by most health-care organizations. In the past, nursing's values have not embraced marketing. Yet developing marketing skills and markets for advanced nursing practice could literally determine the survival of APNs. Always remember the 7-Up "Uncola" and the Avis "we try harder" positioning success stories. APNs can position themselves as the unique provider of certain services so that consumers automatically think of the APN when they seek that service (Smithing & Wiley, 1989a). Examples of marketing niches for APNs can be found in Table 23–1.

Marketing concepts focus on satisfying the needs and desires of consumers. An important marketing concept is that of organizing information about client needs through a marketing survey using two components: service differentia-

TABLE 23–1. EXAMPLES OF MARKETING NICHES FOR ADVANCED PRACTICE NURSES

Adolescent GYN, autonomous or part of another practice	Mammography, breast health counseling
AIDS practice	Medical, nursing, health-care writing
Architectural consultant	Menopause center
Birthing center	Nurse case manager
Breast-feeding counseling, products	Pacemaker center
Brokering services (e.g., elder care)	Pain management
Chronic illness management	Occupational health/workers' compensation consultant
Corporate health consultant	Practice bridging two disciplines
Day care consultant	Practice in mobile van
Diabetic management	Product development: pharmaceutical, toys, personal care, therapeutic devices
Elder care	Psychiatric counseling
Employee cost-containment programs	Radio/TV/media consultant
Environmental consultant	Retirement center
Ethics consultant	Risk management consultant
Family counseling	Same day surgery center
Health policy consultant	School/college health
Health promotion	Stress management consultant
HMO/PPO gatekeeper	Women's health
Homeless shelter	YMCA/YWCA/Boys'/Girls' club
Correctional health care	

tion—that is, identifying aspects of a service valued by clients yet unmatched by competitors—and market segmentation, or dividing clients into groups according to factors that influence selection and use of services (Luckacs, 1984). Service differentiation for an NP survey might include gathering data for a group of people about preferred location, hours of service, or availability of follow-up care. Market segmentation data in the survey might include population, sex, density, age, gender, socioeconomic status, and benefits sought. Graduate curricula for APNs include many skills necessary to function in our changing culture, such as high-level communication and negotiation skills, relationship and teamwork skills, stress management, and mental health skills (James, 1994). As options for health-care services expand, the ability to understand and respond to aspects of service most valued by clients gives APNs a competitive edge (Luckacs, 1984).

Key marketing concepts for advanced nursing practice are to:

- Educate
- Generate income
- Develop support
- Meet existing but unmet client needs
- Make health problems visible

It is helpful for the APN to remember that people usually will not appreciate what a professional does unless they are educated to the facts (Abraham, 1994). People want to know more about unique services. Yet potential employers may have no concept of the expertise APNs could bring to their businesses or practices and would never advertise for one (Weill, Love, Pron, Tesoro, Grey, Hickel, Teti, & Serota, 1989). In fact, once employers work with APNs, they often wonder how they ever got along without one. APNs have many strengths that increase their marketability, and these strengths are rooted in basic nursing practice.

MARKETABLE PROPERTIES OF APNs

Areas of growth in nursing are to be found at the edges of traditional practice. The evolution of health care helps APNs identify areas in which to expand. A new paradigm for care involving the APN at its core demands letting go of old paradigms in which APNs only talk to other nurses or limit professional and educational contacts to the area of specialty. It requires forging unique collaborations among disciplines to create networks and establish partnerships (Shoultz, Hatcher, & Hurrell, 1992) (see Chapter 11). It also includes reading in the economic, political, and marketing literature outside of nursing to learn about issues and strategies.

Realistic self-appraisal of marketable skills is essential, not only for APNs who lose jobs or move to a new area but for all APNs in the current health-care environment. APNs cannot develop markets and sell themselves if they do not clearly recognize their unique skills and how these skills can meet client needs. Such an appraisal also helps APNs to determine what areas of practice need to be developed in order to better position themselves for the marketplace.

In addition to developing the ability to cross settings such as in-patient, out-patient, or home care, research has found certain areas well suited for APN services (Fugate & Tinsley, 1981):

- Coordinating individual or family health needs
- Delivery of more flexible care
- Provision of less expensive care
- Delivery of more personal attention during the encounter
- Provision of health education and counseling

Health-care reform efforts should be seen as opportunities for creating models for innovative services. It is estimated that 85% of all existing job opportunities are not advertised (Ciocci, 1984). Questions that might help APNs identify opportunities for applying these unique skills might include:

1. What motivates me in my practice?
2. What do I do best in my practice?
3. Where do I get the most satisfaction in my practice?
4. What am I most proud of about my practice?
5. Do I have a skill a consumer or organization would pay for?
6. How might I attract a consumer or organization to pay for my skills?

Richard Bolles has written prolifically about how an individual can determine the best fit in a career and then how to market oneself to attain that goal (Bolles, 1990, 1994). Individuals are instructed to formulate a picture of their ideal job by identifying the specific wants and needs that allow them to flourish (Bolles, 1990). By learning how to identify strengths, such as favorite transferable skills, favorite tasks, favorite people with whom to work, and favorite kinds of information with which to work, the APN can identify the unique services they have to offer. This author's experience illustrates the concept of the importance of fit.

> *I was prepared as a clinical nurse specialist in critical care nursing*
> *with a master's degree in medical surgical nursing in 1975. I found a*
> *great deal of satisfaction establishing a nurse managed center for*
> *patients with pacemakers. I marketed the concept to the hospital*

> *administrators, and it became an excellent revenue source as well as a*
> *marketing source for the hospital (Doughty, 1989). Because work with*
> *pacemaker patients demanded more primary care skills than I learned*
> *in my graduate program, I completed an additional year in the adult*
> *and aging NP track in graduate school. After moving to Maine in 1983,*
> *positions for CNSs were at a minimum. I took a position as a Director*
> *of Critical Care Nursing at a tertiary center and employed a new*
> *repertoire of management skills in this position. However, I missed*
> *direct patient care, and after 4 years as a nurse executive, I realized I*
> *was more creative and satisfied when working directly with patients. I*
> *stated an intention to return to the clinical area and started to identify*
> *what I loved to do. I saw myself listening to my pacemaker patients'*
> *stories and helping them solve problems and create a healthy lifestyle.*
> *Within 1 month I received three job offers. One was as an NP in a*
> *holistic OB-GYN practice with another NP and three gynecologists. The*
> *notion of listening to women's stories and helping them create health*
> *appealed to me to the extent that I volunteered in a family planning*
> *clinic to reactivate my GYN skills. I left my executive position and built*
> *a practice at the holistic center. Today, most of my practice is with*
> *perimenopausal and menopausal women, and I experience a great*
> *deal of satisfaction with what I do. I marketed myself through*
> *community lectures and groups for menopausal women as well as in*
> *newsletter articles and radio interviews, emphasizing my unique*
> *contributions to the public as alternative ways to create health through*
> *menopause. I continue to market myself and our holistic menopause*
> *program through public speaking, interviews, brochures, business*
> *cards, office stationary, legislative lobbying for increased advanced*
> *practice opportunities, and networking with colleagues. I consistently*
> *educate my patients about what an NP is, and refer to myself as an NP*
> *when addressing individuals or groups.*

Levin (1993) wrote of the experience of developing a solo practice born out of the idea that what was needed was not more health care but an alternative type of health care for women that was different from the existing medical model in her community. She identified the specific strengths she possessed that would enable her to succeed. These strengths included self-confidence, comfort in dealing with other health-care providers as colleagues, accountability, enjoyment in marketing herself to the lay and medical communities, flexibility, and patience. She attributed her success to her business plan, which included advantages over the competition, and the uniqueness or her nursing-based practice.

Mimi Secor, NP, nurse entrepreneur, articulated early in her evolving NP practice that to succeed she needed to create a niche for herself in the health-care delivery system. She knew she had to do the "usual unusually well or do the unusual" (Bramble, 1991). Secor developed a women's health-care practice that included holistic personalized care and capitalized on a new market as well: fitting cervical caps for contraception. Ongoing marketing was a top priority as she spoke on radio and television shows and to all types of groups. As she hired new NPs, she expected them to market themselves as well.

Evidence from nursing research (Smithing & Wiley, 1989b) indicates that a family NP's marketing message should emphasize:

- Compatibility of services with personal and family norms
- Advantages of services for this particular group
- Health education capabilities of the family NP
- Training and experience of the family NP
- Unique qualities and position in the health-care system of the family NP
- Clear image of the family NP's scope of practice, enhancing the potential of partnership between the consumer and the family NP based on informed choice

BARRIERS TO EFFECTIVE MARKETING OF APNs

Certain overriding issues need to be overcome if marketing for APN services is to be successful. One such obstacle is the image of the nurse as handmaiden to physicians. The media has perpetuated this image of nurses as mindless maidens preoccupied with sexuality (Kalisch & Kalisch, 1980). Some nurses have spoken out, most have not. The public needs to be oriented toward the concepts of nurses functioning in many settings; promoting health, and diagnosing and treating common illness; delivering anesthesia and providing pain management; providing safe prenatal, obstetrical, and postpartum care as well as brokering services for the elderly or chronically ill. It also includes consulting with architects, environmentalists, and health policy writers; and managing nurse-managed centers for those in menopause or with diabetes mellitus. The American Nurses Association (ANA) as well as many of the specialty organizations for APNs have developed public relations videotapes and brochures that help obliterate the old paradigm of handmaiden and that present a more realistic picture of current advanced nursing practice. Baker and Pulcini (1990) wrote that APNs have taken the status quo and re-evaluated, adopted, and re-configured it to form new patterns of practice that identify new ways of interacting with the health-care system, the consumer, and each other.

Although all of this may be true about APNs, much of their public does not know it. Kalisch and Kalisch in 1978 did a content analysis of 3,098 newspaper articles about the treatment of clinical nursing news and found that the quality varied by specialty. Maternity and pediatric nursing was seen as more progressive than community health and medical surgical nursing. Psychiatric nursing had a low level of coverage. They recommended that nursing specialties work with the media to improve their image, that the public be informed that the primary role of the nurse is to promote health and not just serve as handmaiden to the physician, and that nurses are knowledgeable and accountable as well as sympathetic caregivers (Kalisch & Kalisch, 1981). As we move toward the turn of the century, the classic works of these authors remind us that the media has the power to shape the public image and can be a powerful force for change, correction, and action. This is aptly demonstrated by the *Washington Post* on a daily basis. Citing their research since the mid-1970s, the Kalisches remind us that greater attention to the quality of public information about nursing is needed.

Physician dominance in the health-care market has proven to be an obstacle to effective marketing for APNs. Fear of encroachment and lack of understanding about what APNs are educated to do has caused some physicians to attempt to block legislation permitting nurses to practice within their scope. As health-care reform has evolved to over-ride state laws that prohibit APNs from practicing, the barrier of the medical profession itself has become more evident, and the American public has been exposed to "negative marketing." The American Medical Association (AMA) conducted an expensive campaign to convince the public that the quality of health care would be compromised if APNs were "allowed" to provide primary care. The California Medical Association's Political Action Committee distributed posters that showed ducks with stethoscopes quacking messages about non-physician practitioner groups "fowling" up health care by lowering licensing requirements and broadening scopes of practice. In their attempt to discredit APNs and claim ultimate medical responsibility, they revealed a paternalistic attitude that touted the medical establishment's singular ability to be the judge of what constitutes quality health care for the American people (Giordano, 1994). Disseminating misleading information is unethical, an example of negative marketing. The nursing profession had a choice as to how to respond, and in the past might have ignored the smear campaign because it could only reflect on the smearers. The media, however, is powerful in presenting a position, and Virginia Trotter Betts, RN, JD, ANA president, used the opportunity to market APNs' safety records. She responded to the AMA board by pointing out how their accusations against their nurse colleagues were inaccurate and ill-advised in the face of the desperate need for primary health care for all Americans. She did not confine her rebuttal to correspondence with the AMA, but also took her message to the popular press: *The Wall Street Journal* and *USA Today*. Much of marketing is education, and because the AMA claimed that there would be more than enough primary care physicians if the public would just fund their education, it was important for the nursing profession to point out that APNs, working collaboratively with physicians, can provide primary care at times less expensively and sometimes more effectively than physicians alone (Curtin, 1993).

Although the ANA speaks for APNs at the national level, APNs have the responsibility to market themselves at the state and local levels by educating physicians and consumers about what they are equipped to do. It is crucial that APNs support their medical colleagues who value the role of APNs and who refuse to participate in the AMA's campaign to discredit them. It is important to delineate major differences in practice scope and the range of services that nurses and physicians are prepared to provide (DeAngelis, 1994). APNs must educate each other and the public to ensure that the appropriate provider is in place for the most efficient use of that provider's skill, and that appropriate outcomes exist for the client. They also must write to their state and federal representatives and visit them, educating them about nursing's role in health-care reform. There are ANA and other professional services to assist in this process. When one says the word "doctor," everyone knows what is being talked about. The terms nurse-midwife and nurse anesthetist are also clear. But when one says "advanced practice nurse" or "nurse practitioner" or "clinical nurse specialist," many confusing images come to mind unless one has been educated about the role. The media are biased toward physicians, and the more the APNs can educate the consumer about APNs and their unique capabilities, the more effectively they will be able to practice (Smithing and Wiley, 1990a).

A controversial role that has emerged as physician residency positions are deleted is the role of the acute care NP (see Chapter 16). There is a viable argument for "replacing" critical care residents with NPs at the same salary without costs for rotation or turnover (Edmunds, 1991; Keane, Richmond, & Kaiser, 1994). Support for institutional policies, loyalty to the institution, and continuity of care provided by the NP benefit the institution, and the NP typically enjoys the level of skill and responsibility demanded. Graduate programs in nursing to prepare critical care APNs are evolving (Clochesy, Daly, Idemoto, Steel, & Fitzpatrick, 1994), and the success of the role will depend on assertive APNs who insist on practicing nursing rather than medical tasks that the attending physicians don't want to do. In addition, these nurses must command a salary commensurate with their responsibilities (Dracup & Bryan-Brown, 1994; Edmunds & Ruta, 1991). An alternative way to frame this issue that would market acute care APNs is to persuade the institution to put acute care residents who remain in the ICU under the auspices of the department of nursing, so that nursing would control the hospital stay. Entrepreneurial critical care APNs could gather data justifying this concept in terms of benefit to the client and the institution, and APNs could work along with residents, each providing the service that they are best prepared to provide.

As health care evolves, more barriers to effective marketing for APNs will arise. Every profession is requiring creative courage directly proportional to the degree of change the profession is experiencing (Baker & Pulcini, 1990). This implies a willingness to go beyond conventional thinking and to perceive barriers as opportunities to rise to the challenge of placing APNs exactly where the client needs their services. Rosabeth Moss Kantor acknowledges the innovative spirit associated with a way of approaching problems that she calls "integrative" or "a willingness to move beyond received wisdom to combine ideas from unconnected sources, and to embrace change as an opportunity to test limits" (Kantor, 1985).

MARKETING STRATEGIES: MARKETING ONESELF

Critical self-assessment of strengths as well as conceptualizing a desired practice arena are essential first steps in developing a marketing plan. Developing a marketing portfolio is a useful strategy to aid the process. A portfolio differs from a résumé or curriculum vitae in that, in addition to a listing of all previous positions and educational background, a depository for information is developed, much like an artist's portfolio. This portfolio contains a description of skills in a way that provides impressive information to prospective employers, grant writers, or lending institutions so that they might quickly evaluate preparation and fit for a position (Edmunds, 1980) (Table 23–2). When a specific position arises that an APN desires, the APN chooses from the portfolio those promotional tools that best relate to that position, such as a résumé listing previous positions and responsibilities, a curriculum vitae listing academic experience and achievements, articles written by the APN, letters of recommendation from former employers, client and colleague recommendations, credit history, honors, awards, or ideas for research projects.

An APN might also find it useful to include, in a portfolio, information that helps differentiate between what physicians do and what APNs do. Many studies have been published that describe role differentiation and how primary care, for example, differs when provided by an APN (Diers & Molde, 1982; Kassirer, 1994; Safreit, 1992; Scanland, 1990; Weiss, 1983). Professional organizations such as the ANA, the American Academy of Nurse Practitioners, the American College of Nurse Practitioners, the Oncology Nursing Society, the American College of Nurse-Midwifery,

TABLE 23–2. COMPONENTS OF A MARKETING PORTFOLIO FOR APNs

	Scope	**Focus**	**Length**	**Purpose**
Biography	Credentials and experience	Prepares for presentation	One page only	Introduction for presentation
Resume	Work history	Work results	One to two pages (bullets)	Listing how APN made a difference in work setting
Curriculum vitae	• Credentials • Scholarly works • Honors • Publications	Academic communications	Three to five plus pages	Listing of academic accomplishments
Portfolio	Supporting documents of accomplishments	Determined by outcome sought, e.g., grant or position	Varies, multiple documents	Marketing the APN
Video tapes*	Demonstration of skills, expertise	Determined by position sought	30 to 60 minutes	Marketing APN skills to potential partners, employers

*Increasingly, individuals are using video tapes to market themselves. Focus should be on skills that match the position sought. The more professional the product, the better the outcome.

and the American Association of Nurse Anesthetists distribute fact sheets or brochures about advantages of working with particular APNs that might be a useful addition to a marketing portfolio. The purpose of the portfolio is to provide a place for all information about the APN that will serve as a data bank from which the APN can build a current document to convince others of what the APN has to offer.

EXTERNAL AND INTERNAL MARKETING

Two facets of marketing might be useful ways to clarify a business plan: external marketing and internal marketing. External marketing refers to all the techniques that APNs might use to promote themselves or their practice to their consumers or the public at large, such as speaking at community meetings, circulating business cards, writing a column in the newspaper, advertising in the yellow pages, or sending out fliers or brochures about the practice. Internal marketing involves differentiating the unique capabilities of APNs in their practice environment and showing how what they have to offer is different from that provided by anyone else, whether it is of higher quality, more complex, more accessible, or less expensive (Brunk, 1992). Internal marketing is of particular importance to the CNS, whose role is often re-evaluated in the face of budget constraints and position cuts. CNSs have discovered that in order to survive in the current market, they need to be creative in marketing to underserved facilities both within and outside of the institution and to serve as a revenue source for their employer. Hoffman and Fonteyn (1986) see marketing as the key answer to the threat of survival of the CNS role.

Nolan and colleagues studied the marketing strategies of NPs in New York state in the mid-1980s. She and her colleagues believed that in order for APNs to survive the increasing competition in the marketplace, they must use marketing techniques. In the study, 285 NPs (only 19%) responded, and most answered "no" to 10 of 12 marketing strategies listed (Table 23–3). The most common strategy used was verbal identification as an NP at each client visit as well as on the phone. The researchers found that the NP respondents were similar in both demographics and educational preparation. Responses were significantly different if the practitioner had attended a workshop on marketing strategies or if the practitioner had practiced for more than 3 years (Nolan, Conway, Litteer, Peterson-Sweeney, Richardson, Smith, and Stoler, 1988).

In a survey of the marketing activities of 12,000 NPs conducted by the American Academy of Nurse Practitioners (Towers, 1990), only 5,964 responded. Less than half of those responding reported that they marketed themselves; those in rural areas marketed themselves most, those in inner city areas the least. Of those who did market themselves, over 50% used pamphlets. Yellow pages and newspaper advertising were used by less than half of all respondents. A third of all NPs, the highest percentage, had special referral arrangements as a marketing strategy. If, as nurses, we hesitate to promote ourselves, the price we pay is confusion about who we are and what we have to offer, even among ourselves (Nolan et al., 1988).

Scanland (1990) described an excellent example of marketing oneself. She sought a new work environment that provided more flexibility, learning, and growth opportunities and a setting in which she could use both her expertise in geriatrics and her NP skills. She targeted a family practice residency program in the area and gathered data on the gap between the needs of the elderly in that area and the supply of physician services. She contacted the program director and convinced him to hire her to conduct both a clinical practice and resident geriatric education program by matching information from her survey with that from her portfolio.

Another important component of marketing oneself is to pay attention to how the APN is "packaged"—that is, personal attire, personality, self-assurance, professionalism, image—qualities that establish role credibility (Ball, 1990; Smithing & Wiley, 1990b; Stahler-Miller, 1987). When an APN carefully develops a reputation for accessibility, flexibility, and professional demeanor, respect from peers and colleagues follows (Gardner & Weinrauch, 1988).

TABLE 23–3. SELF-TEST—MARKETING STRATEGIES QUESTIONNAIRE

1. Is your name on the door?
2. Do you have a professional listing in the phone book?
3. Do you use business cards?
4. Is your name on office stationery?
5. Do you use pamphlets to explain the role of the primary care practitioner (PCP)?
6. Do you have hospital practice privileges?
7. Have you ever talked to a community group about the role of the PCP?
8. Have you ever talked to a consumer group about services provided by the PCP?
9. Have you ever conducted a needs assessment?
10. Do you introduce yourself as a PCP over the phone?
11. Do you introduce yourself as a PCP at the beginning of the office visit?
12. Have you contacted other health professionals about your role?

Reprinted with permission from "Marketing Strategies of Nurse Practitioners in New York State" by Nolan, Conway, Litteer, et al, August, 1988, edition of *The Nurse Practitioner,* © 1988, Springhouse Corporation.

NEGOTIATING A CONTRACT

Negotiating a contract is an important marketing skill. One of the political-economic realities of the current health-care environment is that there is resistance to recognizing APNs as legitimate providers of care. A contract, written with the expertise of a personal contract attorney, helps the APN to clarify all parameters of a position, including a clause that outlines requirements for ending a professional relationship. When contracting with a health-care institution, APNs should ensure that practice privileges are clearly outlined in the contract to protect the APN-client relationship if the client needs to be admitted to the institution. The contract will vary according to the nature of individual APN practice, but the goal of negotiating a contract is always to protect the APN through outlining expectations, objectives, and the nature of relationships with whom the contract is being formed.

The goal of managed care is to increase pressure on providers to provide more services for less reimbursement (Levin, 1993). When participating in managed care, a contract is essential to clarify commitments of a position. Managed care contracts with providers include an agreement for the APN to provide certain kinds of services for a company, such as pre-employment histories and physical examinations. Provision of education to employees of a company may or may not include the employee's family members and should be clarified by the contract. APNs who work in a health maintenance organization (HMO) have been eliminated by the HMO simply because a large managed care contract refused to recognize the NP as a legitimate provider of care (Baker & Pulcini, 1990). A well-written contract protecting the APN in such a contingency would have prevented the elimination of the role.

An important aspect of professional development also includes making an informal contract with yourself. It is to the APN's advantage to at least review objectives quarterly to determine if he or she is moving along the career path as anticipated and to recommit to the most important criteria of ongoing personal satisfaction in a position. A critical component of this contract includes the balance of the physical, intellectual, emotional, and spiritual quadrants and reviewing whether the position is consuming an unbalanced amount of energy. In that case, neither the APN nor the client benefits.

MARKETING STRATEGIES: MARKETING A SERVICE

Eighty percent of all new products fail in the open market (Gardner & Weinrauch, 1988). Survival of small business depends on several critical factors (Gardner & Weinrauch, 1988):

- Accurate identification of consumer needs
- Financial resources
- Timing of entry into the workplace
- Planning for growth to meet further demands

Accentuation of how a proposed service differs from that provided by others is important. These services include such things as higher quality, more accessibility, or different hours of service. Services targeted toward specific market segmentation data, such as retirement centers, hospital staff, individuals living with chronic pain, or new mothers needing breast-feeding counseling, help the APN to tailor a marketing plan for success based on client need.

Communicating a service is a matter of letting others know about its uniqueness. It is helpful to gather data on how clients discovered that service in order to be able to put future energy and resources into what is known to be successful. Brochures, articles in the newspaper, newsletters, letterhead stationery, business cards, flyers, personal interviews with the media, and group community classes, all help promote a unique service. Yellow pages advertising is expensive, so it is wise to routinely audit how often clients use the yellow pages to initiate contact. Groups such as Rotary, American Association of Retired Persons, American Association of University Women, Junior League, and Kiwanis often invite speakers to address health topics. These opportunities allow the APN not only to promote a service but to clarify misinformation about APNs. Joining professional and civic organizations is an important part of marketing a service as well, and the opportunity to sit on a board of directors or a health-related committee does much to enhance one's professional reputation.

Presenting oneself to the medical community is an important marketing strategy in promoting a service. Having self-confidence about one's skills and knowing one's particular areas of expertise and limits help to communicate a willingness for collaboration. It is important to lay a strong foundation about competency and abilities. Inaccurate reports about NPs taking away paying patients as well as the underinsured are common as well as unsupported accounts of practice errors and poor management of client problems. Successful APN-MD collaboration helps alleviate such fears (see Chapter 11). When one is outlining possible benefits to physicians for including the APN in their referral network, it is important to stress unique areas of expertise: prevention, counseling, education, and the ability to see patients with special, time-consuming needs.

It is important to use every opportunity to remind clients that they are receiving good care because APNs are uniquely prepared to provide this care. Also remember that the office staff who have contact with the public assist the APN in this process by having a critical understanding of the APN's uniqueness and skills and sharing them with the public. When the APN places confidence in a pharmaceutical product, it is helpful to let the sales representative know the difference between what an APN does and what a physician does and to ask to have APNs included as a provider in their patient-oriented brochures. To constantly see the word "doctor," such as "see your doctor with any questions," sends a distinct message to potential clients, health policy decision-makers, and legislators (Smithing & Wiley, 1990a). And finally, a critically important endorsement for the nursing profession is for the APN to be sure to use an APN for personal as well as for family care.

COMMON MARKETING MISTAKES

It is estimated that the biggest obstacle to future viability of the APN's role is lack of consumer awareness and minimal demand for preventive services as a result of inadequate marketing by APN's (Weill et al., 1989). An understanding of this notion, a strong belief in oneself and in the APN role, and a strong understanding of one's own APN philosophy are critical to reversing this tend and enhancing marketing time and energy. When marketing a service, it is important to avoid the common marketing mistakes provided by Abraham (1994).

Research shows that APNs increase their use of marketing strategies after attending a marketing workshop (Nolan et al., 1988). Graduate education would

---

COMMON MARKETING MISTAKES

1. Failure to audit which particular strategies provide the best return (Calmelat, 1993)
2. Failure to continuously ascertain and develop unique services
3. Failure to differentiate from the competition
4. Failure to give clients a reason to return for repeat services
5. Failure to address clients' needs as a priority
6. Failure to educate clients about any changes made, such as an increase in prices
7. Failure to enjoy providing the service

---

do well to incorporate marketing techniques into the curriculum of APNs. Many programs are already providing marketing strategies for students.

Research also indicates that consumers would seek out APN services if they were covered by health insurance and were less costly than covered physician care (Shamansky, Schilling, & Holbrook, 1985). The APN has the perfect opportunity to secure a permanent place in the health-care market in the next century. Being willing to expand into uncharted regions within the scope of advanced nursing practice and the ability to enter into truly collegial relationships with physicians and other professionals are essential to success. Self-directed and self-employed APNs who are in autonomous and accountable positions legitimize the APN as a provider of health care.

CONCLUSION

Marketing oneself and one's services is critical to the survival of APNs and might well influence the future of the nursing profession itself. As the health-care environment changes, clients are becoming sophisticated about what they want as well as about what they need. APNs must become familiar enough with marketing concepts and be flexible enough so that they can position themselves to meet client needs. As a result of successful marketing strategies, clients will not only request APNs, they will demand their services, recognizing the value they receive in the ever-expanding and complex world of health care.

REFERENCES

Abraham, J. (1994). *The Abraham experience*. Rolling Hills Estates, CA: Citation Publishing Group, Inc.

Baker, M. M., & Pulcini, J. A. (1990). Innovation: Nurse practitioners as entrepreneurs. *Nurse Practitioner Forum, 1*(3), 169-174.

Ball, G. B. (1990). Perspectives on developing, marketing, and implementing a new clinical specialist position. *Clinical Nurse Specialist, 4*(1), 33-36.

Bolles, R. N. (1990). *How to create a picture of your ideal job or next career*. Berkeley, CA: Ten Speed Press.

Bolles, R. N. (1994). *What color is your parachute?* Walnut Creek, CA: Ten Speed Press.

Bramble, K. (1991). Mimi Secor: Nurse practitioner entrepreneur. *Nurse Practitioner Forum, 2*(3), 142-143.

Brunk, Q. (1992). The clinical nurse specialist as an external consultant: A framework for practice. *Clinical Nurse Specialist, 6*(1), 2-4.

Calmelat, A. (1993). Tips for starting your own nurse practitioner practice. *Nurse Practitioner, 18*(4), 58, 61, 64, 67-68.

Caveen, W., Cheshire, L., Power, B., & Woolley, D. (1992). Grasping the marketing nettle: A professional development course for nurse practitioners in stoma care. *Professional Nurse, 7*(9), 580, 582, 584-585.

Ciocci, G. (1984). Capitalizing on the hidden job market. *Nurse Practitioner, 9*(12), 31-33.

Clochesy, J. M., Daly, B. J., Idemoto, B. K., Steel, J., & Fitzpatrick, J. J. (1994). Preparing advanced practice nurses for acute care. *American Journal of Critical Care, 3*(4), 255-259.

Curtin, L. (1985). Survival of the slickest. *Nursing Management, 16*(2), 7-8.

Curtin, L. (1993). Barbarians at the gate. *Nursing Management, 24*(12), 9-10.

DeAngelis, C. D. (1994). Nurse practitioner redux. *Journal of the American Medical Association, 271*(11), 868-871.

Diers, D., & Molde, S. (1982). Nurses in primary care. The new gatekeepers? *American Journal of Nursing, 82*(5), 742-745.

Doughty, S. (1989). The CNS in a nurse managed center. In A. Hamric & J. Spross (Eds.), *The CNS in theory and practice.* Philadelphia: WB Saunders, 415-434.

Dracup, K., & Bryan-Brown, C. (1994). The advanced practice nurse in critical care: Yes or no? *American Journal of Critical Care, 3*(31), 163.

Edmunds, M. (1980). Developing a marketing portfolio. *Nurse Practitioner, 5*(3), 41.

Edmunds, M. W. (1991). After 26 years, it's time for "NP" to be a household name. *Nurse Practitioner, 16*(11), 59.

Edmunds, M. W., & Ruta, M. V. (1991). NPs who replace physicians: Role expansion or exploitation? *Nurse Practitioner, 16*(9), 46, 49.

Fugate, D., & Tinsley, D. (1981). Marketing position and promotion for the medical nurse practitioner. *Journal of Health Care Marketing, I*, 8-14.

Gardner, K., & Weinrauch, D. (1988). Marketing strategies for nurse entrepreneurs. *Nurse Practitioner, 13*(5), 46, 48-9.

Giordano, B. P. (1994). Watch out for "friendly fire" from our medical allies! *AORN Journal, 59*(2), 360, 362.

Hoffman, S. E., & Fonteyn, M. E. (1986). Marketing the clinical nurse specialist. *Nursing Economics, 4*(3), 140-144.

James, J. (1994). *Building a twenty-first century mind.* Speech before AACN 1994 NTI. Atlanta, GA.

Johnson, S. H. (1985). *Marketing: Strategies for success.* Workshop, Boston, March 14.

Kalisch, P. A., & Kalisch, B. J. (1980). Perspectives on improving nursing's public image. *Nursing and Health Care, 1*(1), 10-15.

Kalisch, P. A., & Kalisch, B. J. (1981). Communicating clinical nursing issues through the newspaper. *Nursing Research, 30*(3), 132-138.

Kantor, R. M. (1985). Innovation—The only hope for times ahead? *Nursing Economics, 3*, 178-182.

Kassirer, J. P. (1994). What role for nurse practitioners in primary care? *New England Journal of Medicine, 330*(3), 204-205.

Keane, A., Richmond, T., & Kaiser, L. (1994). Critical care nurse practitioner: Evolutions of the advanced practice role. *American Journal of Critical Care, 3*(3), 232-237.

Levin, T. E. (1993). The solo nurse practitioner: A private practice model. *Nurse Practitioner Forum, 4*(3), 158-164.

Luckacs, J. L. (1984). Marketing strategies for competitive advantage. *Nurse Practitioner, 9*(9), 37, 38, 40.

Nolan, C. M., Conway, L. G., Litteer, T. B., Peterson-Sweeney, K., Richardson, K., Smith, S. W., Stoler, Paula M. (1988). Marketing strategies of nurse practitioners in New York State. *Nurse Practitioner, 13*(8), 37, 41-42.

Safreit, B. J. (1992). Health care dollars and regulatory sense: The role of advanced practice nursing. *Yale Journal on Regulation, 9*(2), 417-487.

Scanland, S. (1990). What's happening: The nurse teaches the doc. *Journal of the American Academy of Nurse Practitioners, 2*(4), 174-177.

Shamansky, S. L., Schilling, L. S., & Holbrook, T. L. (1985). Determining the market for nurse practitioner services: The New Haven experience. *Nursing Research, 34*(4), 242-247.

Shoultz, J., Hatcher, P. A., & Hurrell, M. (1992). Growing edges of a new paradigm: The future of nursing in the health of the nation. *Nursing Outlook, 40*(2), 57-61.

Smithing, R. T., & Wiley, M. D. (1989a). Marketing and management. Marketing: An issue of particular relevance to nurse practitioners. *Journal of the American Academy of Nurse Practitioners, 1*(1), 33.

Smithing, R. T., & Wiley, M. D. (1989b). Marketing and management. Marketing techniques in print. *Journal of the American Academy of Nurse Practitioners, 1*(3), 103-104.

Smithing, R. T., & Wiley, M. D. (1990a) Marketing and management. See your physician. *Journal of the American Academy of Nurse Practitioners, 2*(1), 38.

Smithing, R. T., & Wiley, M. D. (1990b). Marketing and management. Marketing techniques in person. *Journal of the American Academy of Nurse Practitioners, 2*(2), 88-89.

Stahler-Miller, K. (1987). *Marketing yourself: How to make your excellence visible.* Workshop held at the Maine Medical Center, Portland, Maine, August.

Towers, J. (1990). Report of the national survey of the American Academy of Nurse Practitioners, Part IV: Practice characteristics and marketing activities of nurse practitioners. *Journal of the American Academy of Nurse Practitioners, 2*(4), 164-167.

Weill, J. A., Love, M. G., Pron, A. L., Tesoro, T. A., Grey, M., Hickel, M., Teti, B. S., & Serota, J. (1989). Future potential, phase I: Nurse practitioners look at themselves. *Journal of Pediatric Health Care, 3*(2), 76-82.

Weiss, S. J. (1983). Role differentiation between nurse and physician: Implications for nursing. *Nursing Research, 32*(3), 133-139.

CHAPTER 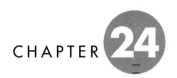 24

Administrative Justification and Support for Advanced Practice Nurses

Sharon L. Krumm

INTRODUCTION

The issues related to advanced nursing practice are among the most challenging faced by nurse administrators (NAds) as well as advanced practice nurses (APNs). In addition, the context in which these issues are addressed is unprecedented. It is one for which there is little history to serve as a guide and one that is constantly changing, thus limiting the ability to test existing theories.

As changes continue to occur in where and how health care is delivered, traditional, and often inflexible, organizational boundaries are disappearing. These boundaries formerly separated practice sites and practitioners, including NAds and APNs. Opportunities exist to create responsive organizations with flexible boundaries. Such organizations will enable NAds, APNs, physicians, and others to build the strong and productive alliances needed to meet society's needs for accessible and affordable health care.

Selected literature on advanced nursing practice (ANP) indicates that administrative support is an important variable (Hamric & Taylor, 1989). The purpose of this chapter is to engage NAds and APNs in alliance-building. At a time when alliances are needed between NAds and APNs, the forces that should bring them together can also drive them apart. NAds face decisions about the economic impact of APNs and how to shape the cultures of their organizations. They have a responsibility to remain knowledgeable about APN roles and to understand clearly what these roles can accomplish for an organization. APNs face decisions about how changes in clinical practice, organizational structure, and policy may affect them now and in the future and about how they can influence these changes. The content for this chapter is derived from the literature, consultation with other administrators, and the author's experiences as an NAd, educator, and clinical nurse specialist (CNS). Aspects of the current health care environment that can bring NAds and APNs together are described. The issues addressed in this chapter include preparing the organization for the addition of APNs, selecting APNs and supporting and positioning them within the organization, and providing the administrative support and resources required for their success. These issues are broadly addressed so that the information can be applied regardless of the practice setting.

THE HEALTH-CARE ENVIRONMENT

Economics is the single driving force behind today's changes in health care. Every nurse, including APNs and NAds, hopes that the rate of change will diminish but must accept that the environment of change will continue. Key economic issues include cost-containment, new forms of payment, consumer preferences, health reform efforts, and technological developments (Shortell, Gillies, & Devers, 1995). The assessment of relevant external and internal factors is important for NAds if they are to use APNs most effectively (Sample, 1989).

Numerous internal and external factors influence how nursing is practiced and how care is delivered in all health care settings: office-based, home health, and institutions. Some of the factors that create opportunities for or impediments to alliance-building are listed in Table 24–1.

TABLE 24–1. FACTORS THAT INFLUENCE NURSING PRACTICE AND DELIVERY OF CARE

External Factors	Internal Factors
Managed care	Reduction in acute-care beds
Global pricing	Increased acuity of in-patients
Emphasis on costs	Restructuring work processes
Demand for outcomes data	Need for standard outcomes data
Interest in patient satisfaction	Creation of new types of workers
Insurers as driving forces regarding clinical decisions	Diminishing resources
Emphasis on primary care	Enhanced training needs
Technological advances	Fewer workers through retirement, buy-out, terminations, etc.
Changing demographics	Application of technology/automation
Shift to less acute/ambulatory/home care	Emphasis on interdisciplinary efforts
Regulatory requirements	Changing organizational structures
Nursing's agenda for health care reform	Job/career insecurity
Licensing/credentialing requirements	New reporting relationships
Changes in the medical profession	Pressure to constrain wages
Better-informed consumers	Multi-site practices/affiliations/networks

EXTERNAL FACTORS

Managed care is pervasive in all sectors of health care because it is seen as a way to save money. The United States Congress may require all Medicare and Medicaid recipients to participate in some type of managed-care program (Grimaldi, 1989). This legislative debate is currently under way, and when resolved, could greatly expand the number of patients covered by this form of health care. The financial cost of an admission, a procedure, or an episode of care is the primary concern of the organization paying for that admission, procedure, or episode of care. Global pricing for expensive or highly technical procedures, such as organ and bone marrow transplantation, and capitation for segments of the population are increasingly important mechanisms of reimbursement. Critical pathways and multidisciplinary guidelines are seen as one way to decrease costs by decreasing duplication and providing closer monitoring of the processes of care. Some reimbursing organizations, especially larger managed-care companies, have established databases related to patient outcomes, including patient satisfaction. However, there is no consensus about the specific data to collect, and few health-care organizations have well-established mechanisms for collecting, analyzing, and presenting these data.

The shift in emphasis to primary care prompted medical schools and residency training programs to redirect their educational programs. There are fewer positions for residents and fellows in medical specialties. In academic medical institutions and affiliated community hospitals, the effect of this change has been fewer house staff and fellows to provide medical care on in-patient units. In some organizations, APNs assume many functions previously performed by these physicians in positions created or modified to respond to the physician shortage.

Physicians' practices are also changing, primarily in response to external factors. Physicians are accepting salary reductions and positions for significantly less money in order to remain employed; managed-care organizations are insisting that physicians care for as many patients as possible in their caseloads while reducing the cost of care for individual patients by reducing utilization of services; and many universities and hospitals are placing conflicting demands on medical faculty to increase the number of patients they care for while maintaining the teaching and research activities required for academic advancement.

Advances in technology and changing demographics enable a shift from delivering care in acute, in-patient settings to delivering it in acute rehabilitation, subacute, transitional, hospice, home, and ambulatory settings. This shift accelerates with each technological advance, including sophisticated automated communications systems. The rapid transfer of technology, electronic communication, consumer access to and demands for the latest therapies, and the organizational and clinicians' abilities to rapidly integrate new therapies into practice, are important factors in a more flexible health care system. Further, individuals with chronic illnesses can receive appropriate care in less acute, primary care settings.

Regulatory agencies, such as the Joint Commission for Accreditation of Health Care Organizations (JCAHO), recently revised their standards to recognize the dynamic nature of health care and reflect the shift in the locus of care. The JCAHO requires consistent standards of care across an organization's care-delivery sites (i.e., in-patient units, ambulatory clinics, and hospital-affiliated physicians' practices or offices). These requirements become especially important as regional and national networks of health care providers form.

INTERNAL FACTORS

The effects of these external factors on health care include reduced need for less acute, non-intensive-care beds. The way work is done within hospitals and other organizations, including reporting relationships and management structures, needs redesigning in light of these changes. Analysis of the activities associated with each care provider and each care process eliminates duplication of effort and as much nonessential work as possible. Re-engineering and restructuring are current buzzwords that describe this process of defining the core competencies of an organization and ensuring that appropriate structures, processes, and resources are consistently available.

Subacute, transitional or skilled nursing, and hospice units exist as free-standing organizations or within hospitals and affiliated practices, such as free-standing surgical centers. The financial goal of these units is to reduce the cost of care by enhancing efficiency, eliminating unnecessary activities, and reducing overhead costs. The ability to provide care at lower costs positions these units to increase revenues by attracting managed-care business.

These changes to reduce costs result in fewer resources for in-patient nursing units, reductions in the overall number of hospital employees, and the introduction of new kinds of workers to provide direct and indirect patient care. These changes are further intensified by the emphasis on automation and the appropriate application of technology. The fierce competition for managed-care contracts among hospitals and other providers increases the pressure for organizations to accelerate these cost reductions.

The distribution of revenue within health-care organizations is also changing. Administrators reward employees for their contributions to a positive financial situation. For example, hospitals value a reduction in the number of acute, in-patient days and reward employees who help achieve these goals. The evolution of the role of nurse case manager in hospitals is one example of how organizations are responding to the need to ensure effective and efficient care across traditional institutional boundaries in order to remain competitive.

Interdisciplinary approaches to care are essential in virtually every area of health care. This requires effective models of collaboration among diverse professional and support personnel and the application of interpersonal skills to ensure their success. Critical pathways and the need to avoid duplication by standardizing care are driving collaboration in ways that could not occur in the past. For example, physicians, nurses, APNs, nutritionists, social workers, pharmacists, physical therapists, and technicians working collaboratively may initiate preoperative teaching and gait training in the home of an individual scheduled for a total hip replacement, follow the patient through the in-patient, subacute, or rehabilitation phase, and return to the patient's home to continue rehabilitation. Detailed, systematic planning and coordination of care across settings are necessary to ensure desired outcomes, patient satisfaction, and financial rewards in such models.

This description of the complex context of modern health care is the stage on which the role of the APN is enacted. Although chaos is often perceived as negative, a closer analysis suggests that the chaotic environment offers unprecedented opportunities to promote the unique qualifications and contributions of APNs. APNs can meet gaps in services, as CNSs, acute-care nurse practitioners (ACNPs), certified nurse-midwives (CNMs), and certified registered nurse anesthetists (CRNAs) can facilitate the integration of nursing into the overall mission of the organization and devise cost-effective and quality clinical program innovations. It is important that APNs and NAds recognize how different the current environment is from that of the recent past and how this difference influences the decisions NAds make regarding APNs. NAds have a vital stake in the successful application of new nursing roles and changes in traditional ones. However, one must keep in mind that the economic incentive to remain viable in a competitive environment overrides most other considerations. The entrance of the APN onto this stage is relatively recent. While some of these roles, such as the CNM and CRNA, have matured, others, such as ACNPs and nurse case managers, are emerging. NAds share this stage with APNs. Both also share responsibility for preserving and enriching nursing's essential values and heritage within the current and emerging environments.

ADMINISTRATIVE STRATEGIES AND ADVANCED NURSING PRACTICE

Although some NAds are cutting APNs from the nursing budget or shifting costs to the department of medicine as a first response to fiscal alarms, there are compelling reasons for NAds to consider APN roles as the answers to many of the important challenges of today's health-care environment. These reasons include extant and historical relevance and the professional attributes of APNs. Among these attributes are expertise in theory-based clinical care; knowledge of clinical practice, including the medical and nursing perspectives; knowledge of health-care systems and the ability to develop and integrate practice within organizations, communities, and systems; the ability to make independent judgments and ethical decisions; the ability to practice in multiple care settings, such as tertiary, hospice, and home care; and flexibility. APNs are able to identify the nature and costs of nursing interventions and their effects on patient outcomes (Minarik, 1993). Additionally, there are specific areas of advanced nursing practice within the domain of nursing, such as pain management and women's health. In addition to the core competencies of APNs described in this text (see Chapter 3 and Section II), APNs possess other attributes that make them invaluable to nurse executives and the organizations in which both practice (Table 24–2). With these reasons as the backdrop for administrative decisions about APN roles, NAds select strategies to implement and ensure the success of these roles.

NAds provide the vision and shape the culture for nursing practice within an organization. This vision is formed by the organization's mission and goals and by the NAd's beliefs about nursing. NAds must embrace and promote a nursing philosophy that recognizes advanced nursing practice as central to quality and access to care and to the advancement of the profession. As it is being formed, this vision should be shaped through dialogue and discussions with APNs and other nursing staff regarding the clinical and professional focus of the vision. This essential collaborative effort between NAds and APNs ensures integration of administrative and advanced clinical thinking and greatly enhances the potential for successful advancement of advanced nursing practice. While achieving organizational goals, NAds interpret organizational issues to APNs and use knowledge gleaned from APNs to influence the larger organization.

To ensure success, NAds need a systematic approach to advanced nursing practice. The following steps are useful: assessing the need for ANP positions, preparing the organization and involving stakeholders in planning for the new position, developing the position description and reporting relationships, recruiting the best APN, and introducing the new APN to the organization.

The vision for advanced nursing practice must be clearly and systematically articulated and promoted throughout the organization. Intradepartmental and interdepartmental meetings, written communication, and press releases are useful for this purpose. The organization's formal and informal leaders will support APNs more readily if the leaders are involved early in the establishment of these positions and, as appropriate, in the interviewing process (Baird & Prouty, 1989). The NAd should identify these leaders and then anticipate and respond to these individuals' needs for specific information. Failure to do so may lead staff to perceive APNs as intruders and undermine collaboration and other processes vital to accomplishing department and organization goals.

The literature supports the significant contributions of the nurse practitioner (NP) role in primary care settings, CNSs in acute and transitional care roles, CNMs in collaborative and private practice, and CRNAs in hospital practices (Brooten &

TABLE 24–2. COMPETENCIES AND ATTRIBUTES OF APNs

Competencies	**Attributes**
Clinical expertise	Self-directed
Consultation	Analytical and questioning
Collaboration	Willing to take risks
Change agency	Visionary
Ethical competence	Articulate
Research skills	Interpersonally competent
Leadership	"Shuttle diplomat" (Brown, 1989)
Teaching/coaching	

Naylor, 1995; Safriet, 1992) (see Chapter 26). Sharing this literature with nurses, other professionals, and administrators is useful for enhancing support within an organization. Roles of NPs in transitional and acute care, the blended CNS/NP role, and the roles of NPs and CNSs as case managers are evolving. Most of the literature about these evolving roles is descriptive, and the effect of these roles on patient outcomes and organizational goals is still being determined.

Gaining physician support for advanced nursing practice is important to the success of the practice. Many physicians acknowledge APNs' contributions to patient care in new and traditional settings and work collaboratively with them to achieve shared patient care goals. Other physicians are less certain about these roles and question the potential difference in their future earning potential that APNs may make. Confusion abounds among physicians and other providers about the specific nature of APN roles, especially in relation to traditional medical education and practice. NAds and APNs can decrease this confusion in a number of ways. These include providing information regarding the attributes of APN roles and the relationship of these roles to enhancing physician practice, such as increasing the number of patients that can be followed in a practice setting, sharing and collaborating in research activities, or freeing up physician time for teaching responsibilities. The positive influence on patient satisfaction and the value added by APNs to physician practices are additional and important considerations. This information can be shared informally through distributing relevant literature or within the context of discussions at clinical and administrative meetings. The importance of using appropriate data to support one's point of view cannot be overemphasized. The demonstration of successful role implementation is the most powerful force for garnering physician support. Building institutional success stories can be most helpful to NAds trying to persuade skeptical physicians.

The emerging focus on advanced nursing practice, especially within the context of work redesign, affects other care providers in different ways. In some organizations, APNs assume functions previously performed by other professionals, including physicians, social workers, and clinical dietitians. "Territorial disputes" may arise. The NAd can minimize the potential for these disputes by maintaining the focus of decision making on patient care requirements and how to address them in the most cost-effective and efficient manner with the best possible outcomes. Sincerely expressed respect for the work of other professionals, coupled with sensitivity and diplomacy, modulates the potential negative effects of these negotiations.

NAds and managers recognize the impact that advanced nursing practice may have on other clinical nursing roles. Nuccio et al. (1993) suggested that role expectations solicited from staff nurses can be useful in developing supportive relationships. Effective relationships must exist among staff nurses, APNs, physicians, and other providers to ensure desired clinical outcomes for patients. Specific, detailed delineation of roles and clear-cut communicating structures and reporting relationships strengthen these relationships. APNs potentially affect the practice of clinical administrators, pharmacists, and nonprofessional direct and indirect care providers. The broadest interpretation of these advanced nursing roles to other staff, well before their introduction, helps ensure their success.

Appropriately expressing the rationale for the placement of the APN within the organization, including reporting relationships, is important. The APN and others in the organization should know the expectations of the position in relation to the organization's goals and objectives. Explicitly stating these expectations is important. NAds are expected to report the extent to which APNs meet anticipated outcomes, including financial objectives.

NAds promote APNs within an organization through formal and informal structures. For example, providing opportunities for APNs to present information to a group of managers and administrators about a clinical program or an aspect of clinical practice displays the contributions of APNs to the organization's goals. This effectively and positively enhances APN visibility. Thus, there is broader recognition of the APNs' skills and contributions within the organization.

Including APNs in an organization's orientation program for clinical and non-clinical employees is another means of promoting their roles. For example, financial personnel benefit from hearing an APN clearly describe the clinical "business" of the organization. When the organization enters contracts with managed-care companies, APNs add significantly to the orientation of external case managers and managed-care personnel.

Additional opportunities for NAds to positively influence the organization regarding APNs include appointing them to departmental or organization-wide committees and task forces in which their knowledge and skills become apparent to NAds, peers, and others and networking through contacts arranged by the NAd. Including APNs in meetings with top NAds communicates a message that APNs are important to and valued by the organization.

Because the primary focus of advanced nursing practice is clinical care for patients, documentation of clinical outcomes is essential. Baird (1985) noted the importance of clinical documentation in ensuring the survival of APN roles. This documentation is also valuable for NAds to show evidence of APNs' contributions to the organization's clinical goals and objectives.

In spite of the profession's efforts, it is still safe to say that the public does not fully understand professional nursing. In particular, the different educational preparations by which nurses enter the profession and the difference this education makes in patient care are unclear and misunderstood. Emerging APN roles and changes in existing roles add to the confusion. Recipients of care and their families need reassurance about the ability of APNs to promote positive outcomes, especially if their care was previously provided by physicians or other professionals. Administrators reassure individuals and families by recruiting APNs qualified through education, certification, licensure, and experience to provide the type and level of care required by specific populations of patients. Attention and responsiveness to anticipated and existing concerns of patients about their care providers is a responsibility shared by NAds.

In addition to shaping the organization's culture to support advanced nursing practice, NAds use other administrative strategies to ensure the APN's success within an organization. Understanding these strategies allows the APN to collaborate more fully with the NAd in their implementation. Promoting the value of advanced nursing practice to the practice mission of an organization is perhaps the most important administrative strategy. Working collaboratively with APNs to delineate the practice is the foremost component of this strategy for NAds. Finally, NAds and APNs working together can influence policy decisions. The development of model state nursing acts, the inclusion of APN services in standard benefits packages and managed-care contracts, differentiated payment rates, and support for nursing education are important policy considerations that require a united effort.

SUPPORTING ADVANCED PRACTICE NURSES

By thoughtfully selecting and introducing the APN to the organization, the NAd prepares the organization for the successful implementation of the role. Many factors are considered in this process (Table 24–3).

The organization's mission is the first consideration. If the education of students and other learners, the discovery of knowledge, and the provision of care are integral to the mission, it is expected that the APN contributes to this mission. An organization's emphasis on research may direct the administrator to select a doctorally prepared APN and influence the placement of the position within the organization's existing structure.

Organizational structure is another influencing factor (Baird & Prouty, 1989; Parrinello, 1995). For example, if the purpose of a position is to directly influence patient-care decisions, a decentralized organization may provide a better fit for a unit-based APN than would a centralized one. A matrix or product-line structure facilitates the consultative role of APNs by supporting their ability to indirectly influence patient-care decisions in more than one clinical setting. Whatever its form, NAds should thoughtfully analyze their organization's structure when placing APN positions. NAds with responsibilities across organizations and within networks of organizations must analyze organizational structures and position placements within and between organizational boundaries. When health-care organizations exist within academic settings, the structural relationships with the appropriate schools of medicine and nursing are also considered. Parrinello (1995) discussed three organizational models that predominate: the physician model, the nursing model, and the joint practice model. Each model has advantages and disadvantages for APNs in relation to decision making, scope of practice, compensation, and collaboration.

The philosophy of nursing and model of care delivery further influence decisions about selecting and implementing APN positions. A nursing philosophy that incorporates the professional development of each staff member supports a traditional CNS role, as do philosophies that include a focus on research and research utilization. Similarly, primary nursing and collaborative practice are care-delivery models with different implications for APNs. For example, an ACNP practicing on an in-patient nursing unit will interact with other caregivers differently than would a CNS who is a member of a collaborative practice in an organization that

TABLE 24–3. ORGANIZATIONAL FACTORS RELATED TO ANP ROLES

Organizational mission
Organizational structure
Philosophy of nursing
Model of nursing care delivery
Organizational strategic plan
Profile of patients
Financial planning
Statutes and regulations governing advanced nursing practice

uses another model of care delivery. The ACNP directs patient care through written orders, whereas the CNS often provides guidance to staff nurses regarding patients' nursing care. A faculty-based practice is another example of a care-delivery model that frequently provides APN primary care services. CNMs are an excellent example of APNs providing primary care within a broad array of clinical settings, including managed-care organizations, free-standing birthing centers, and hospital-based practices. When the organization's philosophy and delivery model support CRNA practices, these practices are enhanced and the organization benefits from the full implementation of these roles.

NAds influence and provide leadership for the achievement of their organization's strategic plans. Once adopted, these plans direct the organization's future activities. The NAd analyzes the organization's strategic plan and associated initiatives for congruency with existing or proposed APN roles. The planning stage of a community-based primary care network is an opportune time to introduce an APN, especially if an APN from the community is recruited for the position. Each APN role must be articulated within the context of these plans, and the relationship of the APN to the organization's strategic plan should be clearly articulated across the organization. It is especially important that upper-level administrators and managers have this knowledge. The more deeply connected the APN is to the organization's strategic plan, the more secure the position is within the organization and the less susceptible it is to adverse effects of external changes and internal budget reductions.

The numbers and profile of patients served by an organization or a unit of the organization are potentially influenced by the adoption of a new APN role. An example is the introduction of a hospital-based CNM program to serve an inner-city population of teenaged mothers for whom existing sources of care are inadequate. An organization may effectively reach new populations of patients this way. Many successful bone marrow transplant programs attribute a great deal of their success to CNSs who practice within these programs. When considering the appropriate role for an APN within an organization, one must analyze patient characteristics such as acuity, chronicity, age, economic status, and ethnicity.

Financial planning for APN positions is primarily an administrative responsibility. Budget projections regarding patient volumes, case mix, relative value units, and income projections are useful in deciding the financial support base for these roles. Salary support for a single position from several sources, such as professional fees, research grants, or the organization's personnel budget, is not unusual. If salary support is provided by more than one source or department, NAds may negotiate on behalf of the APN for this support. It is prudent to provide APNs who are partially or solely supported by grants or other "soft money" with written information about the exact terms and conditions of the support. This includes the expected end-date of the grant and the possibility of continuing the position beyond the grant-funded period. When an APN generates income, negotiations about the appropriation of this income to specific cost centers or budgets may be required. If the organization awards financial incentives for meeting specific targets or criteria, the APN needs assurance of sufficient opportunity to realize these incentives. These fiscal analyses are also required for APNs practicing within nurse-managed centers and nursing networks (Ethridge & Lamb, 1989; Wilcox, Ziegfeld, & Morrison, 1995).

The laws, statutes, and regulations governing APN practices vary among the states. APNs and NAds require working knowledge of these legal and regulatory documents. Please refer to Chapter 22 for a discussion of this information.

An organization's use of critical pathways, the number of managed-care contracts, and the number of existing or planned affiliations are helpful pieces of information for the NAd in deciding to incorporate APNs into an organization or to change existing advanced practice positions, as well as for deciding the number of APNs needed to accomplish the goals of these contracts and affiliations. This information is also useful in gaining organizational support for these positions.

FACTORS IN SELECTING APN POSITIONS

Selection of the appropriate APN position includes consideration of the following (Table 24–4): the goals and objectives of the position; the clinical program; the number and type of other disciplines and professionals within the practice setting; licensure and credential requirements; opportunities for reimbursement of professional fees and third-party payments; the number of APNs required for the practice, such as the need for 24-hour coverage; and the available and potential pool of applicants. Further, the educational preparation and ideally the experience of the APN need to be consistent with the requirements for the position.

The goals and objectives of the position determine the nature of the practice requirements, such as primary care delivery, consultation, program planning, and expansion of physician practices. The nature of the clinical program often determines the selection of the appropriate APN role, as with CRNAs who practice in a surgical procedure area. The number and type of other disciplines and professionals within the practice setting is another consideration. The regulatory restrictions that must be considered include scope of practice, prescriptive authority, and reimbursement. A CNS position may be selected to enhance staff nurses' clinical and communication skills within a clinical program that includes physicians, physician assistants (PAs), and ACNPs. If the purpose of a position is to provide direct patient care in a primary care setting, the licensure and credentialing requirements are different from those of a position designed to provide consultation across care settings.

Further, the educational preparation and previous professional experiences of the APN need to be consistent with the requirements of the position. As organizations seek opportunities to maximize their reimbursement potential, the selection of APN positions such as NPs and CNMs may help achieve this goal. If APN positions are needed to provide services 24 hours a day, seven days a week, the decision about the type of position may differ from what it would be were APN services needed during limited times of the week. Also, there must be an available pool of potential applicants for a position. Newspaper and journal advertisements

TABLE 24–4. FACTORS IN SELECTING APN POSITIONS

Position goals
Clinical program
Other professionals
Licensure/credentialing requirements
Reimbursement potential
Number of positions required
Available pool of applicants

convey the impression that there are significantly more positions for APNs than there are applicants in today's market.

The selection of the appropriate APN for an existing clinical program or nursing unit or with a specific population of patients relates the type of APN position to the organizational structure and the organizational boundaries. For example, a CNS is appropriate when care to complex patients, expert consultation, and staff development for nurses are needed within a single institution's in-patient, ambulatory, and home-care units. A unit-based ACNP can effectively and efficiently care for patients receiving chemotherapy in an acute-care setting or on a bone marrow transplant unit. Examples of patients for whom primary care APNs are well suited include those who are chronically ill, such as persons who are HIV-positive (Diers, 1993), and expectant parents.

ORGANIZATIONAL PLACEMENT AND REPORTING RELATIONSHIPS

There is no one reporting relationship that is correct for all APNs within all organizations. Rather, NAds consider a number of issues when deciding about these relationships. Credentialing and legal requirements for specific APN roles, such as CRNAs and NPs, influence their placement in the organization and their reporting relationships. Medical oversight and credentialing of specific functions are required for CRNAs and NPs. In Dang and Haller's (1995) survey of reporting relationships within academic health centers, departments of medicine and nursing shared reporting relationships in the majority of the responding centers. In most organizations, nursing is responsible for ensuring licensure and adherence to professional standards. The JCAHO's standards support this practice.

The decision of whether to place an APN in a line position or a staff position involves many factors, as noted earlier. An NAd may wish to place an APN in a staff position to mentor the APN into a new position or program. Reporting relationships are visible signals about the importance of a position within an organization and the expected lines of communication. Any anxiety about the long-term viability of line or staff positions and the potential for career advancement in these positions must be recognized and frankly discussed by the NAd and the APN. Discussions of various APN placements are available (Baird & Prouty, 1989; Parrinello, 1995).

Once established, the role, the role objectives and time frame for achieving them, and role expectations must be clearly defined and discussed by the APN and the person or persons to whom the APN is accountable. Any uncertainties about these expectations should be initially discussed and a plan for addressing them agreed upon. As noted by Tierney, Grant, and Mazique (1990), these expectations may include a range of broad categories, such as nurse recruitment and retention, reducing the cost of services, and developing new revenue sources.

APNs require knowledge of the expectations of the person to whom they report regarding their job performance. These expectations should be written and reviewed with the APN at least annually and optimally every six months or whenever an organizational change affects APNs' ability to meet the established expectations. Included in these expectations are the hours and days of work, nonclinical activities such as committee assignments, documentation systems for review of clinical practice, and opportunities for off-site work on projects or professional development activities. When they exist, expectations regarding clinical teaching and research are specified.

Deciding the appropriate number of patients for whom the APN is responsible is based on the context and nature of the clinical practice. In Frampton and Wall's study (1994), NPs and PAs believed that 81 to 91% of the patients they saw were appropriately cared for and did not require the services of a physician. Other factors that influence this number include the organization's standards of practice and the number and diversity of other staff members within the clinical practice. For example, Dang and Haller (1995) found a range of 7 to 16 patients per case manager in the academic hospitals surveyed. Managed-care organizations often have established targets for the numbers of patients seen by NPs or CNMs. Hummel and Pirzada (1994) noted that teams of "non-physician providers" (NPs or PAs) and physicians were extremely cost-effective when the number of patients cared for expanded.

The communication mechanisms and their preferred or required frequency of use need clear definition. These include written reports, certification and license verification, performance improvement targets, and other forms for documenting performance and achievement of objectives.

If the APN does not report directly to the nurse executive but reports to a clinical director or other mid-level nurse administrator, the APN should meet regularly with the nurse executive individually or in a group of other APNs, ideally no less frequently than quarterly. Further, it is useful for APNs and senior-level nurses, including nurse managers, educators, and researchers, to meet as a group with the nurse executive at least semiannually. These meetings provide an opportunity for dialogue, discussion, and information-sharing.

To succeed, APNs need resources, including adequate space for clinical and indirect patient-care activities. They need assurance of appropriate salary support and opportunities for raises or sufficient opportunities to generate income through professional fees. Opportunities for advancement need to be defined. Assistive staff, such as clinical assistants, secretarial support, and data entry personnel, may be required. Access to automated systems is essential in today's environment. Continuing education opportunities, in academic and nonacademic programs, are essential for maintaining one's skills. The organization's support of these activities requires a fiscally responsible and consistently applied approach. Finally, the APN requires the guidance of the NAd to ensure synchrony between the APN and the organization.

SUMMARY

In summary, APNs and NAds should think in terms of the skills that APNs bring to an organization rather than the specific roles they may occupy. This is especially important as changes continue in the provision and the location of care delivery within an organization and within the community. APNs should promote their skills as new opportunities and new relationships emerge, and NAds should assist them in doing so. Further, the community's and the organization's needs and strategic imperatives are the context for the current and future job-related opportunities of APNs. By committing to the mission and objectives of the organization and consistently developing and expanding their skills, APNs ensure their place in the future of health care delivery. Simultaneously, NAds, through creativity and responsible decision making, can create a future for their organizations and the profession in which advanced nursing practice flourishes.

REFERENCES

Baird, S. (1985). Administrative support issues and oncology clinical nurse specialists. *Oncology Nursing Forum, 12* (2), 51–54.

Baird, S., & Prouty, M. P. (1989). Administratively enhancing CNS contributions. In A. Hamric & J. Spross (Eds.), *The clinical nurse specialist in theory and practice* (2nd ed., pp. 261–284). Philadelphia: W. B. Saunders Company.

Brooten, D., & Naylor, M. D. (1995). Nurses' effect on changing patient outcomes. *Image—Journal of Nursing Scholarship, 27* (2), 95–99.

Brown, S. J. (1989). Supportive supervision of the CNS. In A. B. Hamric & J. A. Spross (Eds.), *The clinical nurse specialist in theory and practice* (2nd ed., pp. 285–298). Philadelphia: W. B. Saunders Company.

Dang, D., & Haller, K. (1995). *Analysis of non-physician provider roles.* (Unpublished manuscript) Baltimore: The Johns Hopkins Hospital.

Diers, D. (1993). Advanced practice. *Health Management Quarterly, 15* (12), 16–20.

Ethridge, P., & Lamb, G. S. (1989). Professional nursing case management improves quality, access and costs. *Nursing Management, 20* (3), 30–35.

Frampton, J., & Wall, S. (1994). Exploring the use of NPs and PAs in primary care. *HMO Practice, 4,* 165–170.

Grimaldi, P. L. (1989). Medicaid switch to managed care. *Nursing Management, 26* (7), 12–17.

Hamric, A. B., & Taylor, J. W. (1989). Role development of the CNS. In A. B. Hamric & J. Spross (Eds.), *The clinical nurse specialist in theory and practice* (2nd ed., pp. 41–82). Philadelphia: W. B. Saunders Company.

Hummel, J., & Pirzada, S. (1994). Estimating the cost-effectiveness of nurse practitioner/physician team in long-term care facilities. *HMO Practice, 8* (4), 162–164.

Minarik, P. A. (1993). Legislative and regulatory update: health care reform and managed competition: implications for CNSs. *Clinical Nurse Specialist. 7* (3):105–109.

Nuccio, S., Costa-Lieberthal, K. M., Gunta, K. E., Mackus, M. L., Riesch, S. K., Schmanski, K. M., & Westen, B. A. (1993). A survey of 636 staff nurses' perceptions and factors influencing the CNS role. *Clinical Nurse Specialist, 7* (3), 122–128.

Parrinello, K. M. (1995). Advanced practice nursing: An administrative perspective. *Critical Care Nursing Clinics of North America, 7* (1), 9–16.

Safriet, B. J. (1992). Health care dollars and regulatory sense: The role of the advanced practice nurse. *Yale Journal on Regulation, 9* (2), 417–487.

Sample, S. (1989). Justifying and structuring the CNS role within a nursing organization. In A. B. Hamric & J. A. Spross (Eds.), *The clinical nurse specialist in theory and practice* (2nd ed., pp. 251–260). Philadelphia: W. B. Saunders Company.

Shortell, S. M., Gillies, R. R., & Devers, K. J. (1995). Reinventing the American hospital. *The Milbank Quarterly, 73* (2), 131–158.

Tierney, M. J., Grant, L. E., & Mazique, S. I. (1990). Cost accountability and clinical nurse specialist evaluation. *Nursing Management, 21* (5), 26–31.

Wilcox, P., Ziegfeld, C. R., & Morrison, C. (1995). Advanced practice model response to needs of women at risk for female malignancies. Anaheim, CA: Oncology Nursing Society Congress, April, 1995.

CHAPTER 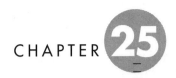 25

Program and Practice Management for the Advanced Practice Nurse

Diane Kaschak Newman

INTRODUCTION

Consumers are demanding health services beyond those that have been tradition-ally available. They are actively selecting health-care providers for particular health problems. Increasingly, consumers are seeking nurses, particularly advanced prac-tice nurses (APNs) who are practicing as nurse practitioners (NPs) in primary care and specialty practices, certified nurse-midwives (CNMs) who are providing childbirth options and women's health services, certified nurse anesthetists (CRNAs) who contract with hospitals and anesthesiologists to provide anesthesia services, and clinical nurse specialists (CNSs) in specialty practices. The practice skills of the APN have been shown to be a cost-effective contribution to health care (Aiken & Sage, 1992). Historically, nurses have practiced under the "medical plan of care." Many nursing decisions have been based on therapeutic measures ordered and directed by physicians, but the medical plan of care is only one part of the provision of health care (Kinlein, 1977). This is an opportune time for the APN to seize the opportunities available for innovative collaborative and indepen-dent practice based on nursing's model of care.

The nursing profession is seeing the growth of the APN through an increase in graduate programs, the availability of direct reimbursement, and the expansion of innovative practice models. Presently, the majority of APNs are in salaried positions with physician practices, provider groups, or institutions in which payment received for their services is applied to practice revenues (Pearson, 1994). As the number of APNs increases, many will seek opportunities outside the traditional job market and opt for independent or collaborative practices. APNs are demonstrating that they can offer service through innovative practice models that deliver health care to defined populations, operate managed-care facilities, consult, and create independent and collaborative practice arrangements. This chapter describes the role of the APN as owner and provider in two specific practice models, an independent practice and in collaboration with other providers. Specific topics include the development, implementation, and management of the practice as well as current reimbursement strategies. The discussion is complemented with over-views of several current private practice models involving APNs.

THE NURSE ENTREPRENEUR

An entrepreneur is defined as a person who is continually searching for and who is receptive to opportunities and change; one who plans, organizes, finances, and operates his or her own business.

A solution to the immediate shortage of primary care providers would be to expand the role of APNs in the health-care system, thus allowing them to function as entrepreneurs in an independent or collaborative private practice setting. Private nursing practice is defined as the practice of nursing within a business framework that is partially or wholly owned by the nurse providing the service (Keller, 1975). Because APNs are uniquely equipped to address many current health-care problems with respect to accessibility, cost, and quality of primary care, many APNs are now venturing into private practice. In this chapter, the models of independent and collaborative private practice for APNs is limited to APNs who work in solo or joint practices providing direct patient care.

CHARACTERISTICS OF AN INNOVATOR

The exciting realization that nurses can provide services in an innovative practice model must be tempered with the reality of starting up a business. There are advantages and disadvantages to starting one's own practice. The advantages include increased freedom, flexibility, independence, income control, continual challenges, and personal and professional growth. The disadvantages include the need to juggle family and work commitments, the need to continually assess and respond to changes in one's marketplace in order to stay in business, and the financial uncertainty inherent in any start-up business venture. APNs must realize that they will be the "boss" and may need to manage not only their own work but a staff as well (Stewart, 1989). Business and managerial skills are not taught in basic nursing programs and will have to be learned. From 1960 to 1980, graduate nursing programs emphasized theories about the profession rather than theories that guide practice. More recently, graduate nursing programs have begun incorporating business and practice concepts into APN education.

Initially, the APN must explore both personal and professional characteristics to determine those qualities that will facilitate starting an independent practice. Several critical examples might include credibility as a nurse expert, interpersonal skills, and business and management knowledge. Calmelat (1993) highlighted the need for individuals to possess the following characteristics prior to opening a nursing practice:

- Unflagging support of those closest, i.e., spouse, children, family
- Well-developed advanced clinical skills
- Financial ability to live without a steady income for at least one year while the practice is growing
- Ability to attend to details; well-honed organizational skills
- Access to capital for start-up expenses
- Relationship with a physician willing to work as a consultant or collaborator

RULES AND REGULATIONS

While in the early planning stages of starting a practice, the APN should review the state's nurse practice act regarding the specific rules and regulations pertaining to scope of practice. State law determines both the scope of practice and regulations about ownership of professional corporations. If one plans to start a business with another health-care professional, such as a physician, physician assistant, or physical therapist, the state board of nursing, state board of medicine, and state board of allied health should be contacted regarding restrictions. Many states require certification in the APN's area of expertise by a national nursing certification organization. Consultation with a legal counsel who has an understanding and background in health-care law is highly recommended and could make the difference in the success of the practice (Stewart, 1989). The APN will also need to contact the Medicare carrier, state Medicaid program, and other insurers to determine the procedure for obtaining provider status and to gather information about these plans and prevailing rates for APNs in the geographical area. If the APN feels that admitting privileges at the local hospital will be a necessary part of the practice, the hospital administration will need to be contacted to determine the procedure.

Usually, this involves submitting an application to the medical board of the hospital, requesting specified privileges in caring for clients.

KEY COMPONENTS OF A BUSINESS

Once a decision is made to provide services through an innovative private practice model, an understanding of the key components of operating a business is essential to success. This identification and understanding of business components will help solidify ideas about operating the practice in an organized, useful format (Newman & Palumbo, 1994). Time and research spent prior to opening the practice forces the individual to consider the myriad of options and to anticipate potential problems. The success of the business will, in part, depend on how well one has researched the components outlined in the following paragraphs. Development of these components will serve a dual purpose: to aid the individual in the preparation of a business plan that can then be used to attract investors, partners, or collaborators and to assist in marketing the practice (Vogel & Doleysh, 1994).

The first component is to develop a *philosophy* or *description of the practice*. Summarize the goals of the practice into a concise statement that includes the specific services to be provided, the target client population, and what type of collaboration has been established with other professionals. When preparing this statement, examples of established APN practices might be helpful. Competing practices in one's geographical area should be identified as should several choices of practice sites and how advertising and promotion of the practice will be handled. Choosing practice sites, specialties, and services with which other providers will not likely compete may be the best opportunity for the APN. The practice models highlighted later in this chapter are for specific services targeting populations not provided for by basic medical models.

The *legal structure* of the practice needs to be carefully considered. However, prior to determining the legal structure, the ownership issue will need to be resolved. Ownership of medical professional practices is dictated by state law; some states have legislation that allows only "like" professionals (i.e., physicians, dentists, psychiatrists) to incorporate. The APN will need to determine if the option of ownership with physicians and other health-care providers is prohibited by state law.

There are three basic ways to structure the practice: a sole proprietorship, a partnership, or a corporation (Vogel & Doleysh, 1994). The primary differences between these structures are tax restrictions and liability. A business can be a *sole proprietorship*, the simplest form of business organization, which involves one owner. It is simple and inexpensive to establish, and control remains with the sole owner. For tax purposes the business income is taxed at the personal tax rate. The major disadvantage of the sole proprietorship is the unlimited liability that accompanies the structure; the owner assumes all liability, including any negligent acts of employees.

A *general partnership* is an association of two or more persons in which each partner retains personal liability. It may be advantageous for the APN to partner with another professional in order to attract venture capital. The unlimited liability remains, as does the personal tax rate on business income. A disadvantage of this structure is the possibility of personality conflicts and disagreements arising between the partners over control and decision-making. As mentioned previously, the legality of partnerships between different professionals is often dictated by state law. CRNAs can join business arrangements as consultants to hospitals and anesthesia groups. Most medical practices are for-profit partnerships.

A *corporation* is a separate legal entity for both tax and liability purposes. Although incorporation protects the owners from some liability (a corporation has limited liability), a medical professional must still have a malpractice policy. A professional corporation can elect a small business ("Sub" S) status, which allows owners to retain the benefit of taxation at the personal rate or, as is sometimes said, to avoid double taxation—first on corporate income and again, second on shareholder dividends. Other advantages of a corporation include the ability to start pension and profit-sharing plans and the possibility of multiple investors. This makes it somewhat easier to attract venture capital. The main disadvantage of a corporation that does not elect small business status is the higher tax cost. A corporation may also be more expensive to establish and operate. A separate but equally important legal issue to consider is defining the association with a collaborating physician through the development of a collaborative practice agreement (CPA). Most state statutes for NPs require some form of medical collaboration. Some states require a copy of the CPA to be on file at the state level. There are three major sections of a CPA: definition of concepts and relationships, delineation of specific clinical issues, and an outline of the contractual business arrangements (Sebas, 1994). The CPA should also include protocols or standards of practice to guide and improve the quality of care offered to patients. The protocols should be based on a minimum safe level; if practice standards are too high to be reasonably met, they may become problematic in a malpractice situation (Moniz, 1992).

Identification of a *management team* and *supporting professional personnel* is part of the initial business planning. Often in a nurse-managed practice, the owner not only provides professional patient services but serves as part of the management team. An organizational chart and job descriptions of the staff should be developed detailing the proposed management team of the corporation. The experience, education, and other qualifications of the APN and other professionals providing services should be described briefly. Supporting professional assistance may be required. Additional ancillary personnel may include an office manager, a receptionist, and a health assistant. The practice will need to contract or consult with an accountant, lawyer, banker, and insurance agent for specific services (Stewart, 1989).

THE MARKETING PLAN

Market research and analysis begins with a feasibility study performed using demographic information about the area served by the practice. This will identify the target population and provide information in order to develop specific strategies to influence clients to use the proposed nursing service rather than that of a competitor. APNs generally serve more than their proportional share of low-income and non-metropolitan patients who lack access to medical care. Serving these populations solely may not be financially feasible for the APN because of poor reimbursement. Market analysis will also assist the APN in continuing identification of prospective clients. It is also helpful to survey other providers, institutions, and agencies in the targeted geographical area to ascertain their perception of the service area. A projection of market penetration over one, three, and five years should be included.

A marketing plan that describes how clients will learn about the service or be referred to the practice will need to be developed. Because most consumers do not understand the role and qualifications of APNs, it is important to articulate exactly what services will be provided in order to educate consumers. How nurses are perceived by the public can have a considerable effect on business; additional effort should be put forth in the area of nurse promotion to groups with whom the professionals will interact. Describe how this will be accomplished (e.g., newspaper advertisements, radio spots, speaking to target institutions and groups, or television spots). In addition, describe the role and qualifications of the professionals in a service brochure to be distributed on site and to all agencies with whom the practice comes in contact (Table 25–1). Another form of advertisement is direct mail. Lists that contain names of people who are most likely to access proposed services can be purchased. An example may be a woman's health practice that purchases a list of woman, aged 20 to 60, who live in adjacent zip code areas that are easily accessible to the practice. Initially, the APN may spend 10 to 20% of gross revenues on marketing.

In addition to marketing to the community and other health-care providers, the APN will need to market to insurers. As managed care dominates the insurer market, APNs must learn how to negotiate exclusivity relationships, capitation rates, and other additional fees available through these insurers (Jenkins & Torrisi, 1995).

A list of possible *providers and specialists who will generate or accept referrals* is an important planning component. To be successful, the APN must maintain a collegial relationship with other health-care providers (Hanson, 1993). The practice will need to find referral sources for patients whose medical problems require additional expertise from a specialist. If the practice is located in an urban setting, locating referrals for indigent patients or the uninsured who need medical care or hospitalization may be difficult because of the lack of provision for this population. This is also true in rural areas in which medical services do not exist or are not easily accessible. In addition, the APN will need to identify laboratories and radiologists who will accept requests for diagnostic tests.

Selecting a name for the practice may be an option worth considering in certain situations. Rather than using an individual's name, a specific practice name may assist in describing the services offered and reflect the business focus—for example, Women's Health Services, Access to Continence Care and Treatment, and The Birth Center. Many professionals use their own name to offer more of a personalized service conception as well as to promote themselves.

THE FINANCIAL PLAN

It is also important to outline an *operating plan*. This plan details the hard and soft assets required to operate the practice. For financial purposes, a list of equipment

TABLE 25–1. EXAMPLE OF A DESCRIPTION OF THE ROLE AND
QUALIFICATIONS OF PROFESSIONALS

Access to Continence Care & Treatment (ACCT) is a group practice of nurse practitioners, clinical nurse specialists, and physicians.

A nurse practitioner or clinical nurse specialist is a registered nurse (RN) who has experience and certification in a health care specialty area.

The staff of ACCT work with people of all ages and their families, providing the information people need to make informed decisions about their health care and lifestyle choices.

Nurse practitioners and clinical nurse specialists practice under the rules and regulations of the nurse practice act of the state in which they work. These nurses hold master's degrees in nursing and practice in collaboration with a medical advisor who is a physician.

---

to be leased or purchased is mandatory. Equipment is not limited to medical equipment and supplies but would also include office equipment, such as computers and a copier. Compiling this list and determining actual specifications of equipment will require decisions on how much administrative (support) work will be done "in house." For example, many practices use off-site facilities for administrative functions such as billing and transcription. Other criteria, such as the need to have patient information in a database, will affect the type and quality of equipment required. Another slant on the equipment purchase/lease list is to determine the cost-effectiveness of taking on the function as opposed to having it performed off-site. The financial plan will incorporate operating decisions and their associated costs.

Development of a *financial plan* is an integral part of business planning. This is clearly the area in which an APN will require assistance from an accountant. Simply put, the financial plan shows, in monetary terms, the amount of capital required to start the practice, the value of the assets and liabilities of the company (balance sheet), projections of profits on revenues over a three- to five-year time span (statement of cash flow), and, generally, a detailed listing of operating expenses (e.g., rent, utilities, phone, malpractice and business insurance, waste disposal, office and medical supplies, advertisements, employee wages and taxes) that are expected to be incurred for each period. These statements together are called proforma financial statements; basically, they are financial projections. Obviously, a proforma that is more detailed, verifiable, and profitable will promote a higher level of confidence in target investors or financial institutions. Depending on the proforma and type of practice, the APN will need to identify funding sources to provide capitalization of the practice. Start-up funds will need to last for at least a year and should include money to renovate and equip an office and cover expenses for at least the first six months. It will take at least four months to establish provider status in major insurance carriers such as Medicare and Medicaid and another two months for the APN to receive payment. The most obvious source of funding would be the individual's personal savings or loans from family and relatives. Outside funding such as banks and small business loans are an additional option, as is federal funding through grants (e.g., Small Business Innovation Research [SBIR] and the National Institute for Nursing Research [NINR]). In addition, APNs may have to work part time in other settings to supplement their income.

MODELS OF INNOVATIVE PRACTICE

The following models of independent practice illustrate several creative ways in which APNs have developed services that are not necessarily addressed by traditional health-care models. For these specific practices, it can be argued that offering these alternative services has been a factor in their success and longevity. The following are examples of innovative private practice models located in Pennsylvania.

NURSE-MANAGED PRIMARY CARE MODEL

The Centers for Family Health at Abbottsford and Schuylkill Falls in Philadelphia are health centers for residents of public housing funded by Public Health Service 340A. Donna Torrisi, RN MSN CFNP, is the director of the centers and has been a major force behind obtaining funding to operate the clinic. The Centers' supervisory board is an active and interested Management Board Tenant Council made up of residents in the public housing project, representatives of the parent corporation, and health center staff. Apartments, for the health-care service, within the public housing complex were donated by the community, allowing the health center to be located on the housing project campus.

The mission of the Centers is to provide primary care to the medically underserved residents of public housing projects in the East Falls section of Philadelphia. Ninety-eight percent of clients are African-Americans. This nurse-managed health center provides primary care to adults and children, prenatal and pediatric care, mental health services, and family planning on-site. A psychologist is on staff to provide group and individual counseling. Specific services, in addition to basic health care, include HIV/AIDS testing and education, tuberculosis screening, routine blood work, preventative health care, evaluation and treatment for drug and alcohol problems, group counseling, teen support, parenting skills, and a support group for grandparents raising grandchildren. The centers are committed to providing health promotion and education through prevention-based programs. In addition to clinical services, outreach workers visit patients in their homes, and free transportation service to the health centers is available. Grant funding enables the Centers to provide extra services such as community outreach and transportation service.

The staff includes three full-time family NPs, a psychologist, an administrative manager, a billing clerk, and office staff. Employees receive benefits that include health insurance for themselves and dependent children and vacation time. The practice has agreements with a collaborating internist and pediatrician, as well as written protocols.

The health center advertises its services through direct mail and word of mouth. Brochures are enclosed in the regional health maintenance organization (HMO) insurer information packet. Methods of payment for services include HMO plans (60%) and Medicaid (40%). Services to the uninsured or "working poor" continue to be funded through the grant.

INDEPENDENT NURSE SPECIALTY PRACTICE MODEL

One example of an independent private practice that targets the problem of urinary incontinence is Access to Continence Care and Treatment, Inc. (ACCT), founded and operated by Diane Newman, RNC, CRNP, FAAN. The practice addresses the growing need for incontinence services, particularly for the elderly in the Philadelphia area.

Since 1986, beginning with a practice called Golden Horizons, Newman and her staff have provided services for persons with urinary incontinence, interstitial cystitis, pelvic pain, and other bowel- and bladder-related disorders. Services are delivered in ambulatory, home care, and extended care settings by APNs who are independent practitioners. Through her practice, Newman and her staff have developed a national reputation for providing state-of-the-art assessment and behavioral treatment of urinary incontinence. The nursing staff all have a Master's Degree in Nursing and collectively have over 8 years of experience in the field of urology and urinary incontinence, 10 years in the field of geriatrics, and 20 years in the field of nursing. Newman has been involved in major research studies, including research funded by the National Institutes of Health on the homebound and industry-supported clinical studies on incontinence products. These studies have shown that in most cases urinary incontinence can be cured or managed by NPs using behavioral methods and alternative measures and devices.

ACCT combines the services of both APNs and physicians and thus is able to offer complete services for urinary incontinence. The staff collaborates with a physician who serves as the medical advisor. In this role, the physician provides medical oversight, additional prescriptive authority, and surgical intervention if absolutely necessary. This structure allows ACCT's services to be completely comprehensive and multifaceted by providing an approach to urinary incontinence that involves prevention, identification, evaluation, treatment, and management.

Since 1987, the staff has provided incontinence care and assessment to the Philadelphia Corporation for Aging (PCA), which serves the frail adult and chronically ill populations of Philadelphia through community-based, long-term care programs. The PCA primarily deals with a minority, underserved, inner-city population. The staff also provides continence consultation to numerous home health agencies and an ambulatory office practice.

Referrals are received from nurses, physicians, NPs, specialists, and social workers, as well as by word of mouth. Reimbursement for services is through several arrangements: contractual, fee-for-service, consultation, and third-party insurance.

Services provided in this independent practice model include evaluation and assessment of urinary incontinence and related problems to include history, modified physical examination, Pap smears, pelvic muscle rehabilitation, and urinalysis; environmental, functional, and mental status assessments; and development of a behavioral training program that offers habit or bladder retraining and pelvic muscle rehabilitation with the use of biofeedback therapy and electrical stimulation. This practice has been successful because it has identified an area of nursing and medicine that is not being served by existing models. The practice targets a specific medical problem that affects a large portion of the population that is not universally helped by standard medical interventions, such as surgery or medication.

THE BIRTH CENTER

The Birth Center in Bryn Mawr, Pennsylvania is an accredited, free-standing birthing center. It was established in 1978 by a community group, which included a CNM and an obstetrician, of women who wanted more control over the birth of their children. It is a nonprofit facility that is run by a community board. The Birth Center is one of 37 centers in the United States accredited through the National Association of Childbearing Centers. There are more than 53 birthing centers in the United States, the majority of which fall into the private for-profit category. Nurse-midwives own the majority (30%) of these centers, with physicians (21%) following second.

The Birth Center is managed by Clinical Director Denise Roy, RN, MSN, CNM, OB/GYN NP. This nurse-managed center provides birthing services, a child education series, and basic gynecological and women's health services, including family planning. The financial area of the practice is managed by a person with a background and experience in hospital administration.

The Center seeks a holistic approach to childbirth and attempts to empower women to be mentally prepared for birth. The center also offers women assistance in making decisions about their pregnancy. During pregnancy, the woman is asked to write a birth plan outlining how she would like to see the birth process evolve. Every birth is attended by a nurse-midwife and RN. Mothers usually stay at The Birth Center for 6 to 12 hours following delivery and are monitored by phone for

48 hours thereafter. Mother and baby receive a home visit by an RN two to three days following the birth. Mothers are scheduled for a six-week postpartum check-up with the midwife who attended the birth.

By design, The Birth Center is a warm and inviting place. It is located in a two-story house and includes two birthing rooms that are furnished like bedrooms, a bathroom with Jacuzzi, and two examination rooms.

The staff includes four full-time CNMs, one of whom is an NP, four RNs, an administrator, a billing clerk, and a receptionist. Employees receive health insurance and paid vacation and can participate in a newly implemented pension plan. The professional staff have a written agreement with an obstetrician and thus function under written protocols for co-management of difficult pregnancies and births. A quality assurance program has been instituted that includes a mandated case review of all complicated and transferred cases. Women identified as ''at risk'' are referred to obstetricians and include those with insulin-dependent diabetes, known cardiac diseases, essential hypertension, psychiatric disorders, cancer, or other severe medical problems. Women who develop complications during birth are transferred to a nearby hospital and the care of the collaborating obstetrician.

The Center advertises its services in local newspapers and through a weekly seminar for mothers interested in birthing centers. Methods of payment for services include HMO plans (50%), Medicaid (5 to 10%), private pay (10 to 15%), and other insurance (10%). A sliding scale called ''birth ships'' has been established for mothers who cannot afford to pay the fee; the balance is subsequently underwritten by private donation.

OVERVIEW OF BARRIERS TO COLLABORATIVE ADVANCED NURSING PRACTICE

Unnecessary restrictions on scope of practice, prescriptive authority, and eligibility for reimbursement prevent APNs with proven ability to safely meet the health-care needs of citizens (Safriet, 1992). In addition, organized medicine has opposed attempts of APNs to establish independent practice because of a fear that it will decrease physician power, control, and income (Birkholz & Walker, 1994). Three issues are central to the expansion of the role of APNs: (1) the legal scope of professional practice, (2) prescriptive authority, and (3) reimbursement privileges. Each of these areas is explored in more detail in the following sections and in Chapter 22.

LEGAL SCOPE OF ADVANCED NURSING PRACTICE

Although the title of APN includes the NP, CNM, CRNA, and CNS, the legal authority and scope of practice differ for these groups (Hanson, 1990). As part of the planning for collegial or independent practice, one should thoroughly review state medical and pharmacy acts and regulations, as well as state health agencies and their restrictions on independent practice. Despite their ability, APNs are constrained from independently practicing by restrictive legal requirements (Safriet, 1992). State nursing laws have expanded to cover APNs in four different approaches. In some states, there is a movement to separate levels of licensure for nurse specialties. The most common approach is to accommodate APN practice by expanding the state's basic definition of professional nurse practice. A second approach is through an amendment to the state's practice act to omit or limit the disclaimer against diagnosis and treatment by APNs. A third approach is to give physicians more delegative powers to APNs. This approach is not beneficial to maintaining APN independence and autonomy. A fourth approach is to separately certify or license APNs.

The definition of specific APNs has been clarified by state and government insurance agencies, specifically Medicare. In order for the APN to be reimbursed for services they must meet the definition of an APN as outlined. The current definition of a certified APN is defined as a registered professional nurse who must:

Be currently licensed to practice as a registered professional nurse in the state in which the services are furnished

Satisfy the applicable state requirements (if any) for qualification of an advanced practice nurse in the state in which the services are furnished

Be currently certified as a APN in a particular specialty by a recognized national certifying body

In order not to disadvantage those CNSs who satisfy all requirements except for state licensure and because many states do not have specific licensure requirements for the CNS, the Health Care Financing Administration (HCFA) is revising the requirements for the CNS. However, until a definition of a CNS is established through rule-making, if a nurse meets the definition of "clinical nurse specialist" as given in the previous list, even where state law does not specifically refer to this term, he or she may be recognized for direct reimbursement.

Most states require some type of relationship between the APN and a physician. This requirement can adversely affect independent nursing practice by imposing unilateral control over the APN regardless of the skill and experience of the APN (Safriet, 1992).

PRESCRIPTIVE AUTHORITY

Prescriptive authority is an integral part of advanced practice nursing that is addressed state by state. Organized medicine has lobbied against any legislative efforts to allow independent prescriptive authority for APNs and in some instances has attempted to limit their authority to certain geographical locations (Wilkin, 1995). Providers in other disciplines have joined organized medicine in opposing prescriptive authority for NPs because of fear of direct competition. Towers (1989), in her report on a national survey of NPs, states that "pharmacologic practices reflect the sites, patients, areas of practice and law of the states in which they reside." There are more APNs with prescriptive authority in the West than any region in the country; Alaska, Washington, and Oregon are currently the only states with a broad licensure, although practice conditions change continuously from state to state (Mahoney, 1992). APNs who have prescriptive authority are more likely to work in non-urban, non-group practice sites. However, a 1989 survey of NPs (Towers, 1989) reported that in all 50 states, NPs managed pharmacological therapies through several different methods. Methods reported are not well defined but include medications signed under the NP's own name, signed jointly with a physician, or prescribed under the physician's name. The majority of NPs prescribe only certain groups of drugs, which include analgesics, antihistamines, antimicrobials, anti-inflammatories, topicals, and vitamins. The majority of studies of NPs and prescriptive authority conclude that NPs with independent prescriptive authority do not prescribe significantly differently than NPs dependent on physician agreement or signature to prescribe (Towers, 1989). Even where APNs are able to remove barriers to their legal scope of practice and prescriptive authority, the impediments to direct reimbursement remain.

DETERMINING REIMBURSEMENT STRATEGIES

When conceptualizing a collaborative nurse practice, understanding the methods for nurse reimbursement are essential. The lack of direct reimbursement is one of the serious impediments to the use of APNs in the health-care system, leading to their under-utilization despite known efficacy, cost-effectiveness, and value (Office of Technology Assessment, 1986). It has also been one of the major reasons why nurses do not view the establishment of a private practice as an attractive option. However, significant changes in the 1980s and early 1990s in federal laws governing health programs have enabled APNs to be directly reimbursed for their services. Almost 80% of providers' reimbursements come from insurance carriers. Third-party payers can be divided into three categories: private health companies, government-sponsored or public health insurance programs, and "independent health plans" such as HMOs. The groups of APNs that have been most successful in obtaining direct third-party reimbursement are nurse-midwives, nurse-anesthetists, and NPs.

The method by which direct third-party reimbursement for services of APNs is accomplished affects the consumer's freedom of choice, access to health care, the cost of health care, and the role of the nurse in the health-care system (Mittelstadt, 1993). APNs must follow specific rules and regulations to be eligible for reimbursement. These rules and regulations are dictated by individual state laws as well as by federal requirements. Many of the changes in federal health programs such as Medicare and Medicaid were made to improve health-care access to underserved populations, such as nursing home residents, low-income women and children, and people in rural areas. Rules and Regulations for APNs under Medicare and Medicaid are under continual review and revision by HCFA and the U.S. Congress.

Medicare

Medicare provides health insurance benefits for all individuals aged 65 years and older, as well as qualified blind and disabled persons. Medicare is regulated by the federal government and financed by employer and employee contributions through payroll taxes and the co-payments and premiums of beneficiaries. Individual medical plans are administered by various commercial carriers, whereas Medicare plans are administrated by state offices of the HCFA. Medicare consists of two parts: Part A, for hospitalization costs, and Part B, a voluntary supplementary medical insurance that covers physicians, medical equipment, out-patient services, NPs, CNMs, CRNAs, and CNSs under certain conditions.

Medicare's allowables are charge-based: they evaluate the cost of a service as the historical price of the service. For example, Medicare profiles are based on the fee schedule that was established 6 to 18 months earlier. Payment by Medicare Part B is usually 80% of the lowest, customary, prevailing, or actual charge for that period. For APNs, the payment for Medicare services is limited to 85% of the participating physicians' fee for the specific service. The American Nurses Association (ANA) is supporting the principle of equal pay for equal work to increase the APN reimbursement to the same rate as that used for physicians.

Currently, providers can either participate in Medicare or be non-participating providers. Many physician providers choose to be non-participators in the Medicare program. They can then collect up to the full limiting charge from the client and secondary carrier. However, the trend is for most providers to participate in Medicare or be penalized. APNs who are Medicare providers must be participating providers, which means they will accept "assignment," the allowable charge determined by Medicare.

Unless specified otherwise, the APN must work in "collaboration" with a physician in order to qualify for reimbursement under Medicare. The HCFA has defined collaboration as a process by which an NP works with a physician to deliver health-care services within the scope of the NP's professional expertise with appropriate medical supervision and direction. There must be jointly developed guidelines or other mechanisms in which the services are performed.

Under the CNS Medicare benefit, coverage is available for CNS services and such "incident to" services if the CNS is legally authorized to perform the services in accordance with state law and the services would otherwise be covered if furnished by a physician. Such CNS coverage is also contingent upon the CNS working in "collaboration" with a physician. As a practical matter, the statutory requirement that the CNS must be "legally authorized to perform the services in accordance with state law" means that a CNS seeking to bill under the new benefit will have to demonstrate to the local Medicare carrier that the CNS meets the definition of a CNS as prescribed in the previous section. This definition allows recognition of CNSs for Medicare coverage purposes, even on an interim basis, although they are not specifically identified as a type of practitioner (or licensed as CNSs) under applicable state law.

Medicare covers APN services in the following areas:

Rural Health Clinics: Congress authorizes NP and CNS services to be covered when provided in rural health clinics. The payment is to the clinic and not directly to the NP. For the purposes of Medicare and Medicaid reimbursement, rural health clinic providers are defined as:

- Services of physician assistants, specialized NPs, and nurse-midwives
- Services and supplies furnished as "incident to" services provided by NPs
- Visiting nurse services on a part-time or intermittent basis to home-bound clients

Rural Areas: To improve access to primary care in rural areas, a law was enacted in 1990 to allow APN services to be reimbursed in rural areas in all settings. The exception is when the services are provided in a hospital setting (in-patient or out-patient), in which case payments must be made to the hospital. A rural area is defined as including any county that is not identified as urbanized by the Bureau of the Census—that is, it is outside of a metropolitan statistical area (MSA). To determine rural areas in a particular state, the APN will need to contact the state health department. Many states have rural health offices within the public health sector. In rural health, the practice or clinic can be privately or publicly owned, can be for-profit or not-for-profit, and need only be under the general direction or collaboration of a physician. At this time it is not necessary for the APN to live in the rural county to be providing services in that county.

Office Practice: Under Medicare, direct reimbursement is not available to NPs or CNSs employed in independent private, non-rural office practice at this time, although Congress is studying such reimbursement. An NP or CNS may, however, be licensed under state law to perform a specific medical procedure and may be able to perform the procedure with direct physician supervision. The service by the nurse must be delivered under the physician's direct supervision, which means that the physician must be in the same room or be present in the office suite. When services are performed outside the office setting, i.e., a home visit to a patient, the physician must make the visit with the APN. The practicing APN must have an employer-employee relationship with a physician. This strict supervision definition severely restricts the APN's practice in an office and home care setting in an urban area.

Hospital Out-Patient Clinics: Direct reimbursement for APNs is reimbursed by Medicare under the "incident to" provision if the APN is an employee of the hospital. Services must be furnished on a physician's order by hospital personnel and under a physician's supervision. Although the presence and availability of a physician is required, the physician's presence is presumed if the clinic is on hospital premises. The physician must see the patient periodically to assess the course of treatment and the patient's progress.

Skilled Nursing Facilities: Because of concern over improving the care of nursing home residents, in 1989 Congress enacted a provision to reimburse APNs for providing services to residents in skilled nursing facilities. Services include Medicare-covered physician services and those that an APN is legally authorized to perform in accordance with state law and regulations. The APN must work in "collaboration" with a physician and meet the individual state's definition of an APN. Payment for the APN services is made to the employer. Therefore, the APN must be an employee or have a contractual relationship with the individual or facility who submits the claim. There must be a valid employment arrangement, and the test used is the common-law test of an employer-employee relationship. The rule requiring collaboration with a physician excludes the ability of APNs to act as the employer. A group of APNs who have incorporated cannot bill for their services; thus, nurses in independent practice cannot bill for services. A team consists of a physician and a physician assistant acting under the supervision of the physician, an NP working in collaboration with the physician, or both. Team cannot be used to describe a medical group that does not employ either physician assistants or APNs. A team of one does not meet the definition of a team. These Medicare rules require close monitoring because yearly Congressional changes to Medicare law could improve the reimbursement status of APN providers.

Medicare Health Maintenance Organizations (HMOs): APN services in Medicare-designated HMOs are covered, with the payment going directly to the HMO in the form of a prepaid capitated payment per beneficiary.

Certified Nurse-Midwives: Services performed by CNMs are covered at 65% of the prevailing charge that would be recognized if the service had been performed by the physician. No supervision by any other health-care professional is needed if not required by the individual state. Services provided by the CNM are not restricted to childbearing but can include other women's health services.

Certified Registered Nurse Anesthetists: Coverage of services performed by CRNAs depends on whether the services are medically directed or non-medically directed. By 1996, payment rates for independent CRNAs will be the same as payment rates for anesthesiologists for the same service.

Community Nursing Organization (CNO): In 1987, Congress authorized CNO demonstration projects to allow the nurse to coordinate and establish the plan of care for Medicare beneficiaries in need of post-acute health-care services, such as home health. Strumpf (1994) states that the CNO combines both community health nursing and managed care into one model with the goals of containing costs and outcomes. Fees are to the CNO as a capitated monthly fee per beneficiary. It is stipulated that the CNO must provide all the post-acute care services needed, which can include nursing care; physical, occupational, or speech therapy; social services; home health care; and durable medical equipment.

Medicaid

Medicaid provides health insurance benefits, as well as other assistance for eligible low-income individuals and families. Medicaid is a jointly funded state/federal insurance program. Coverage varies by state according to federal requirements that stipulate eligibility and basic services covered. Payment is usually lower than is available through other insurance groups. In 1989, Congress mandated that state Medicaid agencies cover certain categories of NPs in order to increase access to care in underserved areas or for certain vulnerable populations. All states, by federal mandate, must cover the services of CNMs, CRNAs, pediatric NPs, and family NPs. APNs receive Medicaid reimbursement in 49 states, 39 of which reimburse at 80 to 100% of a physician's rate (Pearson, 1994). A 1989 ruling required state Medicaid agencies to furnish certified nurse practitioner (CNP) services to all medically needy recipients and to cover services regardless of whether the CNP is supervised by or associated with a physician or other health-care provider. The CNP is paid directly under an independent provider agreement or through the employing provider. To date, all but four states (Illinois, Ohio, Connecticut and Rhode Island) have implemented direct reimbursement to family NPs and pediatric NPs, and many states have opted to include coverage that is broader than mandated and includes all NPs and some categories of CNSs (Keepnews, 1994).

A recent change in the state Medicaid program has been the waiver programs that allow the state to be exempt from one or more federal Medicaid requirements. Many Medicaid programs are implementing "case management" or "gatekeeper" programs in which the recipients must be referred by a "gatekeeper" before a service will be covered. Some states only identify physicians as gatekeepers, thus decreasing the access of NPs and CNSs to the Medicaid population (Keepnews, 1994).

Prior to billing Medicaid, the APN needs to apply for a provider number and become aware of Medicaid rules. Every state publishes a handbook of Medicaid rules complete with updates, and Medicaid payers publish newsletters periodically.

Federal Employee Health Benefit Program (FEHBP)

The FEHBP is the health insurance plan for the approximately 10 million federal employees and their dependents. This is a voluntary, contributory program open to all employees of the federal government. Contracts are held with private health insurance carriers to offer health insurance plans to federal employees. In 1985, Congress mandated that the services of non-physician providers, including NPs, CNSs, CRNAs, and CNMs, be covered in all federal health plans for the medically underserved through Public Law (101–509), enacted November 5, 1990. This law allows federal employees enrolled in the FEHBP direct access to NPs, CNSs, and CNMs, thus reimbursing these health-care providers. Under this provision, insurance carriers for federal plans must make payment directly to these providers if their services are covered under the plan. Collaboration with or supervision by a physician or any other health-care provider is not needed. The payment level is determined by the individual health insurance plan.

Civilian Health and Medical Program of the Uniformed Services (CHAMPUS)

The CHAMPUS program reimburses for health-care services provided to the 7 to 9 million dependents of active duty military personnel and eligible retirees by non-military providers when these people cannot obtain care from a military hospital. CHAMPUS benefits are usually used when the health-care services being provided are only available in the private sector. In 1979, CNMs were covered through direct payment and without a requirement of physician supervision. In 1982, the services of certified NPs, CRNAs, and certified psychiatric NPs were covered with the same provisions. Families of the armed forces and certain civilians receive benefits through various providers who are approved by the headquarters and billing center in South Carolina. The NP must agree to the allowable payment, which is the same rate as that of a physician, and must get provider authorization prior to billing. CHAMPUS is one of the easiest carriers to deal with and a good provider.

Private Health Insurance Programs

Private health insurance plans include carriers such as Blue Cross/Blue Shield, Aetna, Prudential, and Metropolitan. Many of these carriers are merging into larger entities with the move to managed care. NPs receive direct reimbursement by private insurance carriers in 25 states (Pearson, 1994). However, an insurance policy does not explicitly need to include the coverage of nursing services for APNs to be reimbursed for their services. When considering application for third-party reimbursement, the nurse needs to be familiar with the state's nurse practice act, state insurance laws and codes (including reimbursement amendments), judicial decisions, and opinions by the attorney general. State health insurance laws do not necessarily prohibit third-party reimbursement to nurses. In Florida, for instance, direct third-party reimbursement is essentially a 1:1 process. The individual nurse applies to the third-party insurer and requests provider status. If reimbursement is rejected, familiarity with the state's nursing practice act and the state's health insurance laws can assist the nurse in appealing the decision.

Managed-Care Programs

"Managed Care" denotes a spectrum of arrangements that entail some connection between financing and delivery of care, usually with cost-containment (American Academy of Nursing, 1993). Many managed-care companies base their reimbursement on a combination of historical area charge data, relative value scales, and actuarial data. Managed-care entities will usually either discount a physician's fee for services or require that a predetermined fee be charged. However, the majority of managed-care companies pay providers a "capitated" fee, which means the provider cares for a client population for a prearranged amount. Capitation amounts typically vary by "member" age, gender, and risk status and are negotiable. APNs must learn the art of negotiation. Negotiable areas include practice exclusivity, sign-on bonus to the practice for new members recruited to the HMO, and profit-sharing (Jenkins & Torrisi, 1995).

Managed-care programs are offered by commercial insurance carriers and include preferred payment organizations (PPOs) and HMOs among others. HMOs encompass any variety of prepaid group practice arrangements. These programs usually offer health-care services to members enrolled in the plan for a predetermined, prepaid, or discounted fee. Prepaid means that the organization receives a fixed payment or premium to care for members of a certain population and that the organization bears the financial risk for the care that members receive. Participating providers are required to provide services for contracted reimbursement amounts. This reimbursement can range from a discounted fee for service to a lump sum for all services required. There are five main types of HMOs (Mezey & McGivern, 1993):

> *Staff-model HMOs* employ salaried physicians who work in the HMO's own clinics.
> *Group-model HMOs* contract with a large multi-specialty-group practice.
> *Independent Practice Association (IPA) model HMOs* contract with individual physicians or affiliations of independent physicians.
> *Network HMO models* are similar to IPAs except that they contract with several larger physician groups. Some models are *mixed* combinations of group, staff, network, or IPA models.
> *A PPO* is a network of providers, usually physicians and hospitals, that have discounted their fees for an increased volume of patients.

HMOs make extensive use of APNs in order to increase the cost-effectiveness of primary care. Jenkins and Torrisi (1995) state that many private and public HMOs and other managed-care organizations have been slow to enroll primary-care APNs as providers that receive direct capitation payment. California APNs have experienced "lock out" from some managed-care contracts. Once APNs have applied to the insurer for provider status, they will need to become educated concerning billing procedures.

IMPLEMENTING BILLING PROCEDURES AND POLICIES

Development of clear, concise billing procedures and policies will enhance the efficiency of the practice as well as clearly communicate to clients where their responsibilities for payment lie.

Areas Requiring Office Policy

- Cash collection at the time of service
- Acceptance of credit cards

- Assistance in filing insurance claims
- Electronic claim submission
- Fee reduction or sliding scale for low-income patients
- Payment plans
- Interest on unpaid balances
- The practice's level of collection efforts

To bill for medical services, most insurance carriers require that reimbursement codes be used. Reimbursement codes are the standard language used by both insurance carriers and health-care providers. These codes provide a uniform interpretation of medical conditions and identify the billable services of the provider.

Areas of Consideration When Identifying Billing Codes

- Coding all billable procedures, services, and supplies
- Identifying all procedures according to *Physician's Current Procedural Terminology* (CPT) guidelines and codes
- Listing a diagnostic code for all procedures billed
- Using modifiers as necessary

COMMUNICATING CLIENT RESPONSIBILITY

Clients need to assume some level of self-care and financial responsibility for their health care. They should be familiar with their insurance programs, particularly with regard to understanding that most programs do not provide the "blanket insurance" elements that were common in the past. A clearly written client responsibility section should be included in all client information files. This statement should be presented to each client and acknowledged by the client. It may contain a statement of financial responsibility for the account to prevent misunderstandings regarding the client's payment obligation. In addition, it would be advantageous to include a "release of information" and an "assignment of insurance benefits directly to the practitioner" statement as part of the information sheet. These releases expedite the processing of insurance claims when a signature is required and facilitate release or transfer of information should a client request it.

INSURANCE FORMS

To coordinate coverage benefits, many insurance carriers require providers to submit insurance claim forms for clients. These forms must be filled out completely and correctly to receive full reimbursement. Providers must be sure to verify client information for accuracy and obtain current client signatures and pre-authorizations.

To accurately track medical services, the APN should develop a billing form often referred to as a "superbill." Superbills are reserved primarily for office use only and should not be used to bill medical insurance. The use of a well-designed superbill that defines evaluation and management makes it much easier to report services as well as to provide consistency because it allows for accurate identification of services performed (Table 25–2). Some practices print their most common diagnostic codes directly on the superbill; all frequently used procedure codes

TABLE 25–2. SAMPLE SUPERBILL

Office Visit

	New Patient		Subsequent Care Pt.	
1. Low	99201		99211	
2. Moderate	99202		99212	
3. Mod/Complex	99203		99213	
4. High	99204		99214	
5. High/Complex	99205		99215	

E/M codes in the range 99201–99215 are used to report services provided to new and established clients in office and other out-patient facilities. The key coding issues are the extent of history obtained, the extent of examination performed, and the complexity of medical decision-making.

Home Visit

	New Patient		Subsequent Care Pt.	
Low	99341		99351	
Moderate	99342		99352	
Complex/High	99343		99353	

E/M codes in the range of 99341–99353 are used to report services provided to new and established clients in the client's home. The key coding issues are the extent of history obtained, the extent of examination performed, and the complexity of medical decision-making. Additional reporting issues include counseling and/or coordination of care and the nature of presenting problem. Time as a factor in E/M of home visits has not been defined as of *CPT 1993*.

Nursing Home Visit

	New Patient		Subsequent Care Pt.	
Low	99301		99311	
Moderate	99302		99312	
Complex/High	99303		99313	

E/M codes in the range of 99301–99313 are used to report services provided in nursing facilities. The key coding issues are the extent of history obtained, the extent of examination performed, and the complexity of medical decision-making. Additional reporting issues include counseling and/or coordination of care, the nature of presenting problem(s), and the time spent at the bedside and on the resident's facility floor or unit. Assessment of resident's functional capacity should be documented.

should be included. This makes it easy to check the appropriate code, which can then be typed on the form sent to the carrier.

The client information or demographic form used by the practice should specifically ask what insurance the client has. Ask to see the client's insurance card to verify the expiration date and maintain a photocopy in the client's chart. APNs should also develop consistent charging guidelines to be used for all insurance carriers.

UNDERSTANDING BILLING CODES

The APN will need to become knowledgeable about the billing process, the use of billing codes, and how insurance carriers interpret these reimbursement codes. The only nursing services reimbursed are those that insurers consider to be physician services. Therefore, many nursing services that are considered unique to nursing may be excluded (Mezey, 1993). This section outlines the primary coding systems—*International Classification of Disease*, 9th edition (ICD-9-CM), *CPT*, and HCFA Common Procedure Coding System (HCPC) codes—that APNs will use for reimbursement.

The ICD-9-CM codes are diagnostic codes that identify the condition, illness, or injury to be treated. The ICD is a useful tool in the area of classification of morbidity data for indexing medical records, medical care review, ambulatory and other medical care programs, and basic health statistics. The use of these codes is strongly recommended for use when billing insurance carriers (Table 25–3) because services provided in any setting use this diagnostic system. The HCFA has prepared guidelines for using ICD-9 codes and instructions on how to report them on claim forms. Obtain a copy of the guidelines for using these codes from your

TABLE 25–3. SAMPLE OF ICD-9 DIAGNOSIS

110.3	Fungus—groin
112.9	Infection—*Candida*
244.9	Hypothyroidism
250	Diabetes mellitus
250.01	Diabetes mellitus (insulin)
250.6	Diabetes—neuropathy
274.9	Gout—unspecified
290.0	Senile dementia
290.00	Alzheimer disease
309.1	Depression
332	Paralysis agitans (Parkinson's)
401.9	Essential hypertension
401.9	Hypertension—unspecified
413.9	Angina pectoris
414.0	Arteriosclerotic heart disease (ASHD)
427.5	Cardiac arrest
436.0	Cerebrovascular accident (CVA)
440.9	Arteriosclerosis
564.3	Constipation
595.0	Acute cystitis
595.1	Interstitial cystitis
599.5	Urethrocele—male
599.6	Urinary obstruction—unspecified
600	Hematuria
601.0	Acute/chronic prostatitis
618.1	Uterine prolapse (all degrees)
623.1	Vagina/leukoplakia
625.6	Urinary incontinence—stress (female)
626	Pelvic (female) perineum
716.90	Rheumatoid arthritis
728	Muscle wasting tissue
733	Osteoporosis
788.0	Voiding dysfunction

Medicare intermediary. Each service or procedure performed for a client must be represented by a diagnosis that would substantiate those particular services or procedures, such as *dipstick urinalysis* for a diagnosis of urinary tract infection.

CPT codes are those listed in the *Physician's Current Procedural Terminology* (CPT) manual published annually by the American Medical Association (AMA). *CPT* specifies the procedure or medical service given. *CPT* lists over 7,000 descriptive terms used in coding medical services and procedures performed by APNs. All services or procedures paid for by third-party payers are listed in the *CPT* manual. The evaluation and management codes are part of the *CPT* system. Each code is assigned a procedural description, which is referred to as the nomenclature or terminology. The terminology describes procedures consistent with contemporary medical practice performed by multiple providers in many locations.

Medicare and state Medicaid carriers are required by law to use *CPT* codes for the payment of health insurance claims; the majority of insurance carriers recognize and use *CPT* codes. Although there may be a *CPT* code that describes a current medical procedure, an insurance carrier is not obligated to reimburse the provider for that service. The *CPT* codes selected for reimbursement billing should accurately reflect the series or procedures performed.

The HCFA Common Procedure Coding System (HCPC) is used for reporting supplies and medical equipment. To receive full reimbursement, the APN needs to code both diagnosis and service to the greatest possible level of specificity. Inaccurate coding results in partial reimbursement, reimbursement delay, and possible prosecution for fraudulent billing. Medicare and some Medicaid programs also use the HCPC's coding system.

Using Modifiers

Many providers use modifiers to indicate that a service or procedure performed was modified or altered but did not change in its definition or code. For example, modifiers clarify the following components of care:

- Has a technical and professional component
- Was performed by more than one provider and/or in more than one location
- Was partially performed
- Was performed with an adjunctive service or a bilateral procedure
- Was provided more than once
- Involved unusual events or circumstances

Modifier Definition

Understanding the proper use of modifiers substantially affects insurance claim reimbursement. This is particularly true when the APN is the provider. Attaching the appropriate modifier to the *CPT* code tells the insurer the type of provider and the setting in which the service was provided. Examples of modifiers relevant to the APN are:

- **AL** Nurse practitioner/certified nurse-midwife, non-rural, team member
- **AK** Nurse practitioner/certified nurse-midwife, rural, team member
- **AV** Nurse practitioner/certified nurse-midwife, rural, non-team-member

- **AW** Clinical nurse specialist, non-team-member
- **AY** Clinical nurse specialist, team member

The modifier is attached to the end of the *CPT* or HCPC code.

DOCUMENTATION

Proper documentation is essential to the reimbursement process. Insurance carriers will frequently limit or deny reimbursement for services because of insufficient documentation. In addition, they may request refunds after an insurance audit if medical records do not substantiate the reported services. Proper documentation is also important from legal and financial standpoints. Failure to document services rendered translates into non-performance of service. Any billed services must be documented on the client's chart. Notation of unusual services or extenuating circumstances should leave no room for misinterpretation or assumption.

The Evaluation and Management (E/M) services are a new way of classifying and documenting the work of the provider. E/M services are a result of the resource-based relative value scale (RBRVS), which was developed to compensate providers for cognitive effort rather than time expended. The descriptions for the levels of E/M services recognize seven components, six of which are used in defining the levels of E/M services. Two to three components must be documented when an E/M service code is used. Of the seven components, the first three are the key components and have elements that must be part of the documentation on the client's medical record. These seven components are defined as the following:

History should include the client's chief complaint, plus a brief history of present problem or illness and a related system review, as well as family or social history. The comprehensive E/M code visit is the more detailed and thorough history of the client's chief complaint.

Physical examination can be focused and only address the affected body area or organ system or can be comprehensive, including a complete examination of a single system causing the problem, plus multisystem physical examination.

Medical decision-making involves the complexity in establishing a diagnosis and selecting a certain management strategy and should include a list of all possible diagnoses and management options, an analysis of medical records, all diagnostic tests, and other information analyzed.

Counseling is defined as discussions or meetings with client, family, caregivers, and nursing staff (as in long-term care). Counseling can involve discussions about disease process, results of diagnostic tests, prognosis, education and instructions on management, and treatment options.

Coordination of care involves time spent working with other health-care providers and agencies to direct care. This must be well-documented in the client's medical record if it denotes the care.

Nature of the presenting problem is the documentation of the reason for the client's office visit or need to be seen by the provider.

The last component, time, must be included in the client's medical record.

Time is an integral part of the E/M services. Time is defined as "face-to-face" time in the office; time spent reviewing records, tests, arranging further services; or time spent with staff such as in the nursing home. Time should be averaged in minutes and recorded in the client's medical record.

Competence in the use of appropriate billing codes and policies is essential to successful advanced nursing practice. Utilization of state and national resources is necessary for APNs who wish to be health-care providers.

CONCLUSION

This chapter has provided an overview of the development of two private practice models (collaborative and independent) and the tools available to the APN for providing services. Recent changes in reimbursement policies have opened opportunities for the development of successful innovative APN models. The national emphasis on primary care, medical care reform, and preventative health care lends itself to the need for innovative practice delivery systems and the emergence of the APN as a prominent health-care provider. The rapidly aging population has led to a growing need for APN services in home care, community-based programs, and long-term care. APNs are in an optimal position to take on the role of direct providers in the health-care arena. The APN must not lose the opportunity that has become available through changes in state laws and federal reimbursement policies. However, to be successful in a collaborative or independent practice model, the APN must learn about the intricacies of developing a business, understand and be able to financially overcome the barriers to practice, and access the information needed to be reimbursed for services. Collaborative models with nurses and other health-care providers and the development of solo independent practices that target specific underserved areas of medicine are keys to successful private practice in the changing health-care environment. The APN must become not only a nursing expert but an expert in the "art of the deal" to be able to successfully negotiate with insurers, particularly managed-care companies. As the traditional role of the nurse begins to erode, APNs will need to carve out a place in the private practice setting in order to continue to bring high-quality nurse-driven care to clients.

REFERENCES

Aiken, L. H., & Sage, W. M. (1992). Staffing national health care reform: A role for advanced practice nurses. *Akron Law Review, 26,* 187-211.

American Academy of Nursing (1993). *Managed care & national health care reform: Nurses can make it work.* Washington, D.C.: American Academy of Nursing.

Birkholz, G., & Walker, D. (1994). Strategies for state statutory language changes granting fully independent nurse practitioner practice. *Nurse Practitioner, 19*(1), 54-58.

Calmelat, A. (1993). Tips for starting your own nurse practitioner practice. *Nurse Practitioner, 18*(4), 58-68.

Hanson, C. (1990). The nurse practitioner and clinical nurse specialist: Should the roles be merged? *Journal of the American Academy of Nurse Practitioners, 2*(1), 2-9.

Hanson, C. (1993). Our role in health care reform: Collegiality counts. *American Journal of Nursing, 93*(12), 16A–E.

Jenkins, M., & Torrisi, D. (1995). A nurse practitioner, community nursing centers, and contracting for managed care. *Journal of the American Academy of Nurse Practitioners, 7*(3), 119-124.

Keepnews, D. (1994). *The reimbursement manual: How to get paid for your advanced practice nursing services* (Supplement). Washington D.C.: American Nurses Publishing.

Keller, N. S. (1975). The why's and what's of private practice. *Journal of Nursing Administration*, *5*(3), 12-15.

Kinlein, M. L. (1977). *Independent nursing practice with clients* (pp. 2-5, 113). Philadelphia: J. B. Lippincott.

Mahoney, D. F. (1992). A comparative analysis of nurse practitioners with and without prescriptive authority. *Journal of the American Academy of Nurse Practitioners*, *4*(2), 71-76.

Mezey, M. D., & McGivern, D. O. (Eds.) (1993). *Nurses, nurse practitioners: Evolution to advanced practice.* New York: Springer.

Mittelstadt, P. (1993). *The reimbursement manual: How to get paid for your advanced practice nursing services.* Washington D. C.: American Nurses Publishing.

Moniz, D. M. (1992). The legal danger of written protocols and standards of practice. *Nurse Practitioner*, *17*(9), 58-60.

Newman, D. K., & Palumbo, M. V. (1994). Planning an independent nursing practice for continence services. *Nurse Practitioner Forum*, *5*(3), 190-193.

Office of Technology Assessment, U. S. Congress, HCS 37 (1986). *Nurse practitioners, physician assistants, and certified nurse-midwives: A policy analysis (OTA-HCS-37).* Washington, D.C.: U.S. Government Printing Office.

Pearson, L. J. (1994). Annual update of how each state stands on legislative issues affecting advanced nursing practice. *Nurse Practitioner*, *19*(1), 11-13, 17-18, 21-22, 24-27, 31-34, 39-40, 42-44, 50.

Safriet, B. J. (1992). Health care dollars and regulatory sense: The role of advanced practice nursing. *Yale Journal on Regulation*, *9*(2), 417-487.

Sebas, M. B. (1994). Developing a collaborative practice agreement for the primary care setting. *Nurse Practitioner*, *19*(4), 49-51.

Stewart, P. (1989). Program and practice management for the advanced practice nurse. In A. B. Hamric & J. A. Spross (Eds.), *The clinical nurse specialist in theory and practice.* Philadelphia: W. B. Saunders.

Strumpf, N. (1994). Innovative gerontological practices as models for health care delivery. *Nursing & Health Care*, *15*(10), 522-527.

Towers, J. (1989). Report of the National Survey of the American Academy of Nurse Practitioners: Part II, Pharmacologic Management Practices. *Journal of the American of Nurse Practitioners*, *1*, 137-142.

Vogel, G., & Doleysh, N. (1994). *Entrepreneuring: A nurse's guide to starting a business.* New York: National League for Nursing.

Wilken, M. (1995). Nonphysician providers: How regulations affect availability and access to care. *Nursing Policy Forum*, *1*(2), 28-37.

Additional Readings

Badger, F. J., Drummond, M. F., & Isaacs, B. (1993). Some issues in the clinical, social and economic evaluation of new nursing services. *Journal of Advanced Nursing*, *8*, 487-494.

Crowenwett, L. Molding the future of advanced practice nursing. *Nursing Outlook*, *43*(3), 112-118.

Hall, J. K. (1993). How to analyze nurse practitioner licensure laws. *Nurse Practitioner*, *18*(8), 31-34.

Soehren, P. M., & Schymann, L. L. (1994). Enhanced role opportunities available to the CNS/nurse practitioner. *Clinical Nurse Specialist*, *8*(3), 123-127.

Sox, H. C., et al. (1994). Physician assistants and nurse practitioners. *Annals of Internal Medicine*, *121*, 714-716.

Sullivan, E. M. (1992). Nurse practitioner reimbursement. *Nursing & Health Care*, *13*(5), 236-241.

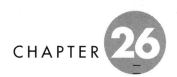

CHAPTER 26

Evaluating Advanced Nursing Practice

Shirley A. Girouard

INTRODUCTION

The advanced practice nurse (APN), as a member of the nursing profession, has a social responsibility to promote the optimal health of individuals, families, and communities. This responsibility to the public includes contributing to the resolution of problems that limit the health-care system's ability to achieve optimal health for individuals. These issues include problems of access to services and concerns about the quality, effectiveness, and cost of interventions. Verification of nursing's contributions to improved health requires the assessment of the structures, processes, and outcomes related to nursing practice. The knowledge gained from these efforts can be used to improve the health of the public by improving the organization, delivery, and financing of health-care services and enhancing the practice, education, and research activities of nurses. Although nursing has always been involved with various aspects of evaluation, both experience and a review of the literature reveal the need for more comprehensive and sound research to fulfill professional obligations and to continue to improve nursing practice.

Advanced nursing practice (APN), as defined in Chapter 3, builds on the foundation of professional nursing practice. By virtue of their educational and practice competencies, APNs must be able to provide society with evidence of their contributions to health care. Changes in the organization, delivery, and financing of health care during the past decade and the continued pressure on the health-care system to be more accountable to policymakers, consumers, and the general public have made evaluation a critical issue for APNs. Employers, consumers, insurers, competing providers, and others are calling on APNs to justify their contributions to health-care outcomes and the health-care system.

Evaluation is the systematic application of research procedures to assess the conceptualization, design, implementation, and utility of health-care interventions. Evaluation procedures make it possible to determine what APN structural and process elements improve access, promote the best quality, contribute to patient outcomes, and provide cost-effective services. Evaluation studies are difficult and documentation is complex because of the context of the evaluation and factors inherent in the APN role. Although some progress has been made, much remains to be done if advanced nursing practice is to be appropriately recognized for its importance and contributions. Rossi and Freeman (1989) identified the types of questions that are typically asked in evaluation research:

- What is the nature and scope of the problem requiring a new, expanded, or modified intervention?
- Where is the intervention provided and whom does it affect?
- What feasible interventions are likely to ameliorate the problem significantly?
- What are the appropriate targets for the intervention?
- Is the intervention reaching the target population?
- Is the intervention being implemented as envisioned?
- Is the intervention effective?
- How much does the intervention cost?
- What are the intervention's costs relative to its effectiveness and benefits?

These and similar questions should guide the APN engaged as a primary evaluator or involved in working with others to evaluate practice. By focusing on practice, the APN uses an understanding of patient issues (Hamric, 1983) to make evaluation meaningful and relevant. The systematic evaluation of APN interventions will contribute to knowledge of nursing practice, and the knowledge thus gained can be interpreted for others to substantiate APNs' contributions to the health-care system. Whether the purpose of the evaluation is to assess individual performance, job satisfaction, a programmatic change, the impact of an institutional or governmental policy, or patient care outcomes, the evaluation must address what difference advanced nursing practice makes in relation to access, quality, or cost if the evaluation results are to have value beyond the individual and the immediate work setting. The underlying question is: So what? That is, what difference does the APN make in the health-care system? Are the APN's contributions unique and valuable, and can this be shown to others? For example:

- In assessing individual performance in a hospital setting, the clinical nurse specialist (CNS) must be able to identify how performance contributes to the patient-focused mission and goals of the organization. Does the CNS's practice reduce length of stay, improve patient outcomes, or enhance the efficiency of staff nurses?
- The certified nurse-midwife (CNM) concerned about job satisfaction needs to link this concept to the practice setting's ability to better meet patient needs or to provide services to groups of clients at a lower cost than those provided by physician specialists.
- A nurse practitioner's (NP's) evaluation of contracted services to a group of chronically ill patients in an out-patient setting would need to document both the quantity and quality of services provided and the NP's ability to reduce hospitalization rates among clients.
- A certified registered nurse anesthetist (CRNA) evaluating anesthesia services in a chronic low back pain clinic would want to clearly document quality of service and patient outcomes.

This chapter discusses why greater attention needs to be given to evaluating the quality and quantity of APN interventions, identifies the problems associated with meaningful evaluation, and describes the content and relevance of Donabedian's model for evaluation activities. The chapter also reviews the related literature and proposes an approach to improve evaluation activities. Finally, the role of APNs in the evaluation process is described.

THE NEED FOR OUTCOME EVALUATION

The evaluation of the APN and the contributions APNs make to patient care is a complex process that can be addressed from a variety of perspectives. The health-care environment has added to the complexity and importance of the issue. Health reform and reimbursement efforts in organizations and government have made the need for evaluation critical to the survival of the APN in all settings. Quality, cost, and productivity issues are paramount. The issues identified by Hamric (1989) regarding cost pressures have clearly escalated. Down-sizing, right-sizing, and new patient care delivery and reimbursement systems require his or her provider to first be more efficient and productive and second to document his or her impact and productivity. Demands by policymakers, third-party payers, employers, and consumers interested in improving health at lower cost are great and place a significant burden on APNs to evaluate practice outcomes. As evidenced by the national debate on health-care reform in 1994 and the ongoing efforts of states to address access, quality, and cost concerns in a climate of fiscal constraint, APNs cannot escape these issues either morally or practically.

Buerhaus (1992, 1994a, 1994b) identified changes in the health-care system in relation to market forces and managed competition that have implications for the evaluation of advanced nursing practice. Traditional market forces and increased competition in health care suggest the need for the innovative use of resources to reduce costs, to maintain or improve quality and satisfaction of payers and clients, and to assess and document care to remain competitive. This results in the demand for cost-related data; assessment of the structures and processes of care to produce cost-effective, quality care; recognition of the contributions of non-nurse providers to care; and understanding what insurers and consumers want from nursing care (Buerhaus, 1992). The implications of these issues are clear for APNs. For example, competition with primary care physicians in managed-care settings (Buerhaus, 1994b) suggests the need for documentation of the contributions and costs of the APN. As Buerhaus (1994a) stated:

> *The possibility that nurses in advanced-practice positions could take on new clinical, economic and managerial roles that strengthen the development of price competition, raise quality and increase access to health care has been neglected by architects of managed competition proposals.*

Federal government programs, such as those of the Agency for Health Care Policy Research (AHCPR) and the Health Care Financing Administration (HCFA), which focus on outcomes and efficacy, highlight the primary importance of evaluation. For example, the HCFA's Health Care Quality Improvement Initiative was undertaken in an effort to improve services to Medicare beneficiaries. This initiative centers on national, uniform criteria to examine patterns of care and outcomes (Jencks & Wilensky, 1992). Medicare, Medicaid, and other categorical federal programs are presently under close scrutiny by Congress, which is demanding information about the efficacy of the health-care programs it funds. Another major indicator of the importance the federal government has given to assessing patient outcomes is the work of the AHCPR, created by Congress in 1989, to study the effectiveness and appropriateness of health-care services used to diagnose, treat, prevent, and manage health problems. As reported by Cummings (1992), the AHCPR, through its Medical Treatment Effectiveness Program, supported grants and contracts for complex projects studying patient outcomes (patient outcome research teams [PORTS]), health status measurement, meta-analysis, and the study of small area variations. Another national effort of particular interest to nurses is the National Institute for Nursing Research's support of research efforts independently and in collaboration with other institutes and agencies of government to promote research related to clinical interventions and outcomes (Hinshaw, 1992).

State governments are involved in similar activities related to their health-care reform efforts and concerns about access, quality, and costs. Approximately 40 states have mandated data collection about the quality of care. Florida, for example, has a quality management system that will establish uniform standards for the certification of centers of excellence and will use practice guidelines, outcome measurements, and peer review approaches to assess quality (Blancett, 1994). Minnesota Care, the state's health-care reform effort, is creating an integrated data system to provide the public with information about the cost, quality, and structure of health-care services, with data being collected from consumers, providers, insurers, employers, policymakers, and others (Josten, 1994). The Oregon Health Plan, a much-watched state initiative to increase access to health-care services and control costs, uses outcome measures such as health status to determine which services will be covered by the Medicaid program (Wegener, 1994). Unfortunately, nursing practice is not a clearly identified component of most of these efforts. Nurses must strive to become involved in federal, state, and private-sector quality initiatives.

APNs working within any organizational setting, particularly those working in hospitals, are well aware of more local efforts engendered by the climate of health-care reform. Hospitals—as well as other organizations—are restructuring, reengineering, and redesigning the way in which they organize and deliver health-care services. Restructuring addresses the architecture of the organization, emphasizing the need to make hospitals lean, decentralized, and self-governing in addition to empowering direct caregivers to make decisions. Revamping the processes by and through which care is delivered—re-engineering—calls forth efforts to be more "user-friendly," efficient, and economical. The concept of redesign deals with who should be doing what, where, for whom, in what quantity, and at what cost. Training and productivity are important components of redesign efforts. Although the quantity and quality of data needed to make these critical decisions are inadequate in most organizations, changes based on existing data are rapidly taking place.

Also contributing to the current emphasis on outcomes are the expectations of accrediting agencies and insurers who are demanding greater information. Insurers and managed-care organizations are concerned about both costs and the services they purchase on behalf of the insured. A recent *New York Times* article (Quint, 1995) reported the results of a study conducted for the National Committee for Quality Assurance on the quality of care provided by large managed-health-care plans. Patients were surveyed to determine satisfaction with their health-care plans, and quality-of-care measures such as immunization rates were assessed. It is important to note that the study did not evaluate how well the health maintenance organizations (HMOs) prevented illness or helped enrollees recover from illness. Through its accreditation procedures, the Joint Commission on Accreditation of Healthcare Organizations (JCAHO) has, since the late 1980s, expected the health-care agencies it accredits to assess patient outcomes. A new JCAHO publication by Global Success Corporation (1995) focuses on ". . . choosing, using and reporting quality indicators." The premier issue of this publication reported to the public its first mandatory "report cards" on the hospitals it accredits.

As this discussion suggests, the context in which health-care decisions are being made at the federal, state, and organizational levels is complex, rapidly changing, and guided by incomplete information. Without better information, the problems faced in relation to access, quality, and costs are unlikely to be well addressed. APNs have much to contribute and much to gain through the application of their knowledge and skill in designing studies, collecting and analyzing data, and disseminating evaluation findings.

PROBLEMS IN EVALUATING ADVANCED NURSING PRACTICE

Addressing the demands for accountability through evaluation of advanced nursing practice remains a difficult task. These problems are both environmental and role-based. As discussed earlier, the environment in which APNs practice and conduct evaluations is constantly shifting, and the focus of health-care delivery systems is changing rapidly. Evaluation is also made more difficult when the program itself changes. For example, an NP evaluating the effect of the NP role on adolescent pregnancy may experience significant problems when a public health department is no longer available to refer patients for pregnancy prevention services. Similarly, the introduction of other programs in a community, such as new home care services, may make it difficult for the pediatric CNS to assess the impact of care on hospital length of stay.

The problems inherent in the role of the APN conducting effective evaluation have been identified by Hamric (1989) and others. Hamric discussed how the independent role of the APN makes it difficult to develop uniform performance criteria for evaluation. In addition, the time and other resources needed to conduct meaningful evaluation may not be at the disposal of the APN. The complexity and difficulties in conducting outcome evaluation, including those mentioned earlier, often result in outcome evaluation that is conceptually and methodologically flawed and thus contributes little to accountability. Hamric also mentioned problems associated with who should evaluate the APN and concerns about role ambiguity of the APN.

Jennings (1991), in a discussion of the challenges facing nurses conducting outcomes research, describes additional problems to be considered, including those related to theory development and model clarity. Outcomes research requires a shift to predictive and prescriptive theories to guide evaluation and to develop hypotheses for testing. These approaches are more difficult than simply exploring or describing a phenomenon. These require advanced levels of knowledge and skill—as well as time—representing a greater challenge for the APN. In addition, to be successful, such approaches often require collaboration with other researchers within and outside the profession. Similarly, clarity of the model for evaluating outcomes is complex because in assessing the APN's contribution to patient outcomes, one must account for intervening variables, such as the effects of changes in health-care reimbursement, which limit services and the impact of other providers on outcomes.

The methodological problems associated with evaluating the impact of the APN, although not unique, are compounded by the fact that the focus of the research is on the APN's contribution to patient care. As Jennings (1991) suggested, defining process, structure, and outcome variables is a demanding task. For example, determining who should identify the outcomes, what the outcomes should be, and the magnitude of these outcomes requires careful attention and is likely to involve a number of stakeholders if the evaluation of outcomes is to be recognized and appreciated. Evaluation of advanced nursing practice is also more challenging because traditional measures of quality, mortality, morbidity, and length of stay are not always sensitive indicators of nursing interventions, and thus the APN must develop methods for assessing more nursing sensitive patient outcomes such as functional status, mental status, satisfaction, and burden of care (Naylor, Munro, & Brooten, 1991).

Additional issues to be considered when evaluating the impact of advanced nursing practice include the requirement to focus primarily on the patient's needs. This focus on patient's needs may preclude thinking about planning an evaluation when a program or intervention is being introduced. It is also difficult to understand the impact of a structure or process of care when baseline data with which to compare the results of the evaluation are not available. For example, assessing the costs of APNs is often difficult because costing-out nursing interventions and nursing's relative contribution to patient outcomes is complex and data are often not available. Compounding the time pressures encountered in evaluating the role of the APN is the need to conduct most evaluation research over a longer time frame in order to determine outcomes. Useful and generalizable evaluation results also require a larger sample and more than one location—often difficult methodological problems for the APN.

EVALUATION RESEARCH

Evaluation research uses the methodological approaches inherent in any research effort. As a form of applied rather than basic research, it focuses on findings that have practical application. Evaluation research is the application of social-science research methods involving collecting, analyzing, and interpreting data to determine the need, implementation, effectiveness, and efficiency of interventions in order to evaluate and improve practice. It is characterized by the formulation of hypotheses, manipulation of variables, and the study of relationships. Evaluation can be both quantitative and qualitative. APNs may be involved with this type of research for a number of reasons: to assess their role, to determine the effectiveness and efficacy of the interventions they directly or indirectly provide, to measure program or organizational quality, to meet accountability standards, or to identify the inputs—structure and processes—related to particular outcomes.

Although there are a number of approaches to conceptualizing evaluation, Donabedian's model for patient care evaluation (1966) is among the best known and most used by nurses as well as other health-care providers and researchers. Donabedian's model has been applied to nursing by Bloch (1975) and applied to the CNS by Hamric (1983, 1989). It provides an excellent framework for evaluating the impact of all categories of APNs (Table 26–1). Structure, process, and outcome variables can be studied as independent or dependent variables. Structural variables relate to the components of a system of care or intervention and would include such elements as numbers and types of providers, agency policies and procedures, characteristics of clients served, practice regulations, and payment sources. Process variables relate to the behavior or actions of the APN. The end-result of the interaction of the structural and process variables is the outcome, the impact of advanced nursing practice on access, quality, or costs. Specific examples of the types of variables that the APN might study are listed in Table 26–2.

The next section of this chapter uses this framework to review the literature related to the evaluation of advanced nursing practice. Because of the volume and variety of studies, none is described or critiqued in detail. The strengths and weaknesses of the overall research are summarized and, given the current climate, outcomes research is emphasized. The reader is encouraged to explore this literature for the APN roles of interest.

TABLE 26–1. A MODEL FOR PATIENT CARE EVALUATION

	Structure	**Process**	**Outcome**
Donabedian & Bloch	Characteristics of: • Setting • System • Care providers	Care processes Appropriateness and completeness of care delivery Coordination of care For nursing, the quality of nursing process	Care recipient End-result of care in terms of change in patient's: • Physical health state • Cognitive state • Psychosocial state • Behavioral state
Hamric & Girouard	APN characteristics: • Education • Certification Institutional characteristics: • APN impact on institutional practices • APN professional activities • APN time documentation	APN role component performance: • Direct practice • Education • Consultation • Research APN impact on staff performance APN evaluation of performance growth Acceptance of APN role Satisfaction with APN: • Staff • Supervisors • Non-nurse providers • Clients	APN impact on patient-related outcomes: • Health status • Knowledge • Psychosocial • Behavioral • Utilization • Costs • Client satisfaction

Adapted from Hamric, A. R. (1989). A model for CNS evaluation. In A. B. Hamric & J. A. Spross (Eds.), *The clinical nurse specialist in theory and practice* (2nd ed., pp. 83–104). Philadelphia: W.B. Saunders.

REVIEW OF THE APN EVALUATION LITERATURE

STRUCTURAL EVALUATION

Structural variables related to the APN, provide information about the role, factors relating to performance, and variables related to outcomes. As Hamric (1989) discussed, structural evaluation can provide a starting point for evaluation of the APN. Structural analysis can describe staffing patterns, indirect patient care actions such as committee and consultative activities of the APN, characteristics of the APN, or the practice setting. These data are relatively easy to obtain and analyze and can provide important information for evaluating the impact of the APN. The literature provides a number of examples and information about the structural characteristics of the APN, both as subgroups of the nursing workforce and within practice settings. APNs should examine and analyze existing data and research findings to determine both substantive and methodological approaches to define relevant structural variables and to clarify structural variables as inputs for outcome measurement.

Structural variables that have received a good deal of attention in the literature relate to amount of time spent on various APN roles, acceptance of the role, and characteristics of the APN. Aradine and Denyes (1972), Nevidjon and Warren (1984), Robichaud and Hamric (1986), and Burge, Crigler, Hurth, Kelly, and Sanborn (1989) focused on how much time CNSs spent in various components of the role. Direct patient care activities, staff education, and consultation consumed the

TABLE 26–2. STRUCTURE, PROCESS, AND OUTCOME VARIABLES—EXAMPLES

Structure	Process	Outcome
• Educational level of APN	• Patient education procedures	• Mortality
• Time spent in role components	• Referral patterns	• Morbidity
• Level of third-party reimbursement	• Prescriptive practice behavior	• Utilization of services
• Organizational characteristics	• APN behavior	• Quality of life
• Mission, goals of organization	• Nurse/APN satisfaction	• Social functioning
• Staffing patterns	• Collaboration	• Costs of care
• Certification	• Staff nurse practices	• Client satisfaction
• Physical environment	• Nursing processes	• Health status
• Regulations, policies		• Activities of daily living
		• Client knowledge

greatest amount of the CNS's time. Research, professional activities, and community service were less important as measured by time spent. Boyd, Staslowski, Catoe, Wells, and co-workers (1991) looked at role components and related activities to document the role of the CNS in meeting organizational needs for supervision as a component of the practice role. Their findings in relation to time spent in practice and education were similar to other research results. They also found that "scholarly" pursuits such as those related to research were allocated less time and importance by the CNSs studied.

A few recent studies have looked at how much time APNs spend with patients. Kearnes (1992) developed a computerized productivity monitor to provide information about how NPs in primary care services allocate time to billable and non-billable activities. The authors plan to implement this as a method to determine time utilization. Another study focused on the amount of time CNSs spent with newborns and their families (Damato, Dill, Gennaro, Brown, et al., 1993), finding that the greater the level of illness of the infant, the more time the CNS spent with the infant and family in the hospital and after discharge. Scupholme, Paine, Lang, Kumar, and DeJoseph (1994), using data from a national study of CNMs, compared CNM practices in a variety of settings. They found that the amount of time spent with clients across ambulatory settings was similar. In exploring the potential for using non-physician providers in place of residents, Knickman, Lipkin, Finkler, Thompson, and Kiel (1992) described the time and provider types needed to meet patient care needs.

Documentation of the time spent in various advanced practice roles gives APNs and prospective employers information about how APNs have functioned in a variety of settings and can form the basis for performance evaluation and role modification to conform with the organization's goals. For example, in light of the present climate in health care, the APN and the employer may need to increase the emphasis on role components relating to outcomes research and billable patient care services. Existing data should help to clearly articulate which role components are valued by the employer. Of interest to those who measure outcomes and issues of productivity are the more recent studies focused on time spent with clients. This type of data can be useful in setting productivity expectations and looking at the variable of time in cost and quality outcomes.

The results of efforts to define the role of the APN are similar to the results of the time studies discussed earlier. For example, Cason and Beck (1982) and Wyers, Grove, and Pastorino (1985) found that CNSs, faculty, and administrators agreed that the role involved expert clinical practice, collaboration, and problem-solving skills. Role characteristics identified by an ethnographic study by Fenton (1985) included collaboration and team-building, the role of change agent, consultation, and patient care monitoring. CNSs and nursing administrators agreed on the importance of the patient care and educational roles of the CNS, but administrators valued research as a role component more highly than CNSs did (Tarsitano, Brophy, & Snyder, 1986). Similarly, Nuccio and associates (1993) surveyed staff nurses, finding that their perceptions of CNS role components included consultation, care of complex patients, staff education, leadership in setting clinical standards, and facilitating and disseminating research. Patient's views were examined in a descriptive study by Cox, Bergen, and Norman (1993). The findings suggested that patients value the expert knowledge and skill of the CNS. Sterling, Noto, and Bowen (1994) described the components of the case management role when performed by the CNS and found that despite the lack of a standard approach to case management, the roles of CNSs were similar. Although most of these studies focused on the CNS, any APN can use these findings.

Other approaches to evaluating the structure of advanced nursing practice include measuring performance in relation to structural standards, such as numbers of meetings and workshops attended and given, numbers of requests for consultation, and numbers and types of clients served (Chambers, Dangel, German, Tripoli, & Jaguar, 1987). In national studies, Draye and Pesznecker (1979) and Repicky, Mendenhall, and Neville (1980) categorized the patient diagnoses treated by NPs. Ramsey, Edwards, Lenz, Odom, and Brown (1993) examined the number of clients and the health problems seen by NPs providing primary care services in a rural setting. Fleming (1992) reported on a study of surgical type, use of anesthetic agents, and pre-existing conditions in relation to type of anesthesia provider. In a study of the practice and educational needs of CRNAs, Dixon (1993) reported the need for more education regarding the use of patient-controlled analgesia, because CRNA practice did not consistently incorporate the best practices. Scupholme, DeJoseph, Strobino, and Paine (1992) reported the results of a national study describing the characteristics and costs of care provided by CNMs. As identified in the health services research literature, organizational characteristics are important variables in patient care outcomes. These types of evaluation may be useful for internal purposes but are not likely to provide the type of information needed regarding the impact of the APN on access, quality, or cost unless they can be identified as having a relationship to other goals. For example, if the outcomes of the APN's practice are better in settings where more RNs are employed, this would provide clear guidance for employers seeking to set high standards of quality.

A few recent studies have looked at organizational variables, such as staffing patterns, agency mission, and governance. Capan, Beard, and Mashburn (1993) described the characteristics of a nurse-managed prenatal clinic and the services it provided. In a study of McKinney Act Clinics, which provide primary care to the homeless, Doblin, Gelberg, and Freeman (1992) described the staffing of these clinics, reporting that 80% employed one or more NPs. In addition, they reported on variation in the role and utilization of NPs and the volume of homeless patients treated in these clinics. Ward and Dracup (1995), in a study of nurse-managed intensive care units (ICUs) in 400 U. S. hospitals, developed a system for determining nursing and medical care needs. They found that 22% of the patients in the study had high nursing and low medical care needs and thus were appropriate patients to receive care in the nurse-managed unit. Smith and Waltman (1994) found that although oncology CNSs believed that they could affect multiple patient outcomes, barriers within the organization, including multiple job expectations, time constraints and other resource issues, the lack of support in an organization, and inadequate policies hindered their ability to achieve their potential. A profile of NPs in the San Francisco Bay area described educational background, certification status, employment characteristics, salary, and practice factors. The study was used to identify barriers that could be overcome to enhance the recruitment and retention of NPs in local agencies (Crabtree, Renwanz-Boyle, Perry, Taylor, & Thrailkill, 1990). The North Carolina Center for Nursing is presently completing a study of all APNs in that state, which will provide similar information.

Acceptance of the APN is a structural variable that was particularly important to assess during the early evolution of APN roles but is now largely irrelevant unless related to other variables. As Shamansky (1985) and Molde and Diers (1985) reported in their reviews of the NP literature, numerous studies have documented the acceptance of NPs. This is also true for other types of APNs. This type of evaluation, as Molde and Diers (1985) suggested, may be useful for purposes of marketing the services of the APN. The issues they raised regarding the need to use traditional market concepts, such as choice of provider, cost, and reimbursement by third-party payers, have not been well studied. This is an opportunity for evaluation research. In addition, this information would be useful for planning and implementing APN programs by suggesting to policymakers the merits of investing in such programs and "selling" APN services to managed-care organizations.

These studies provide information to identify APN roles in meeting organizational needs, articulate position expectations, and serve as a basis for developing job descriptions and performance standards for further evaluation. Given that CNSs, nursing administrators, and others largely agree about role components, with perhaps the exception of the research role, further research related only to the identification of the CNS role may not be needed. Descriptions of the role components of other APN roles would be useful. Further research is needed to assess the impact of all APN roles. As Boyd and associates (1991) suggested after reviewing the literature from 1967 to 1989 regarding CNS practice, there was not "consistent conclusive evidence that there was worth and value of the role of the CNS within the nursing organization." The next generation of research related to advanced nursing practice should assess the effect of the various role components on organizational and client goals, such as access, quality, and costs. Hill, Ellsworth-Wolk, and DeBlase (1993) used the existing literature to guide them in the development of a criterion-based evaluation tool that begins to identify activities that contribute to the goals of the organization and patient outcomes. Their approach illustrates how organizational-level evaluation can begin to move beyond describing roles. The literature also suggests the need to further define and develop the research competencies of the APN. See Chapter 19 for CRNA role evaluation studies.

PROCESS EVALUATION

Process evaluation may focus on what the APN does or on programmatic components—that is, the nature of an intervention. As with structural characteristics, process variables can be examined independently of outcomes to describe what the APN or a program does. One can look at the extent to which a target population is being reached to address access issues or assess the extent to which aspects of the role or program are being undertaken as planned. The literature provides a number of examples of both approaches. Strategies the APN may use to evaluate the process of care include assessments by those supervised directly, such as unit leaders, or indirectly, such as staff nurses; administrative reviews by the APN's supervisor based on goals or job description criteria; evaluation by other health-care providers or clients; reviews of improvements in various components of the nursing process; and peer review (Hamric, 1989).

Hamric, Gresham, and Eccard (1978) and Girouard and Spross (1983) provided examples of how evaluation of APNs' behavior can be assessed in relation to performance of various aspects of the role. Ingersoll (1988) reported that 84% of staff nurses had a favorable impression of the CNS, identifying the CNS as their primary resource in the delivery of care. Interestingly, the APN literature contains few reports of these types of process evaluation. This may mean that such process evaluations are not often used or that they are not viewed as significant methods to assess behavior. APNs might find it beneficial to explore these approaches as one component of their evaluation. Although it does not measure the full scope of effectiveness on outcomes, findings may be useful in justifying the role and clarifying the indirect impact of the role as perceived by those whom the APN seeks to influence.

Administrative assessment of the APN's performance is another useful method for evaluation of APN processes. The most effective way to conduct this type of evaluation is to base it on mutual goals and objectives that are used as an ongoing management tool. Tierney, Grant, and Mazique (1990) described a CNS evaluation tool that includes multidisciplinary review, quality assurance, and time justification to set goals and evaluate the CNS. Houston and Luquire (1991) developed and used 11 performance criteria related to the evaluation of CNS care to specific patient populations, nursing care planning activities, consultative functions, leadership, role modeling, and professional development. They reported that the data substantiated the value of the CNS and enhanced CNS and administrator collaboration. Using patient records, Kearnes (1994) documented the positive effects of a collaborative role for physicians and NPs in caring for hospitalized older patients.

Job satisfaction is an important issue for the APN and the supervisor, because performance and outcomes are likely to be linked to job satisfaction. Numerous studies assess the job satisfaction of the APN; some recent studies examined turnover rates, productivity, and recruitment concerns as well. For example, Collins (1990) found that most CNMs reported they were satisfied with their jobs. Koelbel, Fuller, and Misener (1991a, 1991b) found that, in general, NPs studied were moderately satisfied with their jobs. Age, number of children, urban locations, achievement, company policies and practices, creativity, independence, and compensation were the major predictors of job satisfaction. Tri (1991) studied the job satisfaction of NPs in primary care and the factors contributing to satisfaction and dissatisfaction. Tri reported that overall there was a high level of job satisfaction, with autonomy contributing the most to satisfaction. Salary was the highest dissatisfier. It is unlikely that measuring job satisfaction alone will contribute much to understanding the effect of the APN on patient care. However, the information may be useful for developing and structuring positions within an agency up front and thus reducing the costly effects of recruitment, retention, and performance related to dissatisfaction.

A number of recent studies have used evaluation by other care providers and consumers. Although consumer satisfaction with APN providers will be discussed here, it will also be considered in the discussion of outcomes, because many evaluators include consumer satisfaction as a quality outcome measure. Nemes, Barnaby, and Shamberger (1992) explored the perceptions of surgeons, house staff, and parents regarding the performance of pediatric NPs providing care previously provided by house staff. By an overwhelming majority, all respondents were satisfied with the PNPs' care. Hag (1993) found positive levels of satisfaction among the older adults served in a nurse-managed primary care setting. Clients were most satisfied with the skill level of the geriatric NP and graduate nursing students. In a study of consumer and other provider views of oncology CNS' care, Cox, Bergen, and Norman (1993) reported that patients perceived the CNS as knowledgeable and the interventions as positive. Ramsey, Edwards, Lenz, Odom and Brown (1993) studied the satisfaction of clients in a nurse-managed rural health center. They found that clients were satisfied with the care they received. Trotter and Danaher (1994) found that physicians, other nursing staff, and parents of neonates in the intensive care nursery were satisfied with the clinical expertise, knowledge, and contributions of the neonatal NP.

The process evaluation approach receiving the most attention in the literature deals with the impact of the APN on various aspects of the nursing process. Early work by Georgopoulos and Jackson (1970) and Georgopoulos and Sana (1971) demonstrated the positive impact of the CNS on Kardex documentation and shift reports. Ayers (1971) found that the CNS improved the "clinical insights" of staff nurses on units with CNSs, and Little and Carnevali (1967) reported on positive behavioral differences between the practice of the CNS and that of the staff nurse. Girouard (1978) compared the preoperative teaching performance of staff nurses on units with and without a CNS, finding improved performance on the unit with the CNS. Rogers, Metzger, and Bauman (1984) reported that four of five employers identified improved patient care and staff nurse performance associated with the role modeling and consultation of geriatric NPs. Batey and Holland (1985) described the prescribing behavior of NPs in relation to confidence with prescribing and with physician consultation. Kasch and Knutson (1986) assessed the strengths and limitations of a tool to assess primary care processes of NPs, devising a method for assessing changes in patient function resulting from client education. McBride and associates (1987) studied the impact of the psychiatric CNS on the documentation activities of staff nurses in a state psychiatric hospital. They found that the introduction of the CNS and efforts to improve documentation significantly improved the quality and quantity of documentation.

Other studies provided further evidence of the impact of the APN on various components of the nursing process or described the processes of care used by nurses in APN roles. Ingersoll (1988) found that after the introduction of the CNS, staff nurses gave greater attention to psychosocial needs and the documentation of physiological needs assessment. Martin (1989) described the positive effect of the CNS on a unit-based approach to quality assurance. Geriatric CNS consultation activities resulted in improvements in the implementation of standards of care and clinical judgment by staff nurses (Gurka, 1991). In a study of the effect of a critical care CNS's staff teaching and supervision on preventable pulmonary complications, Hanneman, Bines, and Sajtar (1993) found that the CNS's intervention with staff reduced the number of malpositioned endotracheal tubes and inadvertent extubation. Bell and Mills (1989) described the process of care used by CNMs in an HMO and described collaboration with physicians. Sampselle, Peterson, Murtland, and Oakley (1992) reported that CNMs were more likely to identify clients who were victims of violence than their physician counterparts, suggesting that screening for violence was more likely to be done by the CNM than by the physician.

A study of NPs in nursing homes suggests that the geriatric NPs' processes of care are not substantively different from those of physician providers (Melillo, 1993). Gifford and Stone (1993) documented the ability of NPs to provide colposcopy services that were comparable with those of physicians. Gibson, Martin, Johnson, Blue, and Miller (1994) identified the effect of the CNS on the coordination of community resources and continuity of care through the case management role. The delivery of preventive clinical services by NPs in primary care revealed that although NPs performed a number of the clinical assessments and interventions identified in Healthy People 2000, other criteria were not being met (Lemley, O'Grady, Rouckhorst, Russel, & Small, 1994). In a study of health professionals' adherence to obstetrical practice guidelines, Baldwin, Raine, Jenkins, Hart, and Rosenblatt (1994) found that 90% of all practitioners, including CNMs, adhered to the American College of Obstetricians and Gynecologists prenatal guidelines. Sterling, Noto, and Bowen (1994) reported that the CNS as case manager provided referrals and collaborated with members of other disciplines.

Peer review is an important mechanism for intra-professional development, yet there is little evidence in the literature that APNs use this technique. Winch (1989) discussed the importance of peer evaluation to foster the survival and growth of nurses in advanced practice roles. She reported that although peer review is a concept few would argue with, few APNs practiced peer review. This statement holds true today. One recent article by Caine, Baldwin, Baradell, Earte, and colleagues (1994) described the North Carolina Nurses Association's Council of Psychiatric and Mental Health NPs efforts to develop a formal peer review process. Motivated by the defeat of a legislative initiative to reimburse APNs for their services, they provided an evaluation method for their colleagues in advanced practice. APNs should explore this option because it has much promise for professional support and development. The Nurse Anesthesia Practice model portrayed in Chapter 19 is extremely useful in the application of process evaluation.

OUTCOME EVALUATION

Using Donabedian's model, the evaluation of outcomes involves the measurement of the effects of interventions on patients. Dimensions such as access, quality, and costs are important outcome measures because they directly influence health outcomes. Outcomes reflect the end-result of a treatment or intervention. Given the social responsibility of the nursing profession, improvement in patient outcomes is the reason for nursing's existence. Using Hamric's (1989) rationale, the APN's influence on the behavior, attitudes, and knowledge of non-patients and consumers has been included as a process variable, not as an outcome measure, and discussed earlier. Lang and Marek (1992) identified the outcome indicators used by nurses in quality assurance and research activities. As shown in Table 26–3, they encompass physiological, psychosocial, functional, quality-of-life, service utilization, and patient satisfaction indicators.

The APN can ask a number of questions to evaluate the effect of advanced nursing practice on patient care outcomes. For example:

- What is the APN's impact on patient access to care providers? Does the presence of an APN provider or a program developed by an APN increase

TABLE 26–3. TYPES OF OUTCOME INDICATORS AND EXAMPLES

Physiological status

- Vital signs
- Laboratory values
- Skin integrity
- Wound healing
- Weight
- Symptom control—fatigue, nausea, incontinence

Behavior

- Application of knowledge and skills
- Problem-solving, compliance
- Motivation
- Therapeutic competence
- Self-care

Home/Family

- Family living patterns
- Home environment
- Support
- Role function
- Family strain
- Financial

Psychosocial

- Patterns of behavior
- Communications
- Relationships
- Mentation
- Emotion
- Attitude
- Mood
- Affect
- Coping
- Social contact
- Social functioning
- Occupational functioning
- Spiritual

Knowledge (Client)

- Cognitive understanding:
  - Of nursing problems
  - Of diet, medications, treatment

Utilization of Services

- Length of stay
- Number of clinic visits
- Telephone contacts
- Rehospitalization
- Unnecessary admissions/tests
- Financial costs

Functional Status

- Activities of daily living
- Mobility
- Communications
- Self-care

Quality of Life

- Life satisfaction
- Well-being
- Symptom control
- Standard of living
- Functional capacity
- Safety

Patient Satisfaction

- With care
- With care provider
- Care process
- Scheduling
- Access

From Lang, N. M., & Marek, K. D. (1991). Outcomes that reflect clinical practice. In *Patient outcomes research: Examining the effectiveness of nursing practice.* Proceedings of a conference sponsored by the National Center for Nursing Research, U.S. Department of Health and Human Services, Pub. No. 93-3411, October.

the number of people receiving care? How has this influenced health indicators in the community? Are targeted clients receiving effective interventions?

- Has the APN improved the quality of care in particular settings as measured by changes in the health status of individuals or groups of clients? What impact has the APN had on traditional measures of quality such as mortality and morbidity? Has the physical, functional, or psychosocial health status of clients improved? Are consumers satisfied with care received from the APN?
- What are the costs of providing APN services? Are they less than or more than the costs of similar care provided by other providers? Is the APN cost-effective in delivering care—are the outcomes achieved worth the cost? What is the impact of the APN on rates of service utilization such as unnecessary hospitalizations, length of stay, and readmissions?

Despite the importance of access to health-care services, little has been reported in the literature to assess the impact of APNs on access. This may relate to the difficulties in establishing demand or need for services or the methodological problems in studying the phenomenon. The few studies reported in the literature suggest that this may be an important area for future evaluation. Chambers and West (1978) found that the addition of a family NP to a physician primary care practice increased the volume of patient care provided in the setting. In a study of NP productivity, Holmes, Livingston, and Mills (1976) found that of the two solo practices compared, more services were provided and physician productivity increased by 12% in the practice with the NP. Hastings, Vick, Lee, Sasmar, and co-workers (1980) reported that the volume of primary care services delivered in a large urban jail health service doubled with the introduction of NPs. There is also some evidence that care to homeless patients can be increased with the effective use of NPs (Doblin, Gelberg, & Freeman, 1992). NPs in a community nurse-run clinic were able to provide access to a range of services for prenatal, family, and pediatric clients when a county hospital closed (Capan, Beard, & Mashburn, 1993). Kearnes (1994) reported that an NP-physician collaborative practice resulted in increased access and patient contact for older adults in a large urban hospital. Pickwell (1982, 1989) and Baughan, White-Baughan, Pickwell, Bartlome, and Wong (1990) provided information about NPs working in communities with large minority populations. Because APNs often provide services for underserved populations, further evaluation of their relationship to access would contribute to justification of the role.

A number of studies, including those discussed in relation to process variables, have evaluated patient satisfaction with care, an important outcome measure for the public, policymakers, and insurers. Levy, Wilkinson, and Marine (1971) reported client satisfaction with CNM care. Spitzer and co-workers (1990), in a randomized, controlled trial comparing family physician and NP practice, reported high levels of satisfaction in both the groups of patients cared for by the NPs and those patients cared for by the family practice physicians. Powers, Jalowiec, and Reichelt (1984), in a study of nonurgent emergency room patients, found that 77% of those in the experimental group cared for by the NP were completely satisfied with their care as opposed to 48% in the control group receiving physician care. Similarly, Wright, Erwin, Blanton, and Covington (1992) found high levels of patient satisfaction among patients with minor emergencies served in an emergency-room NP clinic. Rheumatology patients being followed by NPs (Hill, Bird, Harmer, Wright, & Lawton, 1994), post-cesarean section patients receiving CNS care (Brooten, Roncoli, Finkler, Arnold, et al., 1994), renal transplant patients receiving out-patient care from CNSs (Bartucci, 1985), and intrapartum patients of CNMs (Beal, 1984) all reported satisfaction with the care they received from their nurse providers.

A growing body of literature discusses the impact that APNs have had on outcome indicators in a variety of settings. As indicated in Table 23–3, outcome indicators used for the evaluation of the impact of APNs cover a broad range of health status variables related to physiological and psychosocial health, functional status, behavior, knowledge, and quality of life. In a classic study of the impact of NPs, Spitzer and colleagues (1974) demonstrated that physicians and nurses had similar patient results in relation to mortality and that there were no differences in functional status, social function, or emotional status. In addition, CNMs were found to provide care to low-risk maternity patients comparable with that of their physician colleagues in relation to prenatal outcomes, labor and delivery, and early infancy.

NPs managing common respiratory and genitourinary tract infections compared favorably with physicians in relation to diagnosis, and patients reported better symptom relief in the group cared for by the nurse (Komaroff, Sawayer, Flatly, & Browne, 1976). Pozen and co-workers (1977) found that patients receiving care from the CNS returned to work earlier and smoked less after a myocardial infarction than those who received routine physician/nurse care in the coronary care unit. These positive outcomes from this study were attributed to the improved knowledge and counseling by the CNS. Linde and Janz (1979) compared the results of teaching by CNSs with that by staff nurses and found that patients taught by the CNSs had greater knowledge and better compliance than those taught by staff nurses. Little and Carnevali (1967) and Murphy (1971) found no difference in patient outcomes related to CNS intervention. As Hamric (1989) pointed out, this difference in CNS effect on outcomes may be related to the choice of outcome indicators because behavioral and cognitive outcomes, which were not used in earlier studies, are more sensitive to CNS impact.

Other studies have also documented the comparability of APN, physician assistant, and physician care and documented the positive contributions APNs can make to patient outcomes. Hastings and co-workers (1980) found that the primary care delivered to incarcerated patients by medical fellows was comparable with that delivered by NPs. Powers, Jalowiec, and Reichelt (1984) found that nurses and physicians provided equal quality care to non-urgent patients in an emergency-room setting. In a study comparing physician- and NP-managed care for persons infected with HIV, Aiken, Lake, Seman, Lehman, O'Hare, Cole, Dunbar, and Frank (1993) reported that although the patients cared for by NPs were in poorer health than those cared for by physicians, they had comparable functional status and service utilization and had 45% fewer problems with their care. Compared with women cared for by physicians, women cared for by CNMs had lower rates of cesarean section, required fewer pharmacological interventions, and achieved maternal and infant outcomes comparable with those achieved under physician care (Davis, Riedman, Sapiro, Minogue, & Kozer, 1994).

A general study by Knaus, Draper, Wagner, and Zimmerman (1986) relating patient outcomes to processes of care provides further evidence of the value of examining process variables to predict outcomes. In a study of ICUs in 13 hospitals, these authors found that care coordination between physicians and nurses resulted in lower-than-expected rates of mortality. Brooten, Kumar, Brown, Butts, and co-workers (1986) provided one of the best early examples of a sound methodological approach to evaluating the outcomes associated with the intervention of an APN. Brooten and colleagues, using a random clinical trial, demonstrated that patient outcomes following early discharge with follow-up by the APN did not differ in relation to rehospitalizations, acute care visits, or infant growth and development when compared with those hospitalized for the usual and longer time period. Burgess and associates (1987) documented improved psychosocial functioning in myocardial infarction patients followed by the CNS. Crosby, Ventura, and Feldman (1987) reported that patients with peripheral vascular disease had increased levels of exercise when compared with those patients who did not receive care by the NP. Oleske and Hauck (1988) found that home-health-care cancer patients who were provided oncology CNS services and education experienced a significant decrease in cancer mortality during the two-year study period. Alexander, Younger, Cohen, and Crawford (1988) reported that pediatric asthma patients treated in the emergency room by a CNS had fewer emergency-room visits than those not receiving CNS care. CNSs, evaluating their care in one setting, reported that their intervention prevented readmissions, improved comfort and physical condition, and improved patient-family coping (Beyerman, 1989). Patients with advanced lung cancer treated in a home-care program who received care from a CNS had fewer complications, less symptomatic distress, fewer complications, and fewer hospital admissions than those receiving traditional medical out-patient care (McCorkle, Benoliel, Donaldson, Georgiadou, et al., 1989).

The contributions of APNs to the quality of care of patients in long-term-care facilities has been documented in the literature. Studies reported improvements in ADL (Kane, Garrard, Skay, Radosevich, et al., 1989) and decreased hospitalizations, the use of fewer in-dwelling urinary catheters, less incontinence, and reductions in the use of chemical and physical restraints (Shaughnessy, Kramer, & Little, 1990). Kane, Garrard, Buchanan, Rosenfeld, and co-workers (1991) compared the outcomes associated with nursing home care provided by NPs, physician assistants, and physicians. They found no differences in functional status or the use of medications. Both nurses and physician assistants had better outcomes than physicians in relation to congestive heart failure, hypertension, and urinary incontinence. A study by Gurka (1991) found that CNS intervention with intensive care patients prevented complications and reduced the time patients spent in the more costly unit. Kurz-Cringle, Blake, Dunham, Miller, and Annecillo (1994) described a study of a nurse-managed program for patients with chronic mental disorders. The CNS and NP practice program evaluation revealed reductions in the use of medications and a minimization of restraint use.

Studies of APN interventions in perinatal care similarly suggest positive outcomes associated with APN care. Cavero, Fullerton, and Bartlome (1991) found that rates of low-birth-weight infants and cesarean section were lower than county and state rates for patients receiving care in a nurse-midwifery service. Ellings, Newman, Hulser, Bivins, and Keenan (1993) reported that a nurse-run twin clinic had lower rates of very-low-birth-weight infants and fewer neonatal ICU admissions when compared with an obstetrical resident and faculty practice. Compared with national statistics, a nurse-run service was reported to have more favorable outcomes in relation to the number of low-birth-rate infants, complications of hypertension, earlier diagnosis of gestational diabetes, rates of adolescent pregnancy, and emergency-room use by pediatric clients (Capan, Beard, and Mashburn, 1993). Brooten et al. (1994) studied the safety, efficacy, and costs associated with early hospital discharge of babies delivered by unplanned cesarean section and found that patients with CNS follow-up went home earlier and their children had better immunization status than those in the control group.

In a study of infection rates in wounds sutured by nurses in an occupational setting, Ferguson and Sapelli (1992) found favorable infection rates (3.1%) when compared with the overall sutured wound infection rate of 1 to 30% reported in the literature. In a comparison of patients managed by a rheumatology NP and a physician, Hill, Bird, Harmer, Wright, and Lawton (1994) reported better outcomes in relation to pain, morning stiffness, psychological status, and knowledge in the group cared for by the nurse.

COST AS AN OUTCOME MEASURE

The costs of care are of major concern to a number of stakeholders in this country and often drive policy and care decisions. Although the assessment of costs may be difficult, a number of APN evaluations have addressed this outcome. In general, these studies have focused on five areas: reductions in utilization variables such as length of stay, hospital use, and readmissions; the lower costs of using APNs rather than physicians to provide similar services; reductions in the use of diagnostic tests, specific services, or per-visit costs; the lower costs of producing an APN compared with the costs of producing a physician; and reductions in overall costs in the provision of services for a particular condition or problem.

Reduced lengths of hospital stay, less emergency room use, earlier discharge, or earlier discharge from intensive care settings associated with interventions by APNs were reported by Lipman (1988) for children newly diagnosed with diabetes; Brooten et al. (1986); Brooten et al. (1994) for the elderly and other high-risk patients; Alexander, Younger, Cohen, and Crawford (1988), for children with asthma; Gibson, Martin, Blue, and Miller (1994) and Uzark, LeRoy, Callow, Cameron, and Rosenthal (1994) for patients receiving managed care by an APN; Crosby, Ventura, and Feldman (1987) for patients with peripheral vascular disease; Kane et al. (1989, 1991) for nursing home patients; Spisso, O'Callaghan, McKennan, and Holcroft (1990) for trauma care; Garrard and co-workers (1990) for nursing home patients; Gurka (1991) for intensive care patients; and Kearnes (1994) for hospitalized older adults.

Four studies illustrate the lower costs associated with care provided by APNs compared with that provided by physicians. Salkever, Skinner, Steinwachs, and Katz (1982) found that costs per episode of care for patients with otitis media and sore throat were lower for NPs and as effective as physician care. Cherry and Foster (1982) reported that the mean hospital bill for CNM clients was $114 less than the mean hospital charges for a matched group of patients cared for by physicians. In a randomized clinical trial, Brooten et al. (1986) demonstrated lower costs for low-birth-weight babies followed by a CNS. Although infants cared for in a Level III intensive care nursery by neonatal NPs had lower birth weights compared with those cared for by house officers, they averaged 2.4 fewer hospital days and over $3,000 less in total hospital costs (Schultz, Liptak, & Fioravanti, 1994). Additionally, some of the studies discussed in previous sections of this chapter either imply or compare cost differences.

Komaroff, Sawayer, Flatly, and Browne (1976) found that NPs using protocols to manage common respiratory and urinary tract infections ordered 27% fewer tests and medications than physicians did. Reduced utilization of laboratory tests and radiological studies was reported when NPs used algorithms in an ambulatory care setting (Orient, Kettel, Sox Jr., Sox et al., 1983). Weinberg, Liljestrand, and Moore (1983) found reductions in diagnostic tests and reduced length of stay among patients cared for by NPs compared with those cared for by internists in an inpatient rehabilitation setting. In a study of NP-sutured wounds, Ferguson and Sapelli (1992) estimated that wound management costs would be reduced significantly because of lower infection rates in the population served. Graveley and Littlefield (1992) reported lower prenatal per-visit costs for CNM services, and Baradell (1994) found that average per-visit costs for mental health CNSs providing individual psychotherapy were $65 as compared with $80 for psychologists and $100 for psychiatrists. Cromwell and Rosenbach (1988) found that CRNAs were underutilized and that full utilization would offer significant health-care savings.

A few studies have focused on aggregated costs or total costs associated with a particular patient condition. Reid and Morris (1979) reported on the costs of providing perinatal care in four counties in rural Georgia. They found that after the introduction of a CNM program, total perinatal care costs decreased in a population of low- and moderate-income women. Brooten et al. (1986) clearly demonstrated reductions in mean hospital and physician costs for very-low-birth-weight infants discharged early and followed by a CNS compared with the control group. Discharge planning by CNSs was found to decrease hospital costs and increase hospital revenues in a study by Neidlinger, Scroggins, and Kennedy (1987). Buchanan, Bell, Arnold, Witsberger, Kane, and Garrard (1990) reported that although the employment of geriatric NPs in 30 nursing homes did not show evidence of cost savings for continued residents when compared with the control group, the costs for newly admitted patients resulted in cost savings. In addition, geriatric nurse practitioners (GNPs) reduced the use of hospital services for both new and continuing residents. Early hospital discharge of women with unplanned cesarean birth and follow-up by a CNS significantly reduced health costs when compared with the control group (Brooten et al., 1994).

One often-cited analysis of advanced nursing practice was done by the Office of Technology Assessment (OTA) in response to a request from the United States Senate Appropriations Committee (Office of Technology Assessment, 1986). NPs, physician assistants, and CNMs were assessed in relation to their practice and contributions to meeting health-care needs. Using existing reports, the OTA concluded that the quality of care of these providers was satisfactory, comparable with and sometimes exceeding that of physicians. NPs, CNMs, and physician assistants were also found to be cost-effective care providers when compared with physicians. The findings of another major review (Crosby, Ventura, & Feldman, 1987) were similar to those of the OTA. Prescott (1994) provided an excellent analysis of issues related to the education and training of APNs and physicians and the lower salary costs of APNs, suggesting that APNs can be cost-effective alternatives to physicians in a variety of settings. She described how health-care costs could be reduced significantly by using APNs to deliver primary care and other appropriate services. In addition, the author makes a case for the possibility of increasing access without exponential increases in overall costs to the health-care system.

DISCUSSION

The evaluation literature discussed has contributed a great deal to the understanding of the structure, processes, and outcomes associated with advanced nursing practice. Clearly, there is a strong tradition of evaluation on which to base future evaluation and meet nursing's continuing responsibility to demonstrate the important role of APNs in the health-care system. Much, though, remains to be done. Evidence of the need for more and better evaluation is reflected in the threats that many APNs perceive in relation to their job and career security and the demands of employers, third-party payers, and policymakers for professional accountability. The need for more and better evaluation is also reflected in the limited media and public attention given to research findings related to advanced nursing practice. Much of the quality-of-care research focuses on physician care, rarely mentioning the role of nurses in outcomes. When nursing research has identified the contributions of nurses to patient outcomes, it rarely makes the news. By building on knowledge gained from structure, process, and outcome evaluations, these challenges can be met to improve the nation's health and assure a future role for nurses in advanced practice.

Although some of the studies discussed are exemplary, the total quantity and quality of advanced practice evaluation needs to be enhanced. In planning future efforts, the APN should consider the limitations of reported studies in order to improve the design and implementation of evaluations of the APN's impact. The literature provides good information about the roles, activities, and perceived barriers to practice, especially for CNSs. Similar information about NPs and CNMs is also available, but there is little research related to these issues for the CRNA. Although it might be assumed that all APN role activities and barriers are similar, research to confirm these assumptions is desirable. Information about the structure and processes of advanced nursing practice also needs to be enhanced because the reported research generally has used case-study approaches rather than multi-site or multi-role exploration. Although there are a few well-conceptualized studies with good analytic techniques, most research does not use a model or conceptual framework or a rigorously applied research design. Random trials, pre- and post-intervention data, studies over time, and other comparative methods are rare in the research about APNs. Perhaps most significant is the lack of studies that link structures and processes to patient outcomes, particularly those which are nurse-dependent. In addition, greater attention needs to be given to the effect of advanced nursing practice on cost-related variables, such as utilization of services and productivity of the APN. Also desirable are data about the potential of the APN to increase access to services, especially for under-served groups. As suggested, the quality and quantity of evaluation research is improving, but many problems exist in terms of conceptualization of evaluation research and the methods used to assess advanced nursing practice.

Conceptual issues include the focus and scope of evaluation, which must be clear to obtain meaningful results. In the planning phase of evaluation, more careful attention needs to be given to the concept of quality of care, because it is elusive and rarely well conceptualized in the literature. As Hinshaw (1992) noted, more specificity is required about quality of life, functional status, symptom intensity, and patient satisfaction to capture the results of major nursing interventions. In addition, she stated that the focus of many evaluation efforts has been on medical effectiveness rather than nursing concepts such as prevention, health promotion, and symptom management. At the same conference, Abraham and colleagues (1992) reported that only one in nine articles published in six major research journals addressed tests of the effects of nursing interventions on patient care outcomes. Few studies use a conceptual model or link theory and research and thus do not provide a framework for evaluating the impact of the APN. This makes it difficult to generalize the results of individual studies to other settings and to APN practices.

Research design and other methodological problems also contribute to the poor quality of APN evaluation research, thus limiting generalizability. For example, many studies are descriptive rather than evaluative—useful to define variables but not to explain the impact of the role. Studies with a short time frame do not allow for the assessment of many nurse-dependent outcomes, such as changes in health promotion and behaviors. Crosby, Ventura, and Feldman (1987) found that only 14% of the literature they reviewed addressed long-term outcomes. Evaluation of outcomes also requires attention to comparisons—if an outcome is better, it needs to be described in relation to some baseline measure, or an experimental design should be used. Unfortunately, time constraints, data sources, and other factors make this difficult.

Other methodological issues include:

- Sampling inadequacies—Van Cott and associates (1991) reported that 87% of the publications she reviewed used a convenience sample rather than random selection or other more appropriate sampling techniques; small sample size makes impact hard to assess.
- Data sources—large national data sets are rarely used (Hinshaw, 1992); using vital statistics for comparison of outcomes is often not valid because

the populations served by the APN may not be comparable with the general population.

- Measurement tools—not sensitive to the goals of nursing interventions; reliability and validity are rarely addressed.
- Data collection—record reviews do not always reflect the process of an intervention or relevant outcome variables; self-evaluation and other subjective data collection methods may not be easily replicated.
- Data analysis—multivariate techniques, helpful in evaluating complex phenomena, are rarely used in evaluation studies of the impact of advanced nursing practice.

When structural variables are used as the sole criteria for evaluation, how well the APN performs and subsequent effectiveness cannot be determined. When used alone, process evaluation does not evaluate access, quality, or costs. Because there is little evidence that improvements in nursing practice relate to outcomes, process evaluation does not contribute to measuring the impact of the APN on patient care. Additional limitations in the APN evaluation literature include the frequent focus on only one or a few APNs or settings, the lack of multi-disciplinary research, the lack of consistency in the definition of variables, failure to study the impact of the context of care on outcomes, and the lack of replication and extension of evaluation research. Some APN roles, such as the CRNA, have little evaluative data related to their contributions. Peer review should be used more often as an evaluation technique by APNs. Finally, the CNS evaluation literature includes structure and outcome studies related to APN competencies in addition to clinical practice expertise, such as consultation and collaboration. However, other APN studies often neglect these issues, which could be helpful in understanding the distinctive contributions of APNs.

AN APPROACH TO EVALUATING ADVANCED NURSING PRACTICE

CONTRIBUTING TO KNOWLEDGE ABOUT ADVANCED PRACTICE

The APN engaged directly or indirectly in evaluating the impact of practice can use a framework to guide these activities. Where research has been conducted, the research can be used to guide future research efforts (see Chapter 9). The evaluation questions posed by Rossi and Freeman (1990) earlier in this chapter are a good starting point and should be asked in planning phases of an intervention or service. Clarity on these questions will serve to ameliorate many of the problems and issues inherent in the complex evaluation process and practice context. In addition, there are research design and methodological questions to be addressed. As the literature suggests, there is a need for designing studies that link structure, process, and outcomes to determine the impact of the APN on access, quality, and cost. Suggestions from critiques of the literature include using multiple sites, using longer time frames, using comparison groups, focusing on nurse-dependent outcomes, and developing reliable and valid methods to assess outcomes.

Ventura, Crosby, and Feldman (1991) developed a model for assessing NP effectiveness that can be applied to the evaluation of nurses in other advanced practice roles. They created the model with the assistance of a consultant and advisory committee to provide a framework for evaluation and for their review of the evaluation literature. As shown in Figure 26–1, they include "preliminary conditions (predisposing, preparation and enabling)" that influence the APN's ability to perform in the role. These can be considered structural variables and include regulations, educational background, acceptance of the role, and reimbursement issues. In the model, utilization also includes structural variables for evaluation. Delivery of care in this model represents many of the process variables discussed in this chapter. Short-term outcomes, such as patient knowledge at time of hospital discharge and freedom from pain, are those assessed in a time frame close to the delivery of care. Long-term outcomes are those that would be measured longitudinally and might include the patient's ability to return to work, life span,

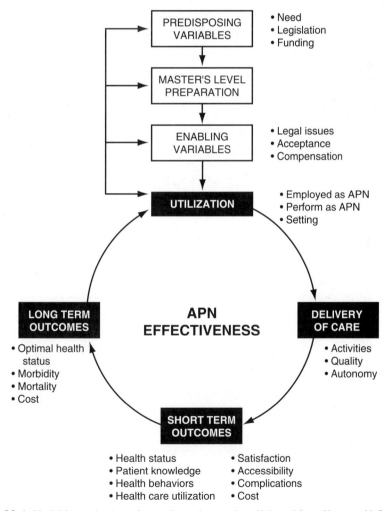

Figure 26–1. Model for evaluating advanced practice nursing. (Adapted from Ventura, M. R., Crosby, F., & Feldman, M. J. (1991). An information synthesis to evaluate nurse practitioner effectiveness. *Military Medicine, 156*(6), 286–291.)

and long-term costs related to what was influenced over time by the delivery of care.

In an article to promote outcomes research in home care agencies, Peters (1994) offered some helpful suggestions for selecting a problem for study and initiating an evaluation effort. The problem should be one:

- About which there is considerable interest or expertise
- For which baseline data exist
- Of high volume, high risk, or high cost
- With which a problem or deficiency has been identified
- That relates to the mission and goals of the agency

Peters also suggests that the nurse go slow, select a manageable area to evaluate, involve all levels of personnel, and be creative. Hamric (1989) had similar recommendations for initiating evaluation. In addition, the APN is advised to discuss with the administrator the components critical to evaluation of the role, to emphasize the importance of collaboration with other nurses and disciplines, to identify the need for planning the evaluation, and to consider the desirability of working with other APNs, faculty, and researchers to implement evaluation efforts.

INDIVIDUAL EVALUATION

Although this chapter has focused on evaluating advanced nursing practice and its impact, APNs may also need to conduct individual performance evaluations of specific activities, competencies, or setting-specific goals related to a role. Such an evaluation may serve as a beginning step in evaluation or as a component of performance review. The framework for individual evaluation of performance is comparable with that used for more broadly conceived evaluation but focuses on job expectations. The APN's position description can be used as a starting point for structuring the performance evaluation. In collaboration with the immediate supervisor and staff with whom the APN works, and with other appropriate colleagues, the APN should identify role expectations and the purpose of the evaluation procedures. For example, the evaluation may be used as a component of annual performance reviews (Girouard & Spross, 1983), to develop annual goals and measure progress in achieving them, or to justify the contributions of the role in a setting (Hamric, 1989).

The steps in the process of individual evaluation (Hamric, 1989) include:

- **Selecting a focus or foci for the evaluation.** For example, the CNS may wish to assess a teaching program developed for preoperative patients (single focus) or may evaluate practice changes associated with the provision of staff in-service education programs on a surgical unit (multiple foci). The CRNA may wish to evaluate the impact of preoperative patient assessment on the perioperative experience of patients (single focus) or assess the volume and effectiveness of services provided (multiple foci). A primary care NP and her physician colleagues decide to determine the volume of laboratory tests that the NP orders for patients with peripheral vascular disease (single focus) or the number and effects of referrals to specialty care by the NP (multiple foci).
- **Determining goals for the evaluation.** The APN would establish the specific outcomes for the activity to be assessed. The goals for the

preoperative patient teaching program might include improvements in post-operative compliance with respiratory regimes and self-care activities. The staff education goal would include participation by 80% of staff in in-service education programs and measures of changes in staff behavior following participation in the programs. Similar goals would be identified by the CRNA or the NP in the examples given.

- **Identify the components of the evaluation.** The APN would determine which structure, process, or outcomes variables, or which combination of these variables, is to be used for the evaluation. Structural variables might include the determination of resources to meet the goal. Process variables, such as participation levels in educational programs for patients or staff, are also to be considered if they are relevant to measuring goal achievement. Outcome variables, such as the quantity of services as a cost indicator or patient outcomes, may also be considered in relation to measuring specific goals.
- **Determine the methodology for assessing goal achievement.** Attendance at in-service education classes, record review, questionnaires, and pre- and post-testing of variables are possible approaches to measuring the APN's performance. The methodology should also include consideration of who will be doing the assessment. Staff, patients, or the APN may provide data for the evaluation. For example, patient and staff satisfaction with educational programs may be assessed through interviews or written questionnaires; the APN may collect data from records or from aggregated data available in reports prepared by medical records. Attention must also be given to the time frame for data collection in relation to the goals and intervention. Whether daily, weekly, monthly, or annual data collection is used depends on the nature of the goals to be evaluated and the resources available to the APN for evaluation activities.
- **Data analysis, interpretation, and reporting.** In planning an individual performance evaluation, the APN should decide how data will be analyzed and interpreted. The APN, the supervisor, or others may be engaged in the process. It is also important to show how the findings of the performance evaluation will be shared. The APN and others may wish to share evaluation findings with administrative personnel, clients, and others within the setting. Whatever the decision, it should be made prior to the evaluation effort so as to provide the APN and others with access to appropriate and useful information. Attention should be given to the use of performance evaluation results for developing future goals and the growth of the APN in the role within the setting and the profession.

A number of case studies in the nursing literature provide examples of how APNs have evaluated their activities. Weilitz and Potter (1993) described the role and impact of six CNSs who led multi-disciplinary teams toward developing and implementing critical paths. They reported improvements in the processes of care and suggested that cost savings and quality improvement were associated with the introduction of the CNS-led critical paths program. Visalli (1994) described positive changes in communications, quality, and practice when psychiatric CNSs combined traditional CNS functions and leadership in the psychiatric hospital's quality improvement program. A number of the studies reported earlier in this chapter also focus on one setting or one aspect of the APN role (e.g., Burgess et al., 1987;

Ferguson & Sapelli, 1992; Girouard & Spross, 1989; Hanneman, Bines, & Sajtar, 1993; Hastings et al., 1980; Ingersoll, 1988; Tierney, 1990; Uzark, LeRoy, Callow, Cameron, & Rosenthal, 1994).

The process of evaluation has been identified as a continuum from episodic, activity-specific assessment and feedback to periodic assessments that contribute to a broader understanding of the contributions of the APN (Hamric, 1985). Regardless of the knowledge, experience, and resources available for evaluation, the APN should be involved in a thoughtful and meaningful assessment of the role and its contributions to patient care.

ROLE OF THE APN IN EVALUATION

The APN has a number of possible roles to play in evaluation, which will be operationalized at different times and to varying degrees. These roles include conducting evaluations of structure, process, and outcome variables and participating in the evaluations of others. In addition, APNs can be involved with quality-assurance activities within their employment settings and with their professional organizations, consult with others conducting evaluations of their practice or of patient care, and disseminate and use study findings to influence institutional and public policy that will affect patient care.

Riccardi and Kuck (1992) identified functions for the APN in quality-assurance programs: developing and implementing standards of care; anticipating, identifying, and prioritizing issues related to practice and the context of care; collaborating in the development of criteria; participating in the design of studies and the analysis of data; facilitating changes in nursing practice based on findings; acting as a liaison to quality-focused and practice committees; and participating in multi-disciplinary studies. To prepare future APNs, Noll and Girard (1993) developed a typology of quality-assurance activities that relate to the role competencies of the APN. For example, in the role of clinician, the APN would establish and promote standards of care, assess practice, identify problems and strategies to address them, and evaluate the effectiveness of interventions. Additional activities relate to the educational, research, leadership, and consultant components of the role. Another role for the APN is to collaborate with researchers to seek and secure financial and other resources needed to conduct evaluations. This is particularly important in order to execute the large-scale studies needed to build a more scientific and relevant data base about the impact of the APN on patient care outcomes.

Two other activities deserve special attention because they are critical to the ability of APNs to fulfill their social responsibility to promote optimal health and assure the place of APNs in the health-care system. Given the amount of evaluation activity going on in the health-care system and the attention being given to patient outcomes, APNs must be actively engaged in planning and implementing state and national government and private-sector evaluation efforts. This requires both political and policy involvement—the APN must seek these opportunities, because they will not come without effort. Related to this is the importance of disseminating findings (and having high-quality findings to disseminate) that will inform policymakers, consumers, and other stakeholders about advanced nursing practice's contributions. Publications in prestigious national and international health-care journals—not just nursing journals—and the use of the media to share findings with the public are strategies that nurses rarely use (see Chapter 23).

CONCLUSION

This chapter has presented a number of compelling arguments to motivate the APN to increase and improve efforts to evaluate the impact of advanced nursing practice in the health-care system. The existing literature has been reviewed, and although it strongly suggests that APNs make a demonstrable difference in the lives of patients, the body and quality of the evidence is by no means definitive. The problems associated with evaluating the impact of the APN and the strengths and weakness of past efforts should help future evaluators improve evaluation conceptualization and methodologies of evaluation. Finally, the frameworks presented can guide the beginning and more experienced evaluator to make increasingly greater contributions to assessing the impact of the APN.

These are challenging times for the APN. There are many exciting opportunities to improve access, enhance quality, and control costs. The data and knowledge gained from evaluation efforts can play a major role in shaping the organization, delivery, and financing of the future health-care system. True today is Hamric's statement made in 1989:

> In the current health care climate, demonstrating positive changes in patients and nursing behavior attributable to [the interventions of APNs] is not only desirable, it is a necessity for survival (p. 103).

Not only will the APN lose, the nursing profession and consumers will lose a great deal if the knowledge, skills, and leadership of APNs is not fully utilized in the evolving health-care system.

REFERENCES

Abraham, I. L, Chalifoux, Z. L., & Evers, G. C. (1992). Conditions, interventions, & outcomes: A quantitative analysis of nursing research (1981–1990). In *Patient outcomes research: Examining the effectiveness of nursing practice*. Proceedings of a conference sponsored by the National Center for Nursing Research, U.S. Department of Health and Human Services, Pub. No. 93-3411, October.

Aiken, L. H., Lake, E. T., Seman, S., Lehman, H. P., O' Hare, P. A., Cole, C. S., Dunbar, D., & Frank, I. (1993). Nurse practitioner managed care for persons with HIV infection. *Image 25*(3), 172-177.

Alexander, J. S., Younger, R. E., Cohen, R. M., & Crawford, L. V. (1988). Effectiveness of a nurse managed program for children with chronic asthma. *Journal of Pediatric Nursing 3*(5), 312-317.

Aradine, C. R., & Denyes, M. J. (1972). Activities and pressures of clinical nurse specialists. *Nursing Research, 21,* 411-418.

Ayers, R. (1971). Effects and development of the role of the clinical nurse specialist. In R. Ayers (Ed.), *The clinical nurse specialist: An experiment in role effectiveness and role development*. Duarte, CA: City of Hope National Medical Center.

Baldwin, L. M., Raine, T., Jenkins, L. D., Hart, L. G., & Rosenblatt, R. (1994). Do providers adhere to ACOG standards? The case of prenatal care. *Obstetrics and Gynecology, 84*(4), 549-556.

Baradell, J. G. (1994). Cost-effectiveness and quality of care provided by clinical nurse specialists. *Journal of Psychosocial Nursing and Mental Health Services, 32*(3), 21-24.

Bartucci, M. R. (1985). A comparative study of outpatient care as perceived by renal transplant patients. *Journal of the American Association of Nephrology Nurses, 12*(2), 119-124.

Batey, M. V., & Holland, J. M. (1985). Prescribing practices among nurse practitioners in adult and family health. *American Journal of Public Health, 75*(3), 258-262.

Baughan, D. M., White-Baughan, J., Pickwell, S., Bartlome, J., & Wong, S. (1990). Primary care needs of Cambodian refugees. *Journal of Family Practice, 30*(5), 565-568.

Beal, M. W. (1984). Nurse-midwifery intrapartum management. *Journal of Nurse-Midwifery, 29*(1), 13-19.

Bell, K. E., & Mills, J. I. (1989). Certified nurse-midwife effectiveness in the health maintenance organization obstetric team. *Obstetrics and Gynecology, 74*(1), 112-116.

Beyerman, K. (1989). Making a difference: The gerontological CNS. *Journal of Gerontologic Nursing, 15*(5), 36-41.

Blancett, S. S. (1994). Florida's health care reform. In *Draft state outlines*, Transformation of the Nursing Workforce, American Academy of Nursing Annual Meeting and Conference, October.

Bloch, D. (1975). Evaluation of nursing care in terms of process and outcomes: Issues in research and quality assurance. *Nursing Research, 24*(4), 256-263.

Boyd, N. J., Staslowski, S. A., Catoe, P. T., Wells, P. R., et al. (1991). The merit and significance of clinical nurse specialists. *Journal of Nursing Administration, 21*(9), 35-43.

Brooten, D., Kumar, S., Brown, L. P., Butts, D., et al. (1986). A randomized clinical trial of early hospital discharge and home follow-up of very low birth weight infants. *New England Journal of Medicine, 315*(15), 934-939.

Brooten, D., Roncoli, M., Finkler, S., Arnold, L., et al. (1994). A randomized trial of early hospital discharge and home follow-up of women having cesarean birth. *Obstetrics and Gynecology, 84*(5), 832-838.

Buchanan, J. L., Bell, R. M., Arnold, S. B., Witsberger, C., Kane, R. L., & Garrard, J. (1990). Assessing cost effects of nursing-home-based geriatric nurse practitioners. *Health Care Financing Review, 11*(3), 67-78.

Buerhaus, P. (1992). Nursing, competition and quality. *Nursing Economics, 10*(1), 21-29.

Buerhaus, P. (1994a). Economics of managed competition and consequences to nurses: Part I. *Nursing Economics, 1*(1), 10-17.

Buerhaus, P. (1994b). Economics of managed competition and consequences to nurses: Part II. *Nursing Economics, 12*(2), 75-80, 106.

Burge, S., Crigler, L., Hurth, L., Kelly, G., & Sanborn, C. (1989). Clinical nurse specialist role development: Quantifying actual practice over three years. *Clinical Nurse Specialist, 3*(1), 33-36.

Burgess, A. W., Lerner, D. J., D'Angostino, R. B., Vokanos, P. S., et al. (1987). A randomized control trial of cardiac rehabilitation. *Social Sciences and Medicine, 24*(4), 359-370.

Caine, D. H., Baldwin, D. S., Baradell, J., Earte, M. M., et al. (1994). Safeguarding the public's trust through the self-governance of peer review. *Journal of Psychosocial Nursing and Mental Health Services, 32*(5), 14-16.

Capan, P., Beard, M., & Mashburn, M. (1993). Nurse-managed clinics provide access and improved health care. *Nurse Practitioner, 18*(5), 50, 53-55.

Cason, C. L., & Beck, C. M. (1982). Clinical nurse specialist role development. *Nursing and Health Care, 3*(1), 25-26, 35-38.

Cavero, C. M., Fullerton, J. T., & Bartlome, J. A. (1991). Assessment of the process and outcomes of the first 1,000 births of a nurse midwifery service. *Journal of Nurse-Midwifery, 36*(2), 104-110.

Chambers, J. K., Dangel, R. B., German, K., Tripoli, V., & Jaguar, C. (1987). Clinical nurse specialist collaboration: Development of a generic job description and standards of performance. *Clinical Nurse Specialist, 1*(3), 124-127.

Chambers, L., & West, A. (1978). Assessment of the role of the family nurse practitioner in urban medical practices. *Canadian Journal of Public Health, 609*, 459-468.

Cherry, J., & Foster, J. C. (1982). Comparison of hospital charges generated by certified nurse-midwives' and physicians' clients. *Journal of Nurse-Midwifery, 27*(1), 7-11.

Collins, C. (1990). Job satisfaction of CNMs. Luxury or necessity? *Journal of Nurse-Midwifery, 35*(4), 237-244.

Cox, K., Bergen, A., & Norman, I. J. (1993). Exploring consumer views of care provided by the Macmillan nurse using critical incident technique. *Journal of Advanced Nursing, 18*(3), 408-415.

Crabtree, M. K., Renwanz-Boyle, A., Perry, B., Taylor, R., & Thrailkill, A. (1990). A collaborative approach to nursing research: Part II, The findings. *Journal of the American Academy of Nurse Practitioners, 2*(4), 146-152.

Cromwell, J. & Rosenbach, M. (1988). The economics of anesthesia delivery. *Health Affairs*, Fall.

Crosby, F., Ventura, M. R., & Feldman, M. J. (1987). Future research recommendations for establishing NP effectiveness. *Nurse Practitioner, 12*(1), 75-76, 78-79.

Cummings, M. A. (1992). Patient outcomes: Research-nursing, an important component. *Journal of Professional Nursing, 8*(6), 318.

Damato, E. G., Dill, P. Z., Gennaro, S., Brown, L. P., et al. (1993). The association between CNS direct care time and total time and very low birth weight infant outcomes. *Clinical Nurse Specialist, 7*(2), 75-79.

Davis, L. G., Riedman, G. L., Sapiro, M., Minogue, J. P., & Kozer, R. R. (1994). Cesarean section rates in low-risk private patients managed by certified nurse-midwives and obstetricians. *Journal of Nurse-Midwifery, 39*(2), 91-97.

Dixon, B. A. (1993). Institutional survey of nurse anesthesia practice in patients receiving opioids via patient-controlled analgesia. *Nurse Anesthetist, 4*(3), 112-117.

Doblin. B. H., Gelberg, L., & Freeman, H. E. (1992). Patient care and professional staffing patterns in McKinney Act Clinics providing primary care to the homeless. *JAMA, 267*(5), 698-701.

Donabedian, A. (1966). Evaluating the quality of medical care. *Milbank Quarterly, 44*, 166-206.

Draye, M. A., & Pesznecker, B. L. (1979). Diagnostic scope and certainty: An analysis of FNP practice. *Nurse Practitioner, 4*(1), 42-43.

Ellings, J. M., Newman, B. B., Hulser, T. C., Bivins, H. A., Jr., & Keenan, A. (1993). Reduction in very low birth weight deliveries and perinatal mortality in a specialized, multidisciplinary twin clinic. *Obstetrics and Gynecology, 81*(3), 387-391.

Fenton, M. V. (1985). Identifying competencies of clinical nurse specialists. *Journal of Nursing Administration, 15*(12), 31-37.

Ferguson, L. A., & Sapelli, D. M. (1992). Nurse practitioner sutured wounds: A quality assurance review. *American Association of Occupational Health Nursing Journal, 40*(12), 577-580.

Fleming, S. T. (1992). Outcomes of care for anesthesia services: A pilot study. *Quality Assurance in Health Care, 4*(4), 289-303.

Garrard, J., Kane, R. L., Radosevich, D. M., Skay, C. L., et al. (1990). Impact of geriatric nurse practitioners on nursing-home residents' functional status, satisfaction and discharge outcomes. *Medical Care, 28*(3), 271-283.

Georgopoulos, B. S., & Jackson, M. M. (1970). Nursing Kardex behavior in an experimental study of patient units with and without clinical nurse specialists. *Nursing Research, 19*(3), 196-218.

Georgopoulos, B. S., & Sana, J. M. (1971). Clinical nursing specialization and intershift report behavior. *American Journal of Nursing, 71*(3), 538-545.

Gibson, S. J., Martin, S. M., Johnson, M. B., Blue, R., & Miller, D. S. (1994). CNS-directed case management. Cost and quality in harmony. *Journal of Nursing Administration, 24*(6), 45-51.

Gifford, M. S., & Stone, I. K. (1993). Quality, access and clinical issues in a nurse practitioner colposcopy outreach program. *Nurse Practitioner, 18*(10), 33-36.

Girouard, S. (1978). The role of the clinical specialist as change agent: An experiment in preoperative teaching. *International Journal of Nursing Studies, 15*(2), 57-65.

Girouard, S., & Spross, J. (1983). Evaluation of the CNS: Using an evaluation tool. In A. B. Hamric & J. A. Spross (Eds.), *The clinical nurse specialist in theory and practice* (pp. 207-218). New York: Grune & Stratton.

Global Success Corporation (1995). Joint Commission issuing first "report cards." *Healthcare Performance Reporting, 1*(1), 1-12.

Graveley, E. A., & Littlefield, J. H. (1992). A cost-effectiveness analysis of three staffing models for the delivery of low-risk prenatal care. *American Journal of Public Health, 82*(2), 180-184.

Gurka, A. M. (1991). Process and outcome components of clinical nurse specialist consultation. *Dimensions in Critical Care, 10*(3), 169-175.

Hag, M. B. (1993). Understanding older adult satisfaction with primary health care services in a nursing center. *Applied Nursing Research, 6*(3), 125-131.

Hamric, A. B. (1983). A model for developing evaluation strategies. In A. B. Hamric & J. A. Spross (Eds.), *The clinical nurse specialist in theory and practice* (pp. 187-206). New York: Grune & Stratton.

Hamric, A. B. (1989). A model for CNS evaluation. In A. B. Hamric & J. A. Spross (Eds.), *The clinical nurse specialist in theory and practice* (2nd ed., pp. 83-104). New York: Grune & Stratton.

Hamric, A. B., Gresham, M. L., & Eccard, M. (1978). Staff evaluation of clinical leaders. *Journal of Nursing Administration, 8*(1), 18-26.

Hanneman, S. G., Bines, A. S., & Sajtar, W. S. (1993). The indirect patient care effect of a unit-based clinical nurse specialist on preventable pulmonary complications. *American Journal of Critical Care, 2*(4), 331-338.

Hastings, G. E., Vick, L., Lee, G., Sasmar, L., et al. (1980). Nurse practitioners in a jailhouse clinic. *Medical Care, 18*(7), 731-744.

Hill, J., Bird, H. A., Harmer, R., Wright, V., & Lawton, C. (1994). An evaluation of the effectiveness, safety and acceptability of a nurse practitioner in a rheumatology outpatient clinic. *British Journal of Rheumatology, 33*(3), 283-288.

Hill, K. M., Ellsworth-Wolk, J., & DeBlase, R. (1993). Capturing the multiple contribution of the CNS role: A criterion-based evaluation tool. *Clinical Nurse Specialist, 7*(5), 267-273.

Hinshaw, A. S. (1992). Welcome: The patient outcomes research conference. Proceedings of a conference sponsored by the National Center for Nursing Research, U.S. Department of Health and Human Services, Pub. No. 93-3411, October.

Holmes, G., Livingston, G., & Mills, E. (1976). Contribution of a nurse clinician to office practice productivity: Comparison of two solo primary care practices. *Health Services Research, 11*(1), 21-33.

Houston, S., & Luquire, R. (1991). Measuring success: CNS performance appraisal. *Clinical Nurse Specialist, 5*(4), 204-209.

Ingersoll, G. L. (1988). Evaluating the impact of the clinical nurse specialist. *Clinical Nurse Specialist, 2*(3), 150-155.

Jencks, S. F., & Wilensky, G. R. (1992). The health care quality improvement initiative: A new approach to quality assurance in Medicare. *JAMA, 268*(7), 900-903.

Jennings, B. M. (1991). Patient outcomes research: Seizing the opportunity. *Advances in Nursing Science, 14*(2), 59-72.

Josten, L. E. (1994). Minnesota state health care reform. In *Draft state outlines*, Transformation of the Nursing Workforce, American Academy of Nursing Annual Meeting and Conference, October.

Kane, R. L., Garrard, J., Buchanan, J. L., Rosenfeld, A., et al. (1991). Improving primary care in nursing homes. *Journal of the American Geriatric Society, 39*(4), 359-367.

Kane, R. L., Garrard, J., Skay, C. L., Radosevich, D. M., et al. (1989). Effects of a geriatric nurse practitioner on process and outcome of nursing home care. *American Journal of Public Health, 79*(9), 1271-1277.

Kasch, C. R., & Knutson, K. (1986). The functional message behavior inventory. Linking nursing action with health care outcomes. *Nurse Practitioner, 11*(6), 61-67.

Kearnes, D. R. (1992). A productivity tool to evaluate NP practice: Monitoring clinical time spent in reimbursable, patient-related activities. *Nurse Practitioner, 17*(4), 50-52, 55.

Kearnes, D. R. (1994). Impact of a nurse practitioner and physician collaborative practice on older adults admitted to a large urban hospital: Differences in treatment and outcome. *Nurse Practitioner, 19*(8), 32, 34-36.

Knaus, W. A., Draper, E. A., Wagner, D. P., & Zimmerman, J. E. (1986). An evaluation of outcome from intensive care in major medical centers. *Annals of Internal Medicine, 104*(3), 410-418.

Knickman, J. R., Lipkin, M., Jr., Finkler, S. A., Thompson, W. G., & Kiel, J. (1992). The potential for using non-physicians to compensate for the reduced availability of residents. *Academic Medicine, 67*(7), 429-438.

Koelbel, P. W., Fuller, S. G., & Misener, T. R. (1991a). An explanatory model of nurse practitioner job satisfaction. *Journal of the American Academy of Nurse Practitioners, 3*(1), 17-24.

Koelbel, P. W., Fuller, S. G., & Misener, T. R. (1991b). Job satisfaction of nurse practitioners: An analysis using Herzberg's theory. *Nurse Practitioner, 16*(4), 43, 46-52, 55-56.

Komaroff, A. L., Sawayer, K., Flatly, M., & Browne, C. (1976). Nurse practitioner management of common respiratory and genitourinary infections, using protocols. *Nursing Research, 25*(2), 84-89.

Kurz-Cringle, R., Blake, L. A., Dunham, D., Miller, M. J., & Annecillo, C. (1994). A nurse-managed inpatient program for patients with chronic mental disorders. *Archives of Psychiatric Nursing, 8*(1), 14-21.

Lang, N. M., & Marek, K. D. (1992). Outcomes that reflect clinical practice. In *Patient outcomes research: Examining the effectiveness of nursing practice*. Proceedings of a conference sponsored by the National Center for Nursing Research, U.S. Department of Health and Human Services, Pub. No. 93-3411, October.

Lemley, K. B., O'Grady, E. T., Rouckhorst, L., Russel, D. D., & Small, N. (1994). Baseline data on the delivery of clinical preventive services provided by nurse practitioners. *Nurse Practitioner, 19*(5), 57-63.

Levy, B. S., Wilkinson, F. S., & Marine, W. M. (1971). Reducing neonatal mortality rate with nurse-midwives. *American Journal of Obstetrics and Gynecology, 109*(1), 50-58.

Linde, B. J., & Janz, N. M. (1979). Effect of a teaching program on knowledge and compliance of cardiac patients. *Nursing Research, 28*(5), 282-286.

Lipman, T. H. (1988). Length of hospitalization of children with diabetes: Effect of a clinical nurse specialist. *Diabetes Education, 14*(1), 41-43.

Little, D. E., & Carnevali, D. (1967). Nurse specialists effect on tuberculosis. *Nursing Research, 16*(4), 321-326.

Martin, J. P. (1989). From implication to reality through a unit-based quality assurance program. *Clinical Nurse Specialist, 3*(4), 192-196.

McBride, A. B., Austin, J. K., Chestnut, E. E., Main, C. S., et al. (1987). Evaluation of the impact of the clinical nurse specialist in a state psychiatric hospital. *Archives of Psychiatric Nursing, 1*(1), 55-61.

McCorkle, R., Benoliel, J. Q., Donaldson, G., Georgiadou, F., et al. (1989). A randomized clinical trial of home nursing care for lung cancer patients. *Cancer, 64*(6), 1375-1382.

Melillo, K. D. (1993). Utilizing nurse practitioners to provide health care for elderly patients in Massachusetts nursing homes. *Journal of the American Academy of Nurse Practitioners, 5*(1), 19-26.

Molde, S., & Diers, D. (1985). Nurse practitioner research: Selected literature review and research agenda. *Nursing Research, 34*(6), 362-367.

Murphy, J. F. (1971). If P (additional nursing care), then Q (quality of patient welfare). *WICHE Community Nursing Research, 4*, 1-12.

Naylor, M. D., Munro, B. H., & Brooten, D. A. (1991). Measuring the effectiveness of nursing practice. *Clinical Nurse Specialist, 5*(4), 210-215.

Neidlinger, S. H., Scroggins, K., & Kennedy, L. M. (1987). Cost evaluation of discharge planning for hospitalized elderly. *Nursing Economics, 5*(5), 225-230.

Nemes, J., Barnaby, K., & Shamberger, R. C. (1992). Experience with a nurse practitioner program in the surgical department of a children's hospital. *Journal of Pediatric Surgery, 27*(8), 1038-1040.

Nevidjon, B., & Warren, B. (1984). Documenting the activities of the oncology clinical nurse specialist. *Oncology Nursing Forum, 11*(3), 54-55.

Noll M. L., & Girard, N. (1993). Preparing the CNS for participation in quality assurance activities. *Clinical Nurse Specialist, 7*(2), 81-84.

Nuccio, S. A., Costa-Lieberthal, K. M., Gunta, K. E., Mackus, M. L., et al. (1993). A survey of 636 staff nurses: Perceptions and factors influencing the CNS role. *Clinical Nurse Specialist, 7*(3), 122-128.

Office of Technology Assessment (1986). *Nurse practitioners, physicians assistants and certified nurse midwives: A policy analysis*. Washington, D. C.: U. S. Congress, HCS 37.

Oleske, D. M., & Hauck, W. W. (1988). A population based evaluation of the impact of interventions for improving care to cancer patients in home settings. *Home Health Services Quarterly, 9*, 45-61.

Orient, J. M., Kettel, L. J., Sox, H. C., Jr., Sox, C. H., et al. (1983). The effect of algorithms on the cost and quality of patient care. *Medical Care, 21*(2), 157-167.

Peters, D. (1994). Strategic directions for using outcomes. *The Remington Report, June/July,* 9-13.

Pickwell, S. M. (1982). Primary health care for Indochinese refugee children. *Pediatric Nursing, 8*(2), 104-107.

Pickwell, S. M. (1989). The incorporation of family primary care for southeast Asian refugees in a community-based mental health facility. *Archives of Psychiatric Nursing, 3*(3), 173-177.

Powers, M. J., Jalowiec, A., & Reichelt, P. A. (1984). Nurse practitioner and physician care compared for nonurgent emergency room patients. *Nurse Practitioner, 9*(2), 39, 42, 44-45.

Pozen, M. W., Stechmiller, J. A., Harris, W., Smith, S., et al. (1977). A nurse rehabilitator's impact on patients with myocardial infarction. *Medical Care, 15*(10), 830-837.

Prescott, P. A. (1994). Cost-effective primary care providers. An important component of health care reform. *International Journal of Technological Assessment in Health Care, 10*(2), 249-257.

Quint, M. (1995). Taking the pulse of HMO care. *The New York Times*, February 25.

Ramsey, P., Edwards, J., Lenz, C., Odom, J. E., & Brown, B. (1993). Types of health problems and satisfaction with services in a rural nurse-managed clinic. *Journal of Community Health Nursing, 10*(3), 161-170.

Reid, M. L., & Morris, J. B. (1979). Prenatal care and cost effectiveness: Changes in health care expenditures and birth outcome following the establishment of a nurse-midwifery program. *Medical Care, 17*(5), 491-500.

Repicky, P. A., Mendenhall, R. C., & Neville, R. E. (1980). Professional activities of nurse practitioners in adult ambulatory care settings. *Nurse Practitioner, 5*(2), 27, 31, 33-34.

Riccardi, E., & Kuck, A. W. (1992). Improving patient outcomes: The role of the clinical nurse specialist in quality assurance. *Journal of Nursing Care Quality, 6*(2), 46-50.

Robichaud, A. M., & Hamric, A. B. (1986). Time documentation of clinical nurse specialist activities. *Journal of Nursing Administration, 16*(1), 31-36.

Rogers, T., Metzger, L., & Bauman, L. (1984). Common concern. Geriatric nurse practitioners: How are they doing? *Geriatric Nursing, 5*(1), 51-54.

Rossi, P. H., & Freeman, H. E. (1989). *Evaluation: A systematic approach (4th ed.)*. Newbury Park, CA: Sage Publications.

Salkever, D. S., Skinner, E. A., Steinwachs, D. M., &

Katz, H. (1982). Episode based efficiency comparisons for physicians and nurse practitioners. *Medical Care, 20*(2), 143-153.

Sampselle, C. M., Peterson, B. A., Murtland, T. L., & Oakley, D. J. (1992). Prevalence of abuse among pregnant women choosing certified nurse-midwife or physician providers. *Journal of Nurse-Midwifery, 37*(4), 269-273.

Schultz, J. M., Liptak, G. S., & Fioravanti, J. (1994). Nurse practitioners' effectiveness in NICU. *Nursing Management, 25*(10), 50-53.

Scupholme, A., DeJoseph, J., Strobino, D. M., & Paine, L. L. (1992). Nurse-midwifery care to vulnerable populations. Phase I: Demographic characteristics of the national CNM Sample. *Journal of Nurse-Midwifery, 37*(5), 341-348.

Scupholme, A., Paine, L. L., Lang, J. M., Kumar, S., & DeJoseph, J. (1994). Time associated with components of clinical services rendered by nurse-midwives. Sample data from Phase II of nurse-midwifery care to vulnerable populations in the United States. *Journal of Nurse-Midwifery, 39*(1), 5-12.

Shamansky, S. L. (1985). Nurse practitioners and primary care research: Promises and pitfalls. *Annual Review of Nursing Research, 3*, 107-125.

Shaughnessy, P., Kramer, A., & Little, D. (1990). *The Teaching Nursing Home Experiment: Its effects and limitations.* Study Paper 6, Center for Health Services Research, the University of Colorado.

Smith, J. E., & Waltman, N. L. (1994). Oncology clinical nurse specialists' perceptions of their influence on patient outcomes. *Oncology Nurse Forum, 21*(5), 887-893.

Spisso, J., O'Callaghan, C., McKennan, M., & Holcroft, J. W. (1990). Improved quality of care and reduction of house staff workload using trauma nurse practitioners. *Journal of Trauma, 30*(6), 660-663.

Spitzer, W. O., Sackett, D. L., Sibley, J. C., Roberts, R. S., et al. (1990). 1965–1990: 25th anniversary of nurse practitioners. A classic manuscript reprinted in celebration of 25 years of progress. The Burlington randomized trial of the nurse practitioner. 1971–1972. *Journal of the American Academy of Nurse Practitioners, 2*(3), 93-99.

Sterling, Y. M., Noto, E. C., & Bowen, M. R. (1994). Case management roles of clinicians: A research case study. *Clinical Nurse Specialist, 8*(4), 195-207.

Tarsitano, B. J., Brophy, E. B., & Snyder, D. J. (1986). A demystification of the clinical nurse specialist role: specialists and nurse administrators. *Journal of Nursing Education, 25*(1), 4-9.

Tierney, M. J., Grant, L. M., & Mazique, S. I. (1990). Cost accountability and clinical nurse specialist evaluation. *Nursing Management, 21*(5), 26-28, 30-31.

Tri, D. L. (1991). The relationship between primary health care practitioners' job satisfaction and

600   ISSUES IN THE CONTINUING EVOLUTION OF ADVANCED NURSING PRACTICE

characteristics of their practice settings. *Nurse Practitioner, 16*(5), 46, 49-52, 55.

Trotter, C., & Danaher, R. (1994). Neonatal nurse practitioners: A descriptive evaluation of an advanced practice role. *Neonatal Network, 13*(1), 39-47.

Uzark, K., LeRoy, S., Callow, L., Cameron, J., & Rosenthal, A. (1994). The pediatric nurse practitioner as case manager in the delivery of services to children with heart disease. *Journal of Pediatric Health Care, 8*(2), 74-78.

Van Cott, M. L., Tittle, M. B., Moody, L. E., & Wilson, M. E. (1991). Analysis of a decade of critical care nursing practice research: 1979 to 1988. *Heart and Lung, 20*(4), 394-397.

Ventura, M. R., Crosby, F., & Feldman, M. J. (1991). An information synthesis to evaluate nurse practitioner effectiveness. *Military Medicine, 156*(6), 286-291.

Visalli, H. N. (1994). Blending clinical nurse specialist functions and quality improvement leadership: A partnership in care. *Journal of Nursing Care Quality, 8*(3), 75-79.

Ward, C., & Dracup, K. (1995). Identifying patients appropriate for nurse-managed ICUs. *American Journal of Critical Care, 4*(3), 255.

Wegener, V. (1994). One state's proposal for reform—The Oregon Health Plan. In *Draft state outlines.* Transformation of the Nursing Workforce, American Academy of Nursing Annual Meeting and Conference, October.

Weilitz, P. B., & Potter, P. A. (1993). A managed care system: Financial and clinical evaluation. *Journal of Nursing Administration, 23*(11), 51-57.

Weinberg, R. M., Liljestrand, J. S., & Moore, S. (1983). Inpatient management by a nurse practitioner: Effectiveness in a rehabilitation setting. *Archives of Physical Medicine and Rehabilitation, 64*(12), 588-590.

Winch, A. E. (1989). Peer support and review. In A. B. Hamric & J. A. Spross (Eds.), *The clinical nurse specialist in theory and practice* (2nd ed., pp. 299-321). New York: Grune & Stratton.

Wright, S. W., Erwin, T. L., Blanton, D. M., & Covington, C. M. (1992). Fast track in the emergency department: A one-year experience with nurse practitioners. *Journal of Emergency Medical Care, 10,* 367-373.

Wyers, M. E., Grove, S. K., & Pastorino, C. (1985). Clinical nurse specialist: In search of the right role. *Nursing and Health Care, 6*(4), 202-207.

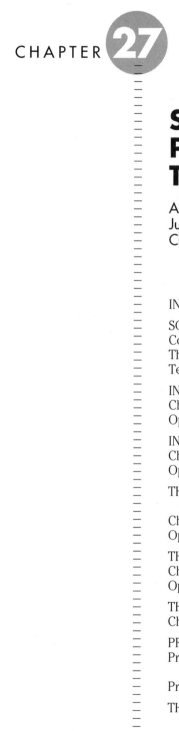

CHAPTER 27

Surviving System and Professional Turbulence

Ann B. Hamric
Judith A. Spross
Charlene M. Hanson

INTRODUCTION

Attempting to predict the future is provocative but hazardous. These are years of unprecedented change and activity in both health care in general and nursing in particular. The pace of change is markedly accelerated, and things that once seemed predictable (remember when the Clinton administration embarked upon health-care reform?) have taken directions different from what anyone could have anticipated. As one of the authors noted previously, "America's healthcare system is facing unprecedented times of massive change, exploding technology, and severe cost-containment pressure. How can we talk of creating the future while contending with the myriad forces that buffet us and call for response?" (Hamric, 1992, p. 11). Yet, in the decisions of the present lie the seeds of the future. By understanding the past and giving careful thought to the swirling trends of the present, nurses are actively making the decisions that will create the profession's future. If this future is to be a preferred one, especially regarding the complete enactment of advanced nursing practice (ANP), it is essential that advanced practice nurses (APNs) be full partners with other providers in the dialogue and debate about the future health-care system.

In general, APNs have fared well in this changing environment. For most APN roles, practice opportunities are plentiful and diverse. APNs' ability to manage system change is essential to their accomplishing a definition of health-care roles that includes APNs as key health-care providers (O'Malley & Cummings, 1995). Within the nursing profession, APNs must be leaders in making visible the work that is uniquely nursing and in strengthening the clinical practice of all nurses.

In this chapter, several forces and issues that will guide changes in the health-care system and nursing profession in the next decade are reviewed. The discussion is structured according to the recurrent themes that Bigbee notes in her historical review of the evolution of advanced nursing practice in Chapter 1. These themes include societal forces; inter- and intra-professional issues; and the importance of organizational, educational, and research development. The implications for advanced nursing practice, in terms of challenges and opportunities, are also discussed. A key conviction of the authors is that although APNs cannot change the chaos or the feeling that they are being buffeted by events over which they have no control, *they can and do choose their responses*. In this important sense, the future is inventible and not inevitable (Malone, 1989). APNs must take leadership, courage, a sense of purpose, and commitment into events and environments that appear to lack opportunities, and they must use problems as opportunities for creativity, organizational development, and personal growth.

SOCIETAL FORCES

COST CONTAINMENT

First and foremost, this is a time of cost containment and retrenchment from overspending in health care at both the federal and state levels. Quality is *not* a major issue in many new proposals for care in today's environment, despite rhetoric to the contrary. Decreasing costs is the driving consideration. Current debates regarding Medicare and Medicaid are complex because of the polarized political views about the government's role in social issues, including access to and financing of health care. Current federal initiatives to change health-care financing are likely to make access to health care even more difficult for vulnerable patient populations than it is now. The move to state control of health-care financing via block grants with restructured reimbursement mechanisms is affecting APNs' practice. Managed competition has made health insurance increasingly complicated for consumers, businesses, and care providers alike. The for-profit hospital industry (e.g., Columbia/HCA and Tenet) is changing the acute care landscape as more and more hospitals are purchased and merged to create large networks of health-care services. These trends do not promise a more accessible, simpler, or more user-friendly system. Changes seem to occur overnight—in providers associated with a given plan, in coverage, and in an agency's membership in a particular network. These changes spill over into community-based care, where many APNs practice. Even those with an avid interest in these issues find it a challenge to stay abreast of the changes.

Further complicating the pressures of cost containment are troubling social issues that directly affect the health of individuals in the United States. Dysfunctional families, escalating crime, family violence, and substance abuse are among a myriad of negative conditions that seem to be intractable problems, increasing the stress on families, communities, and the health-care system. The high risk and high cost of care provision for persons with AIDS and the increasing numbers of elderly and chronically ill individuals further stress a system that is already overburdened. Even though some persons would argue otherwise, it is clear that health care cannot be separated from the larger social context in which it occurs. An example of the negative interplay of these forces is seen in the effort of some insurers to set higher premiums for or to refuse to insure victims of domestic violence.

Challenges

The deemphasis on quality care is a tremendous concern for APNs, who pride themselves on providing holistic quality care. The payer-driven shortened patient visit is already negatively influencing the nursing component of APNs' care. The times require innovative APN practices that focus on components of care, such as caring, preventive services, and family support, that distinguish APNs from other providers. This is a difficult task when APNs are being offered production bonuses to see more patients within capitated care settings, or when nursing staff reductions increase workloads. Many nurses, including APNs, struggle to reconcile the values of the changing marketplace and the values of nursing. It is difficult to hold fast to person-centered values when the system is focused exclusively on decreasing costs. The overall goals of marketplace reform cannot be turned back. Given the inevitability of these changes, what should be nursing's response?

Opportunities

The growing number of vulnerable persons at high risk of being denied access to care is actually an opportunity for APNs. APNs have historically played a major role in the episodic and chronic care of high-risk clients, and they continue to do so. Many faculty practices have focused on vulnerable patient groups, demonstrating the impact of advanced nursing practice (see Chapter 21).

The current emphasis on cutting costs also provides a tremendous opportunity for APNs. As the American Nurses' Association (ANA, 1993) has stated,

*The more effective utilization of registered nurses to provide primary
health care services is part of the solution to the cost and accessibility
problems in health care today. Studies have shown that 60 to 80
percent of primary and preventive care, traditionally done by doctors,
can be done by a nurse for less money.*

(ANA, 1993, p. 1)

These same cost-cutting efforts provide a favorable environment for collaborative practice arrangements among APNs, physicians, and other health care professionals. The team approach to care enhances the ability of the APN to practice high-level nursing as part of an interdisciplinary team of providers.

At the level of the individual APN's practice, there are many opportunities for demonstrating cost savings. One involves identifying "designer" practices, i.e., practices where different practitioners treat the same problem differently (Spross, 1995b). They may involve different prescription medications, procedures, or treatment protocols. Identifying and studying alternatives can lead to choosing the most cost-effective practice that can be standardized across providers, thus saving money for the consumer, the institution, and the system as a whole. A related opportunity is product evaluation. Clinical nurse specialists (CNSs) are particularly skilled in this area (Lyon, 1996). Cost-benefit evaluations of products save institutions money by enabling data-based decisions regarding equipment and products; they also generate income for the institution when APNs enter into external consulting arrangements to test products (see an example in Malone, 1989).

Lyon (1996) has identified exciting possibilities for CNSs to market their expert services to managed care companies and third party payers. The incentives in capitated pay structures are the reverse of the fee-for-service system (i.e., judicious use of services related to desired outcome achievement is rewarded, rather than indiscriminate use of more and more services). In capitated systems, providers cannot afford to use costly and unnecessary or ineffective medical diagnostic or treatment services. Increasingly, companies are beginning to ask why certain patients consume a disproportionate share of their health-care benefits. The central phenomena of concern to nursing, such as fatigue, pain and discomfort, sleep disturbance, difficulty breathing, nausea, dizziness, symptoms of stress, decisional conflict, incontinence, and skin breakdown, are frequently the reasons for patients' increased utilization of health-care resources. These problems cause patients to experience delayed discharge, frequent readmission, or need for extended care. As experts in dealing with these phenomena, CNSs can develop population profiles to answer such questions as: Why are the 5% of persons who have diabetes in this managed care plan using more than 17% of the resources? CNSs' and other APNs' expertise in diagnosing and treating the non–disease-based causes of illness (Lyon, 1990) will be in high demand in capitated systems.

THE SHIFT IN THE HEALTH-CARE SYSTEM'S FOCUS

The health-care system is clearly moving away from hospital-oriented, very high-tech care and toward a system focused on primary care within the context of community-based managed care (Donley, 1995). This change is being accomplished at the same time that use of high-tech specialized medical care continues unabated. It is time for a more balanced allocation of health-care dollars. The future health of the nation will depend on access to and availability of primary care services.

This shift toward community-based managed care has created unprecedented opportunities for advanced nursing practice. The market is favorable to APNs, especially those specializing in primary care, with ever more states recognizing and legitimizing their practice. Consumers and APNs are more closely aligned regarding the value of the advanced care APNs provide than at any time in memory. However, as APNs achieve more autonomy in clinical practice, their education, credentialing, and competence are increasingly being scrutinized by organized medicine, regulators, insurers, consumers, and other stakeholders.

Challenges

The shift away from hospital-based care has increased the need to redirect some APNs into new specialty areas and to provide educational support for them in this regard. As new models emerge that reflect changes in supply and demand, preparation and policy issues will require the best thinkers in nursing, medicine and the allied health fields in order to meet interdisciplinary workforce challenges. The influences of the growth of managed care, the aging of the U.S. population, the shift to primary care, and the ongoing redefinition of the health-care system infrastructure make workforce predictions very difficult indeed. In addition, whether workforce needs will be met is influenced by funding patterns at the federal level, which are in a dramatic state of flux as this chapter is being written. It is clear, however, that most APNs will need some primary care skills.

Opportunities

The constant change reflective of the 1990s places nurses, and especially APNs, in an excellent position for leadership. Among the major health-care stakeholders (hospitals, physicians, nurses, insurers, and consumers), public perception of the role of nurses seems to be the most unchanged. Nurses are seen as stable, competent providers in an unstable and confusing health-care system. They are viewed as patient advocates who can be counted on to do the right thing. The time is right for APNs to showcase their innovative practice styles to gain needed visibility and acceptance by consumers. This is a tremendous opportunity to be seized by every APN. The movement of APNs into case management positions is an example of this opportunity. Many APNs (particularly CNSs) can and should have case management as part of their practice.

There are other ways in which APNs can seize opportunities in this time of changing health-care focus. The times call for a realignment in thinking toward primary prevention and collaboration. For example, the smoking teenager of today is the emphysema or lung cancer patient of tomorrow. Primary care nurse practitioners (NPs) and pulmonary or oncology CNSs can collaborate to intervene at the primary care level to avoid this negative outcome. The changes in and inadequacies of the present system should fuel APNs' creativity in practice innovations.

TECHNOLOGY TRANSFER ISSUES

The transfer of technology and innovations from the laboratory to the clinical setting and between and among disciplines has been a considerable force in the evolution of advanced nursing practice. For example, the development of ANP specialties in oncology and critical care nursing was fostered by the use of new treatments and technologies that required knowledgeable clinicians to administer and monitor them.

Skills, knowledge, and technology usually have been transferred from physicians to nurses in a not necessarily deliberate or planned process. When something became routine for physicians or nurses believed they could do some skill (e.g., chemotherapy administration) as well as, if not better than, physicians, the knowledge and skill became part of nursing practice. The social structures of health care and the slower pace of knowledge development led to a rather haphazard process of knowledge and skill diffusion. (It is important to note that technology transfer occurs in other disciplines as well. For example, physical therapists listen to heart and lung sounds, and emergency medical technicians have skills that overlap with critical care.) The development of the NP role as a primary care provider is one of the few examples in which some joint nursing-medicine deliberation led to the transfer of skills.

Challenges and Opportunities

Several factors argue for a more deliberative approach to the transfer of technology. The issue of cost containment is an ongoing concern. The use of unlicensed personnel is seen by some administrators as one way of controlling costs. However, decisions need to be made as to what can be safely delegated to such personnel, and APNs must be involved in these decisions.

APNs must also be clear about the technologies that should not be transferred. Deciding which knowledge and skills may be transferred from medicine to nursing requires considerable judgment. Having an APN do a particular task is not a reflection of the task's being routine. In work redesign efforts to increase access and decrease costs, two types of transfer may need to be considered. The first is transfer of tasks that can be done by rules, including guidelines for common deviations. This involves defining practices for which rules can be listed and taught. When these rules or procedures are followed, the desired outcomes are reliably reproduced. APNs who can anticipate the need for such transfers and develop proposals to test and implement them will be valuable. The second type of transfer is transfer of knowledge and skills that require abstraction and judgment. Such transfers occur across disciplines in which the practitioners in each of the disciplines are accustomed to dealing with uncertainty and exercising clinical judgment. For example, an APN, physician, and psychologist may all be able to do an adequate pain assessment, initiate interventions within their scope of practice, and recognize the need for another discipline's intervention. Having professionals in a number of disciplines who can begin intervening with important clinical problems while activating the involvement of other team members can benefit patients as well as result in cost savings.

APNs can encourage organizations to develop deliberative approaches to the transfer of knowledge and skills within and across disciplines. By being involved, they can help focus decisions on what is best for patients while meeting fiscal and system goals.

INTER-PROFESSIONAL ISSUES

The historical opposition of organized medicine to expanding roles for nurses is discussed thoroughly in Chapters 1 and 23. Two relatively recent developments are a presumed oversupply of physicians and the increasing emphasis in schools of medicine on preparing primary care physicians. The major threat these developments represent to advanced nursing practice is the competition for scarce health-care dollars for both education funding and clinical practice. Physicians may become threatened by nurses' expansion into primary and outpatient care. Unfortunately, nurses are only beginning to establish an independent claim to provide direct, reimbursable care. Such a task is even more difficult during a time of physician oversupply (Hamric, 1992). In addition, workforce issues also greatly affect the direction of ANP graduate education, the numbers of new APNs who are prepared for practice, and the specialties for which they are prepared.

In too many settings and in public discussions about health care, advanced nursing practice is invisible. The critical role nurses play in the health of the nation is similarly invisible. Patients receive bills for services provided by a physician when, in fact, it was an NP, CNS, or other APN who saw the patient for most or all of the visit. When the bill does not accurately reflect the real ANP services provided, the strength of advanced nursing practice and its influence on patient outcomes are rendered invisible. Likewise, marketers persist in promoting physician services when a large proportion of direct care in health maintenance organizations is provided by APNs and other nurses.

CHALLENGES

The issue of APNs' control of their practices continues to be a challenging one in the regulatory arena. State statutes and regulations requiring on-site consultation or direct supervision by physicians for APN practice are unacceptable and need to be changed (Safriet, 1992). Legislative efforts to secure authority for practice in state statutes, appropriate and fair reimbursement for services, and the ability to provide needed diagnostic and therapeutic interventions for clients must continue until every state recognizes and supports APN practice. Sustaining and promoting effective interdisciplinary practices in a competitive climate is another challenge. Clearly, interdisciplinary practice works—organized medicine thwarts it at its own peril.

OPPORTUNITIES

This is a time for partnerships. The emphasis of managed care and interdisciplinary models is on team efforts. The successful transition to less costly, community-based care requires genuine high-level collaboration among all clinicians, and among teams that include the client. APNs especially will need to refine their collaboration skills if they are to be full partners in the health-care configurations of the future (see Chapter 11). The need for productive alliances between APNs, nurses, nurse administrators, chief executive and operating officers, and physicians has never been greater. Interestingly, some of the threats imposed by managed care—encroachment on physician autonomy, treatment authorizations made by remote individuals without clinical backgrounds, and bureaucratic procedures that ignore client-provider relationships—can enable APNs and physicians to find common ground on which useful, collaborative relationships can be forged.

INTRA-PROFESSIONAL ISSUES

Many nurses do not understand or actively promote advanced nursing practice. Moreover, APNs have not always supported one another or acknowledged the link between different APN roles. For example, the NP role may have been able to develop because of precedents established by certified nurse-midwives (CNMs). CNMs may have been able to expand their practices into primary care because of precedents set by NPs. The movement of NPs into acute care was probably influenced by the contributions of CNSs.

Another intra-professional problem is that few nurse administrators consider advanced nursing practice or APNs as a solution to the demands inherent in today's health-care environment. A disturbing example is evident in a recent article by the Executive Director of the American Organization of Nurse Executives (Beyers, 1995). Writing on the future of nursing, the author did not mention advanced nursing practice or *any* ANP role. With organizations now merging and creating networks of services, nurse administrators and APNs need to work collaboratively and creatively to identify and promote networks of ANP services (see Chapter 24). Nurse administrators need to assess and anticipate organizational needs and help APNs get the continuing education and cross-training they need to be able to respond flexibly. When faced with a new or complex demand or challenge, some of the first questions an administrator should ask are, Is advanced nursing practice a solution? What kind of APN is needed? Can I delegate this to an APN? At the same time, APNs must ensure that administrators in their organizations know who they are and what they do. Nurse administrators have a responsibility to ensure that APN positions are filled with fully qualified APNs and that titles are used appropriately.

CHALLENGES

The definition of advanced nursing practice used throughout this book has not been universally agreed on by the nursing profession. There are important voices in nursing's leadership calling for a singular title of advanced practice nurse. Cronenwett (1995) has stated,

All segments of our profession need to work together toward a common goal, a future in which the legal and professional regulation and education of nurses at the graduate level are aligned so that one educational product, the advanced practice nurse, is prepared to fill a variety of roles in the health care system.

(Cronenwell, 1995, p. 112)

Although this argument has been debated mostly in terms of only two APN roles, namely the NP and the CNS, the clear implication is that all APNs should have the same educational preparation and title. This, indeed, is one direction that advanced nursing practice may take in the next decade. Interest in the blended CNS/NP role is increasing and many believe that this is the preferred ANP role of the future (Snyder & Mirr, 1995).

To an extent, this perspective is useful. There is an immediate need to standardize the definition and competencies of advanced nursing practice, so that all nurses functioning in ANP roles meet these expectations. In terms of regulation and legislative initiatives, use of the common definition and title of APN will promote clarity in public arenas. This clarity will be particularly vital over the next 2 to 3 years as APNs attempt to standardize education and practice during a time of unprecedented growth of the ANP segment of the profession. Individual APNs working at local levels will play key roles in defining the direction of advanced nursing practice. The issue of graduate education for all APNs will be a priority topic, as will the work in progress with the National Council of State Boards of Nursing (NCSBN). Program standards and curricula will be implemented to support eligibility requirements for national certification. In all of these initiatives, a uniform definition of advanced nursing practice, as proposed in this book, is highly desirable.

However, in the authors' view, the "one size fits all" approach, whereby only a generic APN is prepared and all ANP roles are homogenized into one APN title, is not supportable. Realistically, a nurse could not feasibly be prepared to function interchangeably in any APN role, especially if nurse-midwifery practice and nurse anesthesia practice are to be considered advanced nursing practice. In addition, there is a need to make room for emerging ANP roles, which may differ in focus from current roles. Evidence exists that there are real differences in the actual practices of NPs and CNSs (Fenton & Brykczynski, 1993; Williams & Valdivieso, 1994). It is also apparent that actual practices differ significantly according to the needs of the patient population served and the organizational framework within which the role is performed (see Chapter 3 and Part III). Consequently, it is necessary and desirable to retain varied job titles that reflect these actual practices. In reality, it is a strength of advanced nursing practice that APNs use diverse knowledge and skills to meet varied and complex patient needs. Specific titles reflecting specific practices decrease confusion and enhance role clarity, especially when the role incumbents can clearly explain their practice and differentiate it from other APN practices. The public and policymakers can understand this distinction, just as they understand the term *physician* to be the overall descriptor of a medical professional, and *neurologist* or *cardiac surgeon* the descriptor of a physician in a particular specialty (see also Safriet, 1992). The distinctions reflect differences in actual practices. As one of the authors has noted elsewhere, "Would we want electrical engineers building bridges?" (Spross, 1995a, p. 2).

It is critically important to emphasize that evolution and change are the order of the day for advanced nursing practice. As roles change, actual practices may become blended and merged, as is currently occurring with the blended CNS/NP (see Chapter 17). In these situations, job titles should also merge, again reflecting the actual practice.

Another issue confounding role clarity is the effort to certify anyone prepared at the master's level or beyond as an APN, regardless of practice focus. The Oncology Nursing Society has begun offering an advanced certification examination (Oncology Nursing Certification Corporation, 1996). This examination is open to any nurse with a master's (or higher) degree, regardless of whether the nurse is practicing in an ANP role. Consequently, a researcher, educator or administrator can obtain the advanced oncology certified nurse (AOCN) credential as well as an APN. In the authors' opinion, this confuses the meaning of certification for advanced practice, especially in regard to its regulation. The focus on direct clinical practice is a defining characteristic of advanced nursing practice. It distinguishes the practice from the work of an administrator, researcher, or educator. The purpose of certification is to assure the public that the individual can safely practice as an APN. Allowing individuals who do not practice as APNs to become certified as APNs will only confuse regulators, policymakers, and the public. In addition, certifying non-APNs with an APN credential implies that ongoing development of

ANP expertise can be acquired without a patient focus, which is clearly not the case.

OPPORTUNITIES

As other specialties develop credentialing for advanced nursing practice, leaders in this process need to ensure that all the primary criteria and competencies for advanced nursing practice are met. Certification at an ANP level is an important goal for incumbents practicing in all ANP roles.

Advanced nursing practice is powerful. APNs help patients, families, and communities realize the goal of health. The real work of nursing, and especially of advanced nursing practice, must be made visible. In this light, nurse case management and care coordination may be real benefits to nursing. Putting a nurse in charge of managing the process of care makes the contributions of nurses more visible. Nurses' clinical, interpersonal, and coordinating skills are clarified in ways that are meaningful to patients and to payers.

Collaboration between APNs across specialties and roles can also increase the visibility and power of advanced nursing practice. For example, the CNM with expertise in management of labor pain and the fatigue of childbearing can collaborate with an oncology CNS who has expertise in management of cancer pain and fatigue to identify a fuller range of interventions that may benefit both patient populations.

THE IMPORTANCE OF ORGANIZATIONAL DEVELOPMENT

In Chapter 1, Bigbee notes the importance of APNs having a strong, national organizational leadership that confronts issues in a unified and assertive fashion. The specialty organizations of CNMs and certified registered nurse anesthetists (CRNAs) are excellent models of such organizational leadership.

On the basis of her analysis, Styles (1990) argued that three conditions must exist if specialty differentiation is to occur without causing the disintegration of nursing. The conditions are authority, homogeneity, and unity. Well-established specialties are characterized by

- *"explicit statements of scope of practice, roles, curricula and standards;*
- *graduate programs in the specialty;*
- *certification procedures;*
- *mechanisms to support research;*
- *large, vigorous specialty organizations that pull all of these together and move the specialty forward in a systematic, unified manner."*

(Styles, 1990, p. 280)

Currently, specialties are "self-declared and self-ordained" (Styles, p. 281). The absence of a single, central authority for designating specialties deprives the profession of a source of authority for its specialties. As a result, there is considerable heterogeneity among specialty standards for education and practice. Together, these factors keep specialties relatively isolated and foster a professional impotence when specialties have opposing or competing interests that are pursued aggressively and alone (Styles, 1990).

CHALLENGES

Clearly, different ANP specialty groups must overcome their competing and opposing interests in order to unite around issues that will further advance nursing practice. A major breakthrough in organizational leadership is the current joint effort to build an approval mechanism for NP education within the framework of National League for Nursing (NLN) graduate nursing program accreditation. CRNA and CNM documents are being used as models. This joint work in progress, which includes the NLN, the American Association of Colleges of Nursing, the National Organization of Nurse Practitioner Faculties, the several specialty organizations, the four certifying bodies who credential NPs, and the NCSBN, is gratifying and unprecedented. This type of high-level dialogue and consensus building provides important momentum for APN education and practice and should pave the way for a similar structure for CNSs.

OPPORTUNITIES

If all organized ANP groups support legislation that will ensure homogeneity and a common meaning of advanced nursing practice, they could collectively make a great impact (see Chapter 22).

The time is right for a coalition of all ANP groups, such as the Task Force on Advanced Nursing Practice that the ANA convened in 1993. This group, through continuing dialogue, was able to clarify misunderstandings about specialties and agree on many important issues. The ability of ANP groups to work collectively on policy and regulatory issues, even though they may not agree in all instances, will assure a high level of achievement of ANP goals.

THE IMPORTANCE OF EDUCATIONAL DEVELOPMENT

With the exception of the CNS role, which was initially developed as a master's-prepared clinical role, all of the ANP specialties began as informal training programs and have progressed to certificate and, more recently, graduate programs. The graduates of these programs have been the trailblazers of advanced nursing practice, and the profession owes them a profound debt of gratitude. It is increasingly clear that a strong national commitment is developing to have all ANP roles prepared at the graduate level. This is reflective of the expansion of knowledge, the realization that ANP competencies are best taught at the graduate level, the need to achieve parity among APNs, and the need for ANP roles to have legitimacy with those outside the profession.

CHALLENGES

There are several current challenges to the education of APNs. First and foremost is the unprecedented increase in ANP programs as part of the change occurring in health care. Rapid increases in numbers of new programs and changes within existing programs that prepare APNs have led to a lack of qualified faculty to teach, especially in the area of primary care NPs. Strategies such as post-master's tracks with scholarships that allow master's-prepared faculty in other specialties to pursue the appropriate APN credential are imperative.

A second issue is the continuing bilevel educational process for NPs and CNMs. The coexistence of certificate and graduate programs raises questions about the meaning of certification and credentialing and makes it difficult and confusing to explain to non-nurse educators and policy makers how two different educational programs can prepare the same, equivalent provider. The new consensus statement by women's health NP leaders (Consensus Statement on Women's Health NP Education, November 1995), which confirms matriculation to the master's degree within a reasonable time frame, is heartening and will benefit both the profession and advanced nursing practice.

A third challenge is the American College of Nurse-Midwives' initiative to expand the pool of midwives by recruiting non-nurses, a move that will undoubtedly affect nurse-midwifery practice. Although a CNM may be the product of education in two "separate" disciplines (i.e., nursing and midwifery), the extension of nurse-midwifery practice into non–maternity-related areas, such as primary care, has undoubtedly relied heavily on the nursing backgrounds of CNMs. It seems improbable that such non–maternity-related privileges will be accorded to midwives who are not nurses. If this initiative continues, it will be essential to track outcome data, because the extent to which the excellent outcomes of CNM care depend on a nursing background is unknown.

OPPORTUNITIES

Developing credible and stable educational programs using a standardized core curriculum with role-specific preparation (see Chapter 4) is a powerful strategy for strengthening advanced nursing practice. Ensuring consistency and quality across programs is required for advanced nursing practice to obtain the legitimacy it needs to continue to grow. Developing post–master's programs for APNs who want to change ANP jobs is another important initiative, currently seen most frequently in post–master's NP programs. Such programs are also important for NPs who want to move into blended roles and need CNS skills, for APNs who wish to move into case management, and for women's health NPs who wish to develop CNM skills, to name a few possibilities. APNs should view expanding their repertoire of skills as an investment in preparing for an uncertain future.

THE IMPORTANCE OF RESEARCH DEVELOPMENT

The need for sound research data documenting the impact of APN care on patient outcomes is as critical today as it was in the early years of each ANP specialty's development. Research is needed to validate that APNs use the competencies that are the critical components of advanced nursing practice. For example, research is needed to validate the explication of ANP coaching provided by Clarke and Spross in Chapter 7 and to differentiate ANP coaching from that done by nurses who are experts by experience. Demonstrating differences due to unique ANP competencies is also necessary to differentiate ANP roles from those of non-nurse providers, such as physicians, physician house officers, non-nurse case managers, and physician assistants (some of whom claim to be indistinguishable from NPs—however, if the practices are truly indistinguishable, we would argue that the NP is not practicing as an APN).

CHALLENGES AND OPPORTUNITIES

There is a dearth of data about APNs, especially patient outcomes attributable to their interventions (see Chapter 26). This fact makes it difficult for organized nursing to defend the expansion of ANP roles. New partnerships and new technologies that allow for sophisticated databases to be developed need to be the norm for the ensuing decades. These data should include research generated by APNs about their practices so that policymakers, consumers, and others can better understand the dimensions and strength of the care provided by APNs. Funds for research on and development and implementation of technology need to be spent judiciously on areas that offer the most promise for a healthier future.

The development of outcome measures to evaluate advanced nursing practice is critically important (Hamric, 1989; see also Chapter 26). ANP roles require a serious focus on research and the development of innovative, research-based nursing interventions. The critical body of knowledge surrounding ANP interventions and outcomes should be developed (Buchanan, 1994). This will require close collaboration among ANP educators, researchers, and practicing APNs.

PRIORITIES

This analysis reveals several challenges to advanced nursing practice. The chaotic nature of the health-care system is unlikely to settle down and expectations that it will are naive. The rapidity with which change occurs requires a clear vision of the future of advanced nursing practice to guide the profession, organizations, and individual APNs. However, vision alone is not enough if the contributions of APNs to the health of individuals, families, and communities are to be fully realized. Attention must be paid to the process of shaping this vision. From the outset, it must be acknowledged that all nurses will not agree on every criterion, credential, or regulatory point. A commitment to the broader goals of legitimacy for all APNs and full participation in the present and future health-care system are needed to ensure that the profession speaks with one voice when negotiating with policy makers. The failure to engender this commitment will roll back the progress that has been made—non-nurse stakeholders will be able to divide and conquer, and nurses and patients alike will lose. This commitment is the *sine qua non* on which the other priorities are based.

PRIORITIES FOR THE PROFESSION AND SPECIALTY ORGANIZATIONS

The *first* priority is to ensure a uniform definition of advanced nursing practice, as proposed in this book, for use in federal and state legislation and regulation and to develop and implement a plan to see that its adoption is expedited. To promulgate public understanding of advanced nursing practice, a fact sheet or brochure on advanced nursing practice and the various ANP roles is needed. It follows from this first priority that focused attention should be directed to standardizing graduate curricula for advanced nursing practice and strengthening existing and needed credentialing mechanisms. The profession must ensure that graduates meet the criteria for advanced nursing practice and that they can be credentialed as APNs. The *second* priority is the collaborative development of an easily updated and readily retrievable database on advanced nursing practice and its outcomes. The speed with which change occurs and the need for a rapid and flexible response to policy makers and administrators demands that the profession have such data at its fingertips. The *third* priority is to develop a reasoned approach to the transfer of technology and skills to and from nursing and among different levels of nursing personnel. Such a process needs to be able to be accomplished quickly and communicated clearly, and will often need to be interdisciplinary. The process needs to attend to both clinical outcomes and costs.

As nursing leaders and groups address issues related to advanced nursing practice, creative approaches to analysis and discussion are needed. Brainstorming strategies developed by von Oech (1988) were applied to some of the pressing ANP challenges identified in this chapter (Spross, 1995a) and are illustrated in Table 27–1. The five strategies in the table are a selection of the 64 found in the *Creative Whack Pack* (von Oech, 1988). These strategies can uncover values, attitudes, and beliefs that may interfere with productive problem solving. They can also help to reframe problems and enable group members to see the need for a particular solution.

TABLE 27–1. STRATEGIES FOR REFRAMING A PROBLEM

1. SOLVE THE RIGHT PROBLEM.
   - Is the real problem whether to merge the clinical nurse specialist (CNS) and nurse practitioner (NP) roles? Or is it clarifying and agreeing on a common definition of advanced nursing practice (ANP) and advanced practice nurse (APN) for promulgation to policymakers and the public?
   - Rather than dwell on the system's shortcomings and our own disappointments, could we invest our energies in identifying opportunities and strategies for dealing with these changes?
   - If states are going to regulate advanced nursing practice, what laws and regulations will best support the full implementation of all ANP roles?
2. CHANGE THE QUESTION.
   - Will the practice of experienced CNSs who return for their NP credential differ from that of NPs with similar years of experience? How will their clinical judgments be similar? How will they differ?
   - What mix and depth of content in core competencies are needed for various ANP positions?
3. ASK "WHAT IF?"
   - What if the Office of Technology Assessment had done a study of CNS practice?
   - What if the American College of Nurse-Midwives is successful in certifying midwives from other health-care disciplines? What transdisciplinary future awaits us?
   - What if all APNs had some case management skills.
   - What would happen to organizational costs if APNs were held accountable for clinical and fiscal outcomes?
4. LOOK TO THE PAST.
   - What do we learn from looking at the knowledge and technology transfer issue more closely?
   - If technology transfer is a recurring theme of our history, what will that mean for APNs 10 years from now?
   - What can we learn from the entry-into-practice issue to help unify the profession and all APNs?
5. DON'T FORCE IT.
   - If the overall goals of marketplace reform are inevitable, what are the opportunities such changes offer?
   - What if we rally around titling for policy/media purposes but let the market, APNs, and employers drive what happens in organizations?

Strategy items adapted from von Oech, R. (1988). *Creative whack pack.* Stamford, CT: U.S. Games System.

PRIORITIES FOR INDIVIDUAL APNs

Individual APNs must work in concert with their colleagues and their professional organizations to achieve the first priority identified above—uniform regulatory definition of advanced nursing practice.

The current health-care environment can be both exciting and discouraging. Having clearly sanctioned autonomy and accountability for one's practice offers APNs many opportunities for satisfying work. However, the emphases on cost effectiveness, efficiency, and productivity can dehumanize the delivery of health care. Prouty's (1983) advice for creating an environment supportive of CNS practice remains timely for APNs today. Spross (1995b), applying Prouty's advice to today's turbulent environment, offered survival strategies for APNs (Table 27–2). Selected points from this table are emphasized as priorities for APNs: making advanced

TABLE 27–2. STRATEGIES FOR DEALING WITH TURBULENCE: HOW TO IMPLEMENT PROUTY'S (1983) LEADERSHIP MAXIMS

Innovation requires commitment, not magic.
- Think globally and act locally. For example,
  - Propose programs that will meet some gap in care that save money or cost less than alternatives.
  - Make a commitment to action and stay informed about health-care changes. Evaluate the impact of health-care policy proposals on your patient population.
  - Get involved in organization and task redesign efforts in your setting. Evaluate redesigns for their ability to promote advanced practice nurses (APNs) *and* interdisciplinary work.
  - Document failures of managed care and report them to your agency, the managed care providers, and more widely if necessary (i.e., legislators and the media). Present testimony to legislators on the impact to consumers of proposed laws and policies.
  - Select APNs for your own and your family's health care. Encourage friends and colleagues to use APNs.

Opportunities often appear in disguise. Nurses must identify and seize them.
- Learn about the economics of your practice. Learn about billing procedures; if your advanced practice is invisible, work to change the billing practices so that bills reflect your actual services.
- Systematically incorporate simple, inexpensive treatments (such as relaxation) into your practice. Evaluate their clinical and cost outcomes.
- Identify "designer" practices in your setting; identify alternatives and choose the most cost-effective one for standardized implementation.
- Develop and evaluate a critical path for a particular patient group.
- Cross-train in another area to increase your repertoire of strategies to benefit patients.
- Lead continuous quality improvement projects so that nursing and advanced nursing practice become visible.
- Identify and promote the skills you possess that cut across medical specialties and across disciplines (e.g., pain management).
- Collaborate with your administrator to evaluate your agency's marketing practices, particularly those geared to consumers. If your practice is one of the institution's "value-added services," educate your marketing department.
- Identify the values to which you are committed, stay informed, and make a commitment to action. Make a decision, take a risk, pay the price. (Chapter 11)
- Make sure that office staff refer to you as an APN; display your APN credentials.

Create productive alliances.
- Seek out colleagues from other disciplines in your setting. Identify common concerns and clinical problems. Develop supportive interdisciplinary relationships from which improved communication and problem-solving can emerge.
- Identify clinicians who offer complementary modalities (the "healing underground"), and build alliances and environments in which these therapies (e.g., therapeutic touch) can be documented and evaluated.
- Get to know your physician colleagues. Talk about the American Medical Association's opposition to advanced nursing practice and ask them whether they support it. Educate them and ask them to take action.

Adapted from Spross, J. (1995b, November). *Managed care and health care reform: Opportunities for promoting nursing's values.* Paper presented at the 7th M. P. Prouty Lectureship, Dartmouth Hitchcock Medical Center, Hanover, NH.

nursing practice visible, including making explicit the healing underground, and creating productive alliances. These strategies can also be used by graduate educators and administrators who prepare and supervise APNs.

Throughout this book, the invisibility of advanced nursing practice has been a recurrent theme. A key priority for APNs is to make visible what Spross (1995b) called the "healing underground." The research on advanced nursing practice (see Chapter 26) as well as the descriptions of the direct care provided by APNs (Chapters 6, 7, and 14 through 20) suggest that one of the reasons for the positive outcomes of APN care is the processes of care used by APNs. This healing underground must be made explicit. APNs must learn from their own patients their perceptions of what made the difference with regard to a particular outcome. APNs should also make explicit to their clients the processes of care—teaching, counseling, assessing, and supporting a client's decision-making. Too many patients interpret these skilled interpersonal interventions as kindness or as being nice. The reflective practice described by Clarke and Spross (Chapter 7) must be brought to bear on advanced nursing practice itself, such that APNs weave opportunities to teach patients, colleagues, and staff about nursing and advanced nursing practice. APNs are in a position to influence their own, their friends' and their families' choices of providers. It is axiomatic that some of the successes of nurse-midwifery can be attributed to their education of clients, the spread by word-of-mouth of the effectiveness of CNMs, and the use of CNMs by other CNMs for their own pregnancy and primary care needs.

APNs must, as individuals and as groups, address the structures that make APNs shadow providers. In organizations where APNs work, structures such as standards of care, documentation systems, and critical pathways should capture processes as well as outcomes of APN practice. Bills should reflect the name of the APN and all of the services provided. HMO network directories should not be silent when it comes to APNs; APNs should be listed along with physicians, social workers, and psychologists.

The perceptions of nurses and nursing are so uniform that it will be difficult to modify the social environments in which different types of nurses work. While organizational documents may claim the existence of differentiated nursing practice, everyday language and interactions may suggest that a nurse is a nurse. For example, over the course of two years, one APN (a CNM) known to the authors deliberately used everyday interactions with staff and her committee participation to "institutionalize" the term APN and socialize the staff to its use. Until APN became common parlance, staff RNs, NPs, and CNMs were all called nurses. This need to differentiate and make visible advanced nursing practice is by no means a devaluing of any nurse. All nurses are important and valuable, but they are not all the same. Understanding advanced practice and the different and distinct roles APNs assume benefits both the practice environment and the nursing profession.

The need for collaborative relationships and productive alliances among and between APNs, nurses, nurse administrators, chief executive and operating officers, and physicians has been another recurrent theme throughout this book. The current environment will not be supportive of turf protection and battles. The expert interpersonal competence of APNs puts them in an excellent position to shape collaborative environments that will benefit patients, clinicians, and administrators.

THE FUTURE IS NOW—SURVIVING SYSTEM AND PROFESSIONAL TURBULENCE

Graduate students and novice APNs may feel overwhelmed by the preceding discussion of system and professional challenges and opportunities. Where does one start to tackle these enormous issues? It is important to remember that advanced nursing practice truly exists at the individual practice level. The future is ensured by APNs who demonstrate the strength and diversity of advanced nursing practice in their day-to-day work. Both Tables 27–1 and 27–2 focus on questions and strategies individual APNs can use to evolve and strengthen their practices in times of turbulence.

Given the increased attention being paid to advanced nursing practice both within and outside the profession, it is imperative that APNs clearly demonstrate the eight core competencies discussed in Part II. Although all APNs must be prepared for beginning practice with these eight competencies, time and practice are required to truly develop them. In addition to possessing these competencies, the APN who possesses the following attributes will continue to be valuable regardless of changes in the health-care scene.

The most critical attribute is clinical competence in all the facets of advanced nursing practice. APNs must demonstrate the ability to care safely and surely for whatever specialty patient population they choose. They must understand their own limits and know how and from whom to seek help. In addition, ANP educators, certifiers, and regulators must demand competent practice by APNs in all areas of practice.

Caring is the second critical attribute. As Smith (1995) noted,

Advanced practice nursing is not filling the gap with medical care where it does not exist; it is filling the existing gap in health care with the core of nursing practice. . . . The core of advanced practice nursing lies within nursing's disciplinary perspective on human-environment and caring interrelationships that facilitate health and healing.

(Smith, 1995, pp. 2–3)

Patients and families are looking for stable, caring providers in an unstable, intimidating health-care system. The comprehensiveness of nursing's model for health care (the ANA's, 1991, *Nursing Agenda for Health Care Reform* is an example) and its holistic approach to care make APNs very marketable commodities.

Communication skill is another essential attribute. APNs need to excel in communication. Managed care and new partnerships are moving APNs into a team model with new interdisciplinary modalities based on collaboration and colleagueship. As discussed in Chapter 11, successful teamwork requires that all team members (a) have a high degree of competence, in order to engender trust; (b) have excellent communication skills; and (c) have a common understanding of the purpose and goals of the team. In addition, the rapid advances in information technology require skills enabling communication from great distances. These are new skills for many APNs.

Business acumen is another essential attribute (see Chapters 23 and 25). APNs now need to understand the cost of providing health care to a wide variety of individuals and families. Historically, nurses negotiated for set salaried positions and did not have to concern themselves about the costs of providing health care. In today's capitated systems, where providers are prepaid for care rendered to a group of clients, it is extremely important that APNs clearly understand the cost of the care they personally or through a team effort provide to patients. In addition to direct care cost oversight, it will be necessary for APNs to be articulate about programming that supports their clients so that programs are not deleted in organizational efforts to balance institutional budgets. Closely related to the issue of cost is impact on patient outcome. If, in a given agency, the APN's role is not structured to affect patient outcomes in some clearly demonstrable ways, the role "is *a priori* in trouble and vulnerable to budget cuts" (Hamric, 1992, p. 14).

Finally, flexibility always has been and must continue to be a hallmark of the APN. The ability to retrain or change direction as required to meet changing client and institution needs will be extremely useful for APNs over the ensuing decades. In the course of its history, advanced nursing practice has been characterized by its flexibility and creativity in responding to changing health-care needs (see Chapter 1). APN specialties will continue to evolve and diversify as the changes continue.

These are years of great promise and great risk for APNs. The vision of advanced practice that has been promoted throughout this book is not yet fully realized in the health-care system. Close collaboration and support among individual APNs and among all the ANP specialties will allow this vision to become a reality.

REFERENCES

American Nurses' Association. (1991). *Nursing's agenda for health care reform.* Washington, DC: Author.

American Nurses' Association. (1993). Primary health care: The nurse solution. *Nursing facts.* Washington, DC: Author.

Beyers, M. (1995). The future of nursing. *Journal of Nursing Administration, 25,* 8, 10–11.

Buchanan, L. M. (1994). Therapeutic nursing intervention knowledge development and outcome measures for advanced practice. *Nursing and Health Care, 15,* 190–196.

The Consensus Statement on Women's Health NP Education (Nov. 1995). Developed by Association of Women's Health, Obstetrics, & Neonatal Nurses, National Association of NPs in Reproductive Health, the Planned Parenthood Federation of America, and the National Certification Corporation of Obstetric, Gynecologic & Neonatal Nurse Specialists. Chicago, IL: National Certification Corporation, Convener.

Cronenwett, L. R. (1995). Molding the future of advanced practice nursing. *Nursing Outlook, 43,* 112–118.

Donley, S. R. (1995). Advanced practice nursing after health care reform. *Nursing Economics, 13,* 84–88.

Fenton, M. V., & Brykczynski, K. A. (1993). Qualitative distinctions and similarities in the practice of clinical nurse specialists and nurse practitioners. *Journal of Professional Nursing, 9,* 313–326.

Hamric, A. B. (1989). A model for CNS evaluation. In A. B. Hamric & J. A. Spross (Eds.), *The clinical nurse specialist in theory and practice* (2nd ed., pp 83–106). Philadelphia: W. B. Saunders.

Hamric, A. B. (1992). Creating our future: Challenges and opportunities for the clinical nurse specialist. *Oncology Nursing Forum, 19*(1, Suppl.), 11–15.

Lyon, B. L. (1990). Getting back on track: Nursing's autonomous scope of practice. In N. Chaska (Ed.), *The nursing profession: Turning points.* St. Louis: C. V. Mosby.

Lyon, B. L. (February, 1996). Personal communication. Indianapolis, IN: Indiana University School of Nursing.

Malone, B. L. (1989). The CNS in a consultation department. In A. B. Hamric & J. A. Spross (Eds.), *The clinical nurse specialist in theory and practice* (2nd ed., pp 397–413). Philadelphia, PA: W. B. Saunders.

O'Malley, J., & Cummings, S. H. (1995). Change . . . more change . . . and change again!!! *Advanced Practice Nursing Quarterly, 1*(1), 1–6.

Oncology Nursing Certification Corporation. (1996). *Test bulletin.* Pittsburgh, PA: Author.

Prouty, M. P. (1983). Contributions and organizational role of the CNS: An administrator's viewpoint. In A. B. Hamric & J. Spross (Eds.), *The clinical nurse specialist in theory and practice* (pp. 171–184). New York: Grune & Stratton.

Safriet, B. J. (1992). Health care dollars and regulatory sense: The role of advanced practice nursing. *Yale Journal of Regulation, 9,* 417–487.

Smith, M. C. (1995). The core of advanced practice nursing. *Nursing Science Quarterly, 8,* 1, 2–3.

Snyder, M. & Mirr, M. P. (Eds.). (1995). *Advanced practice nursing: A guide to professional development.* New York: Springer Publishing Company.

Spross, J. (1995a, September). *Advanced nursing practice in transition: Core competencies and diverse roles.* Paper presented at the 25th anniversary of the Alpha Chi Chapter of Sigma Theta Tau, Boston College, Chestnut Hill, MA.

Spross, J. (1995b, November). *Managed care and healthcare reform: Opportunities for promoting nursing's values.* Paper presented at the 7th M. P. Prouty Lectureship, Dartmouth Hitchcock Medical Center, Hanover, NH.

Styles, M. (1990). Clinical nurse specialists and the future of nursing. In P. Sparacino, D. Cooper, & P. Minarik (Eds.), *The clinical nurse specialist: Implementation and impact* (pp. 279–284). Norwalk, CT: Appleton & Lange.

Von Oech, R. (1988). *Creative whack pack.* Stamford, CT: U.S. Games System.

Williams, C. A., & Valdivieso, G. C. (1994). Advanced practice models: A comparison of clinical nurse specialist and nurse practitioner activities. *Clinical Nurse Specialist, 8,* 311–318.

INDEX

Page numbers in *italics* refer to illustrations; numbers followed by t indicate tables; numbers followed by n indicate notes.

ISBN 0-7216-5894-6

90016

9 780721 658940